SCHILDDRÜSENHORMONE UND KÖRPERPERIPHERIE
REGULATION DER SCHILDDRÜSENFUNKTION

SCHILDDRÜSENHORMONE UND KÖRPERPERIPHERIE

REGULATION DER SCHILDDRÜSENFUNKTION

ZEHNTES SYMPOSION
DER DEUTSCHEN GESELLSCHAFT FÜR ENDOKRINOLOGIE
IN WIEN VOM 7. BIS 9. MÄRZ 1963

SCHRIFTLEITUNG

PROFESSOR DR. ERICH KLEIN

2. MED. KLINIK UND POLIKLINIK DER MED. AKADEMIE DÜSSELDORF

MIT 104 ABBILDUNGEN

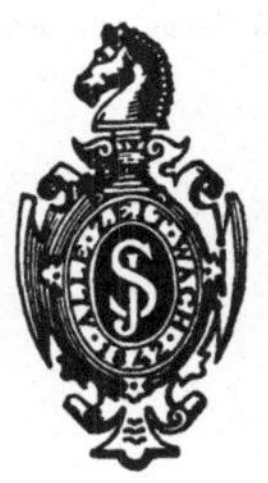

SPRINGER-VERLAG
BERLIN HEIDELBERG GmbH
1964

© Springer-Verlag Berlin Heidelberg 1964

Ursprünglich erschienen bei Springer-Verlag Berlin oHG. Berlin · Göttingen · Heidelberg 1964

Library of Congress Catalog Card Number 55—39230

ISBN 978-3-540-03222-9   ISBN 978-3-662-26787-5 (eBook)
DOI 10.1007/978-3-662-26787-5

Inhaltsverzeichnis

III. Freie Vorträge

Schilddrüse und Schilddrüsenhormone

Hormone und Bluteiweiß

Nebennierenrinde und ihre Hormone

Insulin und Kohlenhydratstoffwechsel

Gonadotrope HVL-Hormone

Keimdrüsen und Keimdrüsenhormone

Alphabetisches Verzeichnis der Referenten und Diskussionsredner

Apostolakis, M., Dr. med., 2. Med. Klinik und Poliklinik der Universität Hamburg, Martinistraße 52.

Bahner, F., Prof. Dr. med., Med. Universitäts-Poliklinik, Heidelberg.

Bansi, H. W., Prof. Dr. med., Allgemeines Krankenhaus St. Georg, 1. Med. Abteilung, Hamburg, Lohmühlenstraße 5.

Bay, V., Dr. med., Chirurgische Universitätsklinik Hamburg, Martinistraße 52.

Beckers, C., Doz. Dr. med., Laboratoire de Pathologie Générale, Université de Louvain, Belgien.

Bennhold, H., Prof. Dr. med., Med. Universitätsklinik Tübingen.

Bergner, D., Dr. med., Med. Universitätsklinik Erlangen.

Börner, W., Doz. Dr. med., Med. Universitäts-Poliklinik Würzburg, Klinikgasse 8.

Bottermann, P., Dr. med., 2. Med. Universitätsklinik München, Ziemssenstraße 1.

Brand, K., Dr. med., Med. Universitätsklinik Heidelberg.

Brücke, F., Prof. Dr. med., Pharmakologisches Institut der Universität Wien.

Buchholz, R., Prof. Dr. med., Frauenklinik der Medizinischen Akademie Düsseldorf, Moorenstraße 5.

Christmann, A., Dr. med., Medizinische Universitätsklinik Erlangen.

Daume, E., Dr. med., Universitäts-Frauenklinik München.

Decker, W., Dr. med., 1. Med. Universitätsklinik München, Ziemssenstraße 1.

Dhom, G., Prof. Dr. med., Pathologisches Institut der Universität Würzburg, Luitpold-
Krankenhaus.

Ditschuneit, H., Dr. med., 1. Med. Universitätsklinik Frankfurt (Main).

Ditschuneit, H. H., Dr. med., 1. Med. Universitätsklinik Frankfurt (Main).

Dolff, E., Prof. Dr. med., Städtische Frauenklinik Essen.

Eickhoff, W., Prof. Dr. med., Pathologisches Institut Duisburg, Bethesda-Krankenhaus.

Emrich, D., Dr. med., Medizinische Universitätsklinik Freiburg/Br.

Englhardt, A., Frau Dr. med., 2. Med. Klinik und Poliklinik der Med. Akademie Düsseldorf,
Moorenstraße 5.

Espinoza, A., Dr. med., 1. Med. Universitätsklinik Frankfurt/Main.

Farkas, K., Dr. med., Staatliches Institut für Rheumatologie, Budapest (Ungarn).

Fellinger, K., Prof. Dr. med., 2. Med. Universitätsklinik, Wien IX, Garnisongasse.

Frahm, H., Doz. Dr. med., 2. Med. Universitätsklinik und Poliklinik Hamburg, Martinistraße 52.

Göbel, P., Dr. med., Med. Universitäts-Poliklinik Tübingen.

Goslar, H.-G., Doz. Dr. med., Anatomisches Institut der Universität Bonn, Nußallee 10.

Goth, E., Prof. Dr. med., János-Krankenhaus Budapest XII (Ungarn).

Greer, M. A., Prof. Dr. med., Division of Endocrinology, Department of Medicine, University
of Oregon Medical School, Portland, Oregon, USA.

Gušić, B., Prof. Dr. med., Universitätsklinik für HNO-Krankheiten, Zagreb (Jugoslawien).

Hamada, H., Dr. med., Schering-AG, Berlin N 65, Müllerstraße 170—172.

Hege, M., Dr. med., Med. Universitätsklinik Heidelberg.

Henning, N., Prof. Dr. med., Med. Universitätsklinik Erlangen.

Herrmann, M., Dr. med., Anatomisches Institut der Universität Bonn, Nußallee 10.

Hess, B., Doz. Dr. med., Med. Universitätsklinik Heidelberg.

Hoeflmayr, J., Dr. med., München 13, Hohenzollernplatz 8.

Höfer, R., Dr. med., 2. Med. Universitätsklinik, Wien IX, Garnisongasse.

Hoff, F., Prof. Dr. med., 1. Med. Universitätsklinik Frankfurt/Main.

Hohlweg, W., Prof. Dr. med., Universitäts-Frauenklinik Graz (Österreich).

Honetz, N., Dr. med., 1. Med. Universitätsklinik, Wien IX.

Horster, F. A., Dr. med., 2. Med. Klinik und Poliklinik der Med. Akademie Düsseldorf,
Moorenstraße 5.

Huber, P., Prof. Dr. med., Chirurgische Universitätsklinik, Innsbruck.

Jöchle, W., Dr. med., Schering-AG, Bergkamen i. W., Postfach 15.

Kaiser, E., Dr. med., Institut für Hygiene und Mikrobiologie der Universität Homburg (Saar).

Karg, H., Doz. Dr. med., München 2, Rheinbergerstraße 1/0.

Karl, H. J., Priv.-Doz. Dr. med., 1. Med. Universitätsklinik München, Ziemssenstraße 1.

Kemeny, V., Dr. med., Staatliches Institut für Rheumatologie, Budapest (Ungarn).

Kemper, F., Doz. Dr. med., Pharmakologisches Institut der Universität Münster, Westring 12.

Kirschner, H., Dr. med., Pathologisches Institut der Universität Hamburg, Martinistraße 52.

Klein, E., Prof. Dr. med., 2. Med. Klinik und Poliklinik der Med. Akademie Düsseldorf, Moorenstraße 5.

Kleyensteiber, G., Dr. med., Med. Universitätsklinik Erlangen.

Kolb, H., Dr. med., 1. Med. Universitätsklinik Frankfurt/Main.

Kopetz, K., Dr. med., 2. Med. Universitätsklinik München, Ziemssenstr. 1.

Kotzaurek, R., Dr. med., 1. Med. Universitätsklinik Wien IX, Garnisongasse.

Kracht, J., Prof. Dr. med., Pathologisches Institut der Universität Hamburg, Martinistraße 52.

Lachnit, V., Prof. Dr. med., 1. Innere Abteilung des Allgemeinen öffentl. Krankenhauses Wiener Neustadt, Wien.

Lemarchand-Béraud, Th., Frau Dr. med., Clinique médicale universitaire de Lausanne (Schweiz).

Lissitzky, S., Prof. Dr. med., Laboratoire de Biochimie Médicale, Faculté de Médecine et de Pharmacie, Boulevard d'Alès, Marseille 5e (Frankreich).

Macht, G., Dr. med., 1. Med. Universitätsklinik Frankfurt/Main.

Marx, K. H., Dr. med., 1. Med. Universitätsklinik Frankfurt/Main.

Matzelt, D., Dr. med., 2. Med. Klinik und Poliklinik der Universität Hamburg, Martinistraße 52.

Melani, F., Dr. med., 1. Med. Universitätsklinik Frankfurt/Main.

Morcos, R., Dr. med., 1. Med. Universitätsklinik Frankfurt/Main.

Mucci, A., Dr. med., 1. Med. Universitätsklinik Frankfurt/Main.

Neumann, F., Dr. med., Schering-AG Berlin N 65, Müllerstr. 170—172.

Nocke, W., Dr. med., Frauenklinik der Med. Akademie Düsseldorf, Moorenstr. 5.

Oberdisse, K., Prof. Dr. med., 2. Med. Klinik und Poliklinik der Med. Akademie Düsseldorf, Moorenstraße 5.

Oertel, G. W., Doz. Dr. med., Institut für Hygiene und Mikrobiologie der Universität Homburg (Saar).

Petersen, F., Dr. med., Therapeutisches Strahlen-Institut, Allgemeines Krankenhanhaus St. Georg, Hamburg.

Petersen, U., Dr. med., 2. Med. Klinik und Poliklinik der Universität Hamburg, Martinistr. 52.

Petzoldt, R., Dr. med., 1. Med. Universitätsklinik Frankfurt/Main.

Pfeiffer, E. F., Prof. Dr. med., 1. Med. Universitätsklinik Frankfurt/Main.

Pfeiffer, G., Frau Dr. med., 2. Med. Universitätsklinik Wien IX, Garnisongasse.

Pitt-Rivers, Rosalind, Frau Prof. Dr. med., National Institute for Medical Research, London, N. W. 7. (England).

Poche, R., Prof. Dr. med., Pathologisches Institut der Med. Akademie Düsseldorf, Moorenstr. 5.

Poser, G., Dr. med., Med. Universitätsklinik Erlangen.

Pražić, M., Prof. Dr. med., Universitätsklinik für HNO-Krankheiten, Zagreb (Jugoslawien).

Rahman, A., Dr. med., 1. Med. Universitätsklinik Frankfurt/Main.

Rausch-Stroomann, J.-G., Dr. med., 1. Med. Universitätsklinik Hamburg, Martinistraße 52.

Reinwein, D., Doz. Dr. med., 2. Med. Klinik und Poliklinik der Med. Akademie Düsseldorf, Moorenstraße 5.

Retiene, K., Dr. med., 1. Med. Universitätsklinik Frankfurt/Main.

Rockenschaub, A., Dr. med., 1. Univ. Frauenklinik, Wien.

Rott, W. H., Dr. med., 1. Med. Universitätsklinik Frankfurt/Main.

Sacks, I. B., Dr. med., University College Hospital Medical School, London, W. C. 1. (England).

Seelich, F., Prof. Dr. med., Physiologisch-chemisches Institut der Universität Wien.

Seuken, A., Frau Dipl. Chem., Frauenklinik der Med. Akademie Düsseldorf, Moorenstraße 5.

Scheibe, O., Dr. med., Chirurgische Universitätsklinik Hamburg, Martinistraße 52.

Scheiffarth, F., Prof. Dr. med., Med. Universitätsklinik Erlangen.

Schild, W., Doz. Dr. med., Frauenklinik der Med. Akademie Düsseldorf, Moorenstraße 5.

Schmidt, H. J., Dr. med., Med. Universitätsklinik Erlangen.

Schmidt-Elmendorff, H., Dr. med., Frauenklinik der Med. Akademie Düsseldorf, Moorenstr. 5.
Schönthal, H., Dr. med., Med. Universitäts-Poliklinik Heidelberg.
Schürholz, K., Dr. med., 1. Med. Klinik der Med. Akademie Düsseldorf, Moorenstraße 5.
Schwarz, G., Doz. Dr. med., Med. Universitäts-Poliklinik Heidelberg.
Schwarz, K., Doz. Dr. med., 2. Med. Universitätsklinik München, Ziemssenstraße 1.
Sturm, A., Prof. Dr. med., Med. Klinik der Städt. Krankenanstalten Wuppertal-Barmen.
Tanka, D., Dr. med., Staatliches Institut für Rheumatologie, Budapest (Ungarn).
Teller, W., Dr. med., Universitäts-Kinderklinik Marburg (Lahn).
Tonutti, E., Prof. Dr. med., Anatomisches Institut der Universität Bonn, Nußallee 10.
Vannotti, A., Prof. Dr. med., Clinique médicale universitaire de Lausanne (Schweiz).
Vecsei/Weisz, P., Dr. med., Staatliches Institut für Rheumatologie, Budapest (Ungarn).
Visscher, M. de, Prof. Dr. med., Laboratoire de Pathologie Générale, Université de Louvain (Belgien).
Vogel, G., Dr. med., Farbwerke Hoechst, Frankfurt-Main-Hoechst, Pharmakologisches Laboratorium.
Voigt, K. D., Prof. Dr. med., 2. Med. Klinik und Poliklinik der Universität Hamburg, Martinistraße 52.
Volkmer, K., Dr. med., 2. Med. Universitätsklinik München, Ziemssenstraße 1.
Wahl, Ch., Dr. med., 1. Med. Universitätsklinik Frankfurt/Main.
Walter, K., Doz. Dr. med., Med. Universitätsklinik Heidelberg.
Wernze, H., Dr. med., Med. Universitätsklinik Würzburg, Luitpold-Krankenhaus.
Witte, S., Prof. Dr. med., Med. Universitätsklinik Erlangen.
Wolf, F., Dr. med., Med. Universitätsklinik Erlangen.
Wyss, F., Priv.-Doz. Dr. med., Med. Abteilung des Insel-Spitals Bern (Schweiz).
Zicha, L., Dr. med., Med. Universitätsklinik Erlangen.
Zimmermann, H., Doz. Dr. med., 2. Med. Klinik und Poliklinik der Med. Akademie Düsseldorf, Moorenstraße 5.

National Institute for Medical Research, London, N. W. 7
University College Hospital Medical School, London, W. C. 1

The Thyroid Hormones and Their Transport in Blood

By

ROSALIND PITT-RIVERS and B. I. SACKS[1]

With 2 figures

Referat

1. Biosynthesis

The thyroid gland concentrates iodide ion from the circulation and converts it to hormonal iodine. This is believed to occur in the following steps:

Formation of 3-monoiodotyrosine (MIT) and 3,5-diiodotyrosine (DIT). Coupling of iodotyrosine molecules to give thyroxine (T_4) and 3,5,3 -triiodothyronine (T_3). It is almost certain that these reactions occur in tyrosine that is covalently bound in the thyroglobulin molecule.

The thyroid contains proteolytic enzymes that can break down thyroglobulin; the T_4 and T_3 so formed are secreted into the circulation and represent the only thyroid hormones in the body (although some metabolites of the thyroid hormones may have physiological activity). The free iodotyrosines are normally dehalogenated in the gland, and the iodide thus obtained either passes into the circulation or is reutilized for hormone biosynthesis [PITT-RIVERS and TATA (66)].

2. The circulating thyroid hormones

The T_4 and T_3 that are secreted into the circulation are not in fact "free"; in 1939, TREVORROW (97) showed that thyroxine added to blood was precipitated by protein precipitants, and behaved like the natural hormone. This protein binding of thyroid hormones differs from the binding in thyroglobin; in the latter the covalent bonds can only be broken by hydrolytic procedures. The protein binding in serum is looser, and the forces can be broken by extraction with organic solvents. This binding, which will be more fully discussed later, is mentioned now, since the thyroid hormone content is generally measured as protein bound iodine (PBI). For details of the analytical procedures used, the reader is referred to articles by PETERS and MAN (64) and BARKER (7).

Since iodoprotein is sometimes found in the blood in certain pathological conditions (see below), the estimation of hormonal iodine in blood has also been made on butanol extracts of serum (BEI) (64). However, another interfering factor in PBI measurements is the occasional presence in serum of organic iodine

---

[1] In receipt of a grant from the British Empire Cancer Campaign.

X-ray contrast media, which may raise the PBI to 30 times the normal value. These compounds will be included in BEI determinations; so far no analytical method has been described which separates hormonal I and I in contrast media.

In normal humans, the PBI ranges between 4 and 8 μg/100 ml serum, with a mean value of about 5 μg (*64, 99*). This represents total hormonal iodine; the contribution of T_3 has so far been the subject of only a few quantitative studies in man. A number of workers have failed to find ^{131}I-labelled T_3 in the blood of normal human subjects. It was first shown in the sera of patients with hyper-thyroidism or thyroid cancer (*32*). This problem requires further investigation.

In the rat, the relative amounts of T_4 and T_3 in thyroid and serum were determined by PITT-RIVERS and RALL (*65*) by isotopic equilibrium studies. After a period of 25 days equilibration, the T_4/T_3 was about 6:1 in the thyroid, and 20:1 in the serum. No such assessment has been made in any other animal.

3. Thyroid hormone turnover

As has been pointed out by RIGGS (*70, 71*), the absolute amount of thyroid hormone secreted daily from the gland is of the greatest importance, since it represents the supply of hormone necessary to maintain the animal in a euthyroid state.

In the past, the rate of secretion of hormone from the gland was generally calculated by determining the amount of exogenous hormone required to maintain athyreotic subjects in a euthyroid state; this gave values of 116 μg hormonal I daily when DL$-T_4$ was given, and 87 μg hormonal I after ingestion of desiccated thyroid. This method has been criticized on the grounds that thyroid or T_4 taken orally are not entirely absorbed or efficiently utilized, and will therefore give rise to requirement values that are too high. Another method depends on the meas-urement of ^{131}I uptake, the ^{127}I excreted and the ^{127}I entering the thyroid per day;

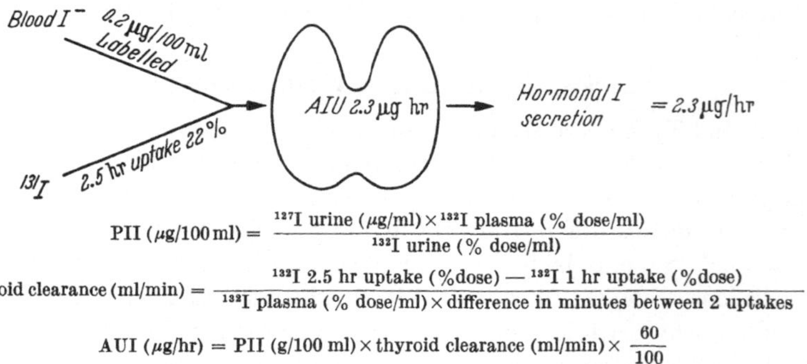

$$\text{PII } (\mu\text{g}/100\,\text{ml}) = \frac{^{127}\text{I urine } (\mu\text{g/ml}) \times {}^{132}\text{I plasma } (\%\ \text{dose/ml})}{^{132}\text{I urine } (\%\ \text{dose/ml})}$$

$$\text{Thyroid clearance (ml/min)} = \frac{^{132}\text{I 2.5 hr uptake } (\%\text{dose}) - {}^{132}\text{I 1 hr uptake } (\%\text{dose})}{^{132}\text{I plasma } (\%\ \text{dose/ml}) \times \text{difference in minutes between 2 uptakes}}$$

$$\text{AUI } (\mu\text{g/hr}) = \text{PII (g/100 ml)} \times \text{thyroid clearance (ml/min)} \times \frac{60}{100}$$

Fig. 1. Calculation of hormonal I secretion by Alexander et al. (*2*).

this method, according to RIGGS (*71*) probably gives daily secretion values that are too low. BERSON and YALOW (*8a*) measured ^{131}I uptake and excretion and calculated that the rate of hormonal I turnover ranged between 40—110 μg per day in subjects with a normal PBI.

ALEXANDER and coworkers (*2*) have used a modification of the method des-cribed by RIGGS (*71*) to determine hormonal I secretion in normal and pathological states. They gave ^{131}I or ^{132}I and measured thyroidal uptake at 1 and 2.5 hr. They calculated the thyroid clearance rate and the absolute iodine uptake from the formulae shown in Fig. 1. Plasma inorganic iodide (PII) was obtained from the determination of ^{132}I in plasma and both ^{127}I and ^{132}I in urine.

Substituting actual experimental data they obtained, we see that in normal subjects the AIU was 2.3 μg/hour, whence the hormonal I secretion was 2.3 μg/hr or 55 μg/day.

Some of the data summarized by these authors are shown in Table 1.

Table 1. *PBI and absolute iodine uptake in different states*

	Normal	Thyrotoxic	Hypo-thyroid	Simple goitre with high uptake	Simple goitre with normal uptake	Hashimoto's disease
^{132}I Uptake in % of dose at 2.5 hr	21.6	66.1	8.2	39.9	27.5	26
Absolute I uptake (μg/hr)	2.3	18.5	0.3	1.9	1.4	2
PBI μg/100 ml	5.0	11.3	0.8	5.0	4.8	2.7

As can be seen, the absolute iodine uptake was greatly increased in thyrotoxicosis and was generally depressed in hypothyroidism, with or without goitre. The thyroid clearance of I was raised to over 12 times the normal value in thyrotoxicosis and to over 3 times the normal value in goitrous patients with high uptakes. It was depressed in hypothyroidism.

These findings are in good agreement with those of other authors (*44*). It has been found that the average secretion of thyroid hormone iodine is normally about 70 μg/day, and may rise to as much as 600 μg/day in hyperthyroidism.

A factor of paramount importance in the regulation of thyroid hormone secretion is the anterior pituitary hormone thyrotrophin (TSH). WOLFF (*106*) showed that in the rat, the normal rate of secretion of labelled hormone was markedly accelerated by TSH injections. Conversely, hypophysectomy or suppression of anterior pituitary activity by thyroxine treatment reduced the discharge of hormonal I from the gland. These findings were soon confirmed by PERRY (*63*).

Hypophysectomy profoundly depresses thyroid hormone biosynthesis in the gland (*96*) while injection of TSH increases the amount of iodothyronines in thyroglobulin, compared with normal values (PITT-RIVERS, unpublished); alterations in hormonal secretion therefore reflect changes in the amounts of hormone present in thyroglobulin.

Thyroid hormone turnover is also dependent upon the rate of its peripheral utilization, metabolism and excretion. This is estimated by measuring the rate of disappearance from the body of ^{131}I labelled T_4 or T_3 after intravenous injection. In order to get meaningful results, it is essential to use labelled hormones of high specific activity, since the rate of disposal of large doses of hormone ist not the same as that of endogenous hormone (*66*). The peripheral turnover is expressed as the half life or 50% retention time, and has been found to vary greatly in different species — some values are shown in Table 2 (*1, 11, 27, 46, 83, 85, 94*).

It will be seen that in man and the rat, the half life of T_4 is longer than that of T_3. In the rabbit and chicken, the half lives of the two hormones are the same; the physiological implications of these findings will be discussed later.

Table 2. *Biological half-lives of thyroxine, triiodothyronine, mono- and di-iodotyrosine in different species*

	Thyroxine	Triiodothyronine	Monoiodotyrosine	Diiodotyrosine
Euthyroid man . .	6.7 days	2.6 days	1.5 hours (approx)	1.5 hours (approx)
Rat	16—19 hours	9—10 hours		
Rabbit	1—2 days	1—2 days		
Chicken.	22.5 hours	22.5 hours		

In hypothyroidism, the half life of T_4 is not much different from the normal but in thyrotoxicosis it falls to between 2 and 4 days (*44*).

The very rapid rate of disappearance of labelled iodotyrosines after intravenous injection in man (*1, 83*) should be noted, since it has a bearing on the problem whether iodotyrosines are normally present in blood (see below).

4. Other iodinated compounds in blood

a) Iodide

In man, the amount of iodide ion in the blood is generally too small to measure, and its value is obtained, as we have seen by measuring radioactive I in the plasma and both radioactive and stable I in the urine. It amounts to only about 1/20 of the total serum iodine.

In the rat, the serum iodide is high; in the isotope equilibrium experiments of Pitt-Rivers and Rall (*65*) the serum PB ^{131}I ranged from 4.5—6.0 μg/100 ml; the serum ^{131}I-iodide was 2.0 μg/100 ml. These results were in fair agreement with chemical analyses which gave PBI and serum I$^-$ as 3.3 and 2.4 μg/100 ml respectively. In the rat, therefore about 40% of the total serum iodine is iodide.

In mammals, the circulating iodide is not bound to protein, as has already been seen. However, Leloup and Fontaine (*53*) have made the interesting observation that in some fish, iodide is bound to protein. This is shown by electrophoretic analysis of salmon and trout sera to which were added [131]I$^-$. There was no protein binding of iodide by rat serum. This binding of I$^-$ is physiologically important; it increases during the migration of salmon, and appears to be a method of conservation of iodide during periods when the fish will have an increased requirement for thyroid hormone.

b) Iodotyrosines

The presence of iodotyrosines has been reported in the blood of normal humans (*104*). The iodide was measured chemically after chromatographic separation of the iodoamino acids.

Certain observations have raised doubts about this finding. The first is that ^{131}I labelled iodotyrosines are not found in blood after tracer doses of [131]I. Pitt-Rivers and Rall (*65*) were only able to detect minute amounts in rat serum after isotope equilibration for 25 days.

Secondly, as we have seen, the biological half lives of the iodotyrosines are very short in man, amounting to 1.5 hours for both compounds. In order to maintain a detectable serum level of iodotyrosines there would have to be a very large pool in the body, for which there is as yet no evidence; the problem awaits clarification.

Iodotyrosines are found in the blood in certain pathological conditions. The most interesting is the syndrome of sporadic goitre with impaired iodotyrosine dehalogenase activity. This has been investigated by STAMBURY, QUERIDO and coworkers (84) by McGIRR and coworkers (54a) and by VAGUE and coworkers (100). These patients are apparently devoid of both thyroidal and peripheral iodotyrosine dejodinase activity and iodotyrosines appear in the urine.

The presence of iodotyrosines has been reported in the blood of thyrotoxic patients (9, 25); the identification of MIT and DIT was made by chromatographic analysis with and without the aid of radioiodine.

Lastly, iodotyrosines have been found in blood after therapeutic doses of ^{131}I. FLETCHER (28) suggests that these probably arise by hydrolysis of thyroglobulin which may leak into the circulation after radiation damage to the gland.

c) Thyroglobulin

Thyroglobulin is not normally present in blood (54, 37). However, it is released into the circulation after surgical trauma, radiation damage and presumably in Hashimoto's thyroiditis (67) although this has not been unequivocally demonstrated (75, 78).

d) Iodinated albumin

A protein has been found in the blood of thyrotoxic patients after the administration of tracer and therapeutic doses of ^{131}I (12, 19, 51, 82) which possesses electrophoretic and immunological properties of an iodoalbumin. A similar protein has been demonstrated in the blood of patients with Hashimoto's thyroiditis and in the blood of a cretin given a tracer dose of ^{131}I (18).

OWEN and coworkers (62) have questioned the part played by radiation damage on the liberation of iodoproteins from the thyroid into the circulation, since they found both thyroglobulin and iodoalbumin in the sera of a number of patients with thyroid cancer whether they had been given tracer or therapeutic doses of ^{131}I.

e) Compound X or serum S-1 iodoprotein

ROBBINS et al. (77) first described a protein containing iodine in the blood of patients with thyroid cancer which was not thyroglobulin. Later studies (67) showed that this protein resembled serum albumin by electrophoresis, solubility and in the ultracentrifuge, but did not react with anti albumin immune serum. Hydrolysis of ^{131}I labelled compound X followed by chromatographic analysis showed that its principal iodinated constituent was MIT. Another compound with the chromatographic mobility of T_4 was also present. That it was in fact T_4 is unlikely owing to the absence of DIT in the hydrolysates.

Because of its physical and chemical properties, ROBBINS and RALL (75) suggest that compound X is related to thyroidal S-1-iodoprotein, a soluble protein found in transplantable thyroid tumours, in normal thyroids of man and sheep and in some thyroid follicular adenomata.

5. Thyroid hormone binding in serum

A number of reviews on the transport of thyroid hormones in the blood have appeared in the past few years (74, 75, 92, 93a, 47); the reader is referred to these for a detailed bibliography.

After the early work of Trevorrow (*97*) previously described, little was done on thyroid hormone transport until 1952-3, when a number of papers appeared on the migration of ^{131}I labelled T_4 added to serum proteins during electrophoresis in veronal buffer at pH 8.6 (*31, 73, 50, 105, 42*). Gordon et al. (*31*) considered that the principal thyroxine binding protein was located on their electrophoretograms near α-1 globulin, but it was soon shown that this protein migrates between α_1 and α_2 globulins. This protein is generally called thyroxine binding globulin (TBG). TBG has not yet been isolated although a partial purification of Cohn fraction IV-6 by ion exchange chromatography has been carried out by Ingbar et al. (*45*) and by Tata (*93, 93a*). Experiments on the electrophoretic migration of TBG at a pH below neutrality suggest that it might be associated with the proteins known as M-2 glycoproteins (*92, 75*). Recently however, Hollander and coworkers (*41*) have found by micro-immunoelectrophoresis in agar gel that the α-globulin that binds T_4 stains as a lipoprotein. Until TBG is isolated in a pure condition these questions remain unsettled.

In 1958, Ingbar (*43*) showed that if paper electrophoresis of labelled T_4 in serum were carried out in tris-maleate buffer at pH 8.6 instead of veronal, nearly half the radioactivity was localized in a position ahead of albumin; this protein has been called thyroxine binding prealbumin (TBPA). TBPA does not bind T_3 in these conditions. Electrophoresis in starch gel also showed strong binding of T_4 by prealbumin (*69, 3*). Binding of T_4 by prealbumin has also been demonstrated by continuous glow electrophoresis (*4*).

Tata (*91*) has shown that the prealbumin isolated by Schulze had a strong affinity for T_4 and that TBPA alone or human serum enriched with TBPA showed binding in the prealbumin zone after electrophoresis in veronal buffer at pH 8.6. No binding in the prealbumin zone was demonstrable after electrophoresis of serum alone.

Factors such as the nature of the buffer used, the pH and the supporting medium during electrophoresis have been shown to modify greatly the binding affinities of TBG and TBPA for T_4 (*95, 56, 16*). The physiological role of TBPA in the transport of thyroid hormone has been questioned, since its binding of T_4 is considerably reduced when electrophoresis is carried out at a physiological pH (*56, 16*). However, Hollander and coworkers (*40, 41*) support the view that TBPA does play a part in the transport of T_4 in the blood. It should also be pointed out that electrophoretic studies of T_4 binding are in themselves "unphysiological", at any pH; nevertheless they have afforded a valuable contribution to our knowledge in this field.

6. Thyroid hormone binding by albumin

Human serum albumin also binds T_4 and T_3, but its affinity for these is lower than that of TBG; however its binding capacity is very great, by virtue of the relatively large amount present in serum (*75*). Early reports indicated that both hormones are bound to the same extent by serum albumin; however, Sterling and coworkers (*86—88*) have found in equilibrium dialysis that at pH 7.4, T_3 has only one tenth of the affinity for albumin as has T_4.

TRITSCH et al. (*98*) measured the T_4 binding capacity of serum albumin by determining the inhibition by albumin of the acceleration by T_4 of the oxidation of DPNH by peroxide in the presence of horse radish peroxidase. They found that a maximum of six molecules of T_4 can be bound by one molecule of albumin.

7. Methods used for quantitating thyroxine binding

a) The saturation method

This involves the addition of increasing amounts of stable T_4 to serum, and measuring the distribution of ^{131}I labelled T_4 after electrophoresis. By this method, the binding capacity of TBG for T_4 has been shown to be between 0.16—0.24 μg/ml serum. The binding capacity of TBG for T_3 is considerably lower.

b) Thyroxine stabilization

TATA (*90*) found that if thyroxine were partitioned between 50% aqueous organic solvent and a large volume of buffer, it exhibited a transient instability, with the apparent formation of iodide. This effect was reversed by addition of human serum protein, and did not occur if the T_4 was present in a protein containing medium. TATA has used this stabilization of T_4 to quantitate the binding of T_4 by Cohn fraction IV-6, and has found that it does not change over a pH range of 7—8.6.

c) Equilibrium dialysis

This method depends upon the transfer of labelled T_4 across a dialysis membrane between 2 chambers containing serum and the same amount of stable T_4 (*14*). The method depends on the amount of free T_4 present in the serum (see below).

d) Erythrocyte uptake test

Another method of estimating thyroid hormone binding depends on the uptake of labelled T_4 or T_3 by erythrocytes from human plasma (*15, 17, 33, 34, 36, 61, 81, 102*). It has been shown that there is good agreement in the results obtained by this method and by dialysis. There is an inverse correlation between TBG capacity and the log of the binding coefficient of uptake of labelled T_3 by erythrocytes.

e) Resin absorption

Absorption studies have been made of labelled T_4 and T_3 by an anion exchange resin (*55*) and by rat diaphragma (*52*). They have not as yet been fully investigated.

8. Thyroxine binding in different species

Electrophoretic studies of T_4-binding have been made in a number of different animals; in the horse, mule, pig, cow, sheep and goat the principal binding of T_4 occurs in the α-globuline zone, although some binding occurs in albumin (*22, 24, 75*). FARER et al. (*24*) have shown that a specific TBG is only found in mammals, but T_4 binding by other proteins can be demonstrated in the sera of birds, fish and reptiles.

An interesting observation has been made on the binding of T_4 and T_3 by serum proteins of the chick and duck by Tata and Shellabarger (*80, 94*). They found that the half lives of ^{131}I-labelled T_4 and T_3 were identical in these birds and that both hormones were bound with the same affinity to serum albumin. TBG binding was absent. Administration of human TBG to cockerels increased the half life of labelled T_4 but did not change that of T_3. The authors postulated that the equipotency of T_4 and T_3 previously described in birds is due to the similarity in their binding by serum proteins, and the relative potency of the two hormones depends upon intensity of serum binding and the consequent rate of distribution to the tissues.

A similar finding has been made in another animal. Brown-Grant (*10*) showed that T_4 and T_3 were equally effective in suppressing TSH secretion in the rabbit. Brown-Grant and Tata (*11*) have since found that the biological half lives of ^{131}I labelled T_4 and T_3 are the same (about 27 hours) in the rabbit.

9. Thyroxine binding in various physiological and pathological conditions

In 1948 Heinemann et al. (*38*) showed that the PBI rose during pregnancy into the thyrotoxic range, although there are normally no signs of hyperthyroidism in pregnant women. It was further shown that in some abnormal pregnancies and abortion, the PBI was low. This problem has since been investigated from the point of view of T_4 binding, and it has been found that in normal pregnancy TBG is considerably increased (*20, 35, 47, 57, 72, 75*), and decreased when abortion occurs. Dowling et al. (*21*) and others have further shown that the administration of oestrogen raises the serum TBG level in men and in non-pregnant women.

In the human (*5*) and rabbit (*56*) foetus, the TBG level is lower than in the adult animal; the rabbit foetus was also shown to contain a T_4 binding protein not found in the adult.

TBG is lowered in certain pathological conditions such as nephrosis, when there is a leakage of protein from the blood (*35, 68, 76*). In infectious hepatitis,

Table 3. *Some factors that affect Thyroxine binding*

Condition	PBI	T_4-binding	Symptoms
Hyperthyroidism	High	Normal	Hyperthyroid
Hypothyroidism	Low	High	Hypothyroid
Pregnancy, normal	High	High	Euthyroid
Pregnancy, abnormal and abortion . .	Low	Low	Euthyroid
Pre-natal	Low	Low	—
Nephrosis	Low	Low	Euthyroid
Liver disease	High or normal	High or normal	Euthyroid
Therapy:			
Oestrogen	High	Normal	Euthyroid
Androgen	Low	Low	Euthyroid
Anabolic steroids	Low	Low	Euthyroid
Salicylate	Low	Low	Euthyroid elevated BMR
Anticonvulsants	Low	Low	Euthyroid

PBI and TBG levels are sometimes elevated, usually in the acute stage of the disease. In cirrhosis, a few cases have shown high PBI and high TBG; in advanced cirrhosis the TBG capacity is usually low (*30, 35, 49, 101*).

Thyroxine binding is depressed by the administration of androgens (*23, 26, 48*), and by anabolic steroids (*79*). It is also depressed by the administration of certain drugs, e. g. salicylates (*6, 39, 60, 107, 108*) and anticonvulsants (*58, 59*). These findings are summarized in Table 3.

10. Abnormal binding of thyroid hormones

TANAKA and STARR (*89*) described a clinically euthyroic man with a PBI of $3.0\,\mu g/100\,ml$ serum, in whose serum there was no detectable TBG. Electrophoresis revealed that T_4 was bound to albumin. A few abnormalities have also been reported in members of the same family. BEIERWALTES and ROBBINS (*8*) investigated several members of a family with elevated PBI and TBG levels; in only one subject was there any indication of hyperthyroidism. FLORSCHEIM et al. (*29*) have also found familial elevation of PBI and TBG capacity without any clinical manifestation of hyperthyroidism.

The opposite situation has been found in 2 sisters studied by CAVALIERI (*13*). The sera of both had normal PBI but low TBG capacity; both sisters showed symptoms of hyperthyroidism. Chromatographic analysis of the sera revealed that about one sixth of the PBI was not extractable with butanol.

A genetically determined defect is thought to be responsible for these abnormalities in thyroxine binding, with or without thyroid dysfunction.

Table 4. *Some effects of abnormal thyroxine binding*

Patient	Relationship	TBG	PBI	Symptoms
W. W.	—	Absent	3.0	Euthyroid
A. H.	} Sisters	Low	5.1	Hyperthyroid
W. R.		Low Normal	6.6	Hyperthyroid
W. W.	Father	High	11.8—16.0	Euthyroid
	Child 2	Normal	25	Euthyroid
	Child 3	High	10.1	Euthyroid
T. W.	Father	High	14.8	? Hyperthyroid
M. H.	Daughter	High	14.8	Euthyroid
H. H.	Granddaughter	High	14.8	Euthyroid
D. L.	Sister of T. W.	High	14.8	Euthyroid

11. Physiological role of thyroid hormone binding; assessment of free thyroxine

It is now generally agreed that the binding of thyroid hormones in the blood serves as a means of regulating the distribution to their target organs (*92, 75, 47*). It is also agreed that the hormones only exhibit their physiological actions in the free state, therefore the level of free T_4 and T_3 will determine the metabolic status of the animal.

Attempts have been made to estimate the amount of free thyroxine in the blood. ROBBINS and RALL (*74*) calculated from the data of BEESON and YALOW (*8a*) the level of free T_4 in normal and pathological subjects; in the normal group the values obtained were between 3.3 and 8.6×10^{-11} M with a mean value of 6.2×10^{-11} M; this means that the free thyroxine was only about 0.06% of the total serum T_4.

Free thyroxine has also been determined using equilibrium dialysis techniques $(14, 86)$. Sterling and Hegedus (86) estimated its concentration to be 1.3×10^{-10} M, or about 0.1% of the total serum T_4. In thyrotoxicosis the value for free thyroxine rose to 0.23% of the total; in hypothyroidism and pregnancy the values found were slightly lower than the normal.

An assessment of free thyroxine has been made using the erythrocyte T_3 uptake test by Walfish et al. (102) and Osorio et al. (61). Although absolute values could not be calculated by this method, the relative T_4 binding capacity was demonstrated in difference states. Fig. 2 is taken from values given by Osorio et al. (61). It can be seen that in spite of the marked elevation of PBI in pregnancy the relative amount of free T_4 parallels the normal range. As has been said before the metabolic status of man and other animals with regard to thyroid hormones depends on the levels of free hormone in the circulation.

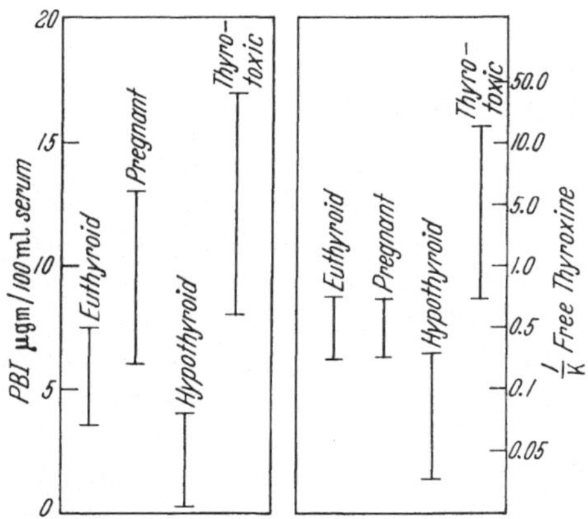

Fig. 2. Hormonal I (PBI) and free thyroxine in different thyroid states [From values given by Osorio et al. (61)].

References

1. Albert, A., and F. R. Keating jr.: J. clin. Endocr. 11, 996 (1951).
2. Alexander, W. D., D. A. Koutras, J. Crooks, W. W. Buchanan, E. M. MacDonald, M. H. Richmond and E. J. Wayne: Quart. J. Med. 31, 281 (1962).
3. Allison, A. C.: Experientia (Basel) 15, 281 (1959).
4. Andreoli, M., e D. Andriani: Minerva nucl. 3, 161 (1959).
5. —, and J. Robbins: J. clin. Invest. 41, 1070 (1962).
6. Austen, F. K., M. E. Rubini, W. H. Meroney and J. Wolff: J. clin. Invest. 37, 1131 (1958).
7. Barker, S. B.: In Methods in Hormone Research, Vol. 1, Chapter 9. E. R. I. Dorfman. New York: Academic Press 1962.
8. Beierwaltes, W. H., and J. Robbins: J. clin. Invest. 38, 1683 (1959).
8a. Berson, S. A., and R. S. Yalow: J. clin. Invest. 33, 1533 (1954).
9. Bird, R., and H. E. A. Farran: J. clin. Endocr. 20, 81 (1960).
10. Brown-Grant, K.: J. Physiol. (Lond.) 127, 352 (1955).
11. —, and J. R. Tata: J. Physiol. (Lond.) 157, 157 (1961).
12. Cameron, C., and K. Fletcher: Nature (Lond.) 183, 116 (1959).
13. Cavalieri, R. R.: J. clin. Endocr. 21, 1455 (1961).
14. Christensen, L. K.: Nature (Lond.) 183, 1189 (1959).
15. — Endocrinology 66, 138 (1960).
16. —, and A. D. Litonjua: J. clin. Endocr. 21, 104 (1961).
17. Crispell, K. R., S. Kahana and H. Hyer: J. clin. Invest. 35, 121 (1956).
18. De Groot, L. J., S. Postel, J. Litvak and J. B. Stanbury: J. clin. Endocr. 15, 1315 (1955).

19. De Groot, L. J., and J. B. Stanbury: Amer. J. Med. **27**, 586 (1959).
20. Dowling, J. T., N. Freinkel and S. H. Ingbar: J. clin. Invest. **35**, 1263 (1956).
21. — — — J. clin. Invest. **39**, 1119 (1960).
22. Dubowitz, L. M. S., N. B. Myant and C. Osorio: J. Physiol. (Lond.) **162**, 358 (1962).
23. Engbring, N. H., and W. W. Engstrom: J. clin. Endocr. **19**, 783 (1959).
24. Farer, L. S., J. Robbins, B. S. Blumberg and J. E. Rall: Endocrinology **70**, 686 (1962).
25. Farran, H. E. A., A. J. Lea, A. W. G. Goolden and J. D. Abbatt: Lancet **1959**, 793.
26. Federman, D. D., J. Robbins and J. E. Rall: J. clin. Invest. **37**, 272 (1958).
27. Feldman, J. D.: Amer. J. Physiol. **188**, 30 (1957).
28. Fletcher, K.: Biochem. J. **67**, 140 (1957).
29. Florscheim, W. H., J. T. Dowling, L. Meister and R. E. Bodfish: J. clin. Endocr. **22**, 735 (1962).
30. Friis, R.: Ugesk. Laeg. **121**, 1311 (1959).
31. Gordon, A. H., J. Cross, D. O'Connor and R. Pitt-Rivers: Nature (Lond.) **169**, 19 (1952).
32. Gross, J., and R. Pitt-Rivers: Lancet **1952**, 593.
33. Hamolsky, M. W.: J. clin. Invest. **34**, 914 (1955).
34. — D. B. Fischer and A. S. Freedberg: Endocrinology **66**, 780 (1960).
35. — A. Golodetz and A. S. Freedberg: J. clin. Endocr. **19**, 103 (1959).
36. — M. Stein and A. S. Freedberg: J. clin. Endocr. **17**, 33 (1957).
37. Harington, C. R.: Proc. roy. Soc. B **132**, 223 (1944).
38. Heinemann, M., C. E. Johnson and E. B. Man: J. clin. Invest. **27**, 91 (1948).
39. Hetzel, B. S., B. F. Good, M. L. Wellby and J. S. Charnock: In Advances in Thyroid Research, p. 56. Ed. R. Pitt-Rivers. New York: Pergamon Press 1961.
40. Hollander, C. S., B. H. Latimer, E. Prout, D. H. Lockwood and S. P. Asper jr.: Metabolism **12**, 45 (1963).
41. — V. V. Odak, T. E. Prout and S. P. Asper jr.: J. clin. Endocr. **22**, 617 (1962).
42. Horst, W., and H. Rösler: Klin. Wschr. **31**, 13 (1953).
43. Ingbar, S. H.: Endocrinology **63**, 256 (1958).
44. — In Clinical Endocrinology. Ed. E. B. Astwood. New York: Grune & Stratton 1960.
45. — J. T. Dowling and N. Freinkel: Endocrinology **61**, 321 (1957).
46. —, and N. Freinkel: J. clin. Invest. **34**, 808 (1955).
47. — — In: Hormones in Human Plasma. Chapter 15. Ed. H. N. Antoniades. London: J. and A. Churchill Ltd. 1960.
48. Keitel, H. G., and M. G. Sherer: J. clin. Endocr. **17**, 854 (1957).
49. Kydd, D. M., and E. B. Man: J. clin. Invest. **30**, 874 (1951).
50. Larson, F. C., W. P. Deiss and E. C. Albright: Science **115**, 626 (1952).
51. — — — J. clin. Invest. **33**, 230 (1954).
52. Lein, A. L., and R. M. Dowben: In: Advances in Thyroid Research. p. 525. Ed. R. Pitt-Rivers. New York: Pergamon Press 1961.
53. Leloup, J., and M. Fontaine: Ann. N. Y. Acad. Sci. **86**, 316 (1960).
54. Lerman, J.: J. clin. Invest. **19**, 555 (1940).
54a. McGirr, E. M.: In: Clinical Endocrinology, I. Part II, Chapter 5. Ed. E. B. Astwood. New York: Grune & Stratton, Inc. 1960.
55. Mitchell, M. L., M. E. O'Rourke and A. B. Harden: In: Advances in Thyroid Research. p. 456. Ed. R. Pitt-Rivers. New York: Pergamon Press 1961.
56. Myant, N. B., and C. Osorio: J. Physiol. (Lond.) **152**, 601 (1960).
57. Nicoloff, J. T., R. Nicoloff and J. T. Dowling: J. clin. Invest. **41**, 1998 (1962).
58. Oppenheimer, J. H., and R. R. Tavernetti: Endocrinology **71**, 496 (1962).
59. — — J. clin. Invest. **41**, 2213 (1962).
60. Osorio, C.: J. Physiol. **163**, 151 (1962).
61. — D. J. Jackson, J. M. Gartside and A. W. G. Goolden: Clin. Sci. **23**, 525 (1962).
62. Owen, C. A. jr., W. M. McConahey, D. S. Childs jr. and B. F. McKenzie: J. clin. Endocr. **20**, 187 (1960).

63. PERRY, W. F.: Endocrinology **48**, 643 (1951).
64. PETERS, J. P., and E. B. MAN: In the Thyroid. p. 137. Ed. S. C. WERNER. New York: Hoeber-Harper 1960.
65. PITT-RIVERS, R., and J. E. RALL: Endocrinology **68**, 309 (1961).
66. —, and J. R. TATA: The Thyroid Hormones. New York: Pergamon Press 1959.
67. — — In: Diseases of the Thyroid. Ed. I. N. KUGELMASS. New York: Charles C. Thomas 1960.
68. RECANT, L.: J. clin. Invest. **35**, 730 (1956).
69. RICH, C., and A. G. BEARN: Endocrinology **62**, 687 (1958).
70. RIGGS, D. S.: Pharmacol. Rev. **4**, 284 (1952).
71. — In: The Thyroid, p. 41. Ed. S. C. WERNER. New York: Hoeber-Harper 1960.
72. ROBBINS, J., and J. H. NELSON: J. clin. Invest. **37**, 153 (1958).
73. —, and J. E. RALL: Proc. Soc. exp. Med. (N. Y.) **81**, 530 (1952).
74. — — Recent Progr. Hormone Res. **13**, 161 (1957).
75. — — Physiol. Rev. **40**, 415 (1960).
76. — — and M. L. PETERMANN: J. clin. Invest. **36**, 1333 (1957).
77. — — and R. W. RAWSON: J. clin. Endocr. **13**, 852 (1953).
78. ROITT, I. M., and D. DONIACH: Brit. med. Bull. **16**, 152 (1960).
79. ROSENBERG, I. N., C. S. AHN and M. L. MITCHELL: J. clin. Endocr. **22**, 612 (1962).
80. SHELLABARGER, C. J., and J. TATA: Endocrinology **68**, 1056 (1961).
81. SILVERSTEIN, J. N., H. L. SCHWARTZ, E. B. FELDMAN, D. M. KYDD and A. C. CARTER: J. clin. Endocr. **22**, 1002 (1962).
82. STANBURY, J. B., and M. A. JANSEN: J. clin. Endocr. **22**, 978 (1962).
83. — A. A. H. KASSENAAR, J. W. A. MEIJER and J. TERPSTRA: J. clin. Endocr. **16**, 735 (1956).
84. —, and A. QUERIDO: J. clin. Endocr. **16**, 1522 (1956).
85. STERLING, K., J. C. LASHOF and E. B. MAN: J. clin. Invest. **33**, 1031 (1954).
86. —, and A. HEGEDUS: J. clin. Invest. **41**, 1031 (1962).
87. — P. ROSEN and M. TABACHNICK: J. clin. Invest. **41**, 1021 (1962).
88. —, and M. TABACHNICK: J. biol. Chem. **236**, 2241 (1961).
89. TANAKA, S., and P. STARR: J. clin. Endocr. **19**, 1485 (1959).
90. TATA, J. R.: Biochem. J. **72**, 214, 222 (1959).
91. — Nature (Lond.) **183**, 877 (1959).
92. — Brit. med. Bull. **16**, 142 (1960).
93. — Clin. chim. Acta **6**, 819 (1961).
93a. — Recent Progr. Hormone Res. 18, 221 (1962).
94. —, and C. J. SHELLABARGER: Biochem. J. **72**, 608 (1959).
95. — C. C. WIDNELL and W. B. GRATZER: Clin. chim. Acta **6**, 597 (1961).
96. TAUROG, A., W. TONG and I. L. CHAIKOFF: Endocrinology **62**, 646, 664 (1958).
97. TREVORROW, V.: J. biol. Chem. **127**, 737 (1939).
98. TRITSCH, G. L., C. E. RATHKE, N. E. TRITSCH and C. M. WEISS: J. biol. Chem. **236**, 3163 (1961).
99. TROTTER, W. R.: Diseases of the Thyroid. Appendix B. Oxford: Blackwell Scientific Publications 1962.
100. VAGUE, J., S. LISSITZKY, J. L. CODACCIONI, R. SIMONIN, G. MILLER, J. BOYER and G. AUDIBERT: Lancet **1962**, 1070.
101. VANOTTI, A., and T. BÉRAUD: J. clin. Endocr. **19**, 466 (1959).
102. WALFISH, P. G., A. BRITTON, R. VOLPÉ and C. EZRIN: J. clin. Endocr. **22**, 178 (1962).
103. WELLBY, M. L., B. S. HETZEL and B. F. GOOD: Brit. med. J. **1963** I, 439.
104. WERNER, S. C., and R. J. BLOCK: Nature (Lond.) **183**, 406 (1959).
105. WINZLER, R. J., and S. R. NOTRICA: Fed. Proc. **11**, 312 (1952).
106. WOLFF, J.: Endocrinology **48**, 284 (1951).
107. —, and F. K. AUSTEN: J. clin. Invest. **37**, 1144 (1958).
108. — M. E. STANDAERT and J. E. RALL: J. clin. Invest. **40**, 1373 (1961).

Diskussion

F. Brücke (Wien):

Können Sie noch einige Worte über die Verhältnisse beim sporadischen Kretinismus sagen?

R. Pitt-Rivers:

In discussing sporadic goitre with iodotyrosine dehalogenase deficiency I think it is evident that this represents wastage of iodine. The second iodide pool of the thyroid (derived from iodotyrosines), shown by Halmi and Pitt-Rivers (1962) to be many times larger than the first iodide pool (from blood) in the rat, may also be very important in iodine economy in man. Vague et al. (1960) have shown that a hypothyroid infant with iodotyrosine dehalogenase deficiency was made completely euthyroid by administration of one drop of Lugols solution per day.

Aus der 2. Medizinischen Klinik und Poliklinik der Medizinischen
Akademie Düsseldorf (Prof. Dr. K. Oberdisse)

Umsatz und Stoffwechsel der Schilddrüsenhormone

Von

Erich Klein

Mit 13 Abbildungen

Referat

Die von der Schilddrüse sezernierten und im Blut von verschiedenen Plasmaeiweißkörpern transportierten oder auch in freier Form vorliegenden Hormone
Thyroxin (T_4) und Trijodthyronin (T_3) müssen schließlich in die Zellen der peripheren Körpergewebe gelangen, um dort ihre spezifischen Wirkungen auszuüben.
Man könnte die Summe dieser Vorgänge als Gewebsphase des endogenen Jod-
haushaltes seiner thyreoidalen Jodid- und Hormonphase gegenüberstellen. Sie ist
im Gegensatz zu den beiden letzteren nur mit Hilfe schwieriger chemischer und
isotopentechnischer Methoden zu erfassen, deshalb kaum erforscht und ohne
diagnostische Bedeutung. Die derzeitigen Kenntnisse darüber beruhen weitgehend auf biochemischen und tierexperimentellen Befunden, die erhebliche
Differenzen von Species zu Species ergeben. Die Unklarheiten mehren sich, wenn,
wie hier, die Verhältnisse beim Menschen in den Mittelpunkt der Betrachtung
rücken sollen. Das ist auf Grund neuerer Untersuchungsergebnisse zwar möglich,
muß aber selbst bei Rückgriffen auf Biochemie und Tierexperiment heute noch
recht lückenhaft bleiben.

Unter dem Aspekt der *Quantität* ihres Verhaltens in der Körperperipherie
spricht man vom *Umsatz*, unter dem der *Qualität* vom *Stoffwechsel* der Schilddrüsenhormone. Beide sind natürlich eng miteinander verknüpft, doch wird sich
herausstellen, daß sowohl der Umsatz wie auch der Stoffwechsel die Führungs-
größe in den wechselseitigen Relationen darstellen kann und es demnach kein
a priori festliegendes Bezugssystem zwischen beiden gibt.

Die Abb. 1 mag vorweg die Positionen von Umsatz und Stoffwechsel der
Schilddrüsenhormone im Organismus erläutern. Dabei sei von der Tatsache
ausgegangen, daß dem thyreoidalen Hormonraum (1) der extrathyreoidale
Hormonraum gegenübersteht, der sich in einen intravasalen (2), extracellulären
(3) und intracellulären (4) Abschnitt unterteilen läßt. 1, 3 und 4 sind virtu-
elle Räume und lassen sich dadurch mit dem intravasalen Volumen vergleichen, daß man bei allen entsprechenden Berechnungen die Hormonkonzentration in ihnen auf die des Plasmas bezieht. Diese Notwendigkeit ergibt
sich daraus, daß zu chemischen Hormon- bzw. Jodanalysen praktisch nur
Blut zur Verfügung steht. Die Messung der Hormonbewegung von 2 über 3 nach 4

gibt Auskunft über den Umsatz, die Analyse von Hormonabbauprodukten da, wo sie zu erfassen sind, gibt Auskunft über den Stoffwechsel der Hormone. Dementsprechend sind die Untersuchungsmethoden für beide Zwecke recht verschieden. Stets aber ist es dazu erforderlich, in einen der extrathyreoidalen Hormonräume ein radioaktiv markiertes Hormon der physiologischen l-Form einzubringen und sein weiteres Verhalten zu verfolgen. Bei älteren Untersuchungen mit inaktiven Hormonen waren wegen des chemischen Nachweises so hohe Dosen nötig, daß jeder physiologische Vorgang gestört wurde.

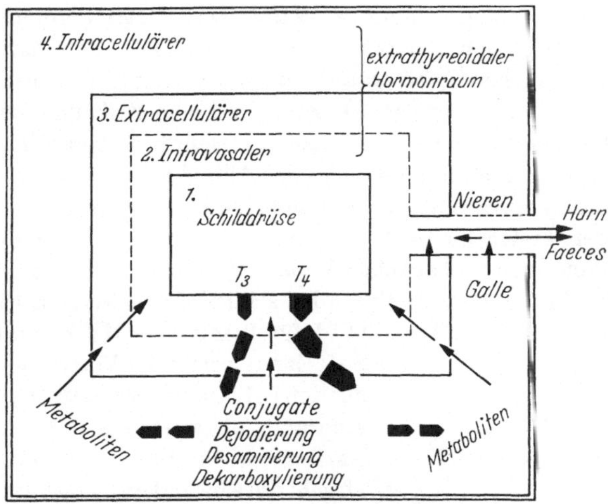

Abb. 1. Die 4 Verteilungsräume der Schilddrüsenhormone. [Der Hormonumsatz bezieht sich auf die Bewegung von 3 nach 4, der Stoffwechsel auf die Vorgänge in 4 mit dem Anfall von Metaboliten in 4, 3, 2, Harn oder Faeces (Galle)]

Auch bei der Verwendung von markierten Hormonen ist jedoch die Beurteilung der Ergebnisse von vornherein durch Einschränkungen belastet:

1. Ihr Nachweis und der ihrer Metaboliten hängt von der Art der radioaktiven Markierung ab. Sie erfolgt meist mit J^{131}, so daß mit der Isotopentechnik nur jodhaltige und keine jodfreien Hormonbruchstücke zu registrieren sind. Für eine Markierung mit C^{14} gilt sinngemäß ein gleicher Vorbehalt, darüber hinaus verhindert die geringe spezifische Aktivität solcher Hormonpräparate eine Anwendung in Spürdosen.

2. Die derzeit verfüg- und beziehbaren markierten Schilddrüsenhormone enthalten J^{131} nur in den Stellungen 3′ (T_3) oder 3′,5′ (T_4), nicht aber an 3 bzw. 3,5. Durch Aktivitätsmessungen ist deshalb nur ein Teil von Veränderungen des Jodgehalts eines Moleküls zu erfassen. In vivo markierte Hormone würden ein Gemisch von an allen Positionen J^{131} enthaltenden Molekülen und beim Verfolgen ihres Stoffwechsels ein anderes Bild ergeben, ohne indessen wesentlich aufschlußreicher zu sein (HAMOLSKI et al. 1953).

3. Die Degradation durch Selbstbestrahlung der Testpräparate (PITT-RIVERS und TATA 1959) macht zwar besondere Aufbewahrungs- und Prüfverfahren vor ihrer Anwendung erforderlich, stört aber den in vivo-Versuch, bei dem das Hormon schnell verdünnt wird, nicht.

Roche et al. (1955, 1956) halten auf Grund von Befunden an Ratten auch 3,3′-Dijodthyronin und 3,3′,5′-Trijodthyronin für echte Schilddrüsenhormone. Abgesehen davon, daß sie beim Menschen bisher nicht gefunden werden konnten, verhalten sie sich in der Körperperipherie weniger wie T_4 oder T_3, sondern eher wie deren Metaboliten (Stanbury und Morris 1957, Dunn und Stanbury 1958). Sie werden deshalb hier nicht als Hormone berücksichtigt.

1. Der Umsatz von Schilddrüsenhormonen

Er ist meßbar als Geschwindigkeit, mit der T_4 und T_3 die Blutbahn verlassen, in die Gewebszellen gelangen und dort täglich verbraucht werden. Als z. Z. optimale Methode bieten sich die Berechnungen des gesamten extrathyreoidalen Hormonjods, der täglichen Umsatzrate davon und des täglichen Umsatzes auf Grund von Messungen des Hormonspiegels im Blut (PBI oder BEI) und der Halbwertzeit (HWZ) der Abwanderung einer i.v. injizierten Spürdosis von $^{131}T_4$ oder $^{131}T_3$ aus dem Blut an (Sterling et al. 1954). Aus der Abb. 2 geht hervor, daß T_3 die Blutbahn und auch den extracellulären Flüssigkeitsraum wesentlich schneller verläßt als T_4. In beiden Fällen bietet der exponentielle Abfall der Blutaktivitäten als Funktion der Zeit einen biphasischen Verlauf. Der anfänglich schnelle Aktivitätsabfall erfolgt anhand von 50 Analysen bei schilddrüsengesunden Personen für T_4 mit einer HWZ von 12−28 (M = 18) Std, für T_3 mit einer HWZ von 1−3 (M = 1,3) Std. Er entspricht der Verteilung der Spürdosis auf den extracellulären extrathyreoidalen Hormonraum, bis sich in ihm die gleiche spezifische Aktivität wie im Blut eingestellt hat. Von dann ab geht die Abwanderung beider Hormone langsamer vor sich, und die sich ergebenden HWZ von 4−8 (M = 5,8) Tagen für T_4 und 1−3 (M = 1,4) Tagen für T_3 werden dem Hormonabbau in den Zellen mit entsprechend mehr oder weniger schnellem Nachschub zugeschrieben (Benua et al. 1952, Sterling et al. 1954). Albert und Keating (1952) konstruierten aus dem Aktivitätsfall sogar 3 anstelle von 2 Phasen und bezogen sie auf die Verteilung in die einzelnen Hormonräume. Alle Autoren sind sich darüber einig, daß T_3 die einzelnen Verteilungs- bzw. Degradationsphasen schneller absolviert als T_4.

Will man aus der HWZ und der ihr zugeordneten Umsatzrate die extrathyreoidale Hormonmenge und den täglichen Hormonumsatz berechnen, so müssen die Serumspiegel von T_4 und T_3 bekannt sein. Sie werden jeweils als Hormonjod chemisch bestimmt. Da die gesunde und auch die kranke Schilddrüse ausschließlich oder überwiegend T_4 sezerniert, haben die meisten Untersucher den als BEI oder PBI ermittelten Hormonjodgehalt des Blutes mit T_4 identifiziert,

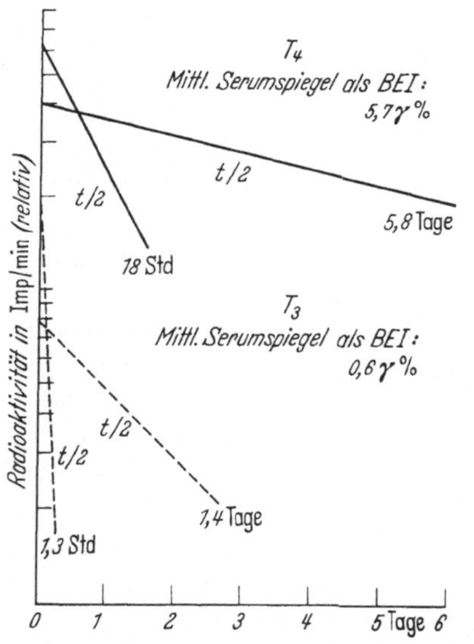

Abb. 2. Die Abwandeiung von radioaktiv markierten Schilddrüsenhormonen aus dem Blut als Grundlage für die Berechnung des Hormonumsatzes (Mittelwerte von 20 Analysen). T_4 = Thyroxin, T_3 = Trijodthyronin. Die 1. Phase mit kurzer Halbwertzeit (HWZ) entspricht der Verteilung auf den extracellulären Hormonraum, die 2. Phase mit längerer HWZ dem cellulären Hormonumsatz

Tabelle 1. *Angaben über den Thyroxin (T_4)-Umsatz beim Menschen*
(Auf Grund von Untersuchungen mit $^{131}T_4$)

	A. HWZ von $^{131}T_4$ (Tg.)	B. Extra-thyr. T_4 Jod (γ)	C. Extra-thyr. T_4-Raum (L)	D. Umsatz-rate von T_4 (% von B/Tg.)	E. T_4-Umsatz (γ/Tag)
INGBAR und FREINKEL (1955)					
Euthyreot (9)	—	508 ± 146	$9,4\pm2,0$	$10,5\pm0,9$	54 ± 17
Hyperthyr. (4)	—	1544 ± 670	$9,1\pm3,5$	$24,4\pm5,6$	359 ± 150
Hypothyr. (5)	—	107 ± 33	$7,5\pm0,6$	$8,8\pm1,4$	11 ± 5
STERLING u. CHODOS (1956)					
Euthyreot (8)	$6,7\pm0,7$	548 ± 107	—	$10,5\pm1,1$	57 ± 11
Hyperthyr. (6)	$4,4\pm1,1$	1021 ± 173	—	$16,9\pm5,0$	179 ± 82
Hypothyr. (9)	$9,7\pm1,4$	238 ± 60	—	$7,3\pm1,1$	17 ± 4
FRIIS (1958)					
Euthyreot (7)	8,0	991	21,0	8,1	85
Hyperthyr. (3)	4,1	2947	20,2	17,7	568
Hypothyr. (1)	10,0	300	6,9	6,9	21
STERLING (1958)					
Euthyreot (10)	$6,6\pm0,7$	557 ± 99	—	$10,7\pm1,1$	59 ± 11
KLEIN (1960)					
Euthyreot					
[Alter 32 Jahre (14)] .	$5,4\pm1,1$	603 ± 200	9,6	$13,5\pm2,6$	81 ± 38
[Alter 70 Jahre (14)] .	$4,3\pm1,5$	610 ± 176	10,2	$17,6\pm6,5$	111 ± 63
Hyperthyr. (21)	3,1	1840	11,0	23,1	432 ± 164
Hypothyr. (12)	11,6	224	12,1	6,2	14 ± 5
HADDAD 1960)					
Euthyreot (12 Kinder) .	$5,0\pm0,1$	$145\pm7,7$	$2,4\pm0,16$	$13,9\pm0,5$	$19,7\pm1,0$
GREGERMAN et al. (1962)					
Euthyreot (73)	$8,4\pm1,4$	714 ± 192	$11,2\pm2,7$	$8,5\pm1,6$	61 ± 21
BASCHIERI et al. (1961)					
Euthyreot (5)	6,7	—	—	—	—
Hyperthyr. (4)	3,5	—	—	—	—
Hypothyr. (3)	8,4	—	—	—	—

so daß sich alle Ergebnisse auf den T_4-Umsatz beziehen (s. Tab. 1). Leicht erhöhte Werte, berechnet pro Kilogramm Körpergewicht, finden sich wegen des Wachstums bei Kindern und Jugendlichen (HADDAD 1960, INGBAR 1960, COTTINO et al. 1961) sowie offenbar wegen Veränderungen des Zellstoffwechsels in höherem Lebensalter (KLEIN 1957, 1960). Stark erhöhte Daten fanden alle Untersucher bei Hyperthyreosen, verringerte Umsätze bei Hypothyreosen. Die Abb. 3 zeigt unsere Ergebnisse von 28 Schilddrüsengesunden, 12 Hypo- und 21 Hyperthyreosen. Mit den außerdem dargestellten normalen Hormonumsätzen bei extrathyreoidalem Hypo- oder Hypermetabolismus stimmen auch Befunde von FRIIS (1958) überein, während STERLING und CHODOS (1956) bei jeder Art von Hypermetabolismus erhöhte Hormonumsätze registrierten, die sie auf einen durch Fieber oder andere Krankheiten vermehrten Hormonbedarf der Peripherie zurückführten. Dagegen lassen sich jedoch manche Einwände erheben.

Obgleich nach den Beobachtungen von BURROW und ROSS (1953), BERSON und YALOW (1954) und INGBAR und FREINKEL (1955) der Hormonumsatz weitgehend vom Hormonspiegel im Blut abhängen soll, läßt sich eine gesetzmäßige Beziehung zwischen beiden nicht belegen. So normalisieren sich unter der ausreichenden Substitution von Hypothyreosen und nach einer erfolgreichen Behandlung von Hyperthyreosen in Übereinstimmung mit dem klinischen Eindruck die Hormonumsätze oft schneller als die dazugehörenden Halbwertzeiten oder Umsatzraten (Ingbar und Freinkel 1958, Sterling 1958, Klein 1960). Es kann auch bei Fällen mit gleichem Bluthormongehalt und gleichen Mengen von extrathyreoidalem Hormonjod der Hormonumsatz durch eine sehr verschiedene Umsatzrate bis in pathologische Bereiche hinein voneinander abweichen. Der Grund für diese Mißverhältnisse dürfte in Eigenarten der peripheren Zellen zu suchen sein. Diese Auffassung wird dadurch gestützt, daß Ingbar et al. (1956) auch bei äußerlich schilddrüsengesunden Familienmitgliedern

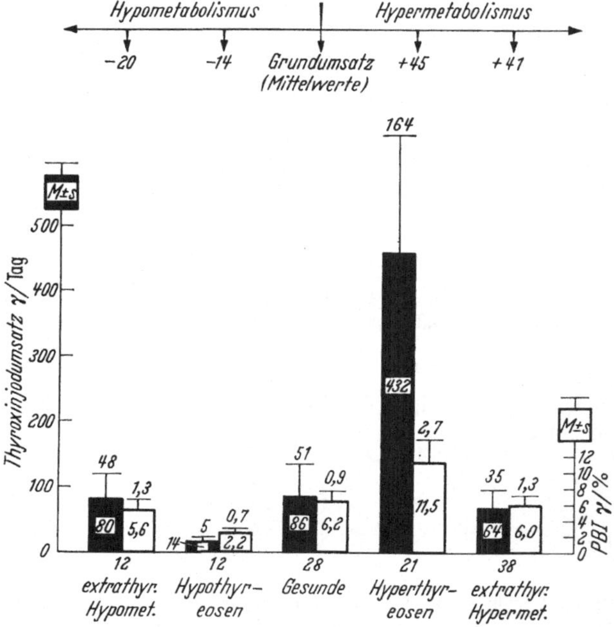

Abb. 3. Hormonjodgehalt des Blutes und peripherer Thyroxinumsatz bei thyreoidalem und extrathyreoidalem Hypo- und Hypermetabolismus (M = Mittelwerte, s = Streuung)

von Hyperthyreosen die dieser Krankheit eigenen erhöhten Hormonumsatzraten als offenbar hereditär fixierte Anlage fanden. Wir haben solche Anomalien des Thyroxinumsatzes mehrfach bei Hyper- und Hypothyreosen (s. Abb. 4) und vor allem beim sporadischen Kretinismus (s. Abb. 5) nachweisen können (Klein 1961, 1962):

Bei 4 von 6 Kretins, 14 von 42 Hyperthyreosen und 10 von 17 Hypothyreosen waren die Hormonumsätze trotz normalen Angebotes vermehrt oder vermindert bzw. die Umsatzraten oder Halbwertzeiten der Hormonabwanderung trotz verminderten oder vermehrten Angebotes normal. Bei den Hyperthyreosen könnte jedoch das Ausmaß eines gleichzeitigen Trijodthyroninumsatzes solche Anomalien vortäuschen.

Berechnungen und Ergebnisse des T_4-Umsatzes stimmen nämlich nur dann mit den untersuchten Vorgängen überein, wenn der Hormonjodgehalt des Blutes tatsächlich in vollem Umfang auf T_4 bezogen werden kann. Schon normalerweise bestehen jedoch bis zu 15% des BEI oder PBI aus T_3, und bei Hyperthyreosen kann der T_3-Anteil 50% und mehr erreichen (Arons und Hydovitz 1959, Klein

1960). Die Relation T_4/T_3 im Blut bzw. im Schilddrüseninkret ist aus methodischen Gründen nur annähernd zu bestimmen. Uns bewährt sich dazu die mehrfache Radiochromatographie nach J^{131}-Gabe (KLEIN 1960, 1962), und bei Vergleichsuntersuchungen stimmten die Ergebnisse gut ($\pm 30\%$) mit denen des Verfahrens

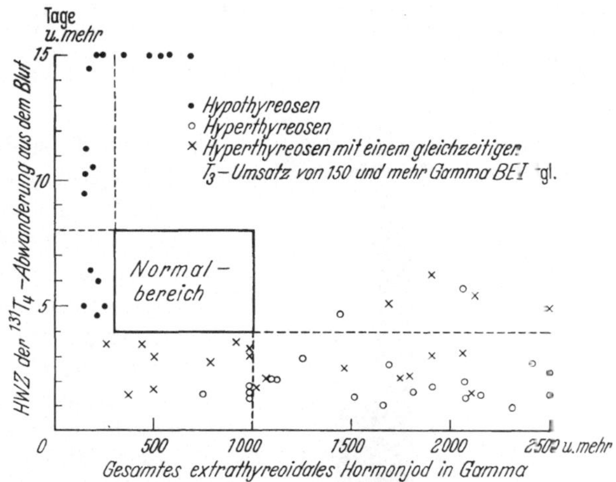

Abb. 4. Die Beziehungen zwischen der Halbwertzeit der Thyroxinabwanderung aus dem Blut und dem gesamten extrathyreoidalen Hormonjod bei Hypo- und Hyperthyreosen. (Bei 14 von 42 Hyperthyreosen und 10 von 17 Hypothyreosen besteht ein Mißverhältnis zwischen beiden Parametern, das bei einem Teil der Hyperthyreosen durch einen hohen gleichzeitigen Trijodthyroninumsatz vorgetäuscht sein könnte)

von PIND (1957) überein. Bei bekanntem T_4/T_3 lassen sich anhand chemischer BEI- oder PBI-Analysen die absoluten Mengen beider Hormone ermitteln und bei

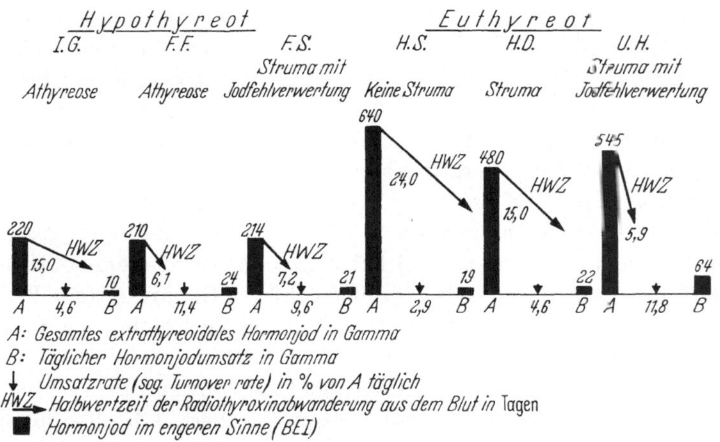

Abb. 5. Der periphere Thyroxinumsatz bei 6 Kranken mit sporadischem Kretinismus. (Mit Ausnahme von I.G. und U.H. bestehen Mißverhältnisse zwischen Hormonangebot und Umsatzrate)

der Umsatzbestimmung in Rechnung stellen. Tab. 2 zeigt die betreffenden Ergebnisse von an 30 schilddrüsengesunden Personen durchgeführten Umsatzuntersuchungen mit $^{131}T_4$ und $^{131}T_3$.

Tabelle 2. *Der Thyroxin(T_4)- und Trijodthyronin (T_3)-Umsatz schildrüsengesunder Menschen* (n = Zahl der Probanden)

	T_4 (n = 30)	T_3 (n = 20)
1. BEI im Blut (γ-%)	5,7±0,8	0,6±0,2
2. HWZ der $^{131}T_4$- bzw. $^{131}T_3$-Abwanderung aus dem Blut (Tage)	5,8±1,1	1,4±0,2
3. Extrathyreoidales T_4- bzw. T_3-Jod (γ)	608±180	42±10
4. Umsatzrate (% von 3/Tag)	12±2,6	49±7,2
5. Umsatz (γ BEI/Tag)	73±21	21±7

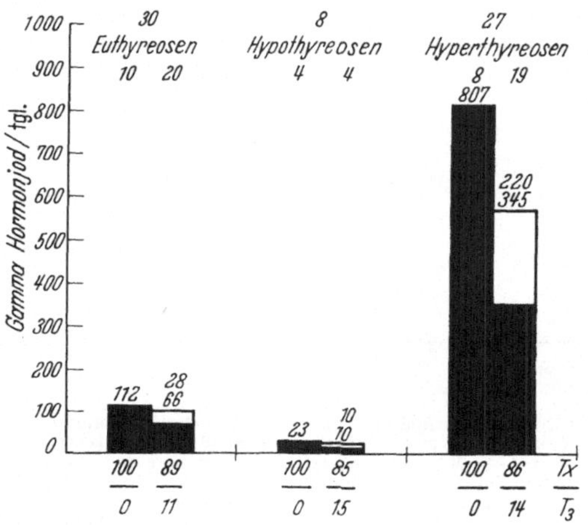

Abb. 6. Die Abhängigkeit des Hormonumsatzes von der Beschaffenheit des Drüseninkretes (T_4/T_3-Relation) bei eu-, hypo- und hyperthyreotischen Probanden. (Bei ausschließlicher Inkretion von Thyroxin wird durchweg mehr Hormonjod umgesetzt als bei gleichzeitigem endogenen Angebot von Trijodthyronin)

Laut Abb. 6 sind im Durchschnitt bei Hyperthyreosen die Umsätze beider Hormone vermehrt, und bei Hypothyreosen trifft das Umgekehrte zu. Zugleich demonstriert die Abbildung, daß bei gleichzeitiger T_3-Inkretion der gesamte Hormonjodumsatz trotz etwa gleicher Schweregrade der Krankheit geringer ist als bei ausschließlicher T_4-Inkretion (KLEIN 1962). HALES et al. (1960) stellten demgegenüber fest, daß T_3 bei Hyperthyreosen die Blutbahn langsamer als normalerweise verläßt und unverändert im Harn erscheint. Sie schließen daraus auf eine thyreogene Leberschädigung, haben aber den quantitativen T_3-Umsatz nicht in Erfahrung gebracht. Wenn nämlich das Blut kein endogenes T_3 enthält, sind Untersuchungen mit $^{131}T_3$ ohne Aussagewert.

Über Veränderungen des Hormonumsatzes durch körperliche Anstrengungen oder bei extremer Außentemperatur ist, abgesehen von unzuverlässigen indirekten Schlußfolgerungen aus PBI-Analysen, nur bekannt, daß Kälte (KASSENAAR et al. 1959) und viele Stunden Arbeitszuwachs bei Tieren den Umsatz steigern, geringe Belastungen indessen keinen Einfluß haben (ESCOBAR und ESCOBAR 1956). Beim gesunden Menschen wandert trotz gleichbleibenden PBI injiziertes $^{131}T_4$ tagsüber schneller aus dem Blut ab als nachts, doch könnten Verschiebungen des Plasmavolumens der Grund dafür sein (WALFISH et al. 1961).

Die, wie geschildert, berechneten Größen sind nur dann auf einen echten Umsatz von Hormonen zu beziehen, wenn diese nicht unverändert, d. h. ohne zur Wirkung gelangt zu sein, den extrathyreoidalen Hormonraum verlassen oder in ihn zurückkehren. Im Harn erscheinen physiologischerweise nur Hormonmetaboliten, vor allem Jodid und vielleicht Spuren von T_3 und T_4. Auch bei Schilddrüsenkrankheiten ändert sich diese Situation nicht wesentlich (FLOCK et al. 1956, 1957, KOT und KLITGAARD 1959, HALES et al. 1960). Im Stuhl hingegen finden sich beim Menschen neben Metaboliten relativ reichlich unveränderte oder konjugierte

Hormone (ALBERT et al. 1949, PITT-RIVERS und TATA 1959). Bei Untersuchungen über die Verteilung der Schilddrüsenhormone auf die verschiedenen Organe hatte sich bald herausgestellt, daß, abgesehen von gewissen Unterschieden zwischen dem Verhalten von T_3 und T_4 (VAN ARSDEL et al. 1954, KUTZIM 1962), ein ungewöhnlich hoher Prozentsatz in der Leber und später in der Galle und im Darm anzutreffen ist (JOHNSON und ALBERT 1951, ALBERT und KEATING 1952, KLITGAARD et al. 1953). Abweichend von den meisten anderen Organen, in denen die Hormonkonzentration nach einer Testdosis langsam ansteigt, erreicht sie in der Leber

schnell ein Maximum, um sogleich wieder abzufallen. Dieses Maximum wird nach T_3 ungleich schneller als nach T_4 registriert, stimmt zeitlich mit der HWZ der kurzen Phase überein (TRIANTAPHYLLIDIS et al. 1955) und fällt somit in den Vorgang der Verteilung einer zugeführten Hormondosis auf den extracellulären Hormonraum – s. Abb.7. Dessen virtuelles Volumen wird also weitgehend durch die Leber repräsentiert und soll bei Tieren ungleich größer als beim Menschen sein (PITT-RIVERS und TATA 1959).

Durch Unterschiede im Sauerstoffverbrauch einzelner Körpergewebe läßt sich diese

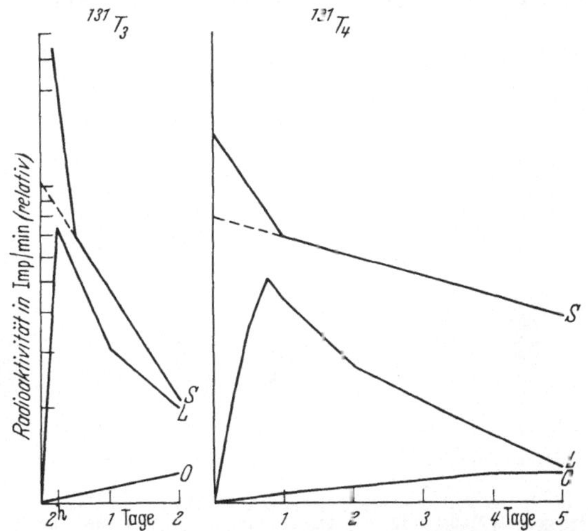

Abb. 7. Das Verhalten der Radioaktivität in Plasma und Leber nach i.v.-Injektion von Radiothyroxin oder Radiotrijodthyronin. (Die Leberaktivität L erreicht in der Phase der Hormonverteilung auf den extracellulären Hormonraum ihr Maximum und sinkt dann parallel zur Plasmaaktivität S wieder ab, während die Aktivität über dem Oberschenkel O wie die der übrigen Organe langsam ansteigt)

Sonderstellung der Leber nicht erklären. Sie beruht vielmehr darauf, daß die Leber T_3 und T_4 lebhaft mit Schwefel- oder Glucuronsäure paart. Die entstehenden Verbindungen sind keine Abbauprodukte im eigentlichen Sinne, sie gelangen zum kleinen Teil direkt in das Blut und zum größeren via Galle in den Darm. Dort hat man sie erstmals identifiziert (TAUROG et al. 1951, 1952, BRIGGS et al. 1953, ROCHE et al. 1953, 1954, FLOCK et al. 1960, 1961). Sie werden hydrolytisch gespalten und weitgehend rückresorbiert. Bei der physiologischen Größenordnung der fäkalen T_4-Clearance von etwa 200–400 cm³ Plasma/Tag und der etwas größeren von T_3 (MYANT 1956) gelangen nur maximal 5% des extrathyreoidalen Hormonjods täglich in den Darm – eine Relation, die auch für Schilddrüsenkrankheiten gilt (BERSON und YALOW 1954, STERLING et al. 1954, FLOCK et al. 1956, TRIANTAPHYLLIDIS et al. 1956).

Die gesamte Ausscheidung von Hormonen ist demnach bei schilddrüsengesunden und -kranken Menschen so gering, daß sie bei Umsatzberechnungen nach den derzeit üblichen Verfahren im allgemeinen vernachlässigt werden kann.

Es gibt indessen einige extrathyreoidale Umstände, unter denen sich diese Verhältnisse ändern. Die klinische Erfahrung lehrt, daß eine exogene Hormonzufuhr nur in Ausnahmefällen eine Hyperthyreosis factitia mit vermehrtem peripheren Hormonumsatz zur Folge hat. Meistens bleibt, unabhängig von der Dosis, die Euthyreose erhalten. Es ist erwiesen, daß selbst hohe Dosen von T_4 oder Thyreoidea sicca den Hormonjodspiegel des Blutes nicht länger als 24 Std zu erhöhen brauchen und offenbar schneller als kleinere Dosen ausgeschieden werden (Joliot et al. 1944, Klein 1960). Bei mit T_4 gefütterten Tieren fanden Premachandra und Turner (1961) die HWZ der $^{131}T_4$-Abwanderung um so langsamer, je höher das PBI anstieg. Sie sahen darin einen Schutzmechanismus. Wir haben an 22 schilddrüsengesunden Probanden den Einfluß von l-T_4 und l-T_3 auf den peripheren T_4-Umsatz geprüft und die Ergebnisse in Abb. 8 dargestellt. Sie zeigen,

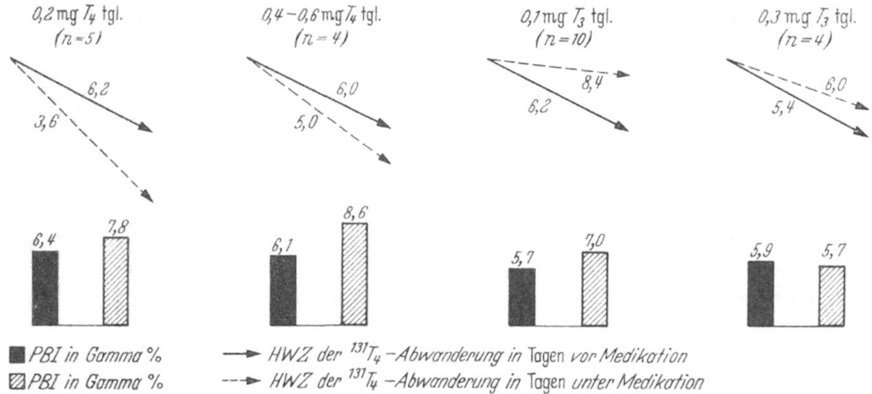

Abb. 8. Das Verhalten der Halbwertzeit der Abwanderung von Radiothyroxin aus dem Blut und des Hormonjodspiegels als Maßstab für den Thyroxinumsatz vor und unter der Medikation von verschiedenen Dosen Thyroxin und Trijodthyronin. (Der Thyroxinumsatz geht nicht dem Angebot parallel und nimmt unter Zufuhr von Trijodthyronin ab)

daß der Hormonumsatz unter geringeren Dosen entsprechend der Zunahme von PBI und Verkürzung der HWZ stärker zunimmt als unter höheren Dosen. Die Medikation von l-T_3 hat im Gegensatz dazu eine Verlangsamung des T_4-Umsatzes zur Folge, weil das exogene Hormon bevorzugt verwendet wird. Diesem unterschiedlichen Verhalten können zugrunde liegen:

1. Eine Rückwirkung der exogenen Hormone auf die TSH-Inkretion des HVL, so daß mit der Produktion auch der Umsatz endogener Hormone reduziert wird (Klein und Berghoff 1960) — ein Problem, das hier nicht näher zu erörtern ist.

2. Eine Intensivierung des enterohepatischen Kreislaufs der Schilddrüsenhormone. Bei Ratten kommt es unter gleichen Umständen zu einer vermehrten T_4-Ausscheidung über die Galle sowie zum Erscheinen mehrerer Hormonmetaboliten (Kot und Klitgaard 1959, Pitt-Rivers und Tata 1959). Beim Menschen fand v. Middlesworth (1960) nach oraler T_4-Zufuhr eine um so viel stärkere T_4-Ausscheidung im Stuhl als nach i.v. Verabreichung, daß der Unterschied nicht allein durch eine mangelhafte Resorption, sondern vornehmlich durch eine Aktivierung des enterohepatischen Kreislaufs mit Reexkretion zu erklären war.

Wenn auf diese Weise mehr Hormone konjugiert, via Galle in den Darm abgesondert und teilweise rückresorbiert werden, so sollten die Hormonester auch im Blut nachzuweisen sein. Laut Abb. 9 ist das zum mindesten bei höheren Hormondosen auch der Fall und fanden sich dann stets Konjugate des durch Zufuhr vermehrten Hormons, nicht aber des endogenen Partners. Dessen Umsatz wird vielmehr auf homöostatischem Wege gedrosselt. Die radiochromatographischen Befunde gleichen denen mancher Hyperthyreosen, so daß der Organismus mit dem enterohepatischen Kreislauf offenbar die Möglichkeit hat, einen exo- oder endogenen Hormonüberschuß partiell zu inaktivieren.

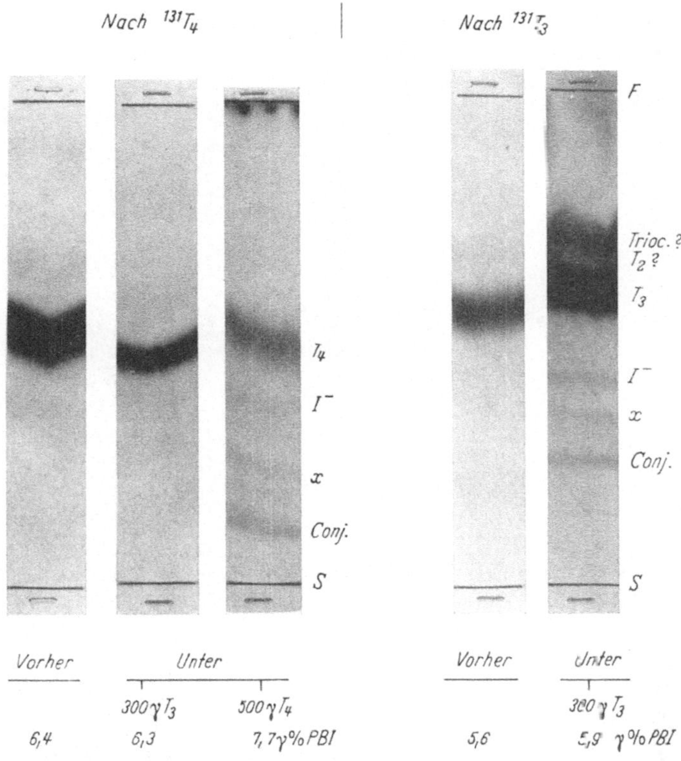

Abb. 9. Hormonkonjugate im menschlichen Blut nach Zufuhr unphysiologischer Dosen von Na-L-Thyroxin und L-Trijodthyronin. (System BDA, aufsteigend. Euthyreosen. Es fallen nur Konjugate des durch Zufuhr vermehrten Hormons und keine des endogenen Partners an)

Weitere Zustände, die trotz erhöhten Hormonspiegels im Blut ohne hyperthyreotische Symptome einhergehen, sind die Gravidität und die Gelbsucht. Im ersteren Fall sorgt der Oestrogenzuwachs für ein festeres Haften der Schilddrüsenhormone an ihren Bluteiweißträgern (DOWLING et al. 1956, VANNOTTI 1957), im zweiten Fall hängen die Verhältnisse von der Grundkrankheit ab. Beim Verschlußikterus kreisen im Blut vermehrt Hormonkonjugate, die durch die Abflußbehinderung in den allgemeinen Kreislauf gelangen und diesen langsamer als nicht konjugierte Hormone verlassen. Bei der akuten Gelbsucht hingegen ist die Leber nicht in der Lage, wie in gesundem Zustand zu dejodieren und zu konjugieren. Die thyreogenen Hormone stauen sich deshalb unverändert vor der Leber an. Weil das Organ für ihren Umsatz ausfällt und offenbar auch Plasmaeiweißverschiebungen den Transport beeinflussen, wandern sie ebenfalls langsamer als normalerweise ab (SCAZZIGA et al. 1955, VANNOTTI und BÉRAUD 1959). Bei

gesunder Schilddrüse ist jedoch das Wechselspiel zwischen ihr und der Körperperipherie so ausgeglichen, daß auch bei vermehrt vorhandenem extrathyreoidalen
Hormonjod durch eine erniedrigte Umsatzrate bzw. verlängerte HWZ nur normale
Hormonmengen zur Wirkung gelangen (RUEGAMER und CHODOS, 1956, VANNOTTI
und BÉRAUD 1959, KLEIN 1960, 1961). Zwei eigene Beispiele zeigt die Abb. 10
links.

Derlei Regulationen gehören in den Bereich der normalen Leistungsbreite der
Homöostase, und es gibt auch immer wieder schilddrüsengesunde Menschen ohne

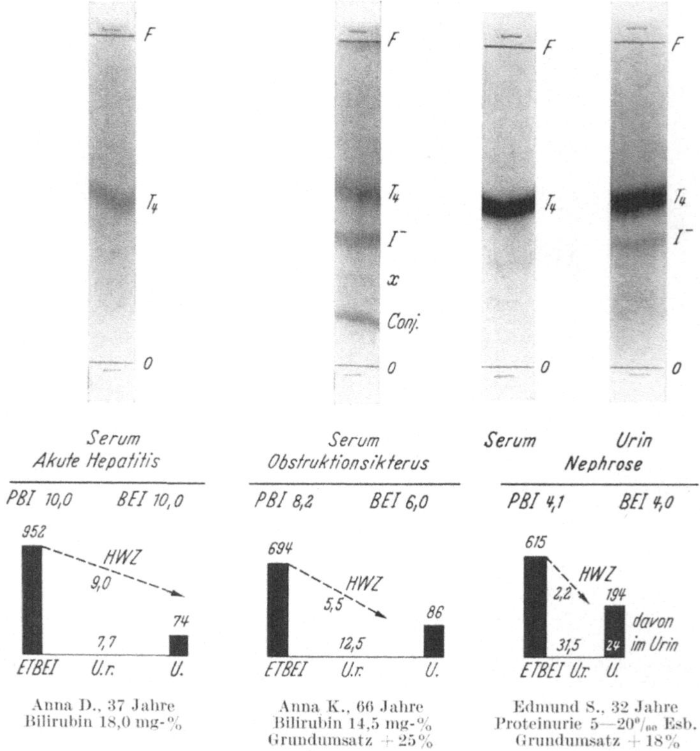

PBI und *BEI:* Hormonjodfraktionen des Blutes in γ-%. *HWZ: HWZ* der $^{131}T_4$-Abwanderung aus dem Blut in
Tagen. *ETBEI:* Extrathyreoidales Hormonjod als *BEI* in γ. *U.r.:* Umsatzrate als % pro Tag vom *ETBEI*.
U.: Umsatz in *BEI* als γ/Tag

Abb. 10. Beispiele für den Umsatz und Stoffwechsel von Thyroxin bei Hepatitis, Verschlußikterus und Nephrose.
(System BDA, aufsteigend. Ein entsprechend der gesunden Schilddrüse normaler Hormonumsatz wird trotz
extrathyreoidaler Ausscheidungsstörungen gewährleistet durch Veränderung der Umsatzrate)

spezielle Familienanamnese, die ein erhöhtes oder erniedrigtes PBI aufweisen und
durch eine entgegengesetzt veränderte Umsatzrate ihren Hormonumsatz regeln
(KLEIN 1960). Ein Spiegelbild der Verhältnisse bei der akuten Hepatitis stellt z. B.
die Nephrose mit Eiweißverlust und konsekutiv erniedrigtem Hormonspiegel im
Blut dar (Abb. 10, rechts). Der eiweißreiche Harn enthält, was normalerweise nie
der Fall ist, reichlich T_4 und die peripheren Gewebe versuchen durch eine stark
beschleunigte Umsatzrate das verringerte Hormonangebot auszunutzen. Gelingt

dies, so bleibt die Euthyreose erhalten, reicht der Kompensationsversuch der Gewebe nicht aus, so stellt sich eine Hypothyreose ein, obgleich die Schilddrüse normal funktioniert.

Wenn bisher ausschließlich vom Umsatz der Schilddrüsenhormone die Rede war, so mögen auch kurz die ihn steuernden Faktoren aufgezählt sein:

1. Die Hormonproduktion bzw. -inkretion, die das Angebot bestimmt. Die Ursachen für krankhafte Veränderungen des Hormonangebots liegen drüsenwärts von intravasalem und extracellulärem Hormonraum und stehen hier nicht zur Debatte (Schilddrüsenkrankheiten).

2. Die Transportverhältnisse der Schilddrüsenhormone im Blut und im extracellulären Flüssigkeitsraum. Sie sind ebenfalls nicht Gegenstand dieser Abhandlung, sondern von PITT-RIVERS und SACKS bereits erörtert worden. Es soll betont sein, daß die transportierenden Eiweißindividuen in Blut und in extracellulärer Flüssigkeit nicht identisch sind und es offenbar für den Übertritt des Hormons vom einen in den anderen Flüssigkeitsraum auf die Relation vom freien zum gebundenen Anteil ankommt. Bei Hypo- oder Hyperthyreosen sowie unter zahlreichen experimentellen Bedingungen, z. B. Gaben von Dinitrophenol oder Salicylaten, finden sich Alterationen des Hormontransportes, die für den Eintritt in die Zellen von entscheidender Bedeutung sind (FREINKEL et al. 1957, INGBAR 1960, BRAVERMAN und INGBAR 1961).

3. Die Vorgänge, die sich beim Eintritt des Hormonmoleküls in die Zellen des Erfolgsorgans abspielen. Sie hängen weitgehend mit den unter 2. genannten Verhältnissen zusammen und sind beim Menschen nicht zu erfassen. Tierexperimentelle Untersuchungen von ROCHE et al. (1960) und MICHEL et al. (1960) haben einigen Aufschluß über dieses für die Hormonverwertung wesentliche Geschehen bringen können. T_3 und T_4 verhalten sich dabei entsprechend ihrer unterschiedlichen Bindung im extracellulären Flüssigkeitsraum zum mindesten in den ersten Stunden ihres Umsatzes sehr verschieden. Nach 5 Std haben bereits 50% einer applizierten T_3-Dosis alle Flüssigkeitsvolumina und auch die Zellmembranen passiert, während T_4 dazu mehr als 15 Std benötigt. Zu jeder späteren Zeit finden sich im extracellulären Hormonraum doppelt so viel T_4 wie T_3. Daraus errechnet sich eine etwa 5fach schnellere Penetrationsgeschwindigkeit des T_3 gegenüber T_4, die wahrscheinlich für die größere Wirksamkeit dieses Hormons verantwortlich ist. Daß T_3 und T_4 als solche die Zellmembranen passieren, ist durch LIPNER et al. (1952), GROS et al. (1957) und FORD et al. (1957) nachgewiesen worden.

Der Übertritt des Hormonmoleküls in die Zelle ist nach LISSITZKY (1960) zugleich eng verknüpft mit seiner ersten metabolischen Alteration durch Dejodierung, so daß sich an diesem Punkt Umsatz und Stoffwechsel der Schilddrüsenhormone direkt berühren.

2. Der Stoffwechsel der Schilddrüsenhormone

Er vollzieht sich in den Zellen der Erfolgsorgane an mehreren Stellen des Hormonmoleküls, wobei grundsätzlich folgende Veränderungs- bzw. Abbaumöglichkeiten bestehen (Abb. 11).

a) Konjugation

Wie alle Phenole können die Schilddrüsenhormone in der Leber und in geringerem Umfang auch in den Nieren mit Schwefel- oder Glucuronsäure gepaart werden (TAUROG et al. 1952, ROCHE et al. 1956). Die Bedeutung dieser Vorgänge wurde bereits beim enterohepatischen Kreislauf besprochen. Nach GROSS et al. (1957) und ROCHE et al. (1960, 1961) kann T_3 in Form seines Sulfatesters nicht so leicht die Zellmembran passieren wie in freier Form, so daß insgesamt die Konjugation keine Degradation der Schilddrüsenhormone, sondern eine vorübergehende Inaktivierung oder Überführung in eine Speicherform bedeutet, die durch Hydrolyse reversibel ist. Neben T_4 und T_3 können auch deren Essigsäurederivate, Dijodthyronin und Thyroxamin konjugiert werden (BARAC 1959, ETLING und BARKER 1959, FLOCK et al. 1960, 1961, DE GREGORIO et al. 1960, GREEN und INGBAR 1961).

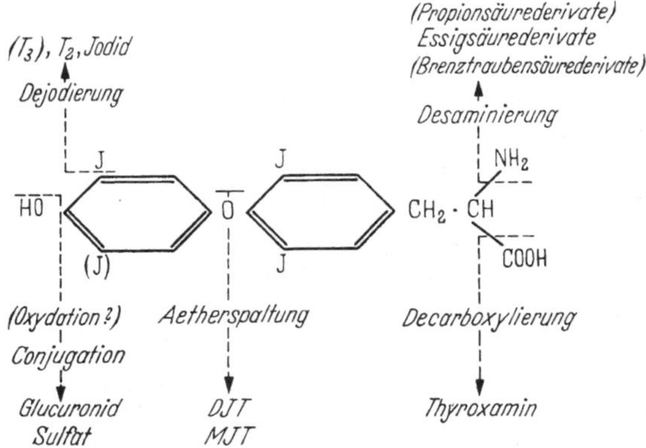

Abb. 11. Abbauwege der Schilddrüsenhormone Thyroxin und Trijodthyronin. [Im letzteren Falle gelten (J) und (T₃) nicht]

b) Dejodierung

Eine Jodabspaltung läßt sich deshalb leicht nachweisen, weil das Verhalten der Schilddrüsenhormone sowohl chemisch wie isotopentechnisch ohnehin nur anhand ihres Jodgehaltes zu verfolgen ist. Dabei war schon immer aufgefallen, daß nach Hormonzufuhr stets vermehrt Jodid in Körpersäften und Exkreten auftritt (BENUA et al. 1952). Vom Jod einer Spürdosis T_4 finden sich innerhalb von 30 Tagen etwa 50% als Jodid im Harn, etwa 35% als Jodid in der Schilddrüse und der Rest im Stuhl, während die Plasmakonzentration in dieser Zeit auf 0 absinkt (INGBAR und FREINKEL 1955). Entsprechend den veränderten Hormonumsätzen sind diese Bewegungen bei Hyperthyreosen beschleunigt und bei Hypothyreosen verlangsamt (TRIANTAPHYLLIDIS et al. 1955, KLEIN 1960, LAMBERG et al. 1962). Bei normaler Schilddrüsenfunktion werden etwa 2—4 % einer bestimmten T_4-Menge täglich dejodiert, und anders als bei den meisten Tieren (MACLAGAN und REID 1957) nimmt dieser Prozentsatz zu, wenn das Hormonangebot exogen oder endogen erhöht wird (TRIANTAPHYLLIDIS et al. 1955, 1956, KLEIN 1960). Interessanterweise hat die Medikation von Salicylaten den gleichen und die von antithyreoidalen Substanzen einen entgegengesetzten Effekt (JONES und v. MIDDLESWORTH 1960, ESCOBAR et al. 1962, HERSHAM und v. MIDDLESWORTH 1962). Da T_3 zwar in vivo, nicht aber in vitro schneller als T_4 sein Jod verliert, scheint die Zelle selber keines der beiden Hormone bevorzugt zu verwerten (WILKINSON und MACLAGAN 1954).

Im Detail sind die Dejodierungsprozesse erst kürzlich näher erkannt worden. ALBRIGHT et al. (1959), STANBURY (1960) und WYNN et al. (1962) verlegen sie in die Mikrosomen, weil sie nach deren Zerstörung sistieren. Unter den von ihnen in Leber und Nieren geprüften Bedingungen erwies sich die Dejodinaseaktivität als hitzestabil bzw. -aktivierbar und $Fe^{\cdot\cdot}$-abhängig, wahrscheinlich wird zugleich der Phenolring des Hormons geöffnet. SPROTT und MACLAGAN (1955) sowie YAMAMOTO et al. (1960, 1961) unterscheiden zwischen einer chemischen und enzymatischen Dejodierung und halten ebenso wie TATA (1959) die Flavinnucleotide für notwendige Coenzyme. Nach LISSITZKY et al. (1960, 1961) hat man sich den Mechanismus bei der Dejodierung so vorzustellen, daß ebenso wie in der Extracellularflüssigkeit auch in der Zelle ein Eiweißkörper existiert, der die Hormone nach der Membranpassage akzeptiert und damit zunächst gegen eine weitere Verwendung schützt. Mit ihm konkurriert um das Hormonmolekül eine Dejodinase. Untersucht an Muskelgewebe, wird sie in die Mitochondrien lokalisiert, weil dieser Zellbestandteil nach Zufuhr von T_4 oder T_3 am meisten abgespaltenes Jod enthält. Zugabe des bindenden Eiweißkörpers verhindert die Dejodierung, die überdies zunächst die Jodatome am β-Ring und nur zögernd die des α-Ringes betrifft (PLASKETT 1961). Ein Teil des in der Zelle abgespaltenen Jodids oder andere jodhaltige Hormonbruchstücke gehen wenigstens passager ebenfalls eine Bindung an noch nicht identifizierte Eiweißindividuen ein, der Komplex bleibt bei papierchromatographischen Analysen wie ein Jodproteid am Start liegen (GALTON und INGBAR 1961, PLASKETT 1961).

Hinsichtlich der Dejodierungsfähigkeit von T_4 und T_3 sowie des Anfalls von Spaltprodukten verhalten sich die menschlichen Organe sehr verschieden. Am intensivsten wirkt die Leber (GEORGI und HARTMANN 1961), die indessen ebensowenig wie Muskulatur und im Gegensatz zu Nieren und Herz aus T_4 kein T_3 bilden soll (ALBRIGHT und LARSON 1959). Die Dejodinaseaktivität von Muskelgewebe ist bei Hypothyreosen gesteigert und bei Hyperthyreosen unverändert (PINCHERA et al. 1962), obgleich für den gesamten Organismus das Umgekehrte zutrifft (RIGGS 1952, KLEIN 1960).

Die entstandenen Metaboliten der Hormone werden sehr unterschiedlich und ebenfalls wieder organabhängig weiter degradiert. Sie können in Blut und Harn erscheinen (LISSITZKY und BOUCHILLOUX 1957, STANBURY 1960). Nachgewiesen sind bisher T_3 (aus T_4), Dijodthyronin, Dijodtyrosin, Jodid und einige auch an der Seitenkette veränderte Produkte (ALBRIGHT et al. 1954, 1959, CRUCHAUD et al. 1955, HOGNESS et al. 1955, PITT-RIVERS et al. 1955, ROCHE et al. 1956, 1957, 1959, TATA et al. 1957, PLASKETT 1958, LARSON et al 1959, FLOCK et al. 1957, 1960). Die meisten von ihnen werden langsamer als die Muttersubstanzen weiter dejodiert (YAMAZAKI und SLINGERLAND 1959). Die Jodtyrosine sind indessen sehr instabil und werden von nahezu allen Geweben schnell und komplett deshalogeniert (ALBERT und KEATING 1951, FLETSCHER et al. 1958, CAMERON 1960, BECKERS und DE VISSCHER 1961). Eine Aktivitätssteigerung der dafür verantwortlichen ubiquitären Dejodase, die wahrscheinlich nicht mit der T_4 und T_3 angreifenden Dejodinase identisch ist, findet sich bei Hyperthyreosen, eine Abnahme bei Hypothyreosen und insbesondere beim sporadischen Kretinismus (STANBURY et al. 1956, STANBURY und LITWAK 1957, CHOFOER et al. 1960, KLEIN 1960, 1961).

Schließlich mag noch eine neue Beobachtung von TATA (1960) erwähnt sein, nach der T_4 bei plötzlich starker Verdünnung in einem wäßrigen Medium reversibel dejodiert wird, sich nach gleichmäßiger Verteilung der Bruchstücke aber wieder in unveränderter Form findet. Ob dieses merkwürdige Phänomen normaler- oder pathologischerweise eine Rolle spielt, ist unbekannt. Bei gewissen Untersuchungstechniken muß es jedoch berücksichtigt werden.

c) Oxydation

In vitro lassen sich ein- bis dreijodierte Thyronine durch Ascorbinsäure-Fe-O_2-Systeme bei lebhafter Dejodierung oxydieren, wobei Semichinone entstehen (LISSITZKY und BOUCHILLOUX 1957). Ob solche schon von NIEMANN (1950) vermuteten Reaktionen im Stoffwechsel eine Rolle spielen, ist bislang nicht erwiesen und auch unwahrscheinlich, denn das wichtigste Schilddrüsenhormon T_4 ließ sich nicht oxydieren und es war bislang auch in Geweben nie eine Thyroninoxydase nachzuweisen.

d) Spaltung der Diphenylätherbindung

Sie war bei Dejodierungsstudien in vitro zu beobachten und führt zur Entstehung von Mono- und Dijodtyrosin einerseits sowie 2,6-Dijod-p-Chinon andererseits (ALLEGRETTI 1954, STANBURY 1960). Auch in vivo finden sich nach $^{131}T_4$ und $^{131}T_3$ auf Papierchromatogrammen Aktivitätsansammlungen im Bereich von Mono- und Dijodtyrosin, die zwar in manchen, aber nicht in allen Systemen den gleichen R_f-Wert wie die Hormonkonjugate haben (KLEIN 1962). Insgesamt scheint mehr für als gegen das Vorkommen von Jodtyrosinen als Abbauprodukten der Schilddrüsenhormone zu sprechen, auch wenn die bekannt schnelle Dejodierbarkeit dieser Aminosäuren ein sehr kritischer Einwand ist (PITT-RIVERS und TATA 1959).

e) Desaminierung

Sie erfolgt oxydativ und führt über die instabilen Brenztraubensäureverbindingen zu den Essigsäurederivaten der Schilddrüsenhormone, die in vitro in Zellpräparaten (ALBRIGHT et al. 1956, ROCHE et al. 1956, LARDY et al. 1957, ETLING und BARKER 1957, TATA et al. 1957, TOMITA et al. 1957, TOMITA und LARDY 1960) und in vivo in Geweben, Galle und Blut nachgewiesen worden sind (MYANT 1956, FLOCK et al. 1957, FORD et al. 1957, ROCHE et al. 1959, BÉNARD et al. 1961). Das dabei agierende Enzym ist von NAKANO und DANOWSKI (1962) näher untersucht worden und unabhängig von den bei der Dejodierung notwendigen Cofaktoren. Nachdem als Metaboliten auch Propionsäurederivate identifiziert wurden, dürfte auch eine reduktive Desaminierung vorkommen (TATA et al. 1957, SLINGERLAND und JOSEPHS 1958).

f) Decarboxylierung

Sie läßt Thyroxamin und Trijodthyronamin entstehen, die wie T_4 und T_3, aber ohne Latenzzeit z. B. die Empfindlichkeit des Darmes gegenüber Adrenalin hochgradig steigern (THIBAULT 1956). Bisher nur tierexperimentell von LACHAZE und THIBAULT (1952) sowie von HILLMANN et al. (1958) in kleinen Mengen bei einem Schilddrüsencarcinom nach Radiojodtherapie idendifiziert, könnten die Amine durchaus regelmäßig anfallende Abbauprodukte sein. Diese Vermutung würde sich bestätigen, wenn die auch in Radiochromatogrammen von menschlichem Serum häufig anzutreffenden Frontbanden nicht, wie bisher angenommen, Artefakten sondern diesen Aminen entsprechen sollten (HILLMANN 1961).

Die soeben besprochenen Abbauwege werden nicht von allen Organen in gleicher Weise benutzt. So weichen Konzentration und Umsatz an Essigsäuremetaboliten in verschiedenen Geweben erheblich voneinander ab (LARSON und ALBRIGHT 1958) und lassen sich Dejodierungsphänomene am besten am Skeletmuskel studieren, weil dort keine Desaminierung und Decarboxylierung stattfindet (TATA 1957). Während Leberbrei durch Kochen seine Fähigkeit, zu dejodieren, nicht aber die zu desaminieren verliert (ALBRIGHT et al. 1959), ist Nierenbrei nach solcher Behandlung sogar stärker wirksam als vorher (ETLING und BARKER 1959). In beiden Geweben bleibt nach Zerstörung der Mitochondrien das Desaminierungsvermögen erhalten, das Dejodierungsvermögen jedoch nicht (LARSON et al. 1957). In Leber, Nieren, Hirn und auch Serum fand man neben inzwischen identifizierten noch eine Reihe von unbekannten Verbindungen, die in der Abb. 11 nicht mit aufgeführt sind (ALBRIGHT et al. 1956, BECKERS und PRUDDEN 1959). Da solche Befunde nicht mit einheitlicher Methodik ermittelt worden sind, lassen sich noch keine verbindlichen Vorstellungen über den qualitativen Hormonstoffwechsel entwickeln.

Trotzdem liegt es nahe, anzunehmen, daß Art und Reihenfolge der Hormondegradation mit der jeweiligen Organfunktion in Zusammenhang stehen. Erst kürzlich sind Beziehungen zwischen der Hormondejodierungsaktivität und dem Sauerstoffverbrauch tierischer Gewebe gefunden worden (TATA 1961). Das Muster der anfallenden Metaboliten kann für den Betrieb einer Zelle nicht gleichgültig sein, wenn deren unterschiedliche biologische Wirkungen in Rechnung gestellt werden. Auf der Suche nach einer ganz bestimmten Wirkform der beiden Schilddrüsenhormone war man eine Zeitlang geneigt, zunächst T_3, später die Amine und Essigsäurederivate dafür zu halten. Kein einzelner Metabolit weist jedoch auch nur annähernd das gleiche breite Wirkungsspektrum der genuinen Hormone auf (LARDY et al. 1957, THIBAULT 1957, PITT-RIVERS und TATA 1959). Die Dissoziation in vielfältige Wirkungsfragmente schließt nahezu aus, daß es eine besondere „aktive" Hormonform gibt. Offenbar produziert die Zelle unter den ihr eigenen und durchaus beeinflußbaren Bedingungen ein bestimmtes Metabolitenmuster, das für sie und damit für einen ganzen Zellverband weitgehend charakteristisch ist.

Der biologische Hormoneffekt läßt sich demnach nur global einerseits auf den Vorgang der Bildung, andererseits auf die Summe der Teilwirkungen von Metaboliten und grundsätzlich nicht auf eine hypothetische spezielle Verbindung zurückführen. Dabei dürfte auch die extracelluläre Verteilung einiger Abbauprodukte von Bedeutung sein, weil sie wiederum das Verhalten der Hormone beeinflussen können: In Modellversuchen hemmt die Zufuhr von T_3,Trijodthyroessig- und Trijodthyropropionsäure den Umsatz von T_4 (KLEIN und BERGHOFF 1960). Neben anderen stützen solche Befunde die Vermutung, daß nicht die Höhe des Hormonjodspiegels im Blut, sondern sein Gehalt an einem oder mehreren Metaboliten im Rahmen der Homöostase die TSH-Inkretion aus dem HVL reguliert (KLEIN 1960, ESCOBAR et al. 1962).

Von allen diesen Erörterungen unberührt bleibt die Bedingung, daß T_3 und T_4 zunächst unverändert in die Zelle gelangen müssen, um wirken zu können. Weil dafür weitgehend das Hormonangebot maßgebend ist, schließt sich hier die Frage an, ob bei Änderungen desselben infolge von Schilddrüsenkrankheiten Abweichungen des Metabolitenanfalls von der Norm nachzuweisen sind. Die Abb. 12

mag demonstrieren, daß sich auf radiochromatographischem Wege nach Injektion von markiertem T_4 oder T_3 im menschlichen Blut neben der Hormonbande entweder keine oder zusätzliche Aktivitätsmaxima darstellen, die unter den gegebenen Bedingungen nur Abbauprodukten entsprechen können (KLEIN 1962).

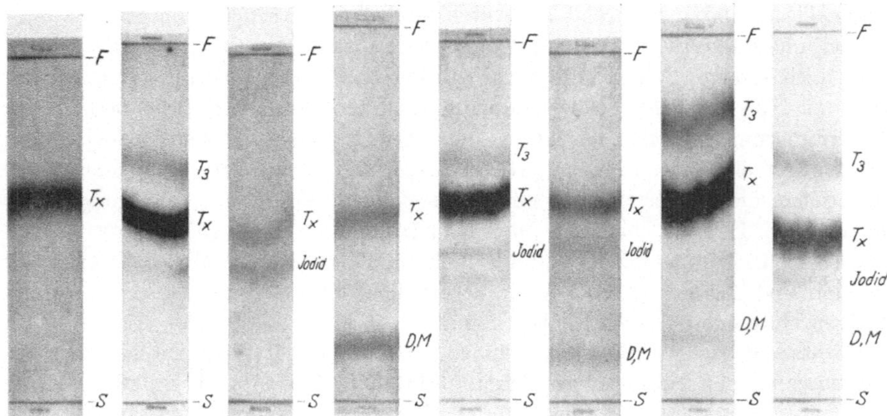

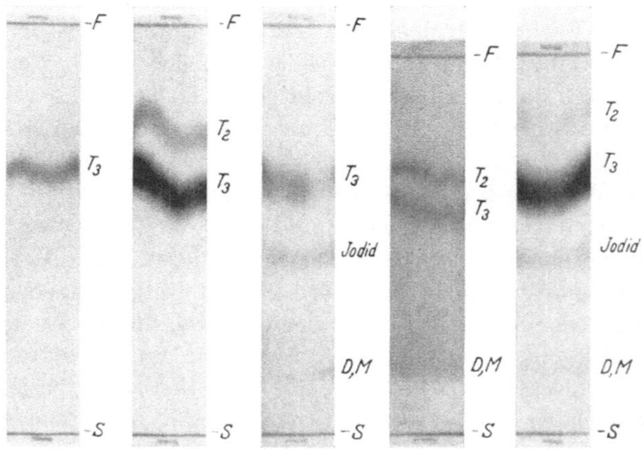

Abb. 12. Im menschlichen Blut nachgewiesene Metaboliten der Schilddrüsenhormone. [Nach Injektion von chromatographisch reinem $^{131}T_4$ (oben) und $^{131}T_3$ (unten). System BDA, aufsteigend. T_4 = Thyroxin, T_3 = Trijodthyronin. Bei der startnahen Aktivitätsbande(D,M) handelt es sich um Dijodtyrosin oder Hormonkonjugate, bei den frontnahen Banden (oben T_3, unten T_2) um T_3 (nur nach T_4), Dijodthyronin sowie Essig- oder Propionsäurederivate]

Ob sie im einzelnen genau identifiziert sind oder nicht, spielt eine geringere Rolle als ihr Nachweis an sich. Bei den startnahen Aktivitätsbanden handelt es sich um Dijodtyrosin oder Hormonkonjugate, bei den frontnahen Banden um T_3 (nach T_4), T_2 (nach T_3) sowie Essig- oder Propionsäurederivate.

Die Abb. 13 zeigt nun anhand von Ergebnissen bei insgesamt 68 Personen, daß das Vorkommen von Metaboliten offenbar weniger vom Ausmaß des Hormonumsatzes abhängt als davon, ob er in Richtung einer Hypo- oder Hyperthyreose verschoben ist. Im einzelnen ergab sich zusätzlich, daß bei eu- und hyperthyreotischen endokrinen Ophthalmopathien häufiger und bei Hyperthyreosen mit starken Grundumsatzsteigerungen seltener als bei einem Vergleichskontingent Metaboliten nachzuweisen waren. Wahrscheinlich spielt in allen diesen Fällen das Sekretionsverhältnis T_4/T_3, das bei Hyperthyreosen und endokrinen Ophthalmopathien in Richtung einer T_3-Zunahme verschoben ist, eine gewisse Rolle (KLEIN 1962).

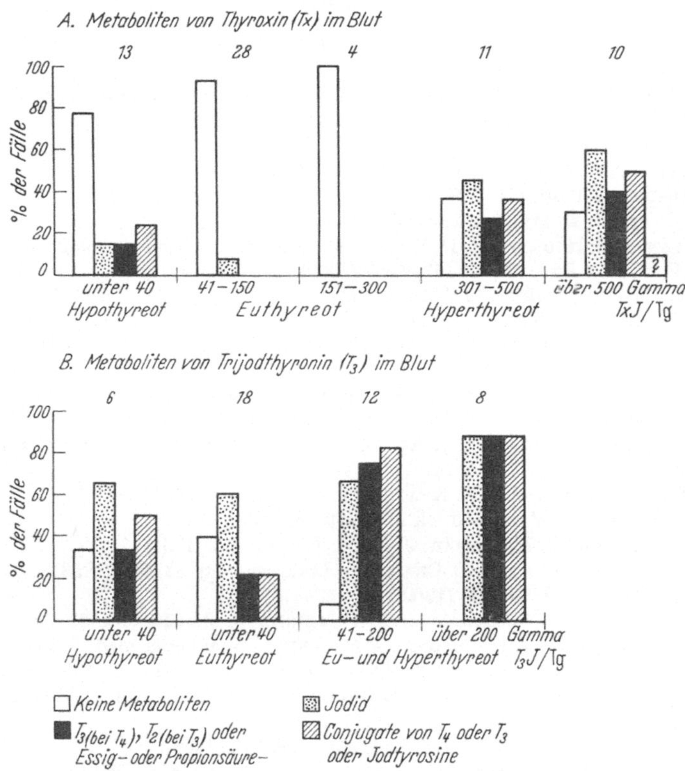

Abb. 13. Die Abhängigkeit des Metabolitenanfalls im Blut vom täglichen Hormonumsatz. A: Metaboliten von T₄. B: Metaboliten von T₃. (T₄-Derivate waren nur bei pathologisch großen oder kleinen Thyroxinumsätzen, T₃-Derivate auch normalerweise nachweisbar) ☐ keine Metaboliten; ▦ Jodid; ■ T₃ oder T₂ oder Essig- oder Propionsäurederivate; ▨ Hormonkonjugate oder Jodtyrosine

Trotz vieler Unklarheiten und Widersprüche zwischen einzelnen Befunden, die weitgehend durch unterschiedliche und nolens volens unzulängliche Methodiken bedingt sind, können die folgenden Feststellungen heute als einigermaßen gesichert gelten:

1. Die Abbauwege der Schilddrüsenhormone überschneiden sich und das Molekül wird dabei meist an mehreren Stellen verändert.

2. Die Abbauwege und die Reihenfolge einzelner Degradationen sind von Organ zu Organ verschieden.

3. Bei Schilddrüsenkrankheiten finden sich Anomalien im Hormonumsatz und Metabolitenanfall, die nicht nur vom Hormonangebot, sondern auch von Eigenarten der Körperperipherie abhängen.

Es kann jedoch keinem Zweifel unterliegen, daß diese Feststellungen recht summarischer Natur und wir von einer Lösung des Stoffwechselproblems der Schilddrüsenhormone noch weit entfernt sind.

Literatur

Albert, A., and F. R. Keating: J. clin. Endocr. 11, 996 (1951).
— — Endocrinology 51, 427 (1952).
— J. Rall, F. R. Keating, M. Power and M. Williams: J. chin. Endocr. 8, 1392 (1949).
Albright, E. C., and F. C. Larson: J. clin. Invest. 38, 1899 (1959).
— — and R. H. Tust: Proc. Soc. exp. Biol. (N. Y.) 86, 137 (1954).
— K. Tomita and F. C. Larson: Endocrinology 64, 208 (1959).
— F. C. Larson, K. Tomita and H. A. Lardy: Endocrilogy 59, 252 (1956).
Arons, W. L., and J. D. Hydovitz: J. clin. Endocr. 19, 548 (1959).
Arsdel, P. van, J. R. Hogness, R. H. Williams and N. Elgee: Endocrinology 55, 332 (1954).
Barac, G.: C. R. Soc. Biol. (Paris) 153, 1285 (1959).
— Arch. int. Physiol. Biochim. 67, 732 (1959).
Baschieri, L., D. Andreani, F. De Luca, M. Negri, G. B. Salabe, A. Pichera and G. Menzinger: In: Advances in Thyroid Research. Ed. by R. Pitt-Rivers, Seite 327. Oxford: Pergamon Press 1961.
Becker, D. V., and J. F. Prudden: Endocrinology 64, 136 (1959).
Beckers, C., and M. de Visscher: Pure and Appl. Chem. 3, 477 (1961).
Bénard, H., A. Cruz, O. Michel, J. Roche et P. Thièblemont: Ann. Endocr. (Paris) 22, 429 (1961).
Benua, R. S., A. Albert and F. R. Keating: J. clin. Endocr. 12, 1461 (1952).
Berson, S. A., and R. S. Yalow: J. clin. Invest. 33, 1533 (1954).
Braverman, L. E., and S. H. Ingbar: J. chron. Dis. 14, 484 (1961).
Briggs, F. N., A. Taurog and I. L Chaikoff: Endocrinology 52, 559 (1953).
Cameron, .C.: Biochem. J. 74, 323 (1960).
Choufoer, J. C., A. A. H. Kassenaar and A. Querido: J. clin. Endocr. 20, 983 (1960).
Cottino, F., G. C. Ferrara, G. Colombo e A. Costa: Panminerva med. 3, 471 (1961).
Cruchaud, S., A. Vannotti, C. Mahaim and J. Deckelmann: Lancet 1955 I, 906.
Dowling, J. Th., N. Freinkel and S. H. Ingbar: J. clin. Invest. 35, 1263 (1956); J. clin. Endocr. 16, 280, 1491 (1956).
Dunn, J. T., and J. B. Stanbury: J. clin. Endocr. 18, 713 (1958).
Escobar, F., and G. M. Escobar: Acta endocr. (Kbh.) 23, 393, 400 (1956).
— — M. D. Garcia Garcia and J. M. Garcia: Acta endocr. (Kbh.) Suppl. 67, 158 (1962).
Etling, N., and S. B. Barker: Ann. endocr. (Paris) 20, 183 (1959).
— — Endocrinology 64, 753 (1959); 65, 95 (1959).
Fletscher, P. E., J. Litvak and J. B. Stanbury: Acta endocr. (Kbh.) 29, 307 (1958).
Flock, E. V., L. J. Bollman and J. H. Grindlay: Endocrinology 67, 419 (1960).
— — — Proc. Mayo Clin. 35, 75 (1960).
— — — and A. L. Orvis: Amer. J. Physiol. 187, 407 (1956).
— — — and B. F. McKenzie: Endocrinology 61, 461 (1957).
— — — and G. H. Stobie: Endocrinology 69, 626 (1961).
Ford, D. H., K. R. Corey and J. Gross: Endocrinology 61, 426 (1957).
Freinkel, N., S. H. Ingbar and J. Th. Dowling: J. clin. Invest. 36, 25 (1957).
Friis, T.: Acta endocr. (Kbh.) 29, 587 (1958).
Galton, V. A., and S. H. Ingbar: Endocrinology 69, 30 (1961).
Georgi, P., and N. Hartmann: Hoppe Seylers Z. physiol. Chem. 325, 173 (1961).
Green, W. L., and S. H. Ingbar: In: Advances in Thyroid Research, herausgegeben von R. Pitt-Rivers, Seite 406. Oxford: Pergamon Press 1961.
Gregerman, R. I., G. W. Gaffney and N. W. Shock: J. clin. Invest. 41, 2065 (1962).

GREGORIO, P. DE, L. C. G. LOBO, R. MICHEL and J. ROCHE: Bull. Soc. chim. Biol. **42**, 1213 (1960).
GROSS, J., D. F. FORD, S. SYMCHOVICZ and J. H. HORTON: In: Ciba Foundation Coll. on Endocrinology, Vol. 10, 182. London: Churchill Ltd. 1957.
HADDAD, H. M.: J. Pediat. **57**, 391 (1960).
— J. clin. Invest. **39**, 1590 (1960).
HALES, I. B., and B. M. DOBYNS: J. clin. Endocr. **20**, 68 (1960).
HERSHMAN, J. M., and L. VON MIDDLESWORTH: Endocrinology **71**, 94 (1962).
HILLMANN, G.: Biosynthese und Stoffwechselwirkungen der Schilddrüsenhormone. Stuttgart: G. Thieme 1961.
— B. KEIL u. P. TASLIMI: Z. Naturforsch. **13b**, 820 (1958).
HOGNESS, J. R., M. BERG, P. VAN ARSDEL and R. H. WILLIAMS: Proc. Soc. exp. Biol. (N.Y.) **90**, 93 (1955).
INGBAR, S. H.: Ann. N. Y. Acad. Sci. **86**, 440 (1960).
— Clinical Endocrinology I, Seite 91. Ed. by E. B. ASTWOOD. New York-London: Grune & Stratton 1960.
—, and N. FREINKEL: J. clin. Invest. **34**, 808 (1955); **37**, 1603 (1958).
— — J. T. DOWLING and L. F. KUMAGAI: J. clin. Invest. **35**, 714 (1956).
JOHNSON, H. W., and A. ALBERT: Endocrinology **48**, 669 (1951).
JOLIOT, F., R. COURRIER, A. HORREAU et P. SÜE: C. R. Soc. Biol. (Paris) **138**, 325 (1944).
JONES, S. L., and L. VAN MIDDLESWORTH: Endocrinology **67**, 855 (1960).
KASSENAAR, A., L. D. F. LAMEYER, and A. QUERIDO: Acta endocr. (Kbh.) **32**, 575 (1959).
KLEIN, E.: Acta endocr. (Kbh.) **34**, 137 (1960).
— In: Advances in Thyroid Research. Ed. by R. Pitt-Rivers. Seite 447. London: Pergamon Press 1961.
— Der endogene Jodhaushalt des Menschen und seine Störungen. Stuttgart: G. Thieme 1960.
— Klin. Wschr. **40**, 3 (1962).
—, u. A. BERGHOFF: In: Radioaktive Isotope in Klinik und Forschung. Band IV, Seite 328. Herausgegeben von K. FELLINGER u. R. HÖFER. München: Urban & Schwarzenberg 1960.
— HJ. HIRCHE u. D. REINWEIN: 7. Symposion Dtsch. Ges. Endokrinologie, Seite 308. Berlin-Göttingen-Heidelberg: Springer Verlag 1961.
KLITGAARD, H. M., H. J. LIPNER, S. B. BARKER and T. WINNICK: Endocrinology **52**, 79 (1953).
KOT, P. A., and H. M. KLITGAARD: Endocrinology **64**, 319 (1959).
KUTZIM, H.: Z. ges. exp. Med. **135**, 377 (1962).
LACHAZE, A., et O. THIBAULT: C. R. Soc. Biol. (Paris) **146**, 393 (1952).
LAMBERG, B.-A., R. GRÄSBECK, F. BJÖRKSTEN and R. KARLSSON: Acta endocr. (Kbh.), Suppl. **67**, 160 (1962).
LARDY, H., K. TOMITA, F. C. LARSON and E. C. ALBRIGHT: In: Ciba Foundation Colloquia on Endocrinology, Band 10, 156. London: Churchill Ltd. 1957.
LARSON, F. C., and E. C. ALBRIGHT: Endocrinology **63**, 183 (1958).
— K. TOMITA and E. C. ALBRIGHT: J. Lab. clin. Med. **50**, 924 (1957).
— — — Endocrinology **65**, 336 (1959).
LIPNER, H. J., S. B. BARKER and T. WINNICK: Endocrinology **51**, 406 (1952).
LISSITZKY, S., and S. BOUCHILLOUX: In: Ciba Foundation Coll. on Endocrinology, Band 10, 135. London: Churchill Ltd. 1957.
— M. ROQUES u. M. TH. BENEVAND: In: Radioaktive Isotope in Klinik und Forschung, Band IV, Seite 301. Herausgegeb. von K. FELLINGER u. R. HÖFER. München: Urban & Schwarzenberg 1960.
— — — In: Advances in Thyroid Research. Ed. by R. PITT-RIVERS. Seite 250. London: Pergamon Press 1961.
MACLAGAN, N. F., and D. REID: In: Ciba Foundation Coll. on Endocrinology. Band 10, 190. London: Churchill Ltd. 1957.
MICHEL, R., J. ROCHE, P. THIEBLEMONT u. O. MICHEL: In: Radioaktive Isotope in Klinik und Forschung, Band IV, Seite 318. Herausgegeben von K. FELLINGER u. R. HÖFER. München: Urban & Schwarzenberg 1960.
MIDDLESWORTH, L. VAN: In: Clinical Endocrinology I, Ed. by E. B. ASTWOOD. Seite 103. New York-London: Grune & Stratton 1960.

Myant, N. B.: Clin. Sci. **15**, 227 (1956).
Nakano, M., and T. S. Danowski: Endocrinology **70**, 340 (1962).
Niemann, C.: Fortschr. org. chem. Naturwiss. **7**, 167 (1950).
Plaskett, L. G.: Nature (Lond.) **181**, 273 (1958).
— Biochem. J. **78**, 652 (1961).
Pinchera, A., G. Menzinger, D. Bellabarba, V. Greco, L. Baschieri e S. Lissitzky: Folia endocr. (Roma) **15**, 338, 376 (1962).
Pind, K.: Acta endocr. (Kbh.) **26**, 263 (1957).
Pitt-Rivers, R., and J. R Tata: The Thyroid Hormones. London: Pergamon Press 1959.
— J. B. Stanbury and B. Rapp: J. clin. Endocr. **15**, 616 (1955).
Premachandra, B. N., and C. W. Turner: Proc. Soc. exp. Biol. (N. Y.) **106**, 818 (1961).
Riggs, D. S.: Pharmacol. Rev. **4**, 284 (1952).
Roche, J., and R. Michel: Ann. N. Y. Acad. Sci. **86**, 454 (1960).
— — et J. Tata: C. R. Soc. Biol. (Paris) **147**, 1574 (1953); **148**, 642 (1954).
— O. Michel, R. Michel et J. Tata: C. R. Soc. Biol. (Paris) **147**, 1243 (1953).
— R. Michel, W. Wolf and J. Nunez: Biochim. biophys. Acta **19**, 308 (1956).
— — — — C. R. Soc. Biol. (Paris) **149**, 884 (1955).
— — J. Closon et O. Michel: C. R. Soc. Biol. (Paris) **150**, 2097 (1956).
— — P. Jouan and W. Wolf: Endocrinology **59**, 425 (1956).
— — N. Etling et P. Jouan: C. R. Soc. Biol. (Paris) **150**, 1320 (1956).
— — et P. Jouan: In: Ciba Foundation Coll. on Endocrinology, Band 10, 168. London: Churchill Ltd. 1957.
— — J. Nunez and C. Jaquemin.: Endocrinology **65**, 402 (1959).
— — J. Closon and O. Michel: Biochim. biophys. Acta **38**, 325 (1960).
— — — In: Advances in Thyroid Research. Seite 497. Ed. by R. Pitt-Rivers. London: Pergamon Press 1961.
Ruegamer, W. R., and R. B. Chodos: Clin. Res. Proc. **4**, 145 (1956).
Scazziga, B. R., L. L. Barbieri u. Th. Beraud: Schweiz. med. Wschr. **1955**, 393 u. 471.
Slingerland, D. W., and R. Josephs: Endocrinology **62**, 853 (1958).
Sprott, W. E., and N. F. Maclagan: Biochem. J. **59**, 288 (1955).
Stanbury, J. B.: Ann. N. Y. Acad. Sci. **86**, 417 (1960).
—, and M. L. Morris: J. clin. Endocr. **17**, 1324 (1957).
— A. A. H. Kassenaar and J. W. A. Meijer: J. clin. Endocr. **16**, 735 (1956).
—, and J. Litvak: J. clin. Endocr. **17**, 654 (1957).
— M. L. Morris, H. J. Corrigan and W. E. Lassiter: Endocrinology **67**, 353 (1960).
Sterling, K.: J. clin. Invest. **37**, 1348 (1958).
— J. C. Lashof and E. B. Man: J. clin. Invest. **33**, 1031 (1954).
—, and R. B. Chodos: J. clin. Invest. **35**, 806 (1956).
Tata, J.: Proc. Soc. exp. Biol. (N. Y.) **95**, 362 (1957).
— Biochem. biophys. Acta **35**, 567 (1959).
— Ann. N. Y. Acad. Sci. **86**, 469 (1960).
— Acta endocr. (Kbh.) **37**, 125 (1961).
— J. E. Rall and R. W. Rawson: Endocrinology **60**, 83 (1957).
Taurog, A., F. N. Briggs and I. L. Chaikoff: J. biol. Chem. **191**, 29 (1951); **194**, 655 (1952).
Thibault, O.: Ann. Endocr. (Paris) **17**, 35 (1956).
— Arch. Sci. Physiol. **10**, 423 (1956).
— In: Ciba Foundation Coll. on Endocrinology, Band 10, 230. London: Churchill Ltd. 1957.
Tomita, K., and H. A. Lardy: J. biol. Chem. **235**, 3292 (1960).
— — F. C. Larson and E. C. Albright: J. biol. Chem. **224**, 387 (1957).
Triantaphyllidis, E., G. Ambrosino, M. Tubiana et R. Cikier: Ann. Endocr. (Paris) **16**, 733 (1955).
— — — — J. Physiol. (Paris) **48**, 726 (1956).
Vannotti, A.: Helv. med. Acta **24**, Suppl. 37 (1957).
—, and Th. Beraud: J. clin. Endocr. **19**, 460 (1959).
Walfish, P. G., A. Britton, P. H. Melville and C. Ezrin: J. clin. Endocr. **21**, 582 (1961).
Wilkinson, J. H., and N. F. Maclagan: J. Endocr. **10**, 15 (1954).
Wynn, J., R. Gibbs and B. Royster: J. biol. Chem. **237**, 1892 (1962).

YAMAMOTO, K., S. SHIMIZU and I. ISHIKAWA: Gunma J. med. Sci. 9, 110 (1960).
— Jap. J. Physiol. 10, 594, 610 (1960).
YAMAZAKI, E., and D. W. SLINGERLAND: Endocrinology 64, 126 (1959).

Diskussion

K. FELLINGER (Wien):

Sie haben gezeigt, daß bei Normalen kaum, bei Hyperthyreosen massiv Metaboliten im Blut nachweisbar werden. Es würde mich wegen der fraglichen Genese der Hyperthyreose sehr interessieren, ob Sie auch untersucht haben, wie sich die Metaboliten bei mit TSH aktivierten Euthyreoten verhalten.

E. KLEIN:

Entsprechende Untersuchungen habe ich nicht durchgeführt und mir sind auch keine von anderen Autoren bekannt.

R. HÖFER (Wien):

Konnten Sie eine Beziehung zwischen Ausmaß und/oder Art des Eiweißverlustes und den von Ihnen untersuchten Veränderungen des Hormonumsatzes feststellen? Ich frage, weil wir einerseits finden, daß bei schweren Nephrosen mit ausgeprägter Hypoproteinämie der Radiojodumsatz (Jodidphase und Hormonphase) oft nicht kompensatorisch gesteigert ist, während bei relativ geringer Hypoproteinämie (wie bei einem Patienten mit Eiweißverlust durch den Darm) der Radiojodumsatz stark gesteigert sein kann. Die beobachteten Patienten waren durchweg metabolisch euthyreot.

E. KLEIN:

Wie Sie und andere Autoren haben auch wir nur wenig einschlägige Fälle hinsichtlich ihres Jodstoffwechsels genauer analysieren können. Ich habe dabei nicht den Eindruck, daß die Unterschiede zwischen Kranken mit Hormonverlust durch die Nieren und solchen mit Hormonverlust durch den Darm anders als zufällig sind. Ob ein kompensatorisch beschleunigter Jodumsatz einsetzt oder nicht, scheint mir eher von der individuellen Regulationsfähigkeit als von grundsätzlichen Differenzen abzuhängen. Belegbare Zusammenhänge der von Ihnen gefragten Art sind bisher nicht erwiesen.

F. WYSS (Bern):

Wir beobachteten (mit KÖNIG und STUDER), daß bei erheblichen Eiweißverlusten durch den Darm der thyreoidale Jodumsatz kaum verändert war und der TSH-Reservetest negativ ausfiel. Wahrscheinlich spielt eine hypophysäre Komponente eine Rolle.

E. KLEIN:

Damit käme ein zusätzlicher pathogenetischer Faktor ins Spiel, nämlich eine vielleicht dysproteinämisch bedingte mangelhafte Synthese von TSH. Die dann registrierten Veränderungen sind nicht mehr homöostatisch zu erklären.

R. KOTZAUREK (Wien):

Wie wurden Thyroxin und Trijodthyronin getrennt bestimmt?

E. KLEIN:

Mit Hilfe chemischer BEI-Analysen und der Radiopapierchromatographie 24 und 48 Std nach einer Dosis von 200 bis 300 micro-C J^{131}. Die Brauchbarkeit dieser Methode, die allerdings langwierig ist, wurde in der Klin. Wschr. 1962, 15 diskutiert.

D. EMRICH (Freiburg):

Eine Einschränkung für die quantitative Beurteilung von Radiochromatogrammen bei Substanzen verschieden hohen Jodierungsgrades besteht vorläufig darin, daß man über die spezifische Aktivität keine Aussagen machen kann.

E. KLEIN:

Der Einwand trifft zweifellos die Hauptschwierigkeit solcher Untersuchungen, wenngleich hinsichtlich der endogen markierten Hormone z. Z. kein Grund für eine über den unterschiedlichen Jodgehalt von Thyroxin und Trijodthyronin hinausgehende Korrektur vorzuliegen scheint.

E. DOLFF (Essen):

Ist Ihre Untersuchungsmethode bei eklamptischen Schwangeren mit schwerem Eiweiß-verlust ohne Gefahr für Mutter und Kind durchzuführen? Sind irgendwelche für die Schwangerschaft prognostischen Ergebnisse zu erwarten.

E. KLEIN:

Beides kann sicher verneint werden, während einer Gravidität sind derartige Methoden kontraindiziert, praktische Konsequenzen haben sie ohnehin nicht.

H. DITSCHUNEIT (Frankfurt):

Die Berechnung des peripheren Hormonumsatzes gründen Sie auf die Bestimmung der HWZ von injiziertem markierten Thyroxin und Trijodthyronin. Hierzu habe ich folgende Fragen:

1. Sind die Halbwertszeiten freien und gebundenen Hormons voneinander verschieden?

2. Ändert sich die HWZ mit der Applikationsart (i.v., per infusionem) und der applizierten Menge?

E. KLEIN:

Zu 1. Da nur freie Hormone die Blutbahn verlassen und dieser Vorgang registriert wird, kann man nicht von der HWZ gebundener Hormone sprechen — obgleich das in diesem Moment noch gebundene Hormon im nächsten Moment frei werden und die Blutbahn verlassen kann. Voraussetzung für die HWZ-Bestimmung ist natürlich die Spür-Methode, d. h. es dürfen nur so große chemische Mengen als markierte Hormone injiziert werden, daß sie die vorliegenden Verhältnisse nicht stören, sondern sich ihnen anschließen. Die Methode hängt von der spezifischen Aktivität der markierten Testsubstanz ab.

Zu 2. Eine HWZ-Bestimmung per infusionem des markierten Hormons wurde bisher nicht unternommen, weil die kontinuierliche Zufuhr bei einer Spür-Methode überflüssig ist. Sie hängt selbstverständlich aus dem unter 1. genannten Grunde von der injizierten Hormonmenge ab. HWZ-Bestimmungen nach Gaben von Hormonmengen, die den Hormonspiegel des Blutes verändern, sind sinnlos. Je höher man den Hormonspiegel bringt, desto kürzer wird bis zu einem bestimmten Grade die HWZ, weil sie unter anderem vom Angebot abhängt.

Clinique Médicale Universitaire, Lausanne
(Directeur: Prof. Dr. A. Vannotti)

Relations entre le transport des hormones thyroïdiennes et des hormones stéroïdes

Th. Lemarchand-Béraud et A. Vannotti
avec la collaboration de M.-R. Assayah

Avec 7 figures

Rapport

I. Introduction

Jusqu'à nos jours, le meilleur critère pour mesurer l'activité hormonale résidait dans la détermination globale du taux plasmatique des hormones. On sait actuellement que la plupart de celles-ci circulent en partie sous forme liée aux protéines et en partie sous forme libre. Le support protidique est plus ou moins spécifique pour chaque hormone. On connaît ainsi la «thyroxine binding globulin» (TBP ou TBG) pour les hormones thyroïdiennes, la transcortine pour les corticostéroïdes, les albumines pour les androgènes, la progestérone et les phénol-stéroïdes (*44*). La force de liaison varie d'un groupe d'hormones à l'autre; si la liaison entre TBP et thyroxine est particulièrement forte, ainsi que celle entre transcortine et cortisol, la testostérone et la progestérone sont en revanche faiblement liées et les phénol-stéroïdes le sont de manière si labile que la majeure partie se trouve sous forme libre (*1*).

Dans un même groupe d'hormones, la force de liaison est d'intensité différente d'une hormone à l'autre. Ainsi, la thyroxine est beaucoup plus fortement liée à la TBP que la triiodothyronine et la cortisol plus fortement que la corticostérone, tandis que l'aldostérone n'est pas ou peu liée. Nous allons considérer plus particulièrement le comportement du transport des hormones thyroïdiennes.

Le support protidique des hormones thyroïdiennes ne joue pas simplement le rôle de transporteur, mais il intervient également dans la régulation hormonale. En effet, on admet actuellement que seule la fraction d'hormone non liée, quoique infiniment faible, pénètre dans la cellule et est biologiquement active. Ce pourcentage d'hormone non liée (estimé à $6 \cdot 10^{-11}$ Mol. par Robbins (*2*) et à 0,11% du PBI total par Sterling (*3*) dépendant, d'une part, du taux d'hormone circulant et, d'autre part, du taux et de la capacité de liaison des protéines plasmatiques (extra-cellulaires) et, semble-t-il également des protéines intra-cellulaires (*4, 5, 6, 7*), on entrevoit le rôle joué par les protéines plasmatiques dans la régulation périphérique des hormones.

On conçoit donc aisément que toute une série de perturbations de la régulation hormonale aient pour cause un trouble du transport. Il est donc indispensable de

Tableau 1

Cas no.	Nom, Age, sexe	Diagnostic	Scinti-graphie	Méta-bolisme basal	Cap-tation I 131 (24 h.)	PBI 131	PBI μg%	Test de HA-MOLSKY	Capacité fixation Mol T 4/1000 ml	Test de saturation		
										TBP	A	TBPA
		Valeurs normales		0% (—10 +10)	40 (15— 50%)	22,1 (10— 50%)	5,0 (4,2— 5,8)	15,7 (13— 18%)	$2,48 \cdot 10^{-7}$ ± 0,25	voir Tableau 5		
1	Bu.G.,15 ans, f.	légère hypo-thyréose	petite	+6%	57,0%	66,3%	6,5	12,1	$2,9 \cdot 10^{-7}$	51,7	20,6	27,6
										23,3	25,1	51,6
										15,6	35,2	49,2
2	Wu.M.,23 ans, f.	euthyréose après opération	normale	—12	51	37,9	8,0	10,8	$2,64 \cdot 10^{-7}$	57,4	17,1	25,5
										29,9	26,8	43,3
										14,9	45,6	34,8
3	Va.S.,41 ans, f.	hypo-thyréose	petite	—15	39,6	93,6	4,1	11,3	$3,84 \cdot 10^{-7}$	50,9	23,1	26,0
										45,7	25,9	28,4
										14,6	30,5	54,9
4	Ca.P.,59 ans, f.	hypo-thyréose	petite	—7	45,6	24,9	4,6	11,3	$2,88 \cdot 10^{-7}$	50,7	14,3	35,0
										20,4	26,7	52,9
										14,4	36,1	49,5
5	Fi.F.,15 ans, f.	hypo-thyréose avec goître	agrandie	+5	49,9	66,6	5,2	10,8	$3,25 \cdot 10^{-7}$	50,9	13,9	35,8
										34,1	25,4	40,0
										14,6	27,2	58,2
6	Ba.S.,39 ans, f.	hyperoestro-génie	isthme élargi	—9	50,0	12,2	7,8	11,6	$3,59 \cdot 10^{-7}$	52,0	13,7	34,3
										40,9	17,4	41,7
										17,7	38,8	46,3
7	Mo.W.,m.	goître nodulaire	2 nodules	—3	51,0	78,0	6,3	8,9	$3,63 \cdot 10^{-7}$	71,3	25,4	3,3
										42,1	30,9	27,0
										21,8	52,0	26,2
8	Gr.L., 44 ans,f.	légère hypo-thyréose	petite	—7	41,0	14,35	5,25	8,9	$3,04 \cdot 10^{-7}$	60,6	15,7	23,7
										35,7	30,8	33,5
										22,4	43,6	34,0

connaître tous les facteurs qui peuvent modifier cette liaison. Cette liaison protéine-hormone peut théoriquement varier du fait du changement soit de la teneur, soit de la structure protéique du support ou sous l'effet de l'altération du mécanisme de la liaison.

Dans l'*hypo-* et l'*hyperthyréose*, la quantité de TBP présente, ainsi que la capacité de liaison semblent peu modifiées; en revanche, le taux d'hormone libre est respectivement diminué ou augmenté selon la quantité d'hormone produite et sécrétée par la glande (*2, 8*).

A côté de ces deux exemples de modification quantitative du rapport TBP-hormone, on connaît aujourd'hui des *troubles primaires du transport* de la thyroxine qui peuvent jouer un rôle en clinique. En effet, Tanaka (*9*), Beierwaltes (*10*) et Florsheim (*11*) ont respectivement montré l'existence d'une élévation congénitale de la TBP, entraînant une augmentation du PBI, mais associée à un état euthyroïdien. A l'inverse, Tanaka et Starr (*12*), Ingbar (*13*), Cavalieri (*14*) et Beisel (*15*) décrivent des cas présentant un taux de PBI et de TBP abaissé accompagné d'un taux normal d'hormone libre et d'un état d'euthyréose.

De plus, nous avons observé des patients *hypo-* et *hyper*métaboliques dont la dysfonction thyroïdienne semble être secondaire à un défaut de transport hormonal (*16*). Chez 8 patients hypométaboliques, cliniquement eu- ou hypothyroïdiens (Tableau 1), nous avons observé un PBI normal ou même élevé, composé essentiellement de thyroxine; cette dernière est neutralisée par l'augmentation de la

Tableau 2

Cas no.	Nom, Age, sexe	Diagnostic	Scinti-graphie	Méta-bolisme basal	Cap-tation I^{131}	PBI 131	PBI $\mu g\%$	Test de HA-MOLSKY	Capacité fixation Mol T4/1000 ml	Test de saturation			
										TBP	A	TB-PA	β
Valeurs hyperthyréose					70% (60—100)	85,3% (60—100)	8,4 (6—12)	26,8% (18—39,2)	1,59 ±0,28 · 10⁻⁷	voir Tableau 5			
9	Cl.A.,32 ans, m.	Dystonie neurovégé-tative	normale	+36	78,2	94,8	2,9	22,8	1,97·10⁻⁷	48,7 23,8 10,8	22,4 30,7 44,8	27,5 45,5 44,4	
10	Ve.P.,50 ans, m.	Dystonie neurovégé-tative	légèrem. élargie	+20	63,5	19,8	4,8	24,0	2,0	50,0 24,7 11,8	18,7 26,0 38,8	31,3 49,3 49,4	
11	Cl.J., 35 ans, m.	Euthyréose	légèrem. élargie	0	53,0	43,0	3,5	20,9	1,52	42,2 18,3 11,6	12,0 17,6 21,3	45,8 64,1 67,1	
12	Du.M.,f.	légère hyper-thyréose	normale	+19	57,9	77,1	4,4	19,3	2,21	56,3 30,1 17,3	36,7 29,5 44,8	9,0 40,4 37,9	
13	La.J.,45 ans, f.	Goître nodulaire	élargie	+29	38,4	47,6	3,8	20,9	1,98	45,9 23,6 16,7	19,9 40,0 36,5	34,2 36,4 46,7	
14	Cr.M.,34 ans, f.	Basedow	élargie	+29	81,5	79,6	2,8	—	1,43	39,3 17,1 11,8	29,8 33,2 42,6	31,0 49,7 45,6	
15	De.H.,48 ans, f.	Basedow	élargie	+32	82,7	98,1	3,5	23,1	1,14	48,2 13,7 11,1	17,3 30,4 43,2	31,0 51,4 40,9	3,1 4,8 4,8
16	Pe.G.,m.	Hyperthy-réose traitée avec l'I^{131}	non homo-gène	+26	49	100	4,4	20,8	2,12	47,3 25,2 18,5	17,3 45,8 36,7	35,4 29,0 50,8	

capacité de la TBP. Ce phénomène s'accompagne d'une diminution du taux d'hormone libre circulant. Tout au contraire, chez 8 patients *hypermétaboliques* présentant des signes cliniques d'hyperthyréose et une hyperactivité glandulaire, mais ayant un taux de PBI abaissé, nous avons mis en évidence une diminution de la capacité de liaison de la TBP correspondant à un pourcentage d'hormone libre élevé (voir Tableau 2).

En plus de ces modifications primaires et essentielles de la capacité de liaison de la TBP d'origine indéterminée, nous savons que différentes conditions peuvent altérer secondairement cette liaison. En effet, une augmentation de la capacité de la TBP accompagnée d'un taux de PBI élevé apparaît au cours de la *grossesse* (*17, 18*) ou lors d'un traitement aux *oestrogènes* (*19, 20*), modification qui semble être due à l'effet anabolique des oestrogènes sur les alpha-globulines, ce qui entraînerait une augmentation de la TBP.

Nous avons observé un tableau similaire au cours de l'*hépatite* épidémique (*21*). L'élévation importante du PBI constatée dans cette affection est secondaire au catabolisme pathologique des hormones thyroïdiennes (absence de glucuro-conjugaison, donc de l'élimination biliaire de la Thyroxine [T4] et diminution de la désiodation de la T4. Cet excès d'hormone circulant reste toutefois sans effet métabolique, car elle est neutralisée par la TBP dont la capacité de liaison est augmentée, observation confirmée par la diminution du taux d'hormone libre

Tableau 3. *Triiodothyronine marqué à l'I^{131} absorbée par les érythrocytes (méthode de* Hamolsky*).*
(Test corrigé pour un hématocrite de 100%; valeurs relatives de l'hormone libre)

Diagnostic	Nombre de cas	%	Amplitude de la dispersion	Déviation standard
Euthyréose	46	15,5	(13,0—18,5)	±0,50
Hypothyréose	8	10,4	(8,7—13,0)	±1,9
Hyperthyréose, Basedow, goîtres nodulaires toxiques	39	26,8	(18—39,2)	±1,76
Goîtres non toxiques	16	15,8	(12,3—18,6)	±0,85
Hépatite virale	17	11,3	(8,0—14,0)	±1,3

(Tableau 3). Au cours de cette affection, on observe également l'absence ou la diminution de la liaison de la thyroxine aux pré-albumines (voir Tabl. 5).

Enfin, on a montré que l'action de certaines drogues telles que le salicylate (*22*), le dinitrophénol (*23*), le diphénylhydantoïne etc. (*24, 25, 26, 27*) qui font abaisser le PBI et dont certaines provoquent une augmentation du métabolisme agissait en déplaçant la thyroxine de sa liaison à la TBP. Ces composés se lient à la TBP et saturent les ponts de jonction; ils déplacent la T4 qui restant principalement sous forme libre entraîne une diminution du taux de TSH, ce qui freine la synthèse hormonale et explique la diminution du PBI observée dans ces cas.

Nous constatons que différentes modifications primaires ou secondaires du transport des hormones thyroïdiennes peuvent altérer la fonction thyroïdienne et tout particulièrement l'activité hormonale périphérique. Devant le rôle joué par ces protéines transporteuses et plus particulièrement la TBP, nous nous sommes demandés si les autres hormones qui circulent également sous forme liée pouvaient influencer le transport des hormones thyroïdiennes en entrant en compétition, interférence périphérique qui pourrait, en partie tout au moins, expliquer certains antagonismes ou relations entre les différentes hormones. Comme la transcortine est très proche de la TBP, nous nous sommes plus particulièrement intéressés aux relations hormones thyroïdiennes-hormones corticoïdes.

On sait que le 70 à 90% des hormones corticoïdes circulent dans le sang sous forme liée à une α-l-globuline nommée par Slaunwhite *transcortine*; elle est de faible capacité estimée à 21 γ/100 ml ou 5 · 10^{-7} Mol (*28, 29*), mais possède une grande affinité. Lorsque la transcortine est saturée, les corticostéroïdes se lient aux albumines. Il y a donc une certaine similitude entre la transcortine et la TBP; aussi nous nous sommes demandés si lors d'une surcharge en l'une ou l'autre hormone, il n'existerait pas des phénomènes de compétition.

II. Méthodes et matériel

Nous avons utilisé pour cette étude des patients examinés à la Clinique Médicale Universitaire de Lausanne. Le diagnostic des cas thyroïdiens a été posé d'après l'examen clinique du patient et les tests thyroïdiens usuels (fixation intra-thyroïdienne de l'iode 131, scintigraphie, indice de conversion, PBI, métabolisme de base et dans certains cas, analyse de l'iode organique circulant par chromatographie) (*30*).

Les tests du transport des hormones thyroïdiennes comportent :

1. Le test de saturation (*31*).

2. Le test d'HAMOLSKY (*32*) mesurant le pourcentage de triiodothyronine marquée se fixant sur les érythrocytes. Ce test indique le pourcent relatif d'hormone libre.

3. Les tests du transport des corticostéroïdes.

En suivant la méthode de dialyse de SLAUNWHITE (*28*), on incube dans un sac à dialyse 2 heures à 4° 1,0 ml de plasma avec 0,5 ml de corticostérone marquée au 14C (0,01 uc/0,14 γ) ; le volume total est ajusté à 5 ml par du tampon phosphate pH 7.4. Après ces deux heures d'équilibre, on plonge le sac de dialyse dans 20 ml de tampon phosphate et dialyse à 4° pendant 18 heures. On prélève ensuite des échantillons de 0,5 ou 1 ml tant de l'intérieur du sac à dialyse que du dialysat lui-même et l'on mesure l'activité dans ces différentes fractions au moyen d'un compteur automatique à flux gazeux, modèle Nuclear. Le pourcentage d'hormone liée est déterminé selon la formule de SLAUNWHITE :

$$\% \text{ lié} = 100 \left(1 - \frac{D - V_i}{I - V_d} \right)$$

D = activité du dialysat
I = activité intérieure du sac
V_d = volume du dialysat
V_i = volume intérieur

Pour déterminer la *capacité de liaison*, on effectue en parallèle une deuxième dialyse dans les mêmes conditions, le sérum ayant été ajusté préalablement par l'adjonction de corticostérone non marquée à 0,50 γ/ml. La diminution du pourcentage de fixation après surcharge de corticostérone est fonction de la capacité de fixation de la transcortine ; plus la diminution est grande, plus la capacité est petite.

Nous avons effectué tous ces tests chez des patients normaux, hypothyroïdiens, hyperthyroïdiens, traités pendant un mois ou plus avec de la prednisone pour diverses affections (polyarthrite asthme, leucémie), dans un groupe de femmes enceintes et, enfin, dans quelques cas d'addisonisme, ainsi que dans un groupe de patients atteints de tuberculose pulmonaire traités avec de l'Isobenzacyl Forte (B-PAS).

III. Résultats

1. Action in vitro des différentes hormones

Nous avons tout d'abord examiné si ces différentes hormones ajoutées in vitro au sérum modifiaient les tests de transport. Les figures 1 et 2 nous montrent que la fixation de la thyroxine aux différentes fractions protidiques n'est changée ni par l'adjonction de corticostérone, ni par celle d'oestradiol, d'ultracortène, ou d'hydrocortisone. La thyroxine qui sature la liaison thyroxine-TBP n'a pas d'action sur la liaison des corticostéroïdes, ni les oestrogènes, ni la testostérone. L'hydrocortisone, la cortisol et la cortisone déplacent, en revanche, la liaison de la corticostérone marquée (Tabl. 4). En conclusion, en dehors des hormones du même groupe, il n'y a pas in vitro de déplacement des liaisons par les autres hormones.

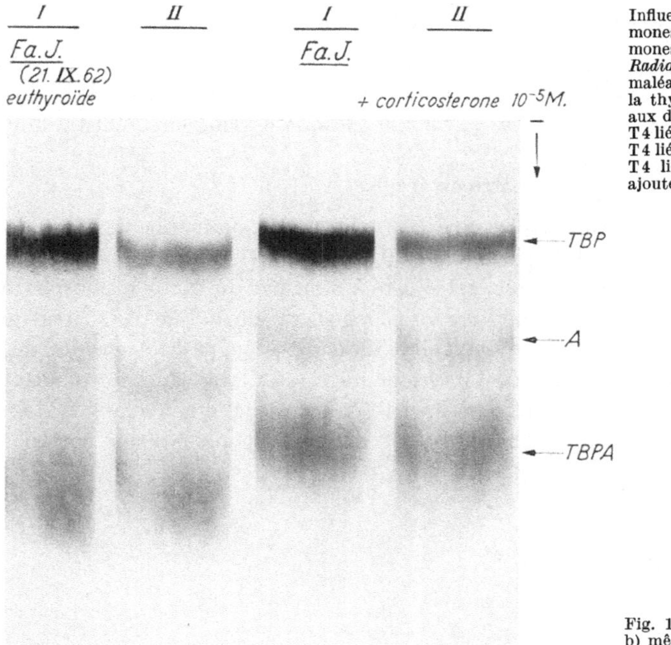

Influence in vitro des diverses hormones sur le transport des hormones thyroïdiennes.
Radioélectrophorèse (tampon trismaléate pH 8.6). Pourcentage de la thyroxine marquée à l'I[131] liée aux différentes protéines: TBP = T 4 liée aux α1-α2-globulines; A = T 4 liée aux albumines; TBPA = T 4 liée aux préalbumines; iode ajouté: I = 10 μg% II = 40 μg%

Fig. 1. a) patient euthyroïdien: b) même sérum + corticostérone 10⁻⁵ M (test normal)

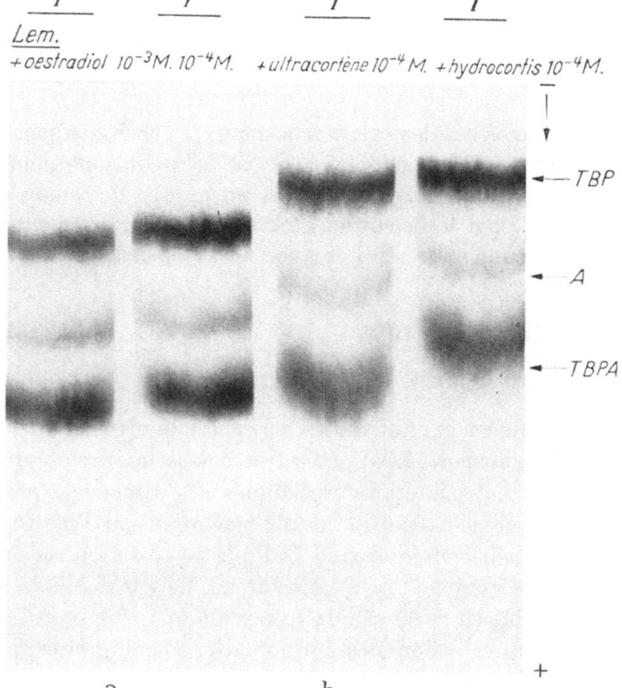

Fig. 2. Même test que celui de la figure 1. a) + oestradiol 10⁻³, 10⁻⁴ M; b) + ultracortène 10⁻⁴ M; c) + hydrocortisone 10⁻⁴ M

Tableau 4. *Influence in vitro des différentes hormones sur le transport*

	a) des hormones thyroïdiennes pourcentage de thyroxine marquée à l'I^{131} liée à (10 μg %)			b) des corticostéroïdes pourcentage de la corticostérone marquée au C^{14} liée (14 μg-%)
	TBP	A	TBPA	
Valeurs normales	45,3	18,4	36,3	73,2
+ thyroxine 10^{-6} M . . .	*16,2* ↓	*33,3* ↑	50,9	67,6
+ oestradiol 10^{-4} M . . .	39,1	17,2	44,7	68,2
+ hydrocortisone 10^{-4} M	43,8	14,5	41,7	*58,5* ↓
+ corticostérone 10^{-4} M .	49,2	11,7	39,1	*46,8* ↓
+ ultracortène 10^{-4} M . .	40,8	13,2	46,0	*49,4* ↓

Chiffres en italiques = différences significatives.

2. Action in vivo

a) Le transport hormonal dans l'hyperthyréose

Dans l'hyperthyréose, l'élévation du PBI est accompagnée d'un pourcentage d'hormone libre élevé et d'une TBP qui n'est pratiquement pas modifiée (Tabl. 5). Toutefois, comme le taux endogène d'hormone est élevé lorsqu'en effectuant le test de saturation, on ajoute encore de la thyroxine exogène, la TBP est plus rapidement saturée, ce qui se traduit par une légère diminution de la capacité. Notons également la modification qualitative, la fixation au niveau des pré-albumines ayant tendance à diminuer en faveur de celle des albumines.

Le transport des corticostéroïdes est normal. Le taux élevé des hormones thyroïdiennes endogènes ne modifie donc en rien le transport des corticostéroïdes et la capacité de la transcortine (Tabl. 6).

Tableau 5. *Répartition de la thyroxine marquée à l'I^{131} dans les différentes protéines plasmatiques*

	Thyroxine ajoutée (μg/100 ml sérum)									Capacité fixation de la TBP (mol. de T 4 liée/1000 ml sérum[1])
	10			40			80			
	TBP %	A %	TBPA %	TBP %	A %	TBPA %	TBP %	A %	TBPA %	
Euthyréose (*21*)	46,8	19,1	34,9	28,5	26,5	44,9	16,2	33,1	50,5	2,48 · 10^{-7}
	±4,1	±3,1	±5,2	±3,1	±3,6	±5,5	±1,8	±4,7	±5,3	±0,25
Hyperthyréose (*18*)	44,6	27,5	22,5	20,2	44,6	34,5	15,7	53,5	30,7	1,81 · 10^{-7}
	±4,6	±4,4	±7,1	±3,6	±6,8	±6,7	±2,2	±6,0	±6,6	±1,06
Hypothyréose (*9*)	63,9	15,9	20,1	35,4	35,4	29,2	18,6	42,4	39,0	2,90 · 10^{-7}
	±6,8	±3,7	±6,4	±6,7	±10,7	±8,9	±2,7	±9,9	±9,0	±0,56
Hépatite virale (*17*)	*81,6*	12,2	6,2	44,8	42,2	10,9	35,3	53,6	10,4	*3,91* · 10^{-7}
	±4,7	±3,6	±2,1	±6,9	±5,2	±4,5	±7,2	±6,9	±4,3	±0,59

[1] Calculée sur la fixation à 40 μg% ± déviation standard.

b) Hypothyréose

Dans l'hypothyréose, le taux endogène d'hormone circulant étant abaissé, on doit ajouter plus d'hormone pour saturer la TBP, d'où une capacité, ainsi qu'une fixation à la TBP légèrement augmentées. Dans cette affection, il semble que la fixation de la corticostérone à la transcortine soit faiblement accrue. Cependant, étant donné que nos cas d'hypothyroïdie sont des hypothyroïdies secondaires, ce phénomène pourrait être expliqué par un hyposurrénalisme (Tableau 6).

Tableau 6. *Influence in vivo de différentes hormones sur le transport*

Diagnostic	a) des hormones thyroïdiennes				b) des corticostéroïdes		
	nombre cas	PBI μg%	Captation T3[1] par les érythrocytes	Capacité fixation TBP (mol. de T4 liée/1.)	Pourcentage corticostérone marquée au C14 liée		Capacité fixation de la transcortine
					14 μg-%	50 μg-%	
Cas normaux	14	4,84	15,8	$2,45 \cdot 10^{-7}$	74,2	46,8	27,4
		$\pm$0,31	$\pm$0,82	$\pm$0,40	$\pm$3,46	$\pm$2,50	$\pm$3,35
Hyperthyréose	13	*12,07*	*24,6*	$1,96 \cdot 10^{-7}$	74,6	55,2	22,4
		$\pm$3,40	$\pm$2,56	$\pm$0,16	$\pm$4,39	$\pm$7,28	$\pm$4,77
Hypothyréose	4	*2,67*	12,1	$2,87 \cdot 10^{-7}$	84,0	60,5	23,5
		$\pm$1,47	$\pm$3,13	$\pm$0,86	$\pm$7,36	$\pm$7,58	$\pm$3,86
Addison	3	4,0	16,3	$2,71 \cdot 10^{-7}$	80,2	53,1	27,1
		$\pm$0,63	$\pm$3,19	$\pm$0,29	$\pm$6,73	$\pm$7,02	$\pm$7,89
Grossesse	"pool"	*8,35*	*9,9*	*4,61 \cdot 10^{-7}*	*86,6*	71,0	*15,6*
		$\pm$2,20	$\pm$1,23	$\pm$0,21	$\pm$6,31	$\pm$6,47	$\pm$0,55
Prednisone: avant traitement	7	5,53	17,2	$2,87 \cdot 10^{-7}$	68,9	51,4	16,9
		$\pm$1,20	$\pm$4,30	$\pm$0,62	$\pm$5,09	$\pm$5,61	$\pm$5,41
Prednisone: pendant traitement	7	4,04	20,3	$1,80 \cdot 10^{-7}$	64,3	51,8	*10,6*
		$\pm$1,07	$\pm$4,81	$\pm$0,55	$\pm$8,47	$\pm$8,27	$\pm$7,63
Tuberculose: avant traitement	18	5,48	15,7	$2,60 \cdot 10^{-7}$	71,2	47,6	24,8
		$\pm$0,72	$\pm$1,13	$\pm$1,86	$\pm$3,95	$\pm$7,13	$\pm$6.28
Tuberculose: pendant traitement (B-PAS)	11	5,01	17,7	$2,18 \cdot 10^{-7}$	*55,3*	38,8	16,5
		$\pm$0,26	$\pm$1,96	$\pm$0,28	$\pm$6,75	$\pm$2,39	$\pm$5,72

Chiffres en italiques = différences significatives.

c) Addison

Chez les trois addisoniens examinés, deux avaient été traités avec la prednisone antérieurement. Toutefois, ces patients montrent une liaison à la transcortine légèrement augmentée, ce qui indique, comme dans l'hypothyréose secondaire, que le peu d'hormone endogène est rendue encore plus inactive par sa liaison à la transcortine. Par contre, le transport des hormones thyroïdiennes est normal, ainsi que le taux de thyroxine libre (Tableau 6).

d) Grossesse ou traitement aux oestrogènes

Les modifications apportées par un traitement aux oestrogènes ou pendant la grossesse sont importantes, le PBI s'élevant dans les valeurs de l'hyperthyréose et la capacité de fixation de la TBP doublant ou triplant. L'effet des oestrogènes sur les corticostéroïdes semble similaire. En effet, le taux des corticostéroïdes sanguin augmente et en parallèle la capacité de fixation, maintenant ainsi un taux d'hormone non liée normal ou même abaissé (*33, 34, 35*). Nous avons examiné deux collectifs de sang provenant d'une trentaine de femmes enceintes chacun (4 ème au 6 ème mois).

Nous constatons que la fixation à la transcortine est nettement plus élevée, accompagnée d'une augmentation de la capacité de la transcortine (Tableau 6). L'action des oestrogènes est donc semblable sur la TBP et la transcortine et confirme les résultats obtenus par de nombreux auteurs (*36, 34, 33, 37, 57*).

e) Patients traités à la prednisone

Il s'agit d'un groupe de malades atteints de différentes affections (leucémie, arthrite, Ca du sein) et étant traités à la prednisone (10—20 mg/jour pendant

3 semaines). Nous les avons groupés, afin de voir si ce traitement modifiait le transport des hormones thyroïdiennes, ainsi que la fonction thyroïdienne. Certains auteurs (*38* à *43*) ont signalé, en effet, que les corticostéroïdes provoquaient une diminution du PBI, associée à une élévation du pourcentage d'hormone libre, variations qui restaient toutefois dans les valeurs normales et qui n'étaient pas constantes.

Avant traitement, la fixation à la transcortine est légèrement abaissée et la capacité faiblement augmentée, modification probablement due aux diverses affections. Pendant le traitement, ces valeurs sont peu modifiées. Toutefois, sous l'effet du traitement, la capacité de la transcortine est encore augmentée. Quant à la fonction thyroïdienne globale, elle reste dans les limites normales. Nous observons cependant une tendance à la diminution du PBI et une augmentation du taux d'hormone libre se reflétant encore dans la diminution de la capacité de la TBP. Ces différences ne sont toutefois pas statistiquement assurées et elles ne sont pas assez importantes pour faire intervenir un phénomène de compétition (Tableau 6).

f) Tuberculose pulmonaire traitée au B-PAS

Enfin, nous avons examiné un groupe de patients atteints de tuberculose pulmonaire avant et pendant un traitement au B-PAS (isobenzacyl forte Wander, composé de Rimifon, de benzacyl et de pyridoxium) (10—12 g par jour pendant un mois); sachant que le salicylate se lie aux α-globulines, nous nous sommes demandés si ce produit influencerait les liaisons hormonales.

Nous constatons, d'une part, que la tuberculose ne modifie ni la fonction, ni le transport des hormones thyroïdiennes, ni celui des corticoïdes, et, d'autre part, que le traitement au B-PAS, s'il n'a pas d'action sur le transport de la thyroxine, fait baisser la fixation des corticostéroïdes. Cette diminution est probablement due au fait que le B-PAS bloque en partie les ponts de liaison de la transcortine (Tableau 6).

IV. Discussion

A la suite de ces différents résultats, nous pouvons conclure qu'il n'y a pas de compétition, ni d'influence entre le transport des hormones corticoïdes et celui des hormones thyroïdiennes. Comme une hyper- ou une hypothyréose ne modifie pas le transport des hormones corticoïdes, de même un hypocorticisme (Addison) n'entraîne pas un trouble du tranport des hormones thyroïdiennes. Un traitement à la prednisone n'a pas un effet aussi marqué sur la fonction thyroïdienne qu'un traitement aux oestrogènes. Toutefois, la prednisone tend nettement à diminuer la fonction thyroïdienne, modification qui selon certains auteurs serait secondaire à l'effet inhibiteur hypophysaire sur la sécrétion de TSH (*41, 45*). Il y a donc absence de compétition. Cette dernière s'explique d'autant mieux que la transcortine et la TBP, tout en étant très proches chimiquement et électrophorétiquement, sont toutefois deux protéines bien différentes.

Outre du problème du support protéique, il est possible que le mécanisme de liaison entre hormone et protéine joue un rôle dans le mode du transport. En ce qui concerne la thyroxine, nous avons essayé de modifier cette liaison en utilisant, d'une part, des inhibiteurs du radical sulfhydril (parahydroximercuribenzoate = HMB, N-éthylmaléimide (NEM) et, d'autre part, des inhibiteurs du groupe

Tableau 7

	TBP *(50, 51, 52, 56)*	Transcortine *(46, 47, 48, 49)*
Nature	α glucoprotéine	α 1 glucoprotéine
Isolé par fraction de COHN	IV 6 IV 9	IV 4
Constante de sédimentation (SVEDBERG) . . .	S = 3,3 3,5	3,0
Poids moléculaire	40.000—45.000	45.000
Capacité de liaison	$2,5 \cdot 10^{-7}$ Mol	$6—25 \cdot 10^{-7}$ Mol

aminé terminal (NH2), dinitrofluorobenzène, (DFB), phénylisothiocyanate (PITH), pensant que ces deux radicaux pouvaient intervenir dans la liaison avec les hormones.

En effet, étudiant la liaison albumine-thyroxine, STERLING (*53*) arrive à la conclusion que cette dernière s'effectue probablement entre le groupe phénolique de la thyroxine et un radical-NH2 de la protéine. De son côté, OPPENHEIMER (*26*), en étudiant l'influence du diphénylhydantoïne sur le déplacement de la thyroxine de son support protidique, montre que ce produit agit par compétition sur la liaison, compétition rendue possible par la similitude de configuration spatiale de ces deux composés. Pour notre part, nous constatons (Fig. 3) que ni le NEM, ni le

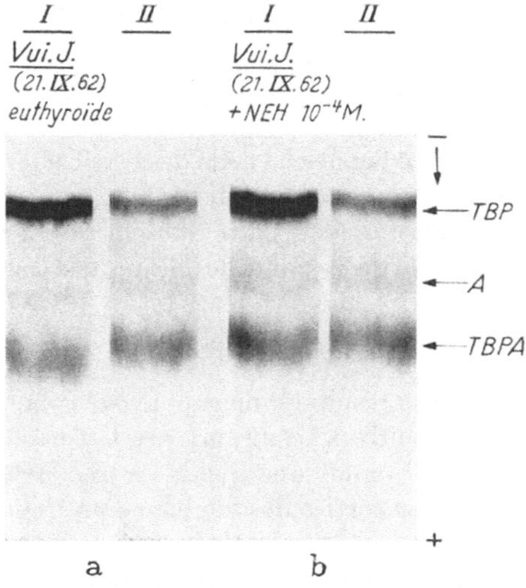

Influence in vitro des substances agissant avec les groupes —SH et —NH₂ sur le transport des hormones thyroïdiennes (hydroxymercuribenzoate = HBM, n-éthylmaléimide = NEM, dinitrofluorobenzol = DFB, phénylisothiocyanate = PITH)
Fig. 3. a) normal, b) blocage du groupe —SH (NEM 10⁻⁴ M)

HMB (Fig. 4a) ne modifient in vitro la liaison TBP-thyroxine, ni celle des albumines et des préalbumines. A plus forte concentration (10^{-2} Mol), on constate une légère diminution de la liaison TBP-thyroxine, diminution qui toutefois n'est pas significative.

Avec le dinitrofluorobenzène, nous observons à partir de 10^{-3} Mol l'inhibition complète de la liaison thyroxine-préalbumine à 10^{-2} Mol, aussi celle de thyroxine-TBP (Fig. 4b). Toutefois, comme ce composé se lie avec la thyroxine par le groupe phénolique de cette dernière, la thyroxine liée au DFB possède en effet des

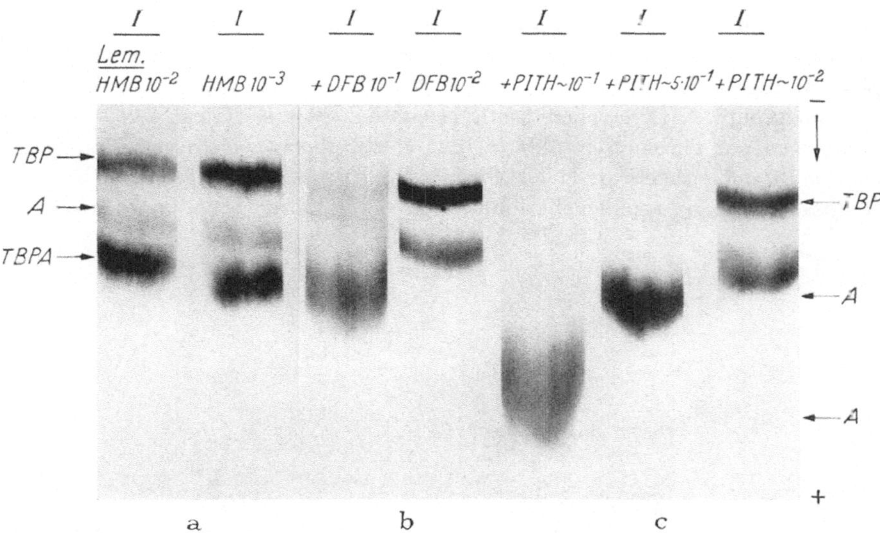

Fig. 4. a) Blocage du groupe —SH (HMB 10⁻³ M, 10⁻² M); b) blocage du groupe —NH₂ (DFB 10⁻¹ M, 10⁻² M); c) blocage du groupe —NH₂ (PITH 10⁻¹ M, 10⁻² M)

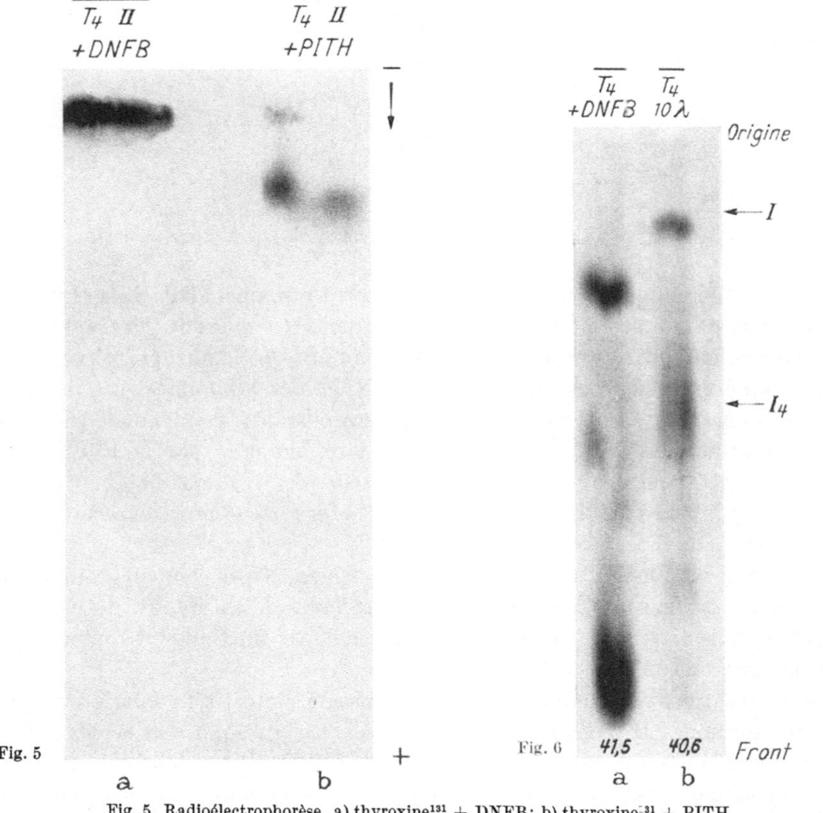

Fig. 5. Radioélectrophorèse. a) thyroxine¹³¹ + DNFB; b) thyroxine¹³¹ + PITH
Fig. 6. Chromatographie (BuOH/NH₄OH2N). a) Thyroxine¹³¹ et I¹³¹; b) thyroxine¹³¹ et I¹³¹ + DNFB

propriétés différentes qui sont mises en évidence par chromatographie (Fig. 6), la thyroxine migrant au front du chromatogramme avec le DFB ou par électrophorèse (Fig. 5), la T_4 restant à l'origine. Nous avons alors utilisé un autre inhibiteur du groupe NH2, le phénylisothyocianate qui ne se lie pas à la thyroxine, puisque ni par chromatographie, ni par électrophorèse, on observe une modification du déplacement de la T4 (Fig. 5). Nous constatons (Fig. 4c et 7b) que ce composé provoque rapidement l'inhibition de la liaison préalbumine-thyroxine

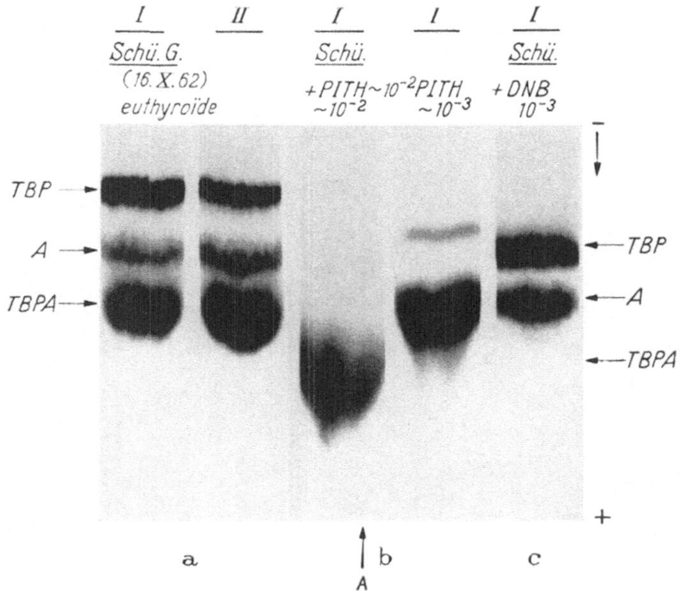

Fig. 7. Radioélectrophorèse. a) test normal (patient euthyroïdien); b) même sérum + PITH 10⁻², 10⁻³ M; c) même sérum + DFB 10⁻³ M

et à 10^{-1} $^{-2}$ Mol supprime entièrement la liaison thyroxine-TBP. Si la thyroxine reste liée aux albumines, nous voyons que ces dernières migrent plus rapidement que normalement, ceci étant dû probablement au fait que le phénylisothyocianate ayant bloqué également quelques radicaux NH2 des albumines, ces dernières sont moins chargées positivement et vont plus rapidement vers l'anode (Fig. 7b).

Les préalbumines étant les premières à être bloquées par le PITH, nous pouvons admettre que cette liaison avec la thyroxine est très sensible. En revanche, celle de la thyroxine à la TBP est probablement plus forte et possède certainement d'autres points de liaison que le groupe NH2.

Quant aux corticoïdes, ni les bloqueurs du groupe SH, ni celui du groupe NH2 n'influencent la liaison transcortine-corticostéroïdes (Tableau 8). Il est donc probable que la liaison de ces hormones se fasse par un tout autre mécanisme que nous ignorons encore.

Ces observations nous montrent qu'il n'y a pas de compétition dans le transport entre les hormones thyroïdiennes et les corticoïdes, puisque non seulement les protéines sont différentes, mais aussi le mode de liaison. Il y a donc une *spécificité des transporteurs hormonaux* et les différentes modifications du transport des hormones semblent rarement dues à des phénomènes de compétition.

Tableau 8. *Action in vitro sur le transport des substances (hydroxymercuribenzoate = HMB, n-ethylmaleimide = NEM, Dinitrofluorobenzol = DFB, phenylisothiocyanate = PITH) réagissant avec les groupes —SH ou —NH$_2$*

	a) des hormones thyroïdiennes Pourcentage de la thyroxine marquée à l'I^{131} liée (10 μg-%)			b) des corticostéroïdes Pourcentage de corticostérone marquée au C^{14} liée (14 μg-%)
	TBP	A	TBPA	
Valeurs normales	45,3	18,4	36,3	73,2
Inhibiteur du groupe —SH				
HMB 10^{-3} M	39,3	14,4	46,3	73,6
NEM 10^{-3} M	40,9	10,8	48,3	72,7
Inhibiteur du groupe —NH$_2$				
DFB ~ 10^{-3} M	24,0 ↓	76,0 ↑	0 ↓	74,4
DFB ~ 10^{-2} M	13,2 ↓	86,8 ↑	0 ↓	
PITH ~ 10^{-3} M	6,6 ↓	93,4 ↑	0 ↓	75,0
PITH ~ 10^{-2} M	0 ↓	100 ↑	0 ↓	65,0

← Différences significatives.

Nous pouvons classer les différents troubles du transport selon les 6 causes probables suivantes:

1. Les *modifications spontanées et primaires*, congénitales ou non du transport des hormones thyroïdiennes qui provoquent soit une élévation de la TBP, soit une diminution de cette dernière, entraînant respectivement une augmentation ou une diminution du PBI, accompagnée le plus souvent d'un état d'euthyréose.

2. Les altérations provoquées par les *oestrogènes* seraient probablement dues à leur action anabolique sur les α-globulines qui en augmentant la quantité de protéine transporteuse et leur capacité provoquent secondairement l'élévation du PBI et des corticoïdes, afin de maintenir un taux d'hormone libre constant.

3. Les composés tels que les *dinitrophénols, les salicylates, les diphénylhydantoïnes* ou les *bleus de Tripan* etc. agissent directement par compétition sur la liaison TBP-T4, en déplaçant la thyroxine qui reste principalement sous forme libre et qui inhibe l'hypophyse et entraîne secondairement une diminution du PBI. Cette compétition est réversible et directement proportionnelle à la concentration des composés. On ne connaît pas encore d'action similaire sur les corticoïdes.

4. *Les androgènes (54)*, ainsi que les stéroïdes anabolisants (55) semblent avoir une action directe sur la capacité de liaison de la TBP, provoquant une diminution de cette dernière et entraînant secondairement une baisse du PBI.

5. *La prednisone et les corticoïdes* agissent sur le transport des hormones thyroïdiennes, mais par un mécanisme encore inconnu. Certains auteurs émettent l'hypothèse d'un freinage hypophysaire. Ces modifications n'altèrent toutefois pas profondément la fonction thyroïdienne.

6. En dehors des différentes hormones et drogues que nous venons de citer, nous savons que *l'hépatite épidémique* est accompagnée d'une élévation du PBI, provenant du trouble du catabolisme des hormones thyroïdiennes et qu'elle entraîne secondairement une augmentation de la capacité de la TBP qui neutralise cet excès d'hormone circulant. Il s'agit donc d'un mécanisme de défense pour maintenir un taux d'hormone libre constant.

Toutes ces altérations du transport des hormones thyroïdiennes apportent le plus souvent une modification du catabolisme périphérique de la thyroxine, de son renouvellement et du taux d'hormone libre. En conséquence, elles sont d'une grande importance dans l'évaluation des observations cliniques. Il semble de plus en plus évident que la seule détermination du taux global des hormones circulantes est insuffisante et qu'il est nécessaire de connaître soit la capacité de fixation des protéines transporteuses, soit le taux d'hormone libre avant d'interpréter l'activité hormonale périphérique.

Remerciements

Ce travail a été effectué grâce à l'aide du Fonds National Suisse de la Recherche Scientifique que nous remercions.

Nous adressons également nos remerciements à Mademoiselle C. Buzzi pour sa précieuse collaboration.

Bibliographie

1. Gray, C. H.: Hormons in blood. New York: Academic Press 1961.
2. Robbins, J., and J. E. Rall: Physiol. Rev. **40**, 415 (1960).
3. Sterling, K., and A. Hegedus: J. clin. Invest. **41**, 1039 (1962).
4. Kallee, E.: En: Leber und Nachbarorgane, p. 64. Bad Mergentheim, Sept. 1961. Stuttgart: Georg Thieme Verlag 1962.
5. — Protides of the biological fluids, p. 161. Amsterdam: Elsevier Publishing Comp. 1960.
6. Tata, J. R.: Recent Progr. Hormone Res. **18**, 221 (1962).
7. — Biochim. biophys. Acta (Amst.) **28**, 91 (1958).
8. Ingbar, S. H., and N. Freinkel: Recent Progr. Hormone Res. **16**, 353 (1960).
9. Tanaka, S., and P. Starr: Metabolism 8, 441 (1959).
10. Beierwaltes, W. H., and J. Robbins: J. clin. Invest. **38**, 1683 (1959).
11. Florscheim, W. H., J. T. Dowling, L. Meister and R. E. Bodfish: J. clin. Endocr. **22**, 735 (1962).
12. Tanaka, S., and P. Starr: J. clin. Endocr. **19**, 485 (1959).
13. Ingbar, S. H.: J. clin. Invest. **40**, 2053 (1961).
14. Cavalieri, R. R.: J. clin. Endocr. **21**, 1455 (1961).
15. Beisel, W. R., H. Zainal, S. Have, V. L. Di Raimondo and P. H. Forsham: J. clin. Endocr. **22**, 1165 (1962).
16. Lemarchand-Béraud, Th., A. Vannotti u. M.-R. Jeanneret: Schweiz. med. Wschr. **93**, 7 (1963).
17. Robbins, J., and J. H. Nelson: J. clin. Invest. **37**, 153 (1958).
18. Dowling, J. T., N. Freinkel and S. H. Ingbar: J. clin. Invest. **35**, 1263 (1956).
19. Engström, W. W., and B. Markardt: J. clin. Endocr. **14**, 215 (1954).
20. Dowling, J. T., N. Freinkel and S. H. Ingbar: J. clin. Endocr. **16**, 1491 (1956).
21. Vannotti, A., and Th. Béraud: J. clin. Endocr. **19**, 466 (1959).
22. Christensen, K.: Nature (Lond.) **183**, 1189 (1959).
23. Koller, E., u. E. Rall: Rdsch. Naturforsch. **10**, 614 (1953).
24. Wolff, J., M. E. Standoert and J. E. Rall: J. clin. Invest. **40**, 1373 (1961).
25. Good, B. F., B. S. Hetzel and L. J. Opit: J. Endocr. **21**, 231 (1960).
26. Oppenheimer, J. H., and R. R. Tavernetti: J. clin. Invest. **41**, 12 (1962).
27. Shimada, S. I., T. Tonizarva, T. Yamada and K. Shichijo: Endocrinology 71, 414 (1962).
28. Slaunwhite, J. R., and A. A. Sandberg: J. clin. Invest. **38**, 384 (1959).
29. Daughaday, W. H.: J. clin. Invest. **37**, 511, 519 (1958).
30. Béraud, Th.: Acta endocr. (Kbh.) **35**, suppl. 55 (1960).
31. Vannotti, A., et Th. Béraud: Expos. ann. Biochim. méd. **21**, 57 (1959).
32. Hamolsky, M. W., M. Stein and A. S. Freedberg: J. clin. Endocr. **17**, 33 (1957).
33. Doe, R. P., H. H. Zinneman, E. B. Flink and R. A. Ulstrom: J. clin. Endocr. **20**, 1484 (1960).

34. SANDBERG, A. A., and W. R. SLAUNWHITE: J. clin. Invest. **38**, 1290 (1959).*
35. WALLACE, E. Z., and A. CARTER: J. clin. Invest. **39**, 601 (1960).
36. DAUGHADAY, W. H., R. E. ADLER, I. K. MARIZ and D. C. RASINSKI: J. clin. Endocr. **22**, 704 (1962).
37. BOOTH, M., P. F. DIXON, C. H. GRAY, J. M. GREENAWAY and N. J. HOLNESS: J. Endocr. **23**, 25 (1961).
38. FRIIS, T., and U. REINICKE: Acta endocr. (Kbh.) **42**, 1 (1963).
39. BERSON, S. A., and R. S. YALOW: J. clin. Endocr. **12**, 407 (1952).
40. BROWN-GRANT, K., G. W. HARRIS and S. REICHLIN: J. Physiol. (Lond.) **126**, 41 (1954).
41. FREDERICKSON, D. S., P. H. FORSHAM and G. W. THORN: J. clin. Endocr. **12**, 541 (1952).
42. MONEY, W. L.: Brookhaven Symposium on Biology 7, 137 (1957).
43. SHERER, M. G., B. N. SIEFRING: J. clin. Endocr. **16**, 643 (1956).
44. SANDBERG, A. A., and W. R. SLAUNWHITE: J. clin. Invest. **36**, 1266 (1957).
45. WERNER, S. C.: Bull. N. Y. Acad. Med. **13**, 712 (1953).
46. SANDBERG, A. A., and W. R. SLAUNWHITE: Recent Progr. Hormone Res. **13**, 209 (1957).
47. DAUGHADAY, W. H.: J. clin. Invest. **35**, 1428, 1434 (1956).
48. SEAL, U. S., and R. P. DOE: J. biol. Chem. **237**, 3136 (1962).
49. GRAY, C. H., and P. F. DIXON: Intern. Symposium on adrenal cortex, Gand, septembre 1962.
50. SCHULTZE, H. E., I. GÖLLNER, K. HEIDE, M. SCHÖNENBERGER u. G. SCHWICK: Z. Naturforsch. **106**, 463 (1955).
51. FREINKEL, N., J. TH. DOWLING and S. H. INGBAR: J. clin. Invest. **34**, 1698 (1955).
52. PETERMAN, M. L., J. ROBBINS and M. G. HAMILTON: J. biol. Chem. **208**, 369 (1954).
53. STERLING, K., P. ROSEN and J. TABACHNIK: J. clin. Invest. **41**, 1021 (1962).
54. FEDERMAN, D. D., J. ROBBINS and J. E. RALL: J. clin. Invest. **37**, 1024 (1958).
55. ROSENBERG, I. N., C. S. AHN and M. L. MITCHELL: J. clin. Endocr. **22**, 612 (1962).
56. TATA, J. R.: Nature (Lond.) **189**, 573 (1961).
57. RASMUSSEN, F.B., O.BUSS, F.LUNDSWAL and D.TROLLE: Acta endocr.(Kbh.)**40**,571(1962).

Aus der 1. Inn. Abt. Allg. Krankenhaus St. Georg, Hamburg

Die klinischen Wirkungen der Schilddrüsenhormone

Von

H. W. Bansi

Mit 4 Abbildungen

Referat

Es liegt nahe, daß sich zum Studium der physiologischen Wirkungen der Schilddrüsenhormone die Vollhypothyreosen anbieten, da hier aus dem Status vor und unter der Substitutionsbehandlung ihre Effekte quantitativ zutage treten. Völliger Ausfall der Schilddrüsenfunktion ist leicht erkennbar. Selbst wenn möglicherweise – was durch den Radiojodtest heutzutage sehr einfach ausgeschlossen werden kann – noch Spuren einer Schilddrüsenhormonsynthese existieren sollten, sind doch die Abweichungen von den normalen „Konstanten" bei Ausfall der Schilddrüsenfunktion absolut eindeutig, und die Umstellungen des Stoffwechsels unter der Therapie in physiologischer Dosierung erfolgen in kurzer Frist in Richtung der Norm. So bietet die Hypothyreose ein fast ideales Bild von der Vielseitigkeit der Schilddrüsenhormonwirkung, und die unter den Augen des Therapeuten sich abspielende „Aufhellung" der meist in einen „Dornröschenschlaf" verfallenen Funktionen gibt den gewaltigen Eindruck wieder, der durch diese jodhaltigen Aminosäuren bewirkt wird. Ein britischer Psychiater, Asher (1949), schlug sehr treffend vor, wenn man sich vom Vorhandensein eines Schilddrüsenhormonmangels überzeugen wolle, daß man ein Photo des zu prüfenden Probanden machen und unter der Substitution die Veränderungen der Gesamtpersönlichkeit auf Grund der Vorlage vor der Behandlung beobachten solle.

Im folgenden soll nicht das Problem des „Wie" dieser Hormonwirkungen kritisch beleuchtet werden, sondern in Beschränkung auf einige wenige Funktionskreise die Wirkungen physiologischer Mengen der beiden bisher als wesentlich anerkannten Schilddrüsenhormone, des L-Tetrajodthyronins, das im Hormonorgan die am meisten vertretene Speicherform darstellt – des L-Thyroxins oder L-T_4- und des L-3,5,3'-Trijodthyronins – L-T_3. Die Bindung dieser beiden Hormone erfolgt, wie wohl bereits von meiner Vorrednerin, Frau Pitt-Rivers, ausführlich diskutiert wurde, an das Thyroxin-bindende Globulin, an Albumin und ein Thyroxin-bindendes Präalbumin (womit letzten Endes die Menge der freien Form der Schilddrüsenhormone reguliert wird). Nur der ungebundene Anteil, das freie Hormon, kann in die Gewebe eindringen und dort in Bindung an vorwiegend subcelluläre Strukturen seine biochemische Aktivität entfalten (Tata 1961).

Absichtlich sei aber auf diese intra- und extracellulären Austauschmechanismen nicht eingegangen, sondern nur über die Gesamtwirkung der beiden Hormone — und gelegentlich auch einmal eines ihrer Analoge — auf den Gesamtorganismus referiert, wobei eine Beschränkung auf folgende Funktionskreise erfolgen soll:

1. Kreislauf und Herz.
2. Wasser- und Elektrolythaushalt, einschließlich der Nierenfunktion.
3. Fett- und Cholesterinhaushalt.
4. Gesamtstoffwechsel und einige spezielle Stoffwechselvorgänge.
5. Wachstum.
6. Beeinflussung des Reglerkreises: Adenohypophyse-Schilddrüse.

An die Spitze der Ausführungen über die Schilddrüsenhormonwirkung am Gesamt-Organismus sei die Einwirkung auf die *Herzfunktion* und damit auf den *Kreislauf* gestellt. Das Myxödemherz, das von meinem verehrten Lehrer ZONDEK (1918) zum ersten Mal beschrieben wurde, zeigt eine allgemeine Dilatation, eine auffallend langsame wurmförmige Herzmuskelkontraktion und sehr häufig auch neben einer gewissen Durchtränkung des gesamten Herzmuskels mit „Myxödem"

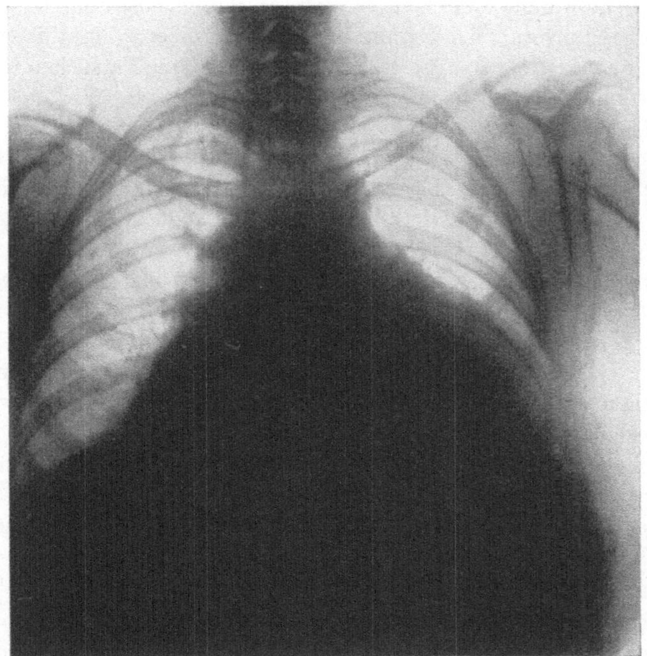

Abb. 1. Durch myxödematösen Perikarderguß enorm erweiterte Herzsilhouette bei Myxödem

(Abb. 1), jener vorwiegend extracellulär gelegenen Flüssigkeit, einen Herzbeutelerguß. Sehr typisch sind die zahlreichen Veränderungen am Myxödem-EKG; ich erinnere nur an die Abflachungen der Nachschwankungen in der Standardableitung, Befunde, die ebenfalls vor mehr als 40 Jahren in der 1. Medizinischen Klinik der Charité durch HERMANN ZONDEK aufgedeckt worden sind und die eine allgemeine Bestätigung gefunden haben. Die Veränderung des Myxödem-EKGs durch

Schilddrüsenhormon-Zufuhr kann man nicht nur als Test für die Schilddrüsenhormone als solche, sondern auch in besonders überzeugender Weise für Hormonanaloge nachweisen, womit man sich leicht von der thyromimetischen Wirkung solcher thyroxin-ähnlichen Substanzen überzeugen kann.

Beim Myxödem ist die Zirkulationsgeschwindigkeit sowie das zirkulatorische Minutenvolumen erheblich herabgesetzt (was sich nach der Fickschen Formel aus dem Gesamtsauerstoffverbrauch/min und aus der relativ hohen arteriovenösen Sauerstoffdifferenz des Blutes zwischen linkem und rechtem Herzen errechnen läßt), wobei die AV-Sauerstoff-Differenz in der Regel stärker vergrößert ist als die Herabsetzung des Gesamtsauerstoffverbrauches. Umgekehrt sieht man unter der Zufuhr von Schilddrüsenhormonen die Zirkulationsgeschwindigkeit sich sehr schnell normalisieren, das Herz erhält seinen normalen Tonus, und bei einem Überschreiten des Normalbedarfs kommt es zu jenen typischen Veränderungen des thyreotoxischen Kreislaufs; abnorm hohes zirkulatorisches Minutenvolumen, solange das Herz noch normal zu arbeiten vermag, abnorm geringe arteriovenöse Sauerstoffdifferenz, eine Blutdruckreaktion, wie sie ähnlich unter Adrenalin zu sehen ist, mit relativ hoher Blutdruckamplitude und eine Herabsetzung der peripheren Gefäßwiderstände. Man hat diese Wirkungen des Schilddrüsenhormons oft durch eine Steigerung der Empfindlichkeit gegenüber sympathicomimetischen Substanzen zu erklären versucht. Eine der auffallendsten Tatsachen in der Klinik und in der experimentellen Medizin ist die synergistische Wirkung der Schilddrüsen- und Nebennierenmark-Hormone, wobei sich gewissermaßen eine Sensibilisierung der Peripherie für adrenergische Impulse abzeichnet. Besonders ABELIN (1956) macht auf zahlreiche sowohl dem Adrenalin als auch dem Thyroxin zukommende Wirkungen aufmerksam und auf sozusagen als komplementär anzusehende Stoffwechseleffekte beider Hormone. Trotzdem muß vor einer „oversimplification" in der Deutung dieser Beobachtungen gewarnt werden. So konnten MACMILLAN und RAND (1962) an Aorten- und Milzstreifen von Kaninchen, die mit erheblichen Dosen Trijodthyronin behandelt waren, zeigen, daß die so vorbehandelten Gefäßstreifen keineswegs gegenüber Noradrenalin empfindlicher waren als die der Kontrolltiere. Auch die Beziehungen der Schilddrüsenhormone zu den Catecholaminen haben noch nicht zu eindeutigen Ergebnissen geführt. Es wäre bestechend, wenn methodische Verbesserungen des Catecholaminnachweises sowie der Serotonine eine Stütze für die klinisch erwiesene antithyreoidale Wirkung z. B. des Reserpin ergäben. Von pharmakologischer Seite wird eine Vermehrung der Dejodierung der Jodthyronine durch Reserpin angenommen (GALTON und INGBAR, 1961), nachdem KUSCHKE und GRUNER (1954) die durch Thyroxin erzielte Steigerung des Sauerstoffverbrauchs bei Ratten durch Reserpin zur Norm zurückführen konnten, was von MONCKE (1957) am hyperthyreotischen Patienten bestätigt wurde. Feststehend ist, daß bei jeder Steigerung der Schilddrüsenfunktion auch eine Steigerung der Sensibilität für die Adrenal- und Noradrenalinkörper vorliegt.

Die Steigerung des zirkulatorischen Minutenvolumens ist ein so eklatanter Effekt der Schilddrüsenhormone, daß gerade diesbezüglich eine Gefährdung des Patienten einsetzt, wenn in planloser Weise Schilddrüsenhormone zugeführt werden.

Unterteilt man die verschiedenen Stromgebiete des Organismus, so ergaben Durchblutungsmessungen des Gehirns, daß dieses weniger minderdurchblutet ist als der Gesamtorganismus (Verminderung um 38% gegenüber 47% des Gesamtkreislaufs). Ferner läßt sich nachweisen, wie SCHEINBERG u. Mitarb. zeigen konnten, daß auch der Gehirnstoffwechsel bei Fehlen der Schilddrüsenhormone herabgemindert ist. Entsprechendes ergaben gleichlaufende Untersuchungen am Traubenzuckerverbrauch des Gehirns.

Die Verminderung des zirkulatorischen Gesamtminutenvolumens führt natürlich auch zu einer *mangelhaften Nierendurchblutung.* Wie OLSEN und ich in gemeinsamen Untersuchungen der Inulin-Clearance zeigen konnten, lag der Mittelwert bei 12 Myxödemkranken bei 65,2 ± 22,8 cm³ pro Minute, berechnet auf den normalen Oberflächenwert von 1,73, und damit signifikant vermindert. Bereits in früheren Untersuchungen war von mehreren Autoren (CORCORAN und PAGE, 1947 — 2 Fälle) mit anderen Methoden eine ungenügende Durchblutung der Nieren und damit die relative Verschlechterung der Nierenfunktion dargelegt worden. Die Filtrations-Fraktion — das ist der Anteil der filtrierten Menge zur Gesamtnierendurchblutung — ist auffallend hoch, was sich allein auch schon aus der langsamen Durchströmung der Glomerula und damit langen Zeit für den Austausch in den Glomerula erklären läßt. Die besonders starke Drosselung der Gesamtnierendurchblutung ergibt sich aus dem auffallend stark reduzierten PAH-Wert, der im Mittel mit 218 ± 89 cm³/min gegenüber unserem Normaldurchschnitt von 586 ± 36,2 cm³/min die Norm um 62,5% unterschritt. Durch Normalisierung der Schilddrüsenfunktion auf dem Wege über eine physiologisch dosierte Schilddrüsenhormonmenge lassen sich diese Ausfallerscheinungen in der Regel recht gut ausgleichen, wobei die Filtrations-Fraktion sich sogar sehr schnell der Norm zu nähern pflegt. Es ist natürlich naheliegend, daß die Schilddrüsenfunktion durch die Beschleunigung der allgemeinen Zirkulationsverhältnisse auch den Wasserstoffwechsel erheblich beschleunigt. Macht man beim Myxödem einen Volhardschen Wasserstoß, so fällt oft eine gewisse Verzögerung der Wasserausscheidung auf. J. H. VOGT hat kürzlich [Acta endocr. (Kbh.) 35, 277 (1960)] nach Wasserbelastung in Anlehnung an den bei uns üblichen Wasserversuch (20 ml/kg Körpergewicht = etwa 1200 cm³) die Wasserausscheidung verzögert gefunden, was er auf eine verminderte Abgabe des ACTH bezog, zumal sich trotz Thyreoidinsubstitution die verzögerte Wasserausscheidung erst langsam wieder normalisierte. Im allgemeinen ist bei mangelnder Schilddrüsenfunktion die ACTH- und Nebennierenrindenfunktion ebenfalls reduziert. Die Bestimmungen der Gesamtwassermenge ergaben beim Myxödem einen Anstieg des Gesamtwassers auf 63 gegenüber 53% KG in der Norm, ein Unterschied, der zwar statistisch nicht signifikant ist, der aber meines Erachtens doch im Rahmen der Klinik recht viel Interessantes besagt. Während sich die extracelluläre Flüssigkeitsmenge kaum von der der Norm unterscheidet, ist beim Vollmyxödem-Kranken doch immerhin eine nicht unerhebliche Durchtränkung der Gewebe mit Wasser festzustellen. Schon lange vor den Studien über die verschiedenen Flüssigkeitsräume wurde mittels Farbstoffmethoden eine Verkleinerung des zirkulierenden Plasmavolumens festgestellt (MEANS, THOMPSON 1926), während WISLITZKY (1932) einen Anstieg des Plasmavolumens unter Thyreoidin beobachtete.

Im Elektrolytbild der Hypothyreosen und nach Zufuhr von Schilddrüsenhormon in physiologischer Dosis lassen sich keinerlei wesentliche Veränderungen feststellen. Eine gewisse Hyponatriämie unter 135 mÄq/l fiel uns in zahlreichen Fällen auf. Anders steht es mit den Eiweißfraktionen der Sera. Die *Hyperproteinämie* ist ein altbekanntes Symptom, und bei Aufgliederung der Fraktionen in der üblichen Elektrophorese fand sich eine Vermehrung der Globulinfraktion (Bansi, Fretwurst und Gronow, Kleinsorg und Krüskemper sowie Weicker 1956).

Die Erhöhung der BSG ist ein regelmäßiges Symptom, das vor allem von Bloomer, Lillington und uns *selbst* betont wird. Unter der Schilddrüsenhormonzufuhr regularisieren sich diese der Hypothyreose zuzuordnenden Symptome. Sie sind aber als Ausdruck einer typischen Schilddrüsenhormonwirkung kaum zu verwerten. Ein Hinweis auf die Umstellung der bei Hypothyreose typisch verschobenen Phärogramme — im Sinne einer „Rechtsverschiebung" der Fettelektrophorese zugunsten des Fettschwanzes und der Fraktion der Lipoproteide — ist schon eher der Ausdruck spezifisch auf den Fettstoffwechsel ausgerichteter Wirkungen der Schilddrüsenhormone, ebenso wie übrigens auch ihrer Analoge (Abb. 2).

Da das Myxödem als eine Ansammlung von Mucoproteinen, die reichlich hexosaminhaltig sind, angesprochen wird,

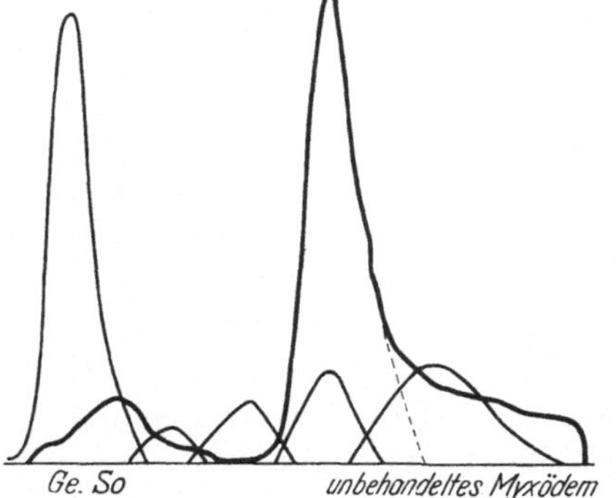

Abb. 2. Eiweiß- und Fettelektrophorese in einem Fall von unbehandeltem Myxödem

liegt es nahe, daß bei Hypothyreosen nach dem Verhalten der Hexosamin-Ausscheidung und ihrer Veränderung nach Schilddrüsenhormonzufuhr gefahndet wird. Mir sind leider bisher nur zwei von Wiener u. Mitarb. näher studierte Fälle bekannt geworden, die einen Anstieg der Harnausscheidung der Hexosamine unter Thyroxin zeigten.

Mit der Normalisierung der Nierendurchblutung und damit ihrer Leistung nach Zufuhr der fehlenden Schilddrüsenhormone beginnt unmittelbar beim Einsetzen ihrer normalen Funktion auch die Ausscheidung jener eigenartigen Flüssigkeitsansammlungen, die der Hypothyreose auch den Namen „Myxödem" (Ord 1878) eingebracht haben. Schon früh hat Schöndorff (1897) unter Pflüger in lang hingestreckten Bilanzversuchen die vermehrte Stickstoffausscheidung im Beginn einer Schilddrüsenhormonzufuhr nicht als Steigerung des Eiweißstoffwechsels, sondern als gesteigerte Ausscheidung gespeicherter Stickstoffschlacken bzw. stickstoffhaltiger Extraktivstoffe erkannt. 1925 fanden die bekannten *USA*-Schilddrüsenforscher Boothby und Sandiford, Sandiford und Slosse — teilweise unter Heranziehung frühester Bilanzversuche meines Lehrers Magnus-

LEVY —, daß bei Athyreoten nach Verabfolgung von Thyreoidin ein Anstieg der N-Ausscheidung im Harn erfolgte, die einer Mobilisierung und Verbrennung eines etwa 2% N-haltigen Proteids entsprach und für das sie das vorwiegend extracellulär gelagerte Myxödem, ein Mucoprotein, verantwortlich machten. Jeweils nach Zufuhr von Schilddrüsenhormonen beobachtet man mit einem deutlichen Abschwellen des Kranken, mit Abnahme des „Myxödems" und dem Anstieg des Grundumsatzes eine überschießende Wasser-, Elektrolyt- und N-Ausscheidung.

In eigenen Versuchen haben wir nach einer 5 tägigen Vorbehandlung bei absolut gleicher Zufuhr einer Vollmyxödemkranken an 2 Tagen 5 mg Thyroxin appliziert und gleichzeitig auch die Elektrolyte mit verfolgt. Während die Na-Ausscheidung von täglich im Mittel 1,67 g auf das Doppelte anstieg, blieb die Kalium-Ausscheidung praktisch unverändert. Die Chloride nehmen bei den Elektrolyten eine Mittelstellung ein. Die Gesamt-N-Ausscheidung im Harn vermehrt sich von 8,13 g pro die auf 11,81 g. Die in der überschießenden Wasserabgabe (+ 638 cm³ Wasser) erscheinende N-Menge beläuft sich somit auf 3,78 g, so daß in unserem Falle die Elimination eines 0,59%igen N-haltigen Proteins errechnet.

Daß anfänglich unter der Thyreoidintherapie nur Natrium vermehrt zur Ausscheidung gelangt, verdient meines Erachtens besondere Beachtung und dürfte zwanglos der rein extracellulär angreifenden Frühwirkung der Schilddrüsenhormone entsprechen: Mobilisierung des „Myxödems". Steigert sich später der sog. Gesamtverbrennungsstoffwechsel, so kommt es zu einem sprunghaften Ansteigen auch der Kaliumausscheidung. Des weiteren interessierte es uns, ob die Relation der Schwefelfraktionen im Harn zum Gesamtstickstoff auf den Abbau einer stark schwefelhaltigen Eiweißsubstanz hinweisen würde und ob gegebenenfalls der sog. Neutralschwefel als Ausdruck des reinen Eiweißabbaus in seiner

Relation zum Gesamtschwefel Veränderungen erfahren würde. In Abb. 3 sind die Relationen Gesamtschwefelausscheidung : Gesamt-N-Ausscheidung für mehrere Fälle aufgezeigt, wobei sich vor und unter der Behandlung kein Unterschied ergibt.

Ziehen wir aus den Versuchen von BYROM und unseren sich ergänzenden Versuchen die Schlüsse, so ergibt sich, daß unmittelbar mit Einsetzen der Thyroxin-

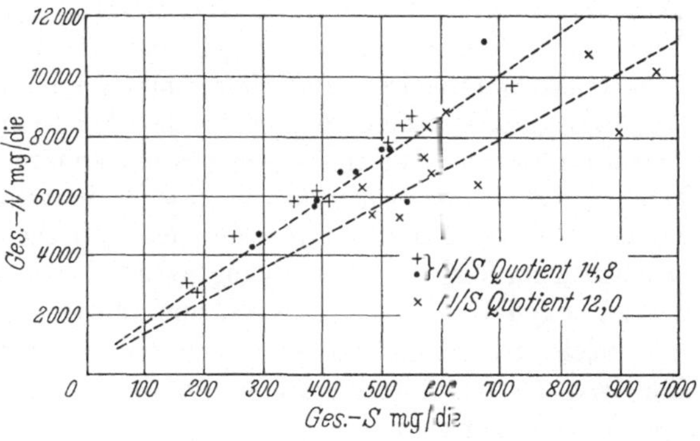

Abb. 3. Relation der Ausscheidungen von N/S bei Myxödem und während der Therapie

wirkung zuerst eine extracellulär gelegene Flüssigkeit, das sog. Myxödem, eliminiert wird. Diese ist vorwiegend natriumhaltig und relativ wenig eiweißarm. Die Ausscheidung erfolgt, ohne daß sich die in diesem Protein befindlichen Schwefelfraktionen — bezüglich ihrer Gesamtmenge und auch hinsichtlich der Relation der

Schwefelfraktionen untereinander — verschieben. Es kann demnach durchaus nicht der Schluß gezogen werden, daß eine besonders schwefelhaltige Proteinfraktion mobilisiert wird.

Die calorigene Wirkung der Schilddrüsenhormone wurde bekanntlich zuerst von Magnus-Levy (1895) an Patienten mit Unterfunktion der Schilddrüse beobachtet. Sie ist in ihrer Wirkungsweise immer noch nicht geklärt, wenn auch die quantitative Relation der Schilddrüsenhormone zu der eintretenden Steigerung der Gesamtverbrennungsvorgänge in toto sehr exakt in sog. Entzugskurven (Boothby, Baldes und Sandiford) erfaßt worden ist, in denen beim Absetzen der Thyreoidinbehandlung gesetzmäßig ein Abfall des Sauerstoffverbrauchs bis zum Minimum erfolgt. Means (1947) gibt bei völligem Fehlen der Schilddrüsenfunktion einen Calorienverbrauch von etwa 23,5 cal/qm Körperoberfläche und Stunde an. Entsprechend sinkt nach eigenen Erfahrungen der Grundumsatz als Integral aller letzten Endes mit Sauerstoffverbrauch ablaufenden Stoffwechselprozesse auf ungefähr −40% der Norm ab.

Das Trijodthyronin hat nach allgemeiner Erfahrung hinsichtlich des in etwa 24 Std einsetzenden calorigenen Effekts ungefähr die 5fache Wirksamkeit gegenüber dem Thyroxin. Verfolgt man eine große Zahl von Patienten mit Überfunktion der Schilddrüse, so fällt ein Absinken des respiratorischen Quotienten bei zunehmender Schwere der Hyperthyreose auf, was sich dadurch erklärt, daß die Glykogen-Reserven mit zunehmender Steigerung der Verbrennungsvorgänge schnell abnehmen, so daß sie zum Zeitpunkt der Grundumsatzbestimmung, die meist nach 12- bis 16stündiger Nahrungskarenz vorgenommen wird, weitgehend erschöpft sind. Wenn wir die Martius-Hesssche Entkoppelungstheorie der Atmungsketten gewissermaßen als Teilerklärung für die calorigene Hormonwirkung anerkennen, so entspricht dies mit den Worten des Klinikers einer Verschiebung der Wärmeproduktion zu Lasten der energetischen Ausbeute von Verbrennungsvorgängen. Diese Feststellung findet auch eine Bestätigung darin, daß im Rahmen der Meyerhof-Hillschen Untersuchungen über die Verbrennung der Kohlenhydrate beim Muskelstoffwechsel, eine Verschiebung im bekannten Meyerhof-Quotienten der Glykogenresynthese zugunsten der Milchsäure, besonders aber auch im Arbeitsstoffwechsel, nachgewiesen werden konnte. Diese kurz nach ihrer Anerkennung durch den Nobelpreis in ihrer Bedeutung zwar wieder eingeschränkte These über die Funktion und den energetischen Wirkungsgrad des Muskels erblickt in der *Resynthese* des Glykogens auf Kosten der verbrennenden Milchsäure, der sog. oxydativen Restitutionswärme, die wesentliche Grundlage der Relation Arbeitsleistungs-Nutzeffekt zu Sauerstoffverbrauch. Bei der Besprechung des Einflusses der Schilddrüsenhormone auf den Arbeitsstoffwechsel wird hierauf noch zurückzukommen sein.

Ganz allgemein ist mit der Steigerung der Verbrennungsvorgänge unter dem Schilddrüsenhormon auch eine Erhöhung des *Stickstoffumsatzes* festzustellen. Diese grundlegende Beobachtung war ja der Ausgangspunkt, der Fr. v. Müller (1893) dazu veranlaßte, für das Schilddrüsenhormon eine allgemeine stoffwechselerhöhende Wirkung anzunehmen. Auch die Harnstoffausscheidung, dessen verminderte Clearance beim Myxödem von Beaumont und Robertson (1943) und von H. Zondek (1952) festgestellt wurde, ist deutlich herabgesetzt und nimmt unter Zufuhr von Schilddrüsenhormonen zu. Mit etikettiertem Glycin durchgeführte Bilanzversuche bei Myxödem ergaben eine wesentlich kleinere Umsatz-rate für die Proteinsynthese als bei Normalpersonen, während diese auf Trijod-thyroninzufuhr bis zu einer übernormalen Umsatzgeschwindigkeit — trotz aus-geglichener N-Bilanz — führte (CRISPELL, WILLIAMS, HOLLIFIELD und PARSON, 1961). Immerhin erscheint die Feststellung nicht unwichtig, daß, wenn ausreichend Calorien in anderer Form zugeführt werden — also nicht als Eiweiß-Calorien, sondern vorwiegend als Fett und Kohlenhydrate —, sich der Stickstoffhaushalt fast auf die Norm zurückdrosseln läßt. LAUTER fand bei den früher üblichen Bilanzversuchen zur Erfassung des endogenen N-Minimums bei überschießender Calorienzufuhr normale N-Verluste. Vor allem bei einem Calorienmangel kommt es also auch zu einem Ansteigen des Stickstoffumsatzes und damit zu einer nega-tiven Bilanz. Diese negative Bilanz hat manche Kliniker veranlaßt (KRÜSKEMPER und KLEINSORG), anabole Hormone in die Therapie der Hyperthyreosen einzuführen. Die Erhöhung der Harnsäureausscheidung, der neuerdings wieder vermehrte Beachtung zur Testung von Schilddrüsenhormonanalogen geschenkt wird, fügt sich gut in die Tatsache der allgemein gesteigerten Stoffwechselabläufe ein (LEEPER und RAWSON).

Ein sehr wichtiges Kapitel der Schilddrüsenhormoneffekte betrifft den *Kreatininhaushalt*. Trotz mancher Einschränkungen ist die Höhe der Gesamt-kreatininurie der Maßstab für die Muskelmasse, wie man auch heute noch die Kon-stanz der endogenen Kreatininurie zur Kontrolle für die Genauigkeit gesammelter Harnportionen verwendet. Kreatin entsteht aus den drei Aminosäuren: *Arginin, Glycin* und dem als Methyldonator dienenden *Methionin*. Es spielt in seiner wechselnden Bindung mit Phosphorsäure eine wesentliche Rolle bei der Muskel-kontraktion und wird im Laufe des Tages in konstantem Verhältnis, unabhängig von der Arbeitsleistung, täglich dehydriert, welches Endprodukt, das *Kreatinin,* im Harn erscheint. Zahlreiche Einflüsse von hormoneller Seite und Erkrankungen der Muskulatur führen zu einer Störung dieser Dehydrierung, weswegen die *Kreatinurie* beim Erwachsenen ein wichtiges Merkmal aller Störungen des Muskel-stoffwechsels darstellt. Beim Kind ist eine gewisse Kreatinurie noch physiologisch und bis zu einem gewissen Grade, wenn auch minimal, bei der gesunden Frau, während beim Manne jede Kreatinurie pathologisch zu bewerten ist. Die Kreatin-urie bei Thyreotoxikose ist ferner ein Hinweis auf die häufige thyreotoxische Myopathie und die dabei typische Adynamie; sie ist ein Prodromalsymptom der thyreotoxischen Krise. Das Auftreten von Kreatin im Harn unter dem Einfluß von Schilddrüsenhormonen ist direkt als Index für eine Schilddrüsenaktivität derartiger Substanzen zu verwerten, wie ich auch bei der Prüfung von Schild-drüsenhormonanalogen feststellen konnte. Welcher Art und auf welchem Wege diese pathologische Störung der Anhydrierung des Muskelkreatinins entsteht, ist noch völlig ungeklärt. In Anlehnung an die Auffassung über die Entkopplung der Atmungskettenphosphorylierung von MARTIUS und HESS möchten wir vermuten, daß infolge einer Hemmung der Kreatinphosphorkinase (ARKONSAS 1951) die Resynthetisierung des Kreatins zu Kreatinphosphorsäure vermindert ist. Nach BENEDICT und ROCHE kann der vermehrte Anteil an deswegen mehr anfallendem Kreatin nicht vom Muskel aufgenommen werden, entgeht der üblichen Anhy-drierung und wird im Harn ausgeschieden. Sicher besteht eine Beziehung zwischen der Schwere der Kreatinurie und der thyreotoxischen Myopathie (BANSI, WALDEN-

STRÖM). Entsprechend ist von uns (BANSI, FRETWURST und MEYER 1957) sowie von RAWSON (1956) auf die *Erhöhung der Phosphatausscheidung* nach Schilddrüsenhormonverabfolgung hingewiesen worden, die im Zusammenhang mit der Kreatinurie steht. Auch diese Feststellung stützt gewissermaßen die Martiussche Entkopplungstheorie, indem bei einer Herabsetzung der normalen Phosphorylierungsrate unter Schilddrüsenhormonzufuhr das Verhältnis zwischen anorganischem Phosphor und ATP zugunsten des ersteren verschoben wird und ebenso wie das sonst überhaupt so gut wie gar nicht auszuscheidende Kreatin nun vermehrt anfällt und im Harn eliminiert wird. Es kann naheliegenderweise bei Beurteilung der Gesamtbilanz im Rahmen der Klinik nichts Bindendes über den Intermediärstoffwechsel ausgesagt werden, zumal die Phosphate auch hinsichtlich des gesteigerten Kohlenhydratstoffwechsels bei Schilddrüsenhormonzufuhr in vermehrtem Maße anfallen könnten. RALL u. Mitarb. (mit RAWSON) (1956) haben diese Probleme ebenfalls anhand von Bilanzstudien an 2 Myxödemkranken diskutiert und neben einer festen Kupplung der Mehrausscheidung von Stickstoff mit Phosphor im Rahmen des P/N-Verhältnisses eine zusätzliche Phosphaturie beobachtet, wobei sie besonders auf die Beziehungen zur Kreatinurie hinweisen. So verbleibt die Phosphatdiurese unter Schilddrüsenhormonen schließlich wohl ein komplexer Vor-

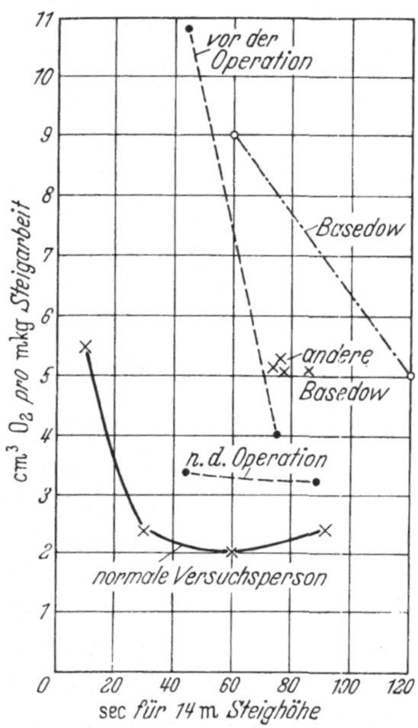

Abb. 4. Arbeitssauerstoffverbrauch pro mkg Steigarbeit bei verschiedenem Arbeitstempo

gang, der aber auf eine gewisse Umstellung der Rationalisierung mancher Verbrennungsvorgänge hinweist (BANSI, FRETWURST und MEYER 1955).

Die *unökonomische* Arbeitsweise des energieverbrauchenden Kraftstoffwechsels wurde in den 20er Jahren an zahlreichen Kliniken studiert. Als erste machten BOOTHBY und SANDIFORD auf eine Erhöhung des Sauerstoffverbrauchs pro mkg geleisteter Arbeit bei Hyperthyreosen aufmerksam. Wir selbst haben seinerzeit in umfangreichen Arbeitsstoffwechselversuchen den je nach Schwere der Thyreotoxikose unökonomisch gesteigerten Energieverbrauch bei einfachen Muskelleistungen verfolgt (Abb. 4). Da gleichzeitig ein gegenüber der Norm erheblich vermehrter Anfall an Milchsäure im Blut erfolgte (BIER 1931), trat die Verschiebung des Meyerhof-Quotienten damit wieder klar zutage.

Daß die Schilddrüsenhormone den *Fetthaushalt* im ganzen und besonders den Serumcholesterinspiegel beeinflussen, ist seit BING und HECKSCHER (1925) bekannt. Die Erhöhung der Spiegel sämtlicher Fettfraktionen, einschließlich der Carotine, bei Unterfunktion der Thyreoidea gilt als wichtiger diagnostischer Hinweis und eines der besten Kriterien, um die Wirksamkeit eines Schilddrüsenpräparates, sowohl der reinen Hormone als auch der zahlreichen Hormonanaloge, zu testen. *Wie* sich dieser Vorgang abspielt, haben Untersuchungen mit markiertem Cholesterin ergeben. FRIEDMAN, BYERS u. Mitarb., sowie THOMPSON und

Vars (1952/53) fanden bei Unterfunktion der Schilddrüsen eine Herabsetzung der Ausscheidung von Cholesterin und Gallensäuren in die Galle, während nach Zufuhr von Schilddrüse die Bildung von Cholesterin aus den Acetatbausteinen in der Leber vermehrt und beschleunigt wurde (Byers, Rosenman, Friedman und Biggs 1952; Dayton und Dayton, Drimmer und Kendall 1954).

Lipsky, Bondy, Man und McGuire (1955) beobachteten die Einverleibung von Acetat 1-C^{14} in das freie und veresterte Cholesterin bei drei myxödematösen Frauen und fanden eine um das 5fache verminderte Ausnützung des Acetats zur Cholesterinsynthese im Vergleich zu 6 Normalpersonen. Von Fletscher und Myant (1962) wird auf Unterschiede im Aufbau des Acetats zur Mevalonsäure hingewiesen, während nach dieser Stufe bei Hypothyreose die Synthese des Cholesterins nicht mehr gehemmt erscheint. Es war dabei in erster Linie die Cholesterinsynthese in der Leber betroffen. Ferner verschwand das markierte Cholesterin langsamer in der Peripherie als bei den Normalpersonen. Wurde durch einen Stoß von 500 γ T_3 der Grundumsatz und das Serumcholesterin normalisiert, so kehrte auch die Syntheserate des Cholesterins zur Norm zurück. Daß beim Hyperthyreotiker das Serumcholesterin sinkt, obwohl seine Synthese gegenüber der Norm beschleunigt ist, ergibt sich aus der gegenüber der Synthese vermehrten Ausscheidung durch die Galle. Hierfür wurden sowohl experimentell als auch am Schnittpräparat zahlreiche Beweise geführt, sowohl mittels Deuterium als auch mit C^{14} markiertem Acetat. Auch Boyd lieferte überzeugende Daten für die Hemmung der Cholesterinsynthese in der Leber durch Thyreoidektomie, während sie nach Thyroxinzufuhr oder Verfütterung zahlreicher Thyroxinanaloge beschleunigt ablief. Kritschewsy faßt die verschiedenen Beobachtungen dahin zusammen, daß beim hyperthyreoidisierten Tier der vermehrte Abbau und die gesteigerte Ausscheidung sich zu der bekannten Senkung der Serumcholesterinwerte kombinieren, obwohl mehr Cholesterin synthetisiert wird. Dasselbe gelte auch für die Phosphorlipide. Trotzdem sollte man nicht zu einer "oversimplification" neigen, denn bei höheren Dosen von Schilddrüsenhormonen scheinen die Verhältnisse in das Gegenteil umzuschlagen (Fletscher und Myant). Außerdem verhalten sich die einzelnen Organe verschieden, besonders was die Ablagerung der Lipide in den Gefäßen betrifft.

Da den Schilddrüsenhormonen sozusagen eine allgemeine, die Stoffwechselvorgänge aktivierende Eigenschaft zuzusprechen ist, ist es eigentlich verwunderlich, daß man dem Zustand von *Fermenten* unter physiologischen Dosen oder abnormer Steigerung der Hormonkonzentration bisher wenig Beachtung geschenkt hat. Gewisse Ansätze lassen aber erkennen, daß Veränderungen gewisser Fermentaktivitäten in Schilddrüsenzellen nach deren Stimulierung beobachtet werden. Es dürften dabei wohl Hemmungen der Fermentaktivitäten als auch Steigerungen vorkommen. Im Hinblick auf die gesteigerte Adrenalinempfindlichkeit nach Thyroxinzufuhr verdienen Bestimmungen der Mono-Oxydaseaktivität, die nach widerspruchsvollen Ergebnissen im Tierexperiment von Wernze u. Mitarb. neuerdings mittels eines Serotoninbelastungsversuchs untersucht wurden, Interesse. Die Autoren, deren Arbeiten noch nicht abgeschlossen sind, vermuten eine übernormale Umwandlung von Serotonin in 5-hydroxy-Indolessigsäure als Ausdruck gesteigerter Aktivität der Amin-abbauenden Enzyme. Von Maley (1957) wurden zahlreiche Fermente in den Mitochondrien thyreotoxisch gemachter

Ratten geprüft und eine Vermehrung der Glutaminase, Succinoxydase, der Cyto-
chromoxydase und der ATP-ase gefunden. Demgegenüber berichten finnische
Autoren (Telkkä, Heikkilä und Hopsu), daß durch Methylthiourazil stimulierte
Schilddrüsenzellen von Meerschweinchen eine vermehrte Fermentaktivität der
Succino-Dehydrogenase aufweisen. Ob man dieses Verhalten nun mit den Schild-
drüsenhormonen in Zusammenhang bringen sollte, erscheint mir zweifelhaft, da
Methylthiourazil durch die Blockierung der eigentlichen Hormonsynthese infolge
gestörter Jodierung und Zusammenlagerung der Tyrosine eher eine vermehrte
TSH-Stimulierung zur Folge hat und die Stimulierung des Wachstums der
Schilddrüsenzellen nicht mit einer Aktivierung der Hormonsynthese einhergeht.
Diese Auffassung wird auch durch histochemische Studien einer Arbeitsgruppe in
San Francisco gestützt (Lindsay und Patricia Jenks), die 21 intracelluläre
Fermente histochemisch untersuchte und keine Beziehung dieser Fermentaktivi-
täten zur Schilddrüsenhormonsynthese antraf, wohl aber zur Stärke der thyreo-
tropen Aktivierung der Schilddrüsenzellen. Labhart betont in seinem Lehrbuch,
daß sich zwischen Schilddrüsenhormonen und Fermentreaktionen keinerlei
Beziehungen im Sinne einer Aktivierung oder des Vorliegens einer als prosthetische
Gruppe aufzeigen lassen. Immerhin erwähnt Rawson in einem programmatischen
Vortrag "Today's thyroidologists and their beckoning frontiers", daß zahlreiche
Fermentsysteme wohl durch Schilddrüsenhormone eine Veränderung erfahren
(Oxydasen, Esterasen, Carbohydrasen, Cathepsins, Amidasen und Transferasen).
Da sich diese Fragestellungen bisher außerhalb der Klinik bewegen und daher
nicht in den Rahmen meines vorwiegend klinisch abgestimmten Referates gehören,
bitte ich, diese Probleme außer Betracht lassen zu dürfen. Interessenten seien auf
die Monographie von Frau Pitt-Rivers und Tata verwiesen, die in bewunderns-
werter Vollständigkeit auch diese Fragestellung behandeln.

Eine hinsichtlich ihres Allgemein-Effektes besonders ins Auge fallende Wirkung
der Schilddrüsenhormone betrifft das *Wachstum*. Ist der Athyreote und der
thyreogene Kretin — ich betone absichtlich das thyreogene im Rahmen des Kretinismus — bzw. das kindliche Myxödem in seinem Wachstum wie stets erheblich
hinter der Norm zurückgeblieben, so sind die mit allen Schilddrüsenwirkstoffen
zu erzielenden Wachstumssteigerungen eine Domäne der klinischen Anwendung
bei im Wachstum gehemmten Kindern. Die durch den Wiener Pädiater Nobel
gesammelten Erfahrungen sind auch heute noch weitgehend richtunggebend.
Gleichzeitige Untersuchungen über den Anstieg der Intelligenz der Hypothyreoten
sind von der Art der Hypothyreose abhängig. Sind neben intrauterinen gleichzeitig mit dem Ausfall der Schilddrüsenentwicklung andere cerebrale Ausfalls-
erscheinungen aufgetreten, so bleibt die Wirkung auf das Gehirn gering. Handelt
es sich aber nur um intrauterin durchgemachte isolierte Störungen der Entwick-
lungsanlage der Thyreoidea oder in utero durchgemachte Thyreoiditiden oder
einen erst in der frühesten Jugend erworbenen Ausfall der Schilddrüsenfunktion,
so ist die Prognose durch eine Schilddrüsenhormontherapie nicht nur wesentlich
besser, sondern manchmal erfreulich gut. Das konnatale Myxödem wird keine
gute Gesamtprognose haben, da die cerebralen Störungen durch die Substitutionstherapie nicht ausgleichbar sind. Ich möchte auf diese für die Pädiater wesentlichen Punkte jedoch nicht näher eingehen. Auffallend ist die gute Verträglichkeit
der Kleinkinder und der im Wachstum zurückgebliebenen Hypothyreoten für

hohe Hormondosen, was auch für das Thybon® von Knorr und Freislederer (1959) bestätigt wurde.

Hier ist wohl auch der Ort, auf die *Beeinflussung des jugendlichen Kropfes* durch Schilddrüsenhormone einzugehen. Die Entstehung jeglicher Schilddrüsenvergrößerung ist — abgesehen von den letztlich als Adenome zu betrachtenden seltenen Wölflerschen kalten und den heißen Adenomen — in erster Linie auf eine Stimulierung des Schilddrüsenwachstums durch das thyreotrope Hormon der Adenohypophyse zu beziehen. Wie weit ein thalamischer Reiz hierbei hineinspielt, wird ein Thema des morgigen Tages sein. Aber wie bei irgendwelchem peripheren Hormonmangel — auf welcher Basis er auch entstanden ist, sei es Jodmangel, Störung des Hormonaufbaus oder chemischer Blockade oder relativem Hormonmangel infolge erhöhter peripheren Bedarfs —, stets wird ein Defizit an Schilddrüsenhormon im Blut den Reglerkreis Adenohypophyse ⇌ Schilddrüse auf den Plan bringen und damit eine vermehrte Absonderung des TSH bedingen. Dadurch erfolgt die histologische Aktivierung der Schilddrüse im Sinne einer Hyperplasie und damit ist der erste Schritt zur Strumabildung getan. Es ist nun eine bereits Reinhold und dem älteren Bruns bekannte Tatsache (1895), daß das Schilddrüsenhormon selbst durch seinen Eingriff in dieses erst 50 Jahre später erkannte Reglersystem den TSH-Reiz aufhebt oder zum mindesten abdämmt. Dadurch hört die thyreotrope Stimulierung des Wachstums der Schilddrüse auf und die Struma geht in ein histologisch typisches Ruhestadium über, indem sie aus der Hyperplasie in eine kolloidspeichernde Ruheschilddrüse übergeführt wird. Es ist eine Eigenart dieses Reglermechanismus, nicht exakt auf das wirkliche Schilddrüsenhormon eingestellt zu sein, sondern auch auf andere Hormonmetaboliten und -analoge zu reagieren. Von dieser Erkenntnis wird bedauerlicherweise bei der Bekämpfung jugendlicher Strumen, die fast als die einzigen Schilddrüsenvergrößerungen noch dem klaren Einfluß dieses Reglersystems unterliegen, viel zu wenig Gebrauch gemacht. Marine sagte schon 1915, zit. nach Langer (1961), daß kaum eine pathologische Situation so leicht zu beeinflussen sei wie die beginnende Hyperplasie der Schilddrüse. Da wir neuerdings eine gewisse Dosis-Wirkungs-Dissoziation der Schilddrüsenhormone und ihrer Analoge kennen und die Hemmung des TSH-Einflusses auf die Schilddrüse anhand der Radiojodidspeicherung der Schilddrüse leicht fast quantitativ erfassen können, bietet sich meines Erachtens die Frühtherapie der juvenilen Struma direkt für die Hemmung des strumigenen TSH-Einflusses an. Hierzu würden sich wohl die Hormonanaloge am meisten eignen, deren Stoffwechseleffekte am geringsten sind, die aber trotzdem die Jodavidität der Schilddrüse verringern, nach meinen Erfahrungen vor allem die Trijodthyropropionsäure und evtl. das Triac. Wieweit Erfolge mit dem wenig stoffwechselaktiven D-Thyroxin (Dethyrona ®) hier vorliegen, entzieht sich leider meiner Erfahrung. Aber schon die jetzt immer mehr in den endemischen Strumengebieten und bei der Recidivprophylaxe sich einbürgernde Therapie mit Schilddrüsenextrakten belegt wohl die Gangbarkeit eines solchen Weges, zumal die jugendliche Struma sehr hormonempfindlich zu sein pflegt.

Ich bitte Sie, mir nicht verübeln zu wollen, daß meine Ausführungen in erster Linie auf die klinische Wirkung der Schilddrüsenhormone abgestellt waren und daß ich, als wohl einer der wenigen Älteren, die noch die große Schule von Magnus-Levy und meinem eigentlichen Lehrer Zondek in der ersten Epoche der

Thyreoidologie aktiv erlebt haben, Ihnen auch die mittels der alten Methoden durchgeführten pathophysiologischen Studien in Erinnerung gebracht habe.

Diskussion

D. Emrich (Freiburg):

Wie könnte man erklären, daß wir in einem Jodmangelgebiet (Südbaden) Erfolge mit der Hormonbehandlung der euthyreoten Struma (Thybon und Vollsalz) vorwiegend bei Jugendlichen bei etwa zum 18. Lebensjahr sahen? Bei älteren Patienten kam es in der Mehrzahl der Fälle nur zu einer geringen Abnahme des Halsumfanges, auch wenn es sich um weiche, diffuse z. T. erst kurze Zeit bestehende Strumen z. B. bei Studenten handelte.

E. Klein (Düsseldorf):

Da die Empfehlung von jodiertem Salz als Behandlungsvorschlag hierzulande nicht ernst genommen wird, bleibt stets unsicher, ob und gar ob genügend Jodid zugeführt wird. Meines Erachtens haben Sie auf die geschilderte Weise eine reine Trijodthyronintherapie betrieben, die bei invenilen Strumen wegen ihrer besonderen Pathogenese — wachstumsbedingtes passageres Mißverhältnis zwischen Hormonbedarf der Peripherie und Hormoninkretion bzw. vermehrte TSH-Inkretion zusammen mit STH bei Wachstumsschüben — wirksam sein kann, bei der Erwachsenenstruma aber erfahrungsgemäß meistens versagt. Ungleich besser werden die Ergebnisse bei Verwendung von Thyreoidea sicca, weil zusammen mit den genuinen Hormonen auch Mono- und Dijodtyrosin zugeführt werden, die nach Dejodierung in vollem Umfang als Jodid zur Wirkung gelangen. Auf diese Weise wird 1. die TSH-Abgabe gehemmt und 2. dem endogenen Jodmangel begegnet. Wir haben bei 234 blanden Strumen eine solche Behandlung regelmäßig kontrollieren und in 80% gute bis genügende Erfolge buchen können. Die kombinierte Hormon-Jodbehandlung der Kröpfe mit Thyreoidea sicca ist der alleinigen Verwendung entweder von Hormonen oder von Jodid auf jeden Fall überlegen, weil sie zwei wesentliche Faktoren der Kropfpathogenese paralysiert.

H.W. Bansi:

Der Vorschlag, anstelle des L-Trijodthyronin das altbewährte Thyreoidin zu verwenden, um nicht nur das wirksamste Hormon, sondern auch die anderen jodhaltigen Bestandteile des Thyreoglobulins zur Verfügung zu haben und damit sozusagen auch Jod zuzuführen, erscheint mir sehr wesentlich. Auch wir hatten mit den Hormonmetaboliten ja stets gewisse Mengen Jod — wenn auch allein in Bindung an den Thyroninrest — zugeführt. Für manche wenig Thyroxin-aktive Verbindungen, wie die Thyroameisensäureverbindungen oder die Dijodthyronine, wo Mengen in einer um mehrere Zehnerpotenzen höheren Konzentration zur Hemmung der Adenohypophyse notwendig sind, möchten wir wegen der relativ leichten Abspaltung von Jod aus diesen Verbindungen eher einen indirekten Jodeffekt vermuten als eine dem Thyroxin entsprechende Wirkung des gesamten Moleküls.

P. Huber (Innsbruck):

Ich habe die gleiche Ansicht wie Bansi und Klein. Durch die Hormontherapie kann man nicht immer eine Verkleinerung euthyreoter diffuser Kröpfe erreichen, wohl aber eine Verhinderung weiteren Größenwachstums. Jodavide Kröpfe eines Endemiegebietes verkleinern sich auch durch Jodid, so daß wir dies zuerst versuchen. Trijodthyronin bevorzugen wir bei Unterfunktionen, Vollhormonpräparate bei ungenügender Wirkung des Jodids.

E. Goth (Budapest):

Wir behandelten etwa 30 Patienten mit euthyreoter Struma mit Thyreoidea sicca und hatten in 60% Erfolg. Nicht nur bei jüngeren, auch bei älteren Patienten. Man muß jedoch 180—200 mg verabreichen. Von Thybon sahen wir keinen Effekt.

Aus dem Pathologischen Institut der Medizinischen Akademie Düsseldorf
(Direktor: Professor Dr. med. H. Meessen)

Die Wirkung der Schilddrüsenhormone auf die Zellstruktur

Von

Reinhard Poche

Mit 3 Abbildungen

Referat

Dem Morphologen zeigt sich die Wirkung der Schilddrüsenhormone entweder in den Veränderungen, die durch den Ausfall der Schilddrüse bewirkt und durch Substitution ihrer Hormone wieder zum Verschwinden gebracht werden, oder in solchen Veränderungen, die nach einem erhöhten Angebot von Schilddrüsenhormonen auftreten. In dem folgenden Referat möchte ich über die Wirkungen einer Überdosierung von Schilddrüsenhormonen berichten und mich dabei auf zwei wichtige Organe beschränken: Die Leber und den Herzmuskel.

Aus der menschlichen Pathologie ist bekannt, daß bei Morbus Basedow und Hyperthyreosen an der Leber ein Glykogenschwund aus dem Cytoplasma der Leberzellen — vereinzelt unter Auftreten von Kernglykogen — eine Verfettung der Parenchymzellen, zentrale Läppchennekrosen sowie eine seröse Hepatitis mit nachfolgender Sklerose, Atrophie und Cirrhose auftreten können (Wegelin 1926, Habán 1933, Rössle 1933, Federlin 1956). Ein Verlust von Glykogen und eine geringe Verfettung (Piper und Poulsen 1947) sowie Kernvacuolen (Movitt, Gerstl und Davis 1953) sind auch in Leberpunktaten von Kranken mit einer Thyreotoxikose nachgewiesen worden. Am Herzmuskel findet man bei Hyperthyreosen und Basedowscher Krankheit eine Hypertrophie, eine fleckige oder diffuse Verfettung, interstitielle Rundzelleninfiltrate sowie eine interstitielle Fibrose und Vernarbungen (Fahr 1916 und 1921, Staemmler 1955, Federlin 1956). Schlesinger und Benchimol (1958) beschreiben Fälle einer „rein thyreotoxischen Herzkrankheit" mit seröser Myokarditis, interstitieller Fibrose, Hypertrophie und Dilatation des linken Ventrikels, bei denen eine Hypertonie, eine Coronarsklerose oder ein Klappenfehler als Ursache oder Teilursache der Veränderungen ausgeschlossen werden konnten.

Im Tierexperiment führt eine vermehrte Zufuhr von Thyroxin zu einem Verschwinden des Glykogens aus den Leberzellen (Habán 1935). Heinlein und Dieckhoff (1936) sahen bei Katzen nach langdauernden intravenösen Gaben von Thyroxin in der Leber eine fleckförmige Blutüberfüllung der Sinusoide, z. T. mit Ausbildung kleiner Blutseen, ein perisinusoidales Ödem, eine mehr oder weniger

starke Verfettung der Leberzellen, eine Auflockerung des Zellverbandes sowie
vereinzelte Leberzellnekrosen. Nach Gaben von thyreotropem Hormon beobachtete EHRENBRAND (1955) beim Meerschweinchen Schwankungen im Gehalt der
Leberzellen an Eiweiß, Fett und Kohlenhydraten, die auffallend eng mit dem
rhythmischen Funktionswandel der Schilddrüse und der Nebennieren korreliert
waren. Die meisten Leberzellen waren aufgehellt und vacuolisiert. Daneben
fanden sich aber auch dunkle Leberzellen, und zwar in den Läppchenzentren solche
mit pyknotischen Kernen (sog. Mauserungszellen) und in der Peripherie der
Läppchen solche mit bläschenförmigen Kernen (sog. Regenerationszellen). Im
Herzmuskel sind die lichtmikroskopisch erfaßbaren Veränderungen nach einer
Überdosierung von Thyroxin im allgemeinen etwas deutlicher ausgeprägt als in
der Leber. Von ZALKA (1935) sah bei Kaninchen und Katzen eine Abnahme des
Glykogens in den Herzmuskelzellen, ferner Herde von akuter bis chronischer
Myokarditis mit Vernarbung und Schwielenbildung. HEINLEIN und DIECKHOFF
(1936) beschrieben bei Katzen eine albuminöse Trübung, Verfettung, Hyalini-
sierung sowie einen scholligen Zerfall von Herzmuskelzellen, ferner herdförmige
und diffuse interstitielle Zellinfiltrate. Diese Veränderungen ähneln manchmal
sehr denen, die BÜCHNER (1933) bei der experimentellen Coronarinsuffizienz
beschrieben hat. Diese Feststellung gewinnt dadurch an Bedeutung, daß HEINLEIN
und DIECKHOFF (1936) bei ihren Versuchstieren auch Wandverquellungen, Media-
nekrosen, Aufsplitterung der Elastica und Lichtungseinengungen an den kleineren
Ästen der Herzkranzarterien beobachteten. Nach Untersuchungen von GEMMILL
(1958) führen eine Verfütterung von Schilddrüsengewebe oder ein Zusatz von
Trijodthyronin zum Trinkwasser bei Ratten und Mäusen unter Anstieg von Puls,
Blutdruck und Grundumsatz zur Ausbildung einer kräftigen Herzhypertrophie.

Die angeführten Beispiele aus der menschlichen und aus der experimentellen
Pathologie gründen sich auf Untersuchungen mit dem Lichtmikroskop, dessen
Auflösungsvermögen im wesentlichen eine Beurteilung der Gewebsstruktur
erlaubt. In den letzten Jahren ist es möglich geworden, mit Hilfe der Elektronenmikroskopie auch Einblicke in die feinere Struktur der Zellen unter der Einwirkung
von Schilddrüsenhormonen zu gewinnen. Die ersten Untersuchungen dieser Art
sind von SCHULZ, LÖW, ERNSTER und SJÖSTRAND (1956) durchgeführt worden.
Sie fanden bei Ratten, die 5 Tage lang täglich eine subcutane Injektion von
0,4 mg Thyroxin bekommen hatten, eine hochgradige Schwellung der Mitochondrien in den Leberzellen. Die Matrix der Mitochondrien war diffus aufgehellt;
die Cristae mitochondriales waren vermindert und verkürzt, so daß ihre Gesamt-
oberfläche im Vergleich zu normalen Mitochondrien um 30% abgenommen hatte.
Dabei war das osmiophobe Spatium der Cristae von 50 Å auf 70 Å verbreitert.
Da die äußeren Membranen trotz der starken Vergrößerung der Mitochondrien
nicht schmäler geworden waren, nahmen die Autoren einen Aufbau von Außen-
membranen auf Kosten der Cristae (Innenmembranen) an. Schwere Veränderungen zeigte auch das Ergastoplasma. Über die ganze Leberzelle verteilt, fanden sich
elektronenoptisch leere Vacuolen, die durch eine starke Schwellung der homogenen
osmiophoben Zwischenschichten der α-Cytomembranen entstanden waren.
Glykogen war nach lichtmikroskopischen Vergleichsuntersuchungen in den Leberzellen nicht nachzuweisen. Die Autoren nehmen an, daß der Verlust von Innenmembranen in den Mitochondrien zu Änderungen der Atmungsintensität der

Mitochondrien führt, und sehen die Ursache der Veränderungen in einer durch Thyroxin bewirkten „Labilisierung der Multienzymsysteme" der Leberzelle.

Die eigenen Untersuchungen erstrecken sich auf die Veränderungen der Ultrastruktur und des Stoffwechsels vom Herzmuskel nach Überdosierung der Schilddrüsenhormone l-Trijodthyronin (POCHE 1957) und l-Thyroxin (PFLEGER, RUMMEL, SEIFEN und TIMP 1959, POCHE 1962) sowie nach Gaben von Dinitrophenol (PFLEGER, RUMMEL, SEIFEN und TIMP 1959, LOCHNER und NASSERI 1960, POCHE 1962, POCHE und LOCHNER 1962).

Bei erwachsenen weißen Ratten, die 6 Tage lang täglich eine intraperitoneale Injektion von 0,4–0,5 mg l-Trijodthyronin bekommen haben, zeigen die Herzmuskelzellen eine Aufhellung des Grundsarkoplasmas infolge Schwundes der kleinen Glykogengranula. Die Zellmembranen sind intakt und zeigen keine vermehrten Membranvesiculationen im Sinne einer Mikropinocytose. Das endoplasmatische Reticulum (sog. longitudinales System des Sarkoplasmareticulums) ist stark geschwollen. Die transversalen Tubuli, die als handschuhfingerförmige Einstülpungen des Sarkolemms die Herzmuskelzelle in Höhe der Z-Streifen der Myofibrillen durchqueren (sog. transversales System des Sarkoplasmareticulums), sind stellenweise auch geschwollen, so daß man in Höhe der Z-Streifen manchmal erweiterte sog. Triaden findet (Abb. 1a). Die Fetttropfen sind im Sarkoplasma etwas vermehrt, ohne daß jedoch lichtmikroskopisch schon eine Verfettung nachweisbar ist. Die Mitochondrien zeigen eine leichte bis mittelgradige Schwellung mit völligem Verlust der Mitochondriengranula, geringer Fragmentierung und leichter Reduzierung der Cristae mitochrondriales, teilweise mit leichter kolbenförmiger Auftreibung des osmiophoben Spatiums der Cristae an den Enden der Fragmente, und mit fleckförmiger Aufhellung der Matrix bei intakten äußeren Membranen. Die Kerne der Herzmuskelzellen sind unauffällig, es findet sich lediglich manchmal eine leichte Erweiterung des perinucleären Raumes zwischen sog. primärer und sekundärer Kernmembran. Die beschriebenen Veränderungen sind nicht in allen Herzmuskelzellen gleichstark entwickelt; es finden sich immer noch unveränderte Herzmuskelzellen. Eine Erhöhung der Dosis von Trijodthyronin führt nicht zu einer stärkeren Ausprägung, sondern nur zu einer größeren Ausdehnung der Veränderungen.

Auch bei Ratten, die 14 Tage lang täglich eine subcutane Injektion von 1 mg/kg Körpergewicht l-Thyroxin erhalten haben, ist das Grundsarkoplasma der Herzmuskelzellen durch Verlust der kleinen Glykogengranula aufgehellt. Die Zellmembranen der Herzmuskelzellen zeigen keine Veränderungen (Abb. 2a), und die transversalen Tubuli sind – im Gegensatz zu den Veränderungen nach l-Trijodthyronin – niemals erweitert (Abb. 1b). Dagegen ist das endoplasmatische Reticulum sehr stark geschwollen. Die Fetttropfen im Sarkoplasma sind gering vermehrt. Die Mitochondrien zeigen eine leichte bis mittelgradige Schwellung mit fleckförmigen Aufhellungen der Matrix und mit einem völligen Verlust der Mitochondriengranula. Die Cristae mitochondriales sind etwas stärker fragmentiert als nach Vorbehandlung mit Trijodthyronin und lassen sehr dichtstehende, umschriebene Erweiterungen des osmiophoben Spatiums von 50 auf 100–150 Å erkennen, so daß ein perlschnur- oder rosenkranzartiges Bild entsteht (Abb.2b). Ganz vereinzelt findet man degenerierte Mitochondrien und beginnende Lipofuscinbildung(Abb.2c).An den Myofibrillen ist das Muster der Myofilamente manchmal etwas aufgelockert und

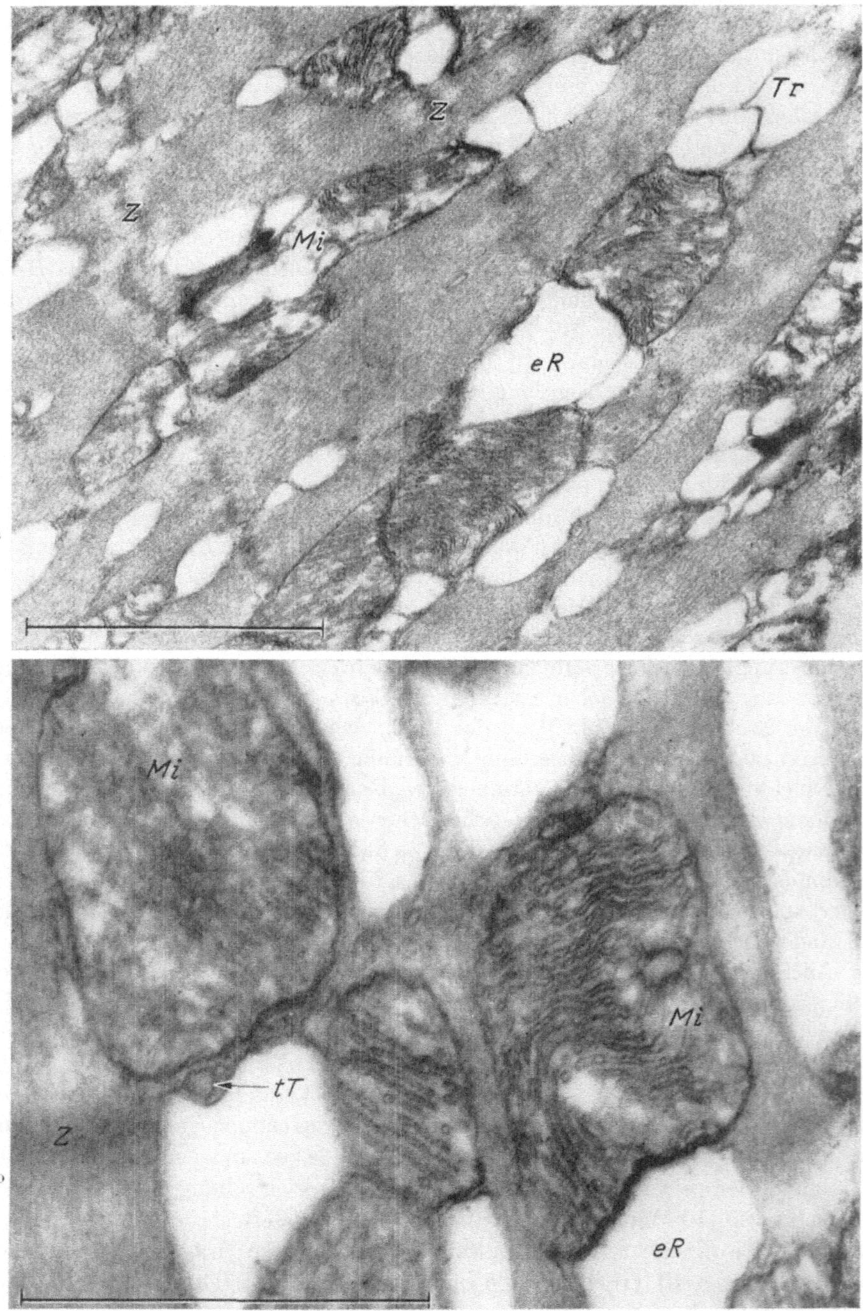

Abb. 1a u. b. a) Ausschnitt aus einer Herzmuskelzelle der Ratte nach Überdosierung von l-Trijodthyronin. Myofibrillen mit Z-Streifen (*Z*). Leicht bis mittelgradig geschwollene Mitochondrien (*Mi*). Starke Erweiterung des endoplasmatischen Reticulums (*eR*). Stark erweiterte sog. Triaden (*Tr*). Elektronenoptisch 16400:1, Endvergrößerung 41000:1 (Arch.-Nr. 6141/57). b) Ausschnitt aus einer Herzmuskelzelle der Ratte nach Überdosierung von l-Thyroxin. Z-Streifen der Myofibrillen (*Z*). Mitochondrien mit leichter bis mittelgradiger Schwellung und Fragmentation der Innenmembranen mit perlschnurartiger Auftreibung des osmiophoben Spatiums (*Mi*). Hochgradige Schwellung des endoplasmatischen Reticulums (*eR*). Die transversalen Tubuli (*tT*) nicht erweitert. Elektronenoptisch 14800:1, Endvergrößerung 56000:1 (Arch.-Nr. 1696 D/60)

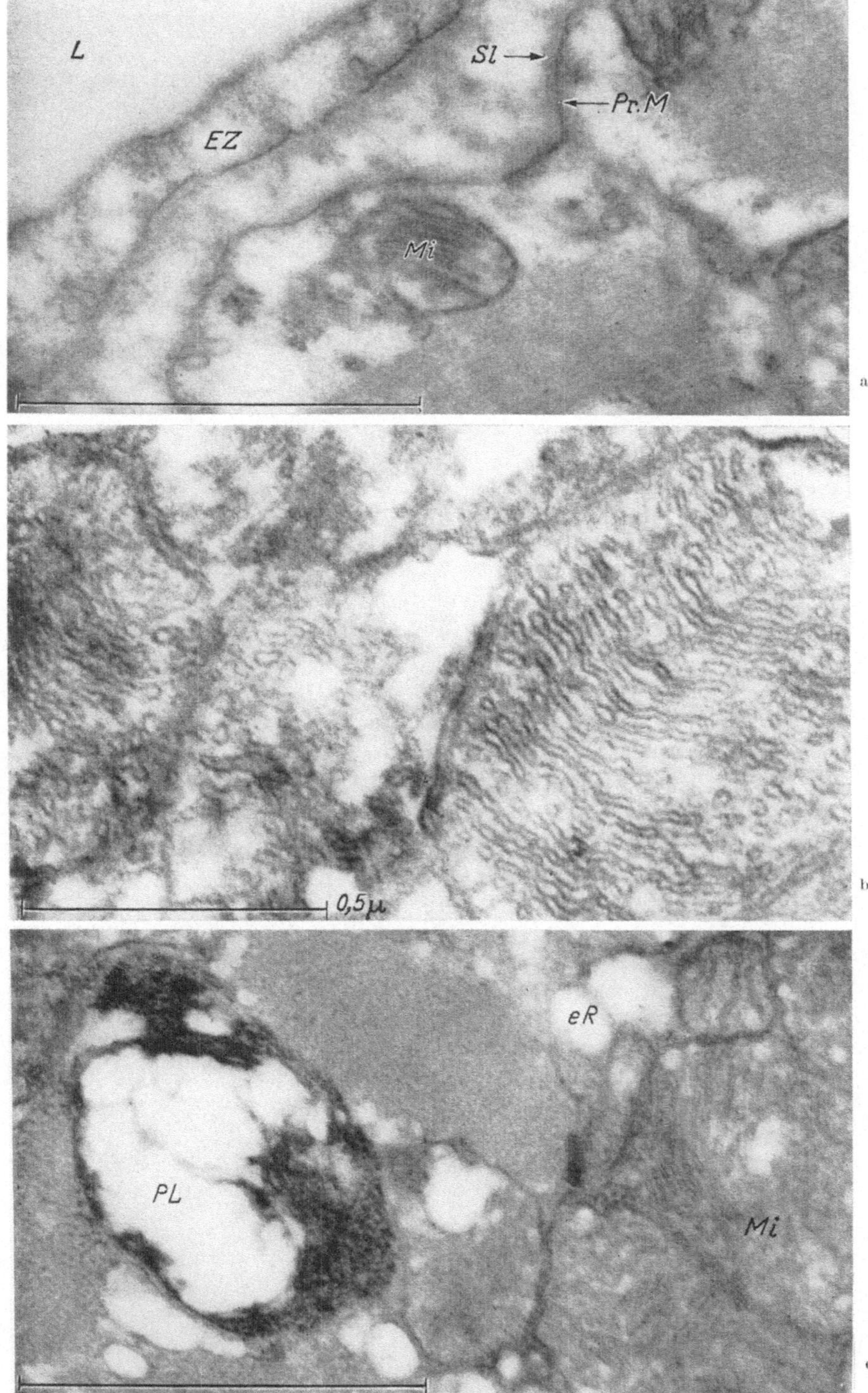

Abb. 2a—c. Herzmuskel der Ratte nach Überdosierung von l-Thyroxin. a) Sarkolemm (*Sl*) mit intakter Protomembran (*PrM*) der Herzmuskelzelle ohne Vermehrung der Membranvesiculationen. Das Grundsarkoplasma unter dem Sarkolemm aufgehellt, die kleinen Glykogengranula verschwunden. Leichte bis mittelgradige Schwellung der Mitochondrien (*Mi*). Neben der Herzmuskelzelle eine Blutcapillare: Lumen (*L*), Endothelzelle (*EZ*). Elektronenoptisch 14800:1, Endvergrößerung 56000:1 (Arch.-Nr. 1886 B/60). b) Mitochondrien mit perlschnurartiger Auftreibung, Schlängelung und Fragmentierung der Innenmembranen. Elektronenoptisch 14800:1, Endvergrößerung 84000:1 (Arch.-Nr. 1654 B/60). c) Schwellung des endoplasmatischen Reticulums (*eR*). Kleinfleckige Matrixschwellung der Mitochondrien (*Mi*). Degeneriertes Mitochondrion mit angelagerter granulärer Substanz: Lipofuscinbildung (*PL*). Elektronenoptisch 14800:1, Endvergrößerung 57000:1 (Arch.-Nr. 1851 B/60)

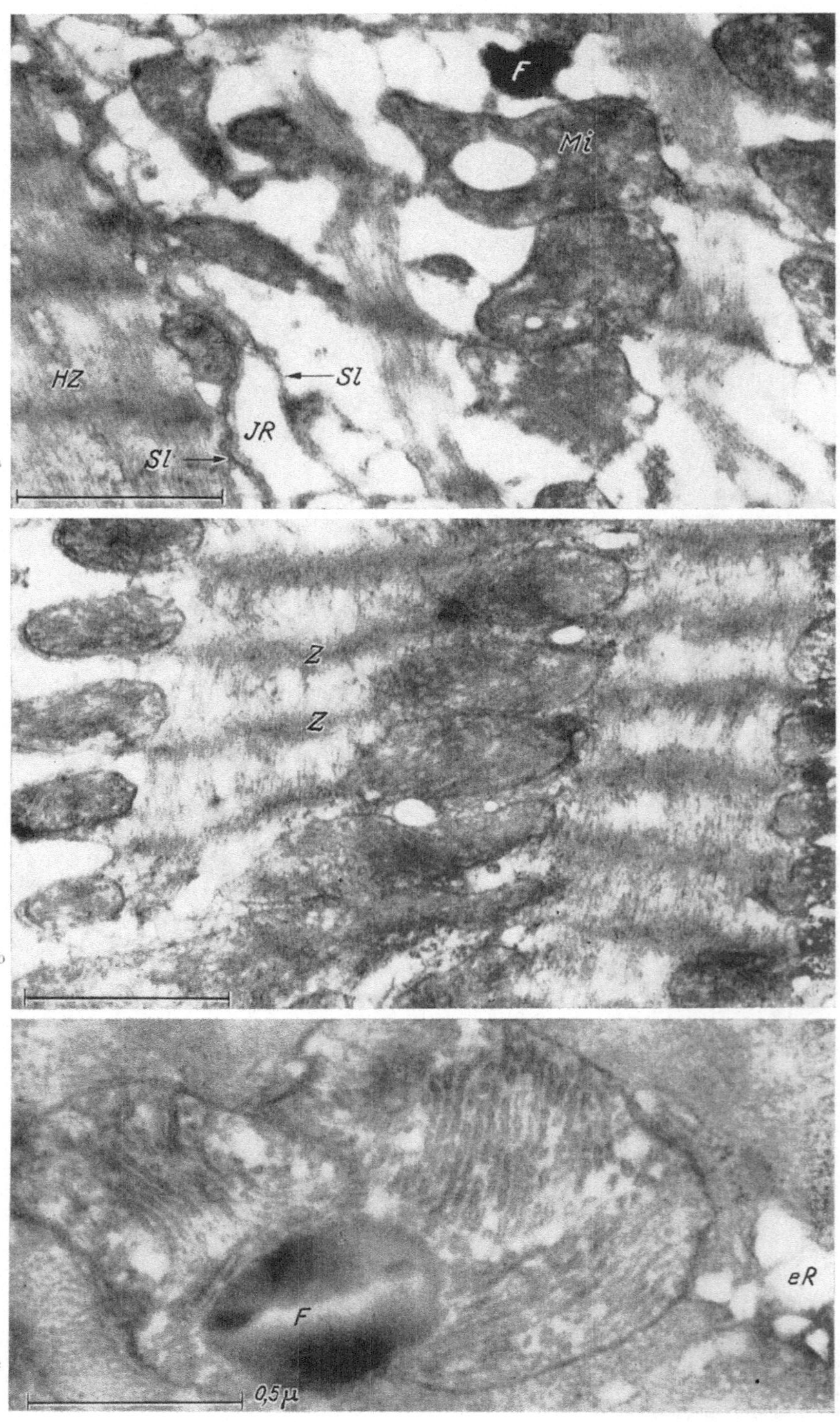
F
Mi
HZ
Sl
JR
Sl
a
Z
Z
b
F
eR
c
0,5 μ

es finden sich Kontrakturen mit Z-Abständen von 0,8 μ gegenüber normalerweise 1–1,3 μ. Die Kerne der Herzmuskelzellen sind unauffällig, lediglich an einzelnen Stellen ist der perinucleäre Raum glanz leicht erweitert. Auch hier erfassen die beschriebenen Veränderungen nicht alle Herzmuskelzellen gleichmäßig, so daß man immer noch intakte, unveränderte Herzmuskelzellen erkennt.

Eine Aufhellung des Grundsarkoplasmas durch Verlust der kleinen Glykogengranula findet sich auch in Herzmuskelzellen von Ratten, die 30 min nach einer subcutanen Injektion von 20mg/kg Körpergewicht 2,4-Dinitrophenol getötet worden sind (Abb. 3). Wie bei den Versuchen mit Schilddrüsenhormonen bleiben auch hier die Zellmembranen der Herzmuskelzellen unauffällig und ohne Vermehrung von Membranvesiculationen. Das transversale Tubulussystem ist nicht erweitert. Die Elemente des endoplasmatischen Reticulums sind dagegen deutlich geschwollen, allerdings nicht ganz so stark wie nach Überdosierung von Thyroxin. Die Fetttropfen sind eben erkennbar vermehrt. Die Mitochondrien haben wie bei den vorhergehenden Versuchen ihre Granula verloren, sind aber im übrigen nur teilweise und im allgemeinen nur leicht geschwollen. Die Matrix der geschwollenen Mitochondrien ist leicht fleckförmig aufgehellt, die Cristae mitochondriales sind manchmal etwas fragmentiert und zeigen gelegentlich einzelne umschriebene Erweiterungen des osmiophoben Spatiums, allerdings nicht so ausgeprägt wie nach Überdosierung von Thyroxin. Andere Mitochondrien konfluieren und erstrecken sich, korkzieherartig geschlängelt, über einige Muskelfächer. Die Myofibrillen zeigen häufig Kontrakturen mit Z-Abständen bis herunter zu 0,4 μ gegenüber normalerweise 1–1,4 μ; in solchen Myofibrillen sind die Myofilamente meistens mehr oder weniger aufgesplittert. Die Zellkerne sind unauffällig, der perinucleäre Raum ist nur ausnahmsweise einmal leicht erweitert. Auch hier betreffen die beschriebenen Veränderungen nicht alle Herzmuskelzellen gleichmäßig, so daß man immer noch Herzmuskelgewebe mit regelrechtem Zellgefüge sieht.

Am Herzmuskel des Hundes findet man nach einer intravenösen Injektion von 10 mg/kg Körpergewicht Dinitrophenol ähnliche Veränderungen wie am Herzmuskel der Ratte; es kommt hier jedoch nicht zu Kontrakturen der Myofibrillen, wenn auch die Abstände der Z-Streifen mit Werten zwischen 1,0 und 1,8 μ außerordentlich schwanken können. Dies unterstreicht, daß die Wirkungen entkoppelnder Substanzen bei verschiedenen Species Unterschiede aufweisen können, und daß demzufolge auch die Übertragung tierexperimenteller Befunde auf den Menschen problematisch ist.

Unsere Experimente an Ratten mit Trijodthyronin, Thyroxin und Dinitrophenol haben gezeigt, daß diese Stoffe am Herzmuskel des selben Versuchstieres wohl gleichsinnige, nicht aber völlig identische Veränderungen der Zellstruktur

---

Abb. 3a—c. Herzmuskel der Ratte nach Vergiftung mit Dinitrophenol. a) Teil einer Herzmuskelzelle mit Aufhellung und Schwellung des Grundsarkoplasmas (leichtes sog. Zellödem) bei weitgehendem Verlust der kleinen Glykogengranula. Die Mitochondrien (*Mi*) teilweise konfluiert; ihre Matrix kleinfleckig aufgehellt. Fetttropfen (*F*). Links im Bild eine intakte Herzmuskelzelle (*HZ*). Der Intercellularraum (*IR*) zwischen beiden Herzmuskelzellen wasserhell. Sarkolemm (*Sl*). Elektronenoptisch 8100:1, Endvergrößerung 29000:1 (Arch.-Nr. 1848 A/60). b) Kontrakturen der Myofibrillen mit verschmierten Z-Streifen (*Z*) und leichter Aufsplitterung der Myofilamente. Elektronenoptisch 8100:1, Endvergrößerung 29000:1 (Arch.-Nr. 1847 D/60). c) Mitochondrien mit geringer fleckförmiger Aufhellung der Matrix und mit leichter perlschnurartiger Auftreibung und Fragmentierung der Innenmembranen, aber wesentlich geringer ausgeprägt als nach Überdosierung von Thyroxin. Fetttropfen (*F*) rings von Mitochondrienmaterial umgeben (Abbauform des Herzmuskelfettes). Das endoplasmatische Reticulum (*eR*) geschwollen [Elektronenoptisch 14800:1, Endvergrößerung 61000:1 (Arch.-Nr. 1563 D/60)]

hervorrufen. *Gleich* sind bei allen drei Versuchsgruppen die Aufhellung des Grundsarkoplasmas durch Schwund der Glykogengranula, der völlige Verlust der Mitochondriengranula, die starke Schwellung des endoplasmatischen Reticulums, die geringe Vermehrung der Fetttropfen im Sarkoplasma und das unauffällige Verhalten der Zellmembranen. *Unterschiede* bestehen dagegen in der Struktur der Mitochondrien; diese sind im allgemeinen nur mittelgradig geschwollen; die geringsten Grade der Schwellung finden sich nach Dinitrophenol und die stärkeren Grade nach Trijodthyronin und Thyroxin. Die perlschnurartige Schwellung und Fragmentierung der Cristae mitochondriales ist nach Thyroxin wesentlich stärker als nach Dinitrophenol und Trijodthyronin. Auch die transversalen Tubuli zeigen ein etwas unterschiedliches Verhalten: Sie sind nur nach Trijodthyronin stellenweise erweitert, nach Thyroxin und Dinitrophenol dagegen nicht. Schließlich erkennt man Kontrakturen der Myofibrillen hauptsächlich nach Dinitrophenol, weniger nach Thyroxin und kaum nach Trijodthyronin. Ein Vergleich unserer Untersuchungen mit denen von Schulz u. Mitarb. (1956) zeigt, daß die Mitochondrien der Leberzellen nach Gaben von Thyroxin viel stärker schwellen, als die der Herzmuskelzellen.

Unterschiede in der Wirkung von Trijodthyronin, Thyroxin und Dinitrophenol sind auch aus der Biochemie bekannt. So werden die biologische Aktivität (Gross und Pitt-Rivers 1953, Gemmill 1953, Tomich und Woollett 1953, Lerman 1953, Anderson 1954, Maclagan und Wilkinson 1954) und die Stoffwechselaktivität (Gross, Pitt-Rivers und Thibault 1953, Asper, Selenkow und Plamondon 1953) von Trijodthyronin 3—5mal stärker als die von Thyroxin angegeben. Andererseits soll Thyroxin aber stärker entkoppelnd wirken als Trijodthyronin (Klemperer 1955). Diesen Angaben stehen die morphologischen Befunde gegenüber, daß es nach Trijodthyronin im Gegensatz zum Thyroxin auch zu einer Schwellung der transversalen Tubuli kommen kann, während nach Thyroxin die perlschnurartige Schwellung und Fragmentation der Cristae mitochondriales stärker ausgeprägt ist. Dinitrophenol unterscheidet sich von den Schilddrüsenhormonen dadurch, daß es unabhängig von seiner Konzentration entkoppelnd wirkt, während Thyroxin nur bei einer Konzentration von 10^{-5} bis 10^{-4} Mol entkoppelt, bei Konzentrationen von weniger als 10^{-6} Mol dagegen die oxydative Phosphorylierung sogar steigern kann (Martius und Hess 1955). Beyer, Löw und Ernster (1956) sprechen bei den Schilddrüsenhormonen von einer „Labilisierung" der Oxydations-Phosphorylierungs-Multienzym-Systeme. Die Apyrase (Adenosintriphosphatase) der Mitochondrien wird — im Gegensatz zur ATPase-Wirkung des Myosins — durch entkoppelnde Substanzen aktiviert, und zwar durch Dinitrophenol wesentlich stärker als durch die Schilddrüsenhormone (Lardy und Maley 1954, Maley und Johnson 1957, Cooper und Lehninger 1957, Klemperer 1957). Hierzu passen unsere morphologischen Befunde am Rattenherzmuskel, daß nach Dinitrophenol die Mitochondrien am wenigsten geschwollen sind, die Myofibrillen jedoch die stärksten Kontrakturen zeigen; denn die Kontraktur charakterisiert einen energiearmen Zustand und läßt auf einen verminderten Gehalt der Herzmuskelzelle an ATP schließen.

Diese wenigen Beispiele zeigen, daß es möglich ist, gewisse Parallelen zwischen Biochemie und submikroskopischer Morphologie zu erkennen. So zeichnet sich ein Weg ab, auf dem es vielleicht eines Tages gelingen wird, durch gezielte Zusammenarbeit biochemischer und morphologischer Forschung auch komplizierte Vorgänge, wie die Wirkung der Schilddrüsenhormone auf Funktion und Struktur der Körperzellen, aufzuklären.

Literatur

1. ANDERSON, B. G.: Potency and duration of action of triiodothyronine and thyroxine in rats and mice. Endocrinology **54**, 659—665 (1954).
2. ASPER JR., S. P., H. A. SELENKOW and C. A. PLAMONDON: A comparison of the metabolic activities of 3,5,3'-l-triiodothyronine and l-thyroxine in myxedema. Bull. Johns Hopk. Hosp. **93**, 164—198 (1953).
3. BÜCHNER, F.: Das morphologische Substrat bei Angina pectoris im Tierexperiment. Beitr. path. Anat. **92**, 311—328 (1933).
4. COOPER, C., and A. L. LEHNINGER: Oxidative phosphorylation by an encyme complex from extracts of mitochondria. IV. Adenosinetriphosphatase activity. J. biol. Chem. **224**, 547—560 (1957).
5. EHRENBRAND, F.: Leberstudien bei experimenteller Hyperthyreose. Anat. Anz. **101**, 315—356 (1955).
6. FAHR, T.: Histologische Befunde an Kropfherzen. Zbl. allg. Path. path. Anat. **27**, 1—5 (1916).
7. FAHR, T.: Zur Frage des Kropfherzens und der Herzveränderungen bei Status thymico-lymphaticus. Verh. dtsch. Ges. Path. **18**, 159—163 (1921).
8. FEDERLIN, K.: Über die Ursache der Verfettungen von Herz, Nieren und Leber bei Thyreotoxikosen. Frankfurt. Z. Path. **67**, 265—271 (1956).
9. GEMMILL, CH. L.: Cardiac hypertrophy in rats and mice given 3,3',5-triiodo-L-thyronine oraly. Amer. J. Physiol. **195**, 385—390 (1958).
10. — Comparison of activity of thyroxine and 3,5,3'-triiodothyronine. Amer. J. Physiol. **172**, 286—290 (1933).
11. GROSS, J., and R. PITT-RIVERS: 3,5,3'-Triiodothyronine. II. physiological activity. Biochem. J. **53**, 652—657 (1953).
12. — — et O. THIBAULT: Recherches sur la nature de la forme d'action directe de l'hormone thyroidienne et de la thyroxine sur les échanges respiratoires du rat. C. R. Soc. Biol. (Paris) **147**, 75—77 (1953).
13. HABÁN, G.: Über Leberveränderungen bei Morbus Basodowii mit besonderer Berücksichtigung der Lebercirrhose. Beitr. path. Anat. **92**, 88—100 (1933).
14. — Leberveränderungen bei experimentellem Hyperthyreoidismus. Beitr. path. Anat. **95**, 573—589 (1935).
15. HEINLEIN, H., u. J. DIECKHOFF: Organveränderungen durch Thyroxin. Virchows Arch. path. Anat. **297**, 252—263 (1936).
16. KLEMPERER, H. G.: The uncoupling of oxidative phosphorylation in rat-liver mitochondria by thyroxine, triiodothyronine and related substances. Biochem. J. **60**, 122—128 (1955).
17. — ATPase activity of rat liver mitochondria. Biochim. biophys. Acta **23**, 404—412 (1957).
18. LARDY, H. A., and G. F. MALEY: Metabolic effects of thyroid hormones in vitro. Recent Progr. Hormone Rec. **10**, 129—145 (1954).
19. LERMAN, J.: The physiologic activity of l-triiodothyronine. J. clin. Endocr. **13**, 1341—1346 (1953).
20. LOCHNER, W., u. M. NASSERI: Untersuchungen über den Herzstoffwechsel und die Coronardurchblutung, insbesondere bei Dinitrophenolvergiftung. Pflügers Arch. ges. Physiol. **271**, 405—419 (1960).
21. MACLAGAN, N. F., and J. H. WILKINSON: Some differences in the metabolism of thyroxine and triiodothyronine in the rat. J. Physiol. (Lond.) **125**, 405—415 (1954).
22. MALEY, G. F., and D. JOHNSON: Adenosine triphosphatase and morphological integrity of mitochondria. Biochim. biophys. Acta **26**, 522—525 (1957).
23. MARTIUS, C., u. B. HESS: Über den Wirkungsmechanismus des Schilddrüsenhormons. Biochem. Z. **326**, 191—203 (1955).

24. Meessen, H., u. R. Poche: Pathomorphologie des Myocards. In: Bargmann-Doerr: Das Herz des Menschen. Stuttgart: G. Thieme 1963.

25. Movitt, E. R., B. Gerstl and A. E. Davis: Needle liver biopsy in thyreotoxicosis. Arch. intern. Med. **91**, 729—739 (1953).

26. Pfleger, K., W. Rummel, E. Seifen u. K. Timp: Der Einfluß von Thyroxin und Dinitrophenol auf die Lactatkonzentration des Blutes. Med. exp. (Basel) **1**, 160—165 (1959).

27. Piper, J., and E. Poulsen: Liver biopsy in thyreotoxicosis. Acta med. scand. **127**, 439—447 (1947).

28. Poche, R.: Das submikroskopische Bild der Herzmuskelveränderungen nach Überdosierung von Schilddrüsenhormon. Beitr. path. Anat. **118**, 407—420 (1957).

29. — Über den Einfluß von Dinitrophenol und Thyroxin auf die Ultrastruktur des Herzmuskels bei der Ratte. Virchows Arch. path. Anat. **335**, 282—297 (1962).

30. —, u. W. Lochner: Ultrastruktur und Stoffwechsel des Herzmuskels vom Hund bei akuter Dinitrophenolvergiftung. Frankf. Z. Path. **72**, 34—49 (1962).

31. Rössle, R.: Über die Veränderungen der Leber bei der Basedowschen Krankheit und ihre Bedeutung für die Entstehung anderer Organsklerosen. Virchows Arch. path. Anat. **291**, 1—46 (1933).

32. Schlesinger, P., and A. B. Benchimol: The pure form of thyreotoxic heart disease A clinical and pathological study. Amer. J. Cardiol. **2**, 430—440 (1958).

33. Schulz, H., H. Löw, L. Ernster u. F. S. Sjöstrand: Elektronenmikroskopische Studien an Leberschnitten von Thyroxin-behandelten Ratten. Proc. Stockholm Conf. Electron Microscopy 1956, S. 134—137. Stockholm: Almqvist & Wiksel 1957.

34. Staemmler, M.: Die Kreislauforgane. In: Kaufmann-Staemmler: Lehrbuch der spez. path. Anat., Bd. I/1, S. 1—380. Berlin: de Gruyter 1955.

35. Tomich, E. G., and E. A. Woollett: The biological activity of triiodothyronine. Lancet **1953 I**, 726.

36. Wegelin, C.: Schilddrüse. In: Henke-Lubarsch: Hdb. allg. u. spez. path. Anat., Bd. VIII, S. 1—547. Berlin: Springer 1926.

37. Zalka, E. v.: Herzmuskelveränderungen bei experimentellem Hyperthyreoidismus. Beitr. path. Anat. **95**, 590—602 (1935).

Diskussion

B. Hess (Heidelberg):

Bei der Diskussion von strukturellen Veränderungen der Mitochondrien unter Bedingungen, die mit einer Grundumsatzsteigerung einhergehen, wie der Hyperthyreose muß man an die sehr interessanten Untersuchungen von Lust und Ernster erinnern, die bei einem euthyreoten Patienten mit Grundumsatzsteigerung in der Skeletmuskulatur Riesenchromosomen gefunden haben. Offenbar gibt es neben der hyperthyreoten Reaktion der Mitochondrien auch noch andere Mechanismen, die zu einer Grundumsatzsteigerung führen können. Da die Mitochondrienschwellung unter den Bedingungen der Hyperthyreose so typisch ist, möchte ich Sie fragen, ob auch Hirnmitochondrien diese Schwellung zeigen. Bekanntlich reagiert das Hirn in vivo auf Zufuhr von Schilddrüsenhormon nicht mit einer Grundumsatzsteigerung. Verschiedene Autoren haben gefunden, daß isolierte Hirnmitochondrien nicht mit Schilddrüsenhormon zur Schwellung zu bringen sind. Es wäre daher interessant zu erfahren, ob auch in situ bei der Hyperthyreose die Schwellung der Hirnmitochondrien ausbleibt.

R. Poche:

Die Wirkung von Schilddrüsenhormonen auf die Ultrastruktur der Zellen des Zentralnervensystems wurde bisher nicht untersucht. Wie vorstehend ausgeführt, kann der Grad der durch Einwirkung von Schilddrüsenhormonen hervorgerufenen Mitochondrienschwellungen in den Parenchymzellen verschiedener Organe, wie beispielsweise Herzmuskel und Leber, unterschiedlich sein. Es wäre deshalb durchaus denkbar, daß die Mitochondrien der Zellen des Zentralnervensystems in vivo durch Schilddrüsenhormone morphologisch nicht oder nur wenig beeinflußt werden.

H. Bennhold (Tübingen):

Ist etwas über die Wirkung von Dinitrophenol auf die Zellstruktur von schilddrüsenlosen Tieren bekannt?

R. Poche:

Elektronenmikroskopische Untersuchungen über die Wirkung von Dinitrophenol auf die Zellstruktur bei schilddrüsenlosen Tieren sind bisher nicht durchgeführt worden. Wir wissen aber nach Untersuchungen von Lindner und Wellensiek (Verh. IV. internat. Kongr. f. Elektronenmikroskopie II, 326, Berlin 1958), daß Dinitrophenol am isolierten Meerschweinchenherzen in einer Konzentration von 10^{-3} Mol in der Perfusionsflüssigkeit zu Kontrakturen führt.

Aus der Medizinischen Universitätsklinik Heidelberg (Prof. Dr. K. Matthes †)

Wirkungsmechanismus des Schilddrüsenhormons

Von

Benno Hess und Karl Brand

Mit 6 Abbildungen

Referat

1. Einleitung

Im Jahre 1924 fand Rohrer (*1*), daß die Zellatmung von Geweben hyperthyreoter Tiere gesteigert ist. Nachdem Otto Warburg (*2*) bereits im Jahre 1913 gezeigt hat, daß die Grana oder Mitochondrien die cellulären Strukturen enthalten, in denen sich die Zellatmung abspielt, ist eine Seite des Problems der biochemischen Wirkung des Schilddrüsenhormons ein Problem des Mitochondrienstoffwechsels. Die folgenden Ausführungen konzentrieren sich daher auf die Funktion und Struktur dieses Zellkompartimentes und lassen vereinfachend viele Einzelheiten über Wirkungen des Hormons auf andere Zellstrukturen und Kompartimente sowie isolierte Enzyme außer acht. Im folgenden sollen zwei verschiedene Erscheinungen besprochen werden, mit denen Mitochondrien auf die Einwirkung des Hormons reagieren:

1. die rasche, innerhalb Sekunden einsetzende Wirkung des Hormons auf die Fließgleichgewichte des mitochondrialen Kompartiments und

2. die langsam anlaufenden Wirkungen auf mitochondriale Enzymaktivitäten.

In der Diskussion wird schließlich versucht, die beiden Erscheinungen unter einem gemeinsamen Gesichtspunkt zu ordnen.

2. Entkopplung

Vor 12 Jahren haben Martius und Hess (*3*) sowie Lardy und Feldott (*4*) in Bilanzuntersuchungen der oxydativen Phosphorylierung die entkoppelnde Wirkung von Thyroxin gefunden. Diese Beobachtung wurde von einer großen Reihe von Autoren bestätigt. Setzt man zu einer Mitochondrienpräparation von Leber, Nieren oder zu Zwerchfellschnitten, zu Sarkosomen der verschiedensten Tiere, Hormon in Form von Trijodthyronin oder Thyroxin in der Größenordnung einer $10^{-6}-10^{-5}$ molaren Lösung hinzu und läßt sie mit bestimmten Substraten atmen, so findet man im Verhältnis zum verbrauchten Sauerstoff eine herabgesetzte Bildung von energiereichem Phosphat, das P/O-Verhältnis sinkt ab [zusammenfassende Darstellung s. (*5*)].

Man beobachtet diese Hormonwirkung nicht nur am isolierten Objekt. Der gleiche Effekt tritt auch in vivo ein, wenn man das Hormon parenteral oder oral zuführt, dann die Tiere tötet und das P/O-Verhältnis in den isolierten Mitochondrien bestimmt. Unter der Einwirkung von Schilddrüsenhormon ist die Ausbeute der Atmung an energiereichem Phosphat verschlechtert, dem Zustand der experimentellen Hyperthyreose entspricht ein herabgesetztes P_i/O-Verhältnis.

Mit dem Fortschritt unseres Wissens über die Struktur der Mitochondrien und die Komponenten der Atmungskette wurden auch vereinfachte Systeme der oxydativen Phosphorylierung untersucht. So kann man mit Digitoninbehandlung oder durch Ultraschall Mitochondrienfragmente darstellen, die noch alle Eigenschaften der oxydativen Phosphorylierung von intakten Mitochondrien besitzen.

Tabelle 1. *Einfluß von Trijodthyronin auf das ATP/ADP-Verhältnis in Rattenlebermitochondrien* [aus(7)]

Exp.-Nr.	Trijod-thyronin 10^{-6} M	ATP + ADP	Verhältnis ATP/ADP	% Abnahme
1	—	0,4	7,6	—
2	1,0	0,4	7,0	8
3	3,0	0,3	6,4	16
4	5,0	0,4	5,6	26
5	7,0	0,3	1,3	83

Auch an diesen Fragmenten läßt sich eindeutig die entkoppelnde Wirkung der Hormone nachweisen. Abb. 1 gibt einen Versuch wieder, bei dem die Wirkung des Hormons auf die letzte Stufe der oxydativen Phosphorylierung zwischen Cytochrom c und dem Warburgschen Atmungsferment geprüft wurde. Man sieht, daß das Hormon nicht nur die Phosphorylierung der gesamten Atmungskette entkoppelt, sondern auch einen isolierten Schritt der oxydativen Phosphorylierung, nämlich ihre Endstufe, unterbrechen kann [HESS und BRAND (6)].

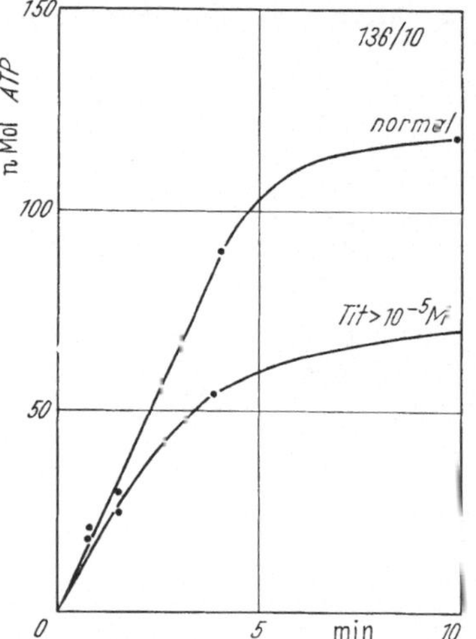

Abb. 1. Wirkung von Trijodthyronin (>10^{-5} molar) auf die oxydative Phosphorylierung der Cytochrom-c-Stufe (Experiment Nr 133/10) (*16*)

Die Folge der entkoppelnden Wirkung ist eine Herabsetzung des ATP/ADP-Verhältnisses der atmenden Mitochondrien, wie sie auf der Tab. 1 dargestellt ist [HESS (7)]. Man sieht, daß mit zunehmender Thyroxin-Konzentration das ATP/ADP-Verhältnis von Leberzellmitochondrien sinkt, eine Erscheinung, die auch in der Klinik unter hyperthyreoten Bedingungen beobachtet wird.

Eng mit der Herabsetzung des ATP/ADP-Verhältnisses hängt der Verlust der sog. Atmungskontrolle der Mitochondrien unter hyperthyreoten Bedingungen zusammen. Unter Atmungskontrolle versteht man die Fähigkeit der oxydativen Phosphorylierung, durch raschen Umsatz den ADP-Spiegel so weit zu senken, daß er den Gesamtumsatz der Atmungskette und damit den Sauerstoffverbrauch limitiert. Diese Fähigkeit geht in Anwesenheit von Schilddrüsenhormon verloren. Die Atmungsfermente werden maximal oxydiert (8), der Sauerstoffverbrauch wird durch die Atmungskette selbst limitiert und ist maximal. Mit der fehlenden Atmungskontrolle hängt weiterhin der mangelnde Acceptor-Effekt zusammen, der von LIPMANN und HOCH (5, 9) beobachtet wurde. Dies besagt, daß ATP-verbrauchende Reaktionen, wie die Hexokinasereaktion, unter hyperthyreoten Bedingungen nicht in der Lage sind, den Sauerstoffverbrauch zu beschleunigen. Dies ist verständlich, da die Atmungskette bereits maximal ausgelastet ist.

3. Umkehr der oxydativen Phosphorylierung unter der Wirkung des Schilddrüsenhormons

Das Studium der Fließgleichgewichte der Atmungskette hat in der letzten Zeit Bedingungen aufgedeckt, die den Eingriff des Hormons auf das mitochondriale Kompartiment und seinen Fließstatus noch wesentlich empfindlicher aufzeichnen als die Messung des P/O-Verhältnisses, nämlich durch Registrierung der sog. Umkehr der oxydativen Phosphorylierung. Was versteht man darunter? Die oxydative Phosphorylierung umfaßt eine Kette von Reaktionen, deren Bilanz

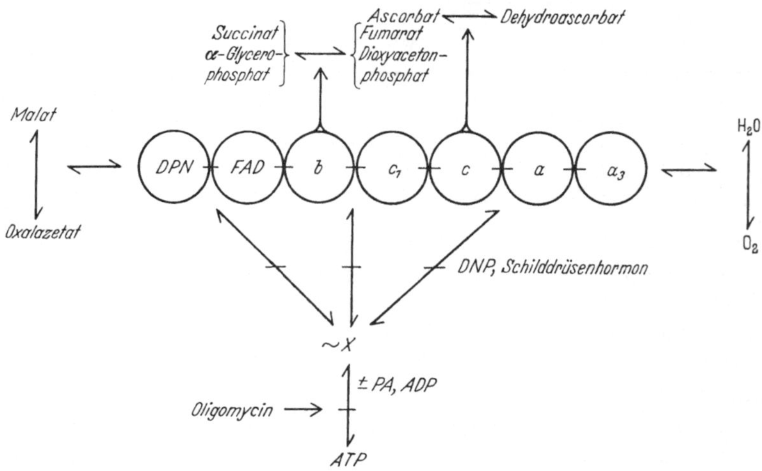

Abb. 2. Hypothetisches Schema der Atmungskettenphosphorylierung

in der Oxydation von Substraten, z. B. von Malat (s. Abb. 2), in einem Elektronentransport über die Atmungskette zum Sauerstoff, sowie in einer Reduktion von Sauerstoff unter Wasserbildung bei gleichzeitigem Aufbau von energiereichem Phosphat in der Form von ATP besteht. Aus thermodynamischen Berechnungen folgt, daß bei einem genügend hohen Phosphorylierungspotential (d. h. bei genügend hoher ATP-Konzentration relativ zur Konzentration von ADP und anorganischem Phosphat) eine Umkehr des Elektronentransportes im Sinne einer Reduktion von DPN- und TPN-abhängigen Substraten bei Oxydation von Cytochrom sowie Substraten positiveren Redoxpotentials oder möglicherweise unter Wasserspaltung möglich sein muß.

Kürzlich wurde von verschiedener Seite der Nachweis einer Umkehr der oxydativen Phosphorylierung im Sinne einer reduktiven Dephosphorylierung an Mitochondrien und Zellen experimentell erbracht [CHANCE und HOLLUNGER (10), CHANCE und HESS (11), KLINGENBERG und SCHOLLMEYER (12, 13), ERNSTER und AZZONE (14)]. Unter den Bedingungen eines hohen Phosphorylierungspotentials läßt sich durch Bernsteinsäure, α-Glycerophosphat, Fettsäuren oder reduziertes Cytochrom c je nach den vorliegenden Mitochondrien-Typen Pyridinnucleotid reduzieren.

Prüft man den Einfluß des Schilddrüsenhormons auf diesen Prozeß, so zeigt sich, daß die Geschwindigkeit der Pyridinnucleotid-Reduktion ein empfindlicher

Indicator der Hormonwirksamkeit ist. CHANCE und HOLLUNGER (*15*) haben an Sarkosomen von Rattenherzen eine halbmaximale hemmende Thyroxinwirkung in der Konzentration von $5 \cdot 10^{-7}$ molar bei Anwesenheit von Bernsteinsäure als Wasserstoffdonator nachgewiesen. Dementsprechend wird Pyridinnucleotid auch durch das Hormon rasch oxydiert. Abb. 3 zeigt einen Versuch, bei dem der Zustand der Pyridinnucleotide von Rattenherzsarkosomen durch Fluorescenz-

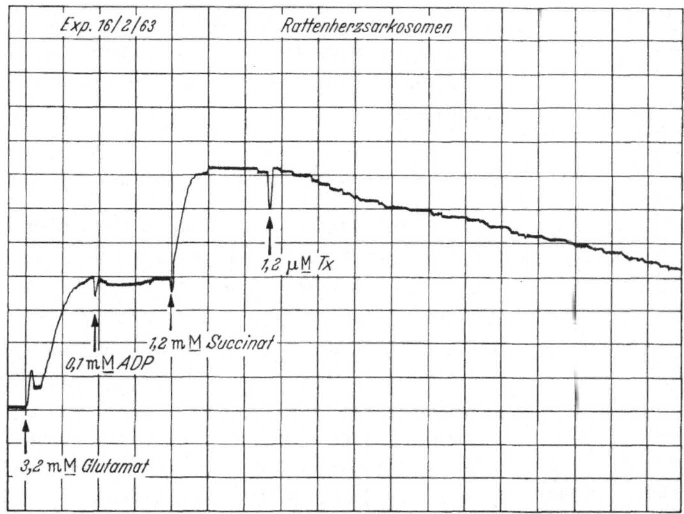

Abb. 3. Registrierung der Pyridinnucleotidfluorescenz (Primärstrahlung 366 mμ, Sekundärstrahlung 420—480 mμ) von gebundenem Pyridinnucleotid in Rattenherzsarkosomen. Eine Abweichung der Kurve nach oben gibt eine Zunahme der Fluorescenz entsprechend einer relativen Zunahme von reduziertem Pyridinnucleotid an. Zeitschreibung 15 sec/Einheit. Konzentrationsangaben: Millimol/l bzw. μMol/l (Experiment 16/2) (*16*)

messung verfolgt wurde [HESS und BRAND (*16*)]. Man sieht, daß durch Zusatz von Thyroxin in 10^{-6} molarer Lösung unmittelbar eine Oxydation vonPyridinnucleotid in Gang gesetzt wird.

Die Versuche zeigen, daß

1. das Hormon die Atmungskette bereits in einem Konzentrationsbereich beeinflußt, in dem das P/O-Verhältnis noch nicht verändert wird und

2. das Hormon die Richtung des Elektronentransports im oberen Teil der Kette kontrolliert, in dem das Fließgleichgewicht zwischen Reduktion von Pyridinnucleotiden einerseits und Oxydation der Kette andererseits beeinflußt wird.

In diesem niedrigen Konzentrationsbereich der hormonalen Wirkung wird bei zunehmender Oxydation der Atmungskette in der Bilanz die Synthese von ATP gefördert. Man beobachtet also eine „Konservierung" von energiereichem Phosphat. Eine „Konservierung" von ATP und eine Steigerung der ATP-Synthese mit kleinen Schilddrüsenhormonkonzentrationen ist durch einfache Messung der ATP-Synthese-Rate schon seit längerer Zeit bekannt [MARTIUS und HESS (*17*), BRONK (*18*), BRAND (*19*)]. Abb. 4 gibt einen Versuch wieder, bei dem die Aktivierung der ATP-Synthese mit kleinen Hormonkonzentrationen beobachtet wurde.

Die aktivierende Wirkung des Hormons auf die ATP-Synthese kommt auch in den Versuchen von Sokoloff und Kaufmann (20) zum Ausdruck. Die Autoren konnten zeigen, daß kleine Hormonkonzentrationen in einem zusammengesetzten System aus Mitochondrien und Mikrosomen den Einbau von Leucin in Eiweiß stark fördern. Da dieser Einbau von der Anwesenheit intakter Mitochondrien mit einer aktiven oxydativen Phosphorylierung abhängt, ist zu schließen, daß die Förderung der ATP-Synthese die Ursache für die Förderung des vermehrten Leucineinbaus in das Eiweiß darstellt. In diesem Befund liegt vielleicht ein Schlüssel für die starke Wirkung des Hormons auf den gesamten Eiweißstoffwechsel.

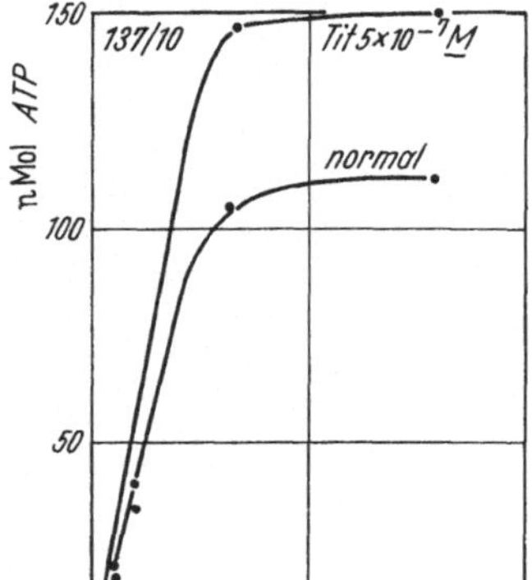

Abb. 4. Aktivierung der ATP-Synthese durch kleine Trijodthyroninkonzentrationen bei Untersuchung der oxydativen Phosphorylierung der Cytochrom-c-Stufe (Experiment 137/10) (16)

4. Morphologische Veränderungen

Eng mit den Verschiebungen der mitochondrialen Fließgleichgewichte hängt eine Erscheinung der Mitochondrien zusammen, die an der Grenze zwischen Biochemie und Morphologie liegt. Es handelt sich um die Schrumpfung oder Kontraktion und Schwellung von Mitochondrien. Schon lange ist bekannt, daß Mitochondrien unter gleichzeitiger Änderung von Volumen und/oder Konsistenz schwellen oder schrumpfen können. Die Erscheinungen wurden zuerst von Raaflaub (21), Packer (22), Lehninger u. Mitarb. (23) sowie vielen anderen Autoren in der letzten Zeit systematisch untersucht [s. (5, 24)]. Durch Trübungsmessung, Messung der Lichtstreuung, Volumenbestimmung und andere Methoden kann gezeigt werden, daß isolierte Mitochondrien je nach den äußeren Bedingungen den verschiedensten Form- und Volumenänderungen unterliegen. Packer (25) wies schließlich nach, daß diese Veränderungen auch in vitro stattfinden.

Raaflaub (26) zeigte als erster, daß die Schwellung der Mitochondrien vom Zustand der Zellatmung abhängt. Tapley und Cooper (27) sowie Klemperer (28) fanden, daß Thyroxin und schilddrüsenaktive analoge Mitochondrien unter Wasseraufnahme zur Schwellung bringen können. Nichtschilddrüsenaktive Hormon-Analoge besitzen diese Fähigkeit nicht. Es handelt sich also um eine spezifische Hormonwirkung. Sie wird in vitro wie in vivo bei der Untersuchung von Mitochondrien hyperthyreoter Tiere beobachtet. Die Schwellung tritt in vitro bereits bei einer Thyroxinkonzentration von 10^{-8}–10^{-7} molar auf und findet sich nur bei den Mitochondrien der Organe, die unter hyperthyreoten Bedingungen mit einem vermehrten Sauerstoffverbrauch reagieren. Maximale Schwellung von Mitochondrien bei höheren Thyroxinkonzentrationen führt zu einer 2–3fachen Volumenzunahme. Die Schwellung setzt nach einer Latenzzeit von 1–2 min ein, ist nach 20 min stationär und kann durch ATP-Zusatz spezifisch im Sinne einer Schrumpfung oder Kontraktion, auch nach langer Zeit, rückgängig gemacht werden. Allerdings geht dabei die oxydative Phosphorylierung irreversibel unter Verlust der Kopplung, der Phosphorylierungsfähigkeit und Freisetzung von DPN aus den Mitochondrien verloren (s. *5, 24*). Die Membran wird durchlässig. Die Organisation der mitochondrialen Enzyme wird zerstört.

Der Mechanismus des Effektes ist ungeklärt. LEHNINGER hat als Angriffspunkt der Hormonwirkung eine direkte Reaktion mit der Mitochondrienmembran diskutiert (*24*). Da jedoch die Atmungsenzyme in die Membran und Cristae der Mitochondrien starr eingebettet sind, ist eine experimentelle Trennung von Membran und Atmungskette und damit eine Prüfung dieser Vorstellung zunächst nicht möglich. Man weiß, daß jede Änderung der Fließgleichgewichte der Atmungskette derartige morphologische Veränderungen mit sich bringt. Es ist daher zu vermuten, daß die Wirkung des Hormons auf die Struktur eine Konsequenz der Reaktion des Hormons mit der Atmungskette darstellt. Eine primäre oder sekundäre Wirkung des Hormons auf die Membran hat für die Koordination von mitochondrialen und cytoplasmatischen Umsetzungen eine große Bedeutung. Wie von verschiedener Seite diskutiert (*24, 29*), wird das Hormon einen regulierenden Einfluß auf den Austausch von niedermolekularen Metaboliten und Substraten zwischen dem extramitochondrialen und intramitochondrialen Kompartiment haben.

5. Lokalisation der Hormonwirkung

Die intracelluläre Verteilung des Schilddrüsenhormons wird durch die starke Bindung des Hormons an fetthaltige Strukturen bestimmt (s. *30*). So nehmen isolierte Mitochondrien oder Sarkosomen das Hormon aus einem Suspensionsmedium zu einem hohen Anteil auf (*5, 9, 31*). In vivo findet man 0,25—0,5 des gesamten Thyroxingehaltes einer Zelle in den Mitochondrien (*5, 32*). Der Mechanismus der Verteilung des Hormons innerhalb der Mitochondrien ist nicht bekannt. Der Gehalt der Mitochondrien an organisch-gebundenem Jod steht etwa in einem stöchiometrischen Verhältnis zu anderen Komponenten der Atmungskette. Rechnet man das organisch gebundene Jod der Mitochondrien als Thyroxin — was hinreichend begründet ist —, so findet sich Thyroxin und Cytochrom a etwa in einem Verhältnis von 1 : 1 (*6*). Nimmt man an, daß das Hormon direkt an dem Umsatz der Atmungskette beteiligt ist, so muß man mit Wechselzahlen von etwa 100 sec^{-1} rechnen. Bei dem Eigenumsatz des Hormons ergibt sich eine katalytische Wirksamkeit von 230000 : 1.

Der chemische Angriffspunkt des Hormons innerhalb der Atmungskette ist nach wie vor ungeklärt. An den Vorstellungen über den molekularen Reaktionsmechanismus hat sich seit den Arbeiten von KENDALL (*33*) sowie NIEMANN (*34*) im Prinzip nichts geändert. Für die hormonelle Wirksamkeit ist eine Mindestkonfiguration erforderlich, die als biochemisch-funktionelle Gruppe ein phenolisches Hydroxyl in einer Position haben muß, die die Ausbildung einer chinoiden Struktur zuläßt. Die chemisch optimale Struktur stellt das Hormon in der tetra- oder trijodsubstituierten Form dar. Man vermutet, daß das Hormon durch Abgabe von einzelnen Elektronen zu einem Semichinon oder Chinonradikal reversibel oxydiert wird (Übersicht s. *35*).

Aus elektrometrischen Titrationen geht das Redoxpotential des Hormons zu $E'_0 = +0,8$ Volt bei p$_H$ 0 hervor (*36*). Mit diesem Potential gehört die Struktur in die Reihe der Cytochrome. Es ist bisher allerdings nicht gelungen, ein Oxydationsprodukt des Hormons durch Reaktion mit dem Cytochromsystem darzustellen.

Nach diesen Vorstellungen sollte man annehmen, daß der Angriffspunkt des Hormons an den Orten der Bildung energiereicher Zwischenverbindungen der oxydativen Phosphorylierung zu suchen ist und mit den phosphatübertragenden Reaktionen und der Bildung von ATP selbst nichts zu tun hat. Dies läßt eindeutig belegen, wenn man den Einfluß des Hormons auf die oben beschriebene Rückreaktion der oxydativen Phosphorylierung in Anwesenheit von Oligomycin untersucht.

Nach den Arbeiten von Lardy (37) gelingt es, mit einem Antibioticum Oligomycin, die Übertragung der primären, energiereichen Phosphatverbindungen auf ADP zur Bildung von ATP zu unterbinden (s. Abb. 2). Unter diesen Bedingungen bleibt die erste Stufe der Atmungsreaktionen intakt, wie aus Beobachtungen der ^{18}O-Austauschrate, des ^{32}P-ATP-Austausches (37) sowie der Rückreaktion der Atmungskette [Ernster (38)] geschlossen wird. Untersucht man nun den Einfluß des Hormons auf die Rückreaktion bei oligomycinbehandelten Mitochondrien von Ratten, so zeigt sich, daß eine starke Hemmung der Umkehr der oxydativen Energiegewinnung zu beobachten ist. Auf Abb. 5 ist die Reduktionsgeschwindigkeit von Pyridinnucleotid, gemessen mit der Fluorescenzmethode, gegen die Mitochondrienkonzentration mit und ohne Trijodthyronin dargestellt. Man sieht eine 65%ige Hemmung der Rückreaktion durch das Hormon (44). L-Thyroxin wirkt in der gleichen Größenordnung. In Gegenwart von Oligomycin wird eine halbmaximale Wirkung bei einer Trijodthyroninkonzentration von $5 \cdot 10^{-7}$ molar gefunden. Die Analyse des DPN/DPNH-Verhältnisses ergibt einen entsprechenden Anstieg der DPN-Konzentration (44). Aus diesen Befunden folgt, daß das Hormon auch bei Blockierung der phosphatübertragenden Reaktionen stark wirksam ist, also in den Mechanismen der Bildung energiereicher Zwischenverbindungen eingreift. Die chemische Natur dieser Reaktionen ist jedoch noch unklar. Möglicherweise wirkt das Hormon im Wettbewerb mit anderen Chinonen der Atmungskette. Eine nähere Lokalisation der Hormonwirkung innerhalb der drei Stufen der Bildung energiereicher Zwischenverbindungen (s. Abb. 2) ist z. Z. noch nicht möglich. Wir vermuten, daß das Hormon in den Bereich der Cytochrom c-Stufe eingreift.

6. Induktive Wirkungen des Schilddrüsenhormons

Seit langem ist bekannt, daß unter den Bewegungen des Schilddrüsenhormons im Serum Enzymaktivitäten der Zelle zu- oder abnehmen. Während bislang die beobachteten Enzymaktivitäten nur relativ kleinen Änderungen unterworfen waren, deren kinetische Signifikanz unverständlich blieb [s. bei (35)], fanden Lardy und seine Mitarbeiter (39) vor kurzem eine starke Aktivitätsänderung eines mitochondrialen Enzyms, der α-Glycero-Phosphat-Oxydase. Es ergab sich, daß nach Injektion von Schilddrüsenhormon das Enzym mit einer Latenzzeit von etwa 12 Std in der Rattenleber um maximal das 22fache an Aktivität zunimmt, um nach Absetzen der Hormonapplikation innerhalb von 8 Tagen wieder normal zu werden.

Das Enzym gehört zu einem vor einigen Jahren von Bücher (40) neu entdeckten Cyclus, der die Aufgabe hat, Wasserstoff in die Mitochondrien mancher Organe ein- und auszuschleusen. Das Enzym ist in der mitochondrialen Struktur fest verankert und oxydiert dort α-Glycero-Phosphat zu Dioxyacetonphosphat.

Es arbeitet im Wechsel mit einem zweiten cytoplasmatischen Enzym, der α-Glycero-Phosphatdehydrogenase, die innerhalb der Kette der Glykolyse das in den Mitochondrien zu Dioxyacetonphosphat umgesetzte α-Glycero-Phosphat wieder aufreduziert. Die beiden Intermediate Dioxyacetonphosphat und α-Glycero-Phosphat diffundieren zwischen den beiden Enzymen und cellulären Räumen hin und her und verschieben den Wasserstoff in die Richtung, die durch den Fließstatus der Zelle gerade bevorzugt wird. Die Arbeitsgruppe in Wisconsin fand nun,

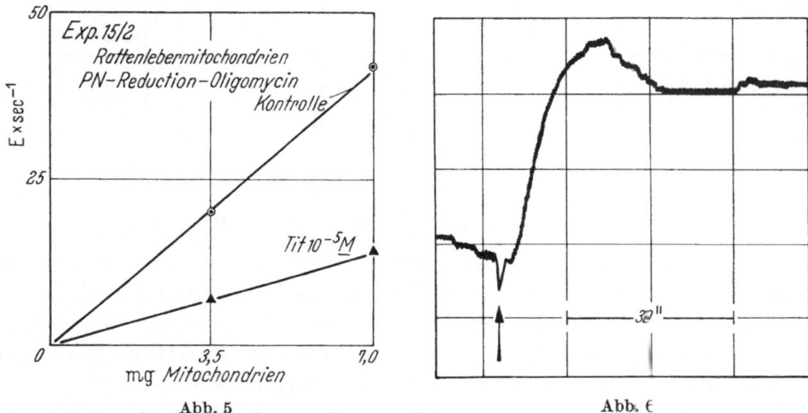

Abb. 5
Abb. 6

Abb. 5. Hemmung der Rückreaktion in Oligomycin behandelten Mitochondrien. Ordinate: Reduktionsgeschwindigkeit von gebundenem Pyridinnucleotid von Rattenlebermitochondrien gemessen an der relativen Fluorescenzänderung pro sec. Abszisse: Mitochondrienkonzentration in mg Biureteiweiß (44)

Abb. 6. Registrierung der Fluorescenz von gebundenen Pyridinnucleotid von Rattenlebermitochondrien (Meßbedingungen s. Abb. 3) Ordinate: relat. Fluorescenzeinheiten. Zugabe von α-Glycero-Phosphat bei ↑ (16)

daß nur das mitochondriale Enzym dieses Cyclus seine Aktivität steigert, nicht dagegen das cytoplasmatische Enzym. Tab. 2 gibt den Sauerstoffverbrauch von submitochondrialen Partikeln bei verschiedenen Substraten wieder. Man sieht die starke Steigerung der α-Glycero-Phosphat-Oxydation im Gegensatz zur Oxydation anderer Substrate. Tab. 3 zeigt schließlich die α-Glycero-Phosphat-Oxydation verschiedener Organe neben den entsprechenden P/O-Verhältnissen. Neben der Steigerung der Sauerstoffaufnahme in der Leber ist hier die Herabsetzung des P/O-Verhältnisses unter hyperthyreoten Bedingungen angegeben.

Die starke Aktivitätssteigerung des mitochondrialen Enzyms ist sinnvoll, da sie die wirksame Überführung von Wasserstoff zur Sättigung der unter den hyperthyreoten Bedingungen stark gesteigerten Zellatmung erst ermöglicht. Der Befund erklärt also die Substratseite der hyperthyreoten Mitochondrien und zeigt, wie der rasche Nachschub an verbrennbaren Intermediaten in die Mitochondrien zustandekommt. Als Quelle des α-Glycero-Phosphats dürfte der beschleunigte Zucker- sowie Fettabbau anzusehen sein.

Die Empfindlichkeit des Phänomens auf Äthionin sowie die lange Latenzperiode des Aktivitätsanstieges zeigen, daß es sich um eine echte Enzymneubildung handelt, die das Hormon auf dem Wege der Enzyminduktion erzeugt.

Die Veränderung der mitochondrialen Fließgleichgewichte durch die Aktivitätssteigerung der α-Glycero-Phosphat-Oxydase geht aus folgendem Experiment hervor: Während unter normalen Bedingungen dieses Enzym in der Leber zu schwach ist, um eine Reduktion der Pyridinnucleotide durch α-Glycero-Phosphat zustandezubringen, wird unter hyperthyreotem Zustand eine rasche Reduktion gefunden, wie auf Abb. 6 dargestellt ist (*16*).

Tabelle 2. *Atmung von submitochondrialen Partikeln nach* Y.-P. LEE, A. E. TAKEMORI *und* H. LARDY (*39*)

Substrat	Q_{O_2}	
	normal	hyper-thyreotisch
α-Glycerophosphat	31	141
β-Oxybutyrat	160	155
Succinat	106	131
Cholin	83	57

Tabelle 3. *Oxydative Phosphorylierung in Anwesenheit von* α-*Glycero-Phosphat nach* Y.-P. LEE, A. E. TAKEMORI *und* H. LARDY (*39*)

Organ	normal		hyperthyreotisch	
	O_2-Aufnahme	P/O	O_2-Aufnahme	P/O
Leber	3,4	2,2	16,4	0,9
Niere	5,2	0,7	14,0	0,3
Hirn	3,8	0,9	4,2	0,7

7. Diskussion und Zusammenstellung

Die Wirkungen des Schilddrüsenhormons auf die Struktur und Funktion von Mitochondrien und Sarkosomen lassen sich in Sofort- und Spätwirkungen in Abhängigkeit zweier Konzentrationsbereiche gliedern. Die Erscheinungen sind auf Tab. 4 halbschematisch zusammengestellt. Bei den Sofortwirkungen haben wir zwischen zwei Konzentrationsbereichen zu unterscheiden.

Tabelle 4. *Schematische Übersicht der Wirkungen des Schilddrüsenhormons auf Sarkosomen und Mitochondrien*

Reaktionszeit	Test	Konzentrationsbereich molar	
		10^{-8}—10^{-6}	10^{-6}—10^{-5}
1 bis 5 sec	Sauerstoffverbrauch	gesteigert	
	Redoxstatus der Atmungsfermente	oxydiert	maximal oxydiert
	ATP-Synthese	gesteigert	gehemmt
	Umkehr der oxydativen	gehemmt	
	P/O-Verhältnis	normal oder gesteigert	ent-koppelt
	Mitochondrienstruktur	geschwollen	
	Wärmebildung	vermehrt	
	Leucineinbau	gesteigert	?
	Acceptoreffekt	fehlt	
12 Std	α-Glycerophosphat-Oxydase-Aktivität	vermehrt	

1. Niedrige Konzentrationen steigern die ATP-Synthese, den Sauerstoffverbrauch bei einem P/O-Verhältnis bis zum Maximum bei gleichzeitiger Oxydation der Pyridinnucleotide. Das Fließgleichgewicht des Elektronentransports wird in Richtung zum Sauerstoff verschoben. Es handelt sich um den physiologischen Regulationsbereich. Die Wirkung ist reversibel.

2. Hohe Konzentrationen führen zur Hemmung der ATP-Synthese, zu maximaler Atmung, zur Entkopplung des P/O-Verhältnisses, zu maximaler Schwellung der Mitochondrien, zu irreversibler Zerstörung der mitochondrialen Koordination.

Bei den langsam einsetzenden Wirkungen tritt mit einer Latenz von 12 Std die Aktivitätssteigerung der α-Glycero-Phosphat-Oxydase ein und verändert das Gleichgewicht der verschiedenen Oxydasen zueinander. Je mehr sich der Zustand der Hyperthyreose einstellt, folgen eine Reihe von Veränderungen des Zellstoffwechsels, die seit langem bekannt sind. Die Erniedrigung der ATP-Konzentrationen und der relative Entkopplungseffekt regen die Glykolyse an. Die Änderung der mitochondrialen Struktur ist gleichbedeutend mit einer veränderten Permeabilität der Mitochondrien. Der Austausch zwischen dem cytoplasmatischen und mitochondrialen Kompartiment ist gesteigert.

Das Nebeneinander von Sofort- und Spätwirkung könnte man durch zwei verschiedene Angriffspunkte des Hormons einmal direkt an der Atmungskette und zweitens nach dem Vorschlag von KARLSON (*41*) an spezifischen Gen-Orten erklären. Einfacher erscheint es uns, eine einheitliche Vorstellung zu haben und die Theorie der Induktion durch Massenwirkung heranzuziehen.

Die Sofortwirkung des Hormons findet danach ihre Grundlage in einer primären chemischen Reaktion mit einer noch unbekannten Komponente des Atmungssystems. Die Folge ist, eine Veränderung des Fließstatus der Atmungskette. Es kommt zu lokalen Änderungen von Metabolitspiegeln und schließlich zu Massenwirkungen, die den Stoffwechsel der Zelle sekundär verändern. Die Spätwirkung findet ihre Grundlage in einer de-novo-Synthese von Enzymen und ändert das Enzymverteilungsmuster. Sie kann einfach durch die obengenannte Massenwirkung im Sinne einer induzierten Enzymsynthese erklärt werden. Die durch das Hormon erzeugte unmittelbare Veränderung von Substratspiegeln stellt den Massenreiz zur Enzymneubildung auf dem Wege der Induktion dar. So findet man in der Tat einen Anstieg der α-Glycero-Phosphat-Konzentration bei entkoppeltem Zellstoffwechsel (*42*).

Man kann annehmen, daß eine Reihe klinisch wichtiger Beobachtungen des hyperthyreoten- und hypothyreoten Zellstoffwechsels ihre Erklärung in den induktiv veränderten Enzymverteilungsmustern finden. Ein interessantes neues Beispiel dieser Art sind die Beobachtungen über die Verschiebung der Aktivität der Hydroxy-Methyl-Glutaryl-Reduktase der Leber, die GRIES, MATSCHINSKY und WIELAND (*43*) beobachtet haben. Die Aktivität des Enzyms ist unter hyperthyreoten Bedingungen etwa 60 mal größer als unter hypothyreoten Bedingungen. Da das Enzym weitgehend die Geschwindigkeit der Cholesterinsynthese limitiert, ist der Befund für das Verständnis des Cholesterinstoffwechsels bei der Hypo- und Hyperthyreose von großer Bedeutung.

Teleologisch gesehen ist diese Folge der Ereignisse sinnvoll. Die rasche chemische Primärwirkung des Hormons regt eine latente Umstellung der Fließgleichgewichte an, die durch Induktion eines neuen Enzymmusters manifest wird.

Wir danken Fräulein G. GEY und Fräulein H. HELFERICH für ihre ausgezeichnete technische Mitarbeit bei der Durchführung unserer Untersuchungen, sowie der Deutschen Forschungsgemeinschaft, Bad Godesberg, und der Research Corporation, New York, für ihre wertvolle Unterstützung unserer Arbeiten.

Literatur

1. ROHRER, A.: Biochem. Z. **145**, 154 (1924).
2. WARBURG, O.: Pflügers Arch. ges. Physiol. **158**, 19, 189 (1914).
3. MARTIUS, C., and B. HESS: Arch. Biochem. **33**, 486 (1951).
4. LARDY, H. A., and G. FELDOTT: Ann. N. Y. Acad. Sci. **54**, 636 (1951).
5. HOCH, F. L.: Physiol. Rev. **42**, 605 (1962).
6. HESS, B., u. K. BRAND: Vortrag vor der Jahrestagung der Gesellschaft für Physiologische Chemie, Zürich 1960.
7. — In G. E. W. WOLSTENHOLME and C. M. O'CONNOR (eds) Ciba Foundation Symposium on the Regulation of Cell Metabolism, S. 124. London: J. and A. Churchill 1959.

8. CHANCE, B.: Proceedings of the Third International Congress of Biochemistry, Brussels 1955.
9. HOCH, F. L., and F. LIPMANN: Proc. Acad. Sci. (Wash.) 40, 909 (1954).
10. CHANCE, B., and G. HOLLUNGER: Fed. Proc. 16, 163 (1957).
11. HESS, B., and B. CHANCE: J. biol. Chem. 234, 2413 (1959).
12. KLINGENBERG, M., W. SLENCZKA u. E. RITT: Biochem. Z. 332, 47 (1959).
13. —, u. P. SCHOLLMEYER: Biochem. Z. 333, 335 (1960).
14. AZZONE, G. F., and L. ERNSTER: Nature (Lond.) 187, 65 (1960).
15. CHANCE, B., and G. HOLLUNGER: Nature (Lond.) 185 666 (1960).
16. HESS, B., u. K. BRAND: Unveröffentlichte Versuche.
17. Martius, C., u. B. HESS: Biochem. Z. 236, 191 (1955).
18. BRONK, I. R.: Biochim. biophys. Acta 37, 327 (1960).
19. BRAND, K.: Inaugural-Dissertation, Heidelberg 1962.
20. SOKOLOFF, L., and S. KAUFMANN: J. biol. Chem. 236. 795 (1961).
21. RAAFLAUB, I.: Helv. physiol. pharmacol. Acta 11, 142 (1953).
22. PACKER, L.: J. biol. Chen. 235, 242 (2960).
23. LEHNINGER, A. L., B. L. RAY and M. SCHNEIDER: J. biophys. biochem. Cytol. 5, 97 (1959).
24. — Physiol. Rev. 42, 467 (1962).
25. PACKER, L., and R. H. GOLDER: J. biol. Chem. 235, 1234 (1960).
26. RAAFLAUB, I.: Helv. physiol. pharmacol. Acta 10, c22 (1952).
27. TAPLEY, D. F., and C. COOPER: Nature (Lond.) 178, 1119 (1956).
28. KLEMPERER, H.: Biochem. J. 60 122 (1955).
29. HESS, B., u. B. CHANCE: Naturwissenschaften 46, 248 (1959).
30. TATA, J. R.: Recent Progr. Hormone Res. 18, 221 (1962).
31. KLEMPERER, H. G.: Biochem. J. 60, 128 (1955).
32. CARR, E. A., JR., and D. S. RIGGS: Biochem. J. 54, 217 (1953).
33. KENDALL, E. C.: Trans. Amer. Ass. Phycns 30, 420 (1915).
34. NIEMANN, C., and C. E. REDEMANN: J. Amer. chem. Soc. 69, 1549 (1941).
35. PITT-RIVERS, R., and J. R. TATA: The Thyroid Hormones, 103. London, New York, Paris, Los Angeles: Pergamon Press 1959.
36. EVERT, H. E.: Fed. Proc. 12, 201 (1953).
37. LARDY, H. A.: Biological Structure and Function. London: Acad. Press 2, 265 (1961).
38. ERNSTER, L.: Oxydative phosphorylation and its reversal. In: Funktionelle und Morphologische Organisation der Zelle. S. 98, Berlin-Göttingen-Heidelberg: Springer 1963.
39. LEE, Y. P., A. E. TAKEMORI and H. LARDY: J. biol. Chem. 234, 3051 (1959).
40. KLINGENBERG, M., and TH. BÜCHER: Ann. Rev. Biochem. 29, 669 (1960).
41. KARLSON, P.: Dtsch. med. Wschr. 86, 668 (1961).
42. HESS, B.: Control of Metabolic rates. In: Control mechanism in respiration and fermentation. 333—350. Herausg. v. B. WRIGHT. New York: Ronald Press 1963.
43. GRIES, F. A., F. MATSCHINSKY and O. WIELAND: Biochim. biophys. Acta 56, 615 (1962).
44. HESS, B., u. K. BRAND: Biochem. Z. 338, 376—380 (1963).

Diskussion

F. SEELICH (Wien):

Nach den Ausführungen von Herrn HESS scheint die Dejodierung und Elektronenaufnahme des organisch gebundenen Jod keine unmittelbare Beziehung zur Wirkung der Schilddrüsenhormone zu haben. Ich wäre für eine etwas ausführliche Begründung dieser Auffassung dankbar.

B. HESS:

Die Dejodierung des Schilddrüsenhormons hat meines Erachtens für die katalytische Funktion des Hormons keine Bedeutung, sondern muß als ein wichtiges Regulativ des Eigenumsatzes des Schilddrüsenhormons in der Zelle angesehen werden. Gegen eine Beteiligung an der Funktion des Hormons sprechen folgende Gesichtspunkte: die Dejodierung ist in den Mikrosomen lokalisiert, sie ist in der Peripherie irreversibel und verläuft schließlich viel zu langsam, um die rasche Wirkung des Hormons auf die oxydative Phosphorylierung erklären zu können.

R. POCHE (Düsseldorf):

Herr HESS sprach davon, daß die Mitochondrien der Gegenstand sind, an dem sich Biochemie und Morphologie berühren, wenn auch die Ausgangspunkte unterschiedlich sind. Der Biochemiker arbeitet an Mitochondrien, die aus dem Milieu der Zelle herausgelöst worden sind, macht also einen in vitro-Versuch; bei unseren morphologischen Untersuchungen handelt es sich dagegen um in vivo-Versuche am ganzen Tier, bei denen das Untersuchungsmaterial in Narkose entnommen und sofort fixiert wird. Um so bemerkenswerter und erfreulicher ist es, daß die Ergebnisse beider Forschungsrichtungen in vielen Punkten gut übereinstimmen. So kann ich die Ausführungen von Herrn HESS, daß sich aus verschiedenen Organen isolierte Mitochondrien unterschiedlich verhalten können, daß also Mitochondrion nicht gleich Mitochondrion gesetzt werden darf, auch vom morphologischen Standpunkt aus nur unterstreichen: Beispielsweise kommt es nach Überdosierung von Thyroxin in den Leberzellen zu viel stärkeren Mitochondrienschwellungen als in den Herzmuskelzellen. Wir haben aber auch am gleichen Organ zwischen einzelnen Tierarten, wie Ratte und Hund, Unterschiede gefunden. Ich möchte deshalb Herrn HESS fragen, ob isolierte Mitochondrien, die aus dem gleichen Organ stammen, ebenfalls bei verschiedenen Tierarten unterschiedlich reagieren.

B. HESS:

Der elektronenoptische Vergleich der Struktur von Mitochondrien und Sarkosomen in situ sowie nach Isolierung zeigt keine wesentlichen Unterschiede. Gleichfalls konnten wir mit biochemischen Methoden den Funktionszustand von Mitochondrien und Sarkosomen in situ sowie nach Isolation vergleichen und nachweisen, daß kein wesentlicher Unterschied zwischen beiden besteht. Man kann also heute ruhig annehmen, daß sich isolierte Mitochondrien strukturell wie funktionell nicht von den intracellulären Mitochondrien unterscheiden.

Laboratoire de Biochimie Médicale
Faculté de Médecine et de Pharmacie
Boulevard d'Alès — Marseille 5e

Désiodation des hormones thyroïdiennes

Par

Serge Lissitzky

Referat

La mise en évidence de la désiodation de la thyroxine in vivo a été réalisée depuis longtemps grâce à des expériences montrant que l'iode de l'hormone administrée à un animal était en grande partie éliminé dans les urines sous forme d'iodure minéral. Par contre, jusqu'en 1954 on ne savait pratiquement rien des systèmes biochimiques cellulaires responsables de cette désiodation. L'intérêt de les mieux connaître était pourtant essentiel en raison de ce que l'iode est un constituant spécifique des hormones thyroïdiennes et que sa présence dans la molécule est une condition nécessaire à leur activité biologique.

Deux problèmes principaux ont été posés conjointement concernant d'une part la nature du (ou des) système biochimique responsable de la désiodation et d'autre part la signification physiologique de cette dernière.

Cet article essaiera de préciser les réponses que, dans l'état actuel des données acquises, on peut donner à ces questions sur la base des résultats obtenus avec les systèmes in vitro[1].

De nombreux systèmes non enzymatiques sont capables de désioder la L-thyroxine[2] et la 3:5:3′-tri-iodo-L-thyronine en solution (Tableau 1).

On peut remarquer qu'ils appartiennent à deux catégories 1. systèmes contenant un métal, insensibles à l'action de la lumière ou 2. systèmes contenant un pigment, photosensibles.

Tous, à des degrès divers sont générateurs de radicaux libres et en particulier de radicaux OH. Outre l'iodure, les autres produits détectables de la réaction de désiodation sont indiqués dans le Tableau 2. La 3:5-di-iodotyrosine est régulière-

Tableau 1. *Systèmes non enzymatiques réalisant la désiodation de T_4 et T_3 en solution*

	Nature	Référence
1	lumière, rayons X	*4*
2	H_2O_2—Fe^{++} (réactif de Fenton)	
3	ascorbate-Fe^{++}—O_2—EDTA	*5*
4	Cu^{++}-biquinoline	*6*
5	FMN (ou bleu de méthylène)-oxygène-lumière	*7, 8, 9, 10*

[1] Quelques articles généraux ont déjà été publiés sur cette question. Ils pourront être utilement consultés par le lecteur qui y trouvera une bibliographie plus complète (*1*) (*2*) (*3*) (*3a*).

[2] Abréviations utilisées : T_4 : L-thyroxine; T_3 : 3 : 5 : 3′-tri-iodo-L-thyronine; DIT : 3 : 5-di-iodo-L-tyrosine; FMN : flavinemononucléotide.

ment formée indiquant que tous ces systèmes produisent une rupture de la liaison diphényléther de la molécule des hormones.

Tableau 2. *Produits formés au cours de la désiodation de T_4 et T_3 par divers systèmes non enzymatiques*

Système	Produits formés à partir de	
	T_4	T_3
lumière (pH 9 à 12)	I^-, DIT	I^-, DIT
ascorbate-Fe^{++}-O_2-EDTA	I^- (traces)	I^-, DIT
Cu^{++}-biquinoline	I^-, DIT	I^- (traces)
FMN BM $\Big\}$ -O_2-lumière	I^-, DIT, 3 : 3' : 5'-tri-iodothyronine	I^-, DIT

Dans le cas du système FMN-oxygène-lumière, la 3:3':5'-tri-iodothyronine a pu être caractérisée avec certitude en petite quantité comme produit de la réaction à côté de DIT prépondérante. Ceci indique la possibilité de deux voies de dégradation désiodante de la thyroxine, l'une majoritaire avec élimination des atomes d'iode en 3':5' sous forme d'iodure minéral et formation de DIT par rupture du pont diphényléther, l'autre, minoritaire, où les atomes d'iode des positions 3 et 5 partiraient en premier puis ceux en 3':5' et aboutissant à la formation de thyronine.

L'étude des systèmes biologiques capables de catalyser la désiodation des hormones sans modifier le radical alanyl, commencée il y a une dizaine d'années, n'a pas encore abouti à des résultats bien clairs quant à la nature du (ou des) système(s) enzymatique(s) fonctionnant in vivo.

On rappelera que des enzymes d'oxydation tels que la polyphénoloxydase de champignon (*11*) ou la peroxydase de raifort (*12*) sont capables de désioder les hormones plus ou moins activement. Jusqu' à présent il n'a pas été possible de rapporter l'activité désiodante des tissus animaux sur les hormones à la présence de l'un ou de l'autre de ces enzymes.

Des coupes, des homogénats ou des extraits par des solutions diluées de KCl de nombreux tissus (froie, rein, cerveau) de mammifères (rat, lapin) désiodent lentement les hormones pour des pH compris entre 6 et 7,5 et à 37°. Une caractéristique remarquable de l'activité désiodante des coupes et des homogénats de foie et de rein de rat est leur grande résistance à l'action inhibitrice de la chaleur. D'une manière générale cette thermostabilité disparaît pour les fractions acellulaires (mitochondries, microsomes) par centrifugation différentielle d'homogénats ou avec les préparations d'enzyme soluble (thyroxine-désiodase).

Trois systèmes enzymatiques principaux ont été décrits au cours de ces dernières années. Leurs caractéristiques essentielles sont résumées dans le Tableau 3.

Des préparations enzymatiques solubles ont été obtenues (*13*) (*15*) à partir des muscles squelettiques ou le foie de lapin. Elles catalysent la désiodation de T_4 et à un moindre degré de T_3 en présence de FMN, d'oxygène et de lumière, chacun de ces facteurs étant indispensable à l'activité de la préparation enzymatique. L'addition d'ions ferreux est sans effet ou inhibitrice à forte concentration. L'activité est essentiellement contenue dans les mitochondries mais les microsomes sont également actifs, à un moindre degré cependant.

Tableau 3. *Systèmes enzymatiques catalysant la désiodation de T_4 et T_3*

Origine	Forme et localisation cellulaire	pH optimum	Facteurs nécessaires	Inhibiteurs	Références
Muscle squelettique, Foie (Lapin, rat)	1) mitochondries (microsomes accessoirement) 2) enzyme soluble (thyroxine-désiodase) obtenu à partir des mitochondries	6,0 à 6,4	FMN, oxygène, lumière	réducteurs, diéthyl-stilbestrol, cytochrome C, TBP, Fe^{++}	LISSITZKY et al. (*14*) (*15*), TATA (*13*), YAMAMOTO et al. (*16*)
Foie, rein (rat)	microsomes	6 à 7	Fe^{++} cystéine ou GSH, acide ascorbique, oxygène, prétraitement par la chaleur,	versène, catéchol, cyanures, p-chloromer-curibenzoate	STANBURY (*17*)
Foie (rat)	microsomes	4,5 à 5	Fe^{++}, Oxygène, pré-incubation	certains agents réducteurs, chélateurs, composés phénoliques (DOPA, hydro-quinone)	WYNN et al. (*18*)

Les deux autres systèmes sont constitués par des microsomes de foie de rat. Celui décrit par STANBURY (*17*) est thermostable, nécessite un préchauffage de deux minutes à 100° et la présence d'ions ferreux, d'oxygène et de glutathion réduit, d'acide ascorbique ou de cystéine. Le versène, le catéchol et les cyanures sont inhibiteurs. WYNN, GIBBS et ROYSTER (*18*) ont confirmé l'activité du système microsomal de foie de rat, le rôle activateur des ions ferreux et celui inhibiteur des chélateurs et de l'absence d'oxygène. Par contre, et en contradiction avec les expériences de STANBURY, ces auteurs n'ont pas pu mettre en évidence le rôle activateur d'aucun composé réducteur.

Malgré quelques différences, il paraît cependant vraisemblable de penser que les réactions observées sont les mêmes, ayant comme caractéristique essentielle l'activation par les ions ferreux et que les différences peuvent s'expliquer du fait d'inhibiteurs ou d'activateurs contaminant les préparations brutes utilisées. Par contre, ces deux systèmes semblent très différents du système mitochondrial activé par le FMN et la lumière.

Récemment (*19*), on a pu obtenir une préparation enzymatique soluble à partir de mitochondries de foie de rat par extraction avec KCl 0,15 M. Une telle préparation est activée par FMN et lumière en présence d'oxygène mais elle est insensible à l'addition d'ions ferreux dans une large zone de concentration et dans différentes conditions de milieu dont celles décrites par WYNN et al (*18*).

D'autre part, si les microsomes de foie de rat sont bien activés par les ions ferreux ou le FMN à la lumière, il n'en est pas de même des mitochondries qui sont totalement insensibles à l'addition des ions ferreux (Tableau 4). De plus si la présence de catalase est indifférente ou même augmente l'activité désiodante des microsomes en présence de FMN, elle inhibe par contre fortement ce même système en présence d'ions ferreux (Tableau 5).

Le système dépendant de FMN est de plus insensible à l'action des formateurs de complexes métalliques. Il apparaît donc que deux systèmes enzymatiques distincts catalysant la désiodation des hormones thyroïdiennes existent dans le foie de rat, l'un mitochondrial dépendant de FMN, insensible à ou activé par la catalase, l'autre microsomal dépendant des ions ferreux et inhibé par la catalase. Tous deux nécessitent de l'oxygène et sont peu ou pas actifs en l'absence de cofacteurs.

Il est à noter que l'activité désiodante spontanée des coupes ou homogénats est toujours très faible et ne peut être mise en évidence qu'après des temps d'incubation prolongés et des concentrations en substrat très élevées par rapport aux concentrations physiologiques en hormones. Ces caractéristiques ne sont pas rencontrées pour les préparations solubles ou les fractions acellulaires.

Cette différence est explicable par la présence dans les cellules et dans le sang de protéines capables de fixer la thyroxine (TBP), l'union des hormones avec les TBP les protégeant vis-à-vis de l'action catalytique des enzymes, proportionnellement à la fraction fixée (3) (20).

Le principal composé iodé formé au cours de la désiodation de T_4 et T_3 par tous les systèmes biologiques étudiés est l'iodure. Cependant il s'accumule toujours concomitamment un matériel iodé de $R_f = 0$ dans la plupart des

Tableau 4. *Désiodation de la* L-*thyroxine par des mitochondries ou des microsomes de foie de rat en présence d'ions ferreux ou de flavinemononucléotide*

Conditions	Nature des particules	Thyroxine dégradée (%)
1	mitochondries	0
	microsomes	20,4
2	mitochondries	14,9
	microsomes	15,7

Conditions 1. [I^{131}]-L-thyroxine, concentration finale $2,5 \times 10^{-6}$ M et 2 μc dans 0,25 ml de propane-1:2-diol à 10%; 0,5 ml de suspension de mitochondries ou de microsomes dans le saccharose 0,25 M correspondant à 50 mg de foie frais; 0,5 ml de $FeSO_4$ 5×10^{-3} M et 3,75 ml de tampon phosphate 0,05 M de pH 6,5.

Préincubation pendant 5 min de tous les éléments du milieu moins les particules puis, après addition de celles-ci, incubation pendant 10 min à 37° à l'air avec agitation de 60 RPM dans l'appareil de WARBURG.

Conditions 2. Même composition du milieu mais $FeSO_4$ est remplacé par FMN à la concentration finale de 5×10^{-6} M. Mêmes conditions d'incubation mais sous illumination très faible. Mesure de la désiodation par précipitation à l'acide trichloracétique (concentration finale 5%) après addition de 1 ml de sérum.

Les témoins contenaient les mêmes constituants à l'exception des particules.

Tableau 5. *Action de la catalase sur la désiodation de la* L-*thyroxine par les microsomes de foie de rat en présence d'ions ferreux ou de flavinemononucléotide*

	L-thyroxine dégradée (%)	
	sans catalase	avec catalase
Système 1 (Fe^{++}, 5×10^{-4} M)	23,3	1,1
Système 2 (FMN, 5×10^{-6} M)	10,0	17,5

Même composition des milieux que dans les expériences décrites dans le Tableau 4 et mêmes conditions d'incubation. Pour les essais avec catalase, 0,1 mg de catalase de boeuf 2 × cristallisée (Sigma, St-Louis, Miss. U.S.A.) a été ajouté au milieu. Les résultats correspondent à la moyenne de trois expériences différentes avec essais en double. Les chiffres extrêmes ne s'éloignent pas de la valeur moyenne de plus de 5%.

solvants chromatographiques et qui correspond à des protéines iodées (*21* (*22*) (*3*) (*23*). Ce matériel se forme avec tous les systèmes utilisés en présence comme en l'absence d'activateurs.

Il vient d'être montré en utilisant comme substrat de la thyroxine marquée en 3:5 ou en 3':5' (*24*) ou doublement marquée par H^3 et I^{131} (*25*) (*26*) que ces protéines iodées sont constituées par l'association de DIT provenant de la dégradation de l'hormone unies par des liaisons non covalentes avec certaines protéines du milieu. La spécificité des protéines intervenant dans la formation de ce matériel reste à établir. Cependant Roche, Nunez et Jacquemin (*27*) viennent de suggérer, en utilisant des préparations très variées comme source d'activité désiodante, que l'hormone se fixerait dans un premier temps à un matériel protéique (probablement l'enzyme); dans un deuxième temps le complexe formé libérerait partiellement l'iodure et retiendrait la totalité du squelette carboné de l'iodothyronine, que l'on pourrait libérer comme Plaskett l'avait montré antérieurement (*24*) sans former de di-iodotyrosine. Tous les travaux récents ont par contre éliminé la possibilité d'une transiodation entre la thyroxine et les protéines du milieu suggérée précédemment (*13*).

Les milieux d'incubation de T_4 avec des préparations de foie ou de muscle squelettique de rat contiennent par ailleurs toujours de petites quantités de DIT libre (*8*). Accessoirement des traces de thyronine ont pu être mises en évidence (*28*).

Tous les auteurs sont d'accord pour éliminer T_3 comme produit intermédiaire de la réaction de désiodation de T_4.

Il semble donc bien que la voie principale de la désiodation des hormones thyroïdiennes par les tissus in vitro s'accompagne de la rupture du pont diphényl-ether de leur molécule avec formation de di-iodotyrosine et d'un complexe protéique intermédiaire dont la signification demeure à préciser.

Si, comme on a pu s'en rendre compte, la nature des systèmes enzymatiques catalysant la désiodation des hormones thyroïdiennes in vitro est encore très mal connue, la situation est encore plus obscure sur la réalité de l'intervention de ces systèmes in vivo.

En ce qui concerne le système activé par FMN et la lumière, il est évidemment exclu que cette source d'énergie puisse entrer en jeu pour les tissus animaux. D'autre part de nombreux travaux ont montré son caractère non spécifique. Des protéines très variées peuvent remplacer les préparations tissulaires (*29*) et même des homogénats de Escherichia Coli chauffés ou non (observations non publiées) catalysent la désiodation de T_4 en présence de FMN, d'oxygène et de lumière selon un mécanisme analogue à celui manifesté par les mitochondries de foie de rat ou la «thyroxine-désiodase» soluble de muscles squelettiques de lapin.

On peut dès lors se demander si un système enzymatique activé par le FMN avec une source d'énergie chimique remplaçant l'énergie lumineuse fonctionne bien in vivo pour catalyser la désiodation des hormones thyroïdiennes. Des expériences récentes (*8*) réalisées à l'obscurité ont montré que dans un milieu permettant la glycolyse aérobie du fructose-1:6-diphosphate, le flavinemono-nucléotide produit une activation de la désiodation de la thyroxine par des homogénats de foie ou de muscle squelettique de rat, ce qui paraît pouvoir être un argument en faveur de ce que l'enzyme soluble isolé à partir de ces tissus pourrait être celui qui assure la désiodation in vivo. Le Tableau 6 montre les résultats obtenus dans une série d'expériences.

Tableau 6. *Effet conjugué du milieu de Reif-Potter-Le Page et de FMN sur la désiodation de la* L-*thyroxine par des homogénats de foie de rat a l'obscurité et à la lumière*

Milieu	FMN (M)	Distribution de la radioactivité sur les chromatogrammes (%)					
		obscurité			lumière		
		MO + I⁻	MO	I⁻	MO + I⁻	MO	I⁻
Phosphate	sans	26,0	6,9	19,1	16,8	4,2	12,3
Reif-Potter-Le Page	5×10^{-5} M	39,1	11,3	27,8	25,7	10,5	15,2
Phosphate	sans	27,6	6,9	20,7	80,4	14,4	66,0
Reif-Potter-Le Page	5×10^{-5} M	62,8	25,0	37,8	50,0	9,2	40,8

0,1 ml d'homogénat au 1/10e dans le saccharose 0,25 M; $[I^{131}]$-L-T_4: $2,5 \times 10^{-6}$ M et 2 μc; volume total: 1 ml; phosphate 0,1 M pH 7,4. Incubation pendant 45 min à 37°.

Mesure de la désiodation par chromatographie en n-butanol-ac. acétique-eau (78:5:17) et mesure de la distribution de la radioactivité sur les bandes chromatographiques à l'aide d'un dispositif automatique enregistreur. Pour les expériences à la lumière, les fioles ont été incubées dans un appareil de Warburg — photosynthèse dont l'illumination était réglée au 1/4 de la puissance totale.

MO = matériel-origine iodé de $R_f = 0$.

Le milieu de REIF-POTTER-LE PAGE (Cancer Research, 1953, *13*, 807) contient fructose-1:6-diphosphate, ATP, DPN, nicotinamide, cytochrome C, $MgCl_2$, $KHCO_3$, KH_2PO_4, Na_2HPO_4 et NaF.

Cependant le diphosphopyridine nucléotide sous forme oxydée ou réduite a le même effet activateur que FMN.

Les systèmes activés par les ions ferreux n'ont pas encore été étudiés sous un aspect intégré. L'impression générale qui ressort de l'ensemble des résultats disponibles est
1) le caractère ubiquitaire de la répartition des systèmes capables de désioder les hormones 2) le manque de données sur la nature de l'enzyme (ou des enzymes) impliqués dans la désiodation des hormones 3) le manque de corrélation entre les observations in vitro et in vivo.

Il est bon de rappeler que les conditions techniques très précises doivent être respectées pour obtenir des résultats significatifs concernant la désiodation eu égard aux nombreuses causes d'erreurs possibles (*15*) (*30*).

Les relations existant entre la désiodation des hormones et leur action physiologique sont encore fort imprécises.

Les principiales possibilités sont les suivantes:

1. la désiodation est liée spécifiquement à l'action des hormones thyroïdiennes sur le métabolisme cellulaire en donnant naissance à des composés plus immédiatement actifs;

2. la désiodation est un mécanisme d'inactivation des hormones thyroïdiennes et de régulation de leur taux cellulaire;

3. la désiodation est une manifestation non spécifique de l'activité métabolique cellulaire.

Ces hypothèses ont été discutées récemment (*1*) (*3a*) (*3*) (*32*).

La première est la plus séduisante. TATA (*31*) dans une étude de la désiodation de la thyroxine par les muscles squelettiques chez le rat normal ou thyroïdectomisé a pu conclure que la désiodation enzymatique des hormones thyroïdiennes devait être liée d'une manière ou d'une autre à leur action calorigénique, bien que la nature exacte de cette relation demeure obscure. Cependant, dans ces expériences, les études de désiodation ont été réalisées en présence de FMN et à la lumière ce qui enlève beaucoup de signification aux valeurs trouvées en raison du caractère non spécifique de l'activation photochimique due au FMN.

GALTON et INGBAR (*32*) ont observé que le foie de têtard désiodait activement les hormones thyroïdiennes alors que cette propriété n'existait plus dans le foie de la grenouille adulte. Ils ont relié cette observation au fait que la grenouille adulte ne répondait plus à l'action des composés à action thyroïdienne, contrairement au têtard. Il apparaitrait ainsi que, chez la grenouille, la transition de la forme larvaire à la forme adulte est associée à une diminution ou une perte de la capacité de désioder les hormones thyroïdiennes. Ces résultats sont en faveur de l'hypothèse que certaines actions métaboliques des hormones pourraient être liées à leur désiodation mais n'en apporte pas la preuve. Il ne semble pas en outre que des composés plus actifs que les hormones se forment au cours de leur désiodation. En particulier la $3:5:3'$-tri-iodothyronine n'est pas un produit ou un intermédiaire de la réaction de désiodation de la thyroxine. De plus la formation de protéines iodées au cours de la désiodation des hormones ne paraît pas être particulièrement spécifique des enzymes de désiodation des hormones, car elle est observée avec de nombreuses protéines banales (*29*) au cours de la désiodation induite par les flavines en présence de lumière.

L'existence de nombreuses protéines cellulaires capables de fixer les hormones et ce faisant de les rendre insensibles à l'action des enzymes de désiodation paraît par contre militer en faveur d'un rôle de la désiodation dans l'inactivation et la régulation de leur taux cellulaire (*1*). Cependant comme on ne sait pas si la désiodation intervient après ou avant que les hormones ait exercé leur activité à l'interieur de la cellule, cette hypothèse, bien que vraisemblable, n'a pas encore pu être démontrée.

Enfin il est possible que la désiodation soit simplement une manifestation non spécifique de l'activité métabolique cellulaire.

Des travaux récents ont montré que, pour des homogénats de foie ou de muscle squelettique de rat, toute augmentation de la consommation d'oxygène liée au maintient ou à l'activation de la glycolyse aérobie, s'accompagne d'une augmentation parallèle de la désiodation de la thyroxine (travaux non publiés).

De plus amples recherches sont nécessaires pour préciser le rôle physiologique de la désiodation des hormones thyroïdiennes et la nature des enzymes responsables. Cependant quelques bases expérimentales existent dès maintenant in vitro dont il serait utile de vérifier le bien fondé in vivo.

Bibliographie

1. LISSITZKY, S.: VIII Congresso Nazionale de la Societa di Endocrinologia. Simposio su gli ipertiroidismi, Napoli 18—19 Déc. 1959, p. 7. Pisa: Giardini Ed.
2. PITT-RIVERS, R., et J. TATA: The Thyroid Hormones, 1 vol. 247 p. Pergamon Press 1959.
3. LISSITZKY, S.: Bull. Soc. Chim. biol. (Paris) **42**, 1187 (1960).
3a. — Exposés Annuels de Biochimie Médicale. Paris: Masson Ed. 1961.
4. LEIN, A., et R. MICHEL: C. R. Soc. Biol. (Paris) **153**, 538 (1959).
5. LISSITZKY, S., et M. ROQUES: Bull. Soc. Chim. biol. (Paris) **39**, 521 (1957).

6. — — C. R. Soc. Biol. (Paris) **152**, 1333 (1958).
7. — M. T. Benevent et M. Roques: Biochim. biophys. Acta **51**, 407 (1961).
8. Benevent, M. T., M. Roques, J. Torresani et S. Lissitzky: Bull. Soc. Chim. biol. (Paris) sous presse.
9. Susuki, M., I. Ishikawa, S. Shimizu et K. Yamamoto: Biochim. biophys. Acta **51**, 402 (1961).
10. Galton, V. A., and S. H. Ingbar: Endocrinology **70**, 210 (1962).
11. Lissitzky, S., et S. Bouchilloux: Ciba Colloquia Endocrinology **10**, 135 (1957).
12. Mayrargue-Kokja, A., S. Bouchilloux et S. Lissitzky: Bull. Soc. Chim. biol. (Paris) **40**, 815 (1958).
13. Tata, J. R.: Biochem. J. **77**, 214 (1960).
14. Lissitzky, S.: Radioaktive Isotope in Klinik und Forschung, in Strahlentherapie 4, 301 (1960).
15. — M. Roques et M. T. Benevent: Bull. Soc. Chim. biol. (Paris) **43**, 727, 743 (1961).
16. Yamamoto, K., S. Shimizu and I. Ishikawa: Jap. J. Physiol. **10**, 610 (1960).
17. Stanbury, J. B.: Ann. N. Y. Acad. Sci. **86**, 417 (1960).
18. Wynn, J., R. Gibbs and B. Royster: J. biol. Chem. **237**, 1892 (1962).
19. Manté, S., et S. Lissitzky: Bull. Soc. biol. (Paris) en préparation.
20. Tata, J. R.: Bull. Soc. Chim. biol. (Paris) **42**, 1171 (1960).
21. Plaskett, L. G.: Nature (Lond.) **181**, 273 (1958).
22. Tata, J. R.: Biochim. biophys. Acta **35**, 567 (1959).
23. Galton, V. A., and S. H. Ingbar: Endocrinology **69**, 30 (1961).
24. Plaskett, L. G.: Biochem. J. **78**, 652 (1961).
25. Nunez, J., et Cl. Jaquemin: C. R. Acad. Sci. (Paris) **249**, 138 (1959).
26. — — C. R. Acad. Sci. (Paris) **252**, 802 (1961).
27. Roche, J., J. Nunez et Cl. Jaquemin: Biochim. biophys. Acta (Amst.) **69**, 271 (1963).
28. Lissitzky, S., M. T. Benevent, M. Roques et J. Roche: Bull. Soc. Chim. biol. (Paris) **41**, 1329 (1959).
29. Morreale de Escobar, G., F. Escobar del Rey et P. Llorente-Rodriguez: J. biol. Chem. **237**, PC 2041 (1962).
30. — P. Llorente-Rodriguez, T. Jolin-Buzo and F. Escobar del Rey: J. biol. Chem., sous presse.
31. Tata, J. R.: Acta endocr. (Kbh.) **37**, 125 (1961).
32. Galton, V. A., and S. H. Ingbar: Endocrinology **68**, 435 (1961).

Aus der 2. Med. Klinik und Poliklinik der Med. Akademie Düsseldorf
(Prof. Dr. K. Oberdisse)

Wirkung von Stoffwechselgiften und Thyroxin auf die Permeabilität intakter Zellen

Von

A. Englhardt

Mit 2 Abbildungen

Untersuchungen von Bruns am intakten Tier und von Zierler am isolierten Muskel hatten gezeigt, daß lebende Zellen unter bestimmten Bedingungen für Enzymeiweiß permeabel sind und daß diese Permeabilität eine Funktion des Zellstoffwechsels ist. Die Erhaltung des Konzentrationsgradienten zwischen enzymreichen Organzellen und dem enzymarmen Extracellulärraum kann nur durch Zufuhr freier Energie erhalten werden [Bruns (1)]. Um diese Gesetzmäßigkeiten weiter aufzuklären, wurden Untersuchungen an intakten lebenden isolierten Zellen (Leukocyten) durchgeführt. Diese führten zu Beobachtungen über die Wirkungsweise des Thyroxin auf die Zellpermeabilität, über die nachstehend berichtet wird.

Methodik. Leukocyten wurden aus dem Blut Gesunder nach einer bereits früher beschriebenen Methode (2) isoliert. Nach Inkubation in verschiedenen isotonen Lösungen über $^1/_2$ bis 8 Std wurden die Zellen durch Zentrifugieren entfernt und Aktivitätsmessungen einzelner Enzyme durchgeführt (LDH, MDH und GAPDH). Enzymtests nach Delbrück, Zebe und Bücher (2a). Inkubation bei 37 Grad. Gasphase 95% O_2 + 5% CO_2, bzw. Luft. Folgende Inkubationslösungen wurden verwendet: Isotone NaCl- bzw. KCL-Lösung, Thyrode, Krebs-Ringer-Bicarbonat, sowie eine isotone Salzlösung, die unter dem Namen Sterisal hergestellt wird. Die Lösungen wurden vor Gebrauch sterilisiert. Folgende Stoffwechselinhibitoren wurden getestet: 2—4 Dinitrophenol 10^{-5}—10^{-3} m, Monojodacetat, Na-Arsenat, NaN_3, NaF, NaCN in Konzentrationen 10^{-4}—10^{-2} m. Der Zusatz von 10^{-7}—10^{-2} L-Thyroxin erfolgte nach Lösen in 0,04 n NaOH zum gepufferten Medium bei p_H 7,5 in sehr kleinem Volumen. In einzelnen Versuchen wurde die Glucoseutilisation der Zellen nach Beck und Valentine (3) sowie die intracelluläre ATP-Konzentration nach Bücher bestimmt. Die Messung der optischen Absorption der Zellsuspensionen erfolgte in Anlehnung an eine von Lehninger für Mitochondrien ausgearbeitete Methode (4) bei 520 mμ am Beckmann-Photometer. Direkte gravimetrische Bestimmung des Feucht- und Trockengewichts zur Analyse des Hydratationszustands der Zellen. In einzelnen Versuchen flammenphotometrische Bestimmung des Na^+- und K^+-Gehalts des Suspensionsmediums.

Abkürzungen. LDH Lactatdehydrogenase, MDH Äpfelsäuredehydrogenase, PGADH Phosphoglycerinaldehyddehydrogenase. Tris: Tris (hydroxymethyl) aminomethan, Trap Triäthanolamin-Puffer.

Ergebnisse

Isolierte Leukocyten geben sowohl im Serum wie in isotonischen Lösungen mit oder ohne Zusatz von Glucose oder O_2-Sättigung zunehmend Enzyme an das Inkubationsmedium ab. Die Glucoseverwertung dieser Zellen sinkt im Lauf von Stunden auf nicht mehr exakt meßbare Werte ab, gleichzeitig sinkt die intracelluläre ATP-Konzentration. Der Enzymaustritt geht dem Zusammenbruch intracellulärer Stoffwechselprozesse zeitlich parallel. Wie frühere Versuche gezeigt hatten, erfolgt der Austritt der Enzyme in das Medium mit einer bestimmten, für das einzelne Enzym charakteristischen Geschwindigkeit. Diese ist unabhängig vom Konzentrationsgradienten des Enzyms zwischen Zelle und Extracellulärraum, steht aber in einer gewissen Relation zum Molekulargewicht (5).

Unter der Wirkung von Stoffwechselinhibitoren treten vermehrt Enzyme in die Inkubationslösung aus. Am wirksamsten waren Monojodacetat und NaF, weniger wirksam NaCN, Na-Arsenat (Na_2AsO_4) und NaN_3. Die Wirkung des

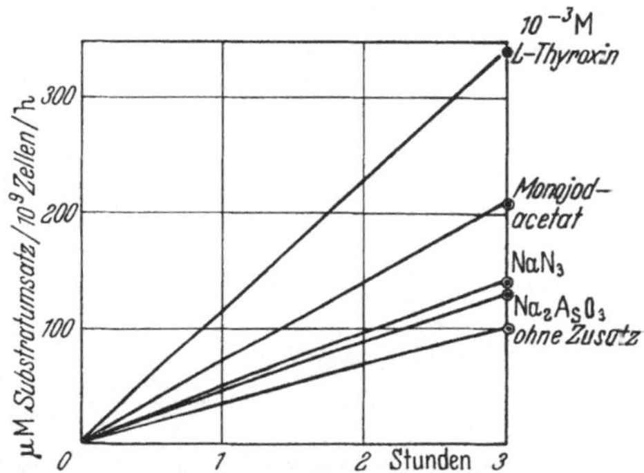

Abb. 1. Schwellung und Permeabilität weißer Blutzellen für Encyme und K^+. Inkubation bei Zimmertemperatur. Zeit 60 min. Messung der Absorption bei Wellenlänge 520 im Beckmannphotometer. Gravimetrische Bestimmung der Wasseraufnahme der Zellen. Abszisse: Zeit in Minuten. Ordinate D 520, LDH, GAPDH und MDH, sowie K^+ im Inkubationsmedium (isotone Salzlösung). Bei t_0 Zusatz von L-Thyroxin 10^{-3} m. Bei $t_{120\,min}$ gravimetrische Bestimmung der Aufnahme von H_2O. K^+-Abgabe und Wasseraufnahme in mMol bzw. µMol/10^6 Zellen

Thyroxin war bei niedrigen Konzentrationen ähnlich der der Stoffwechselgifte, wurde aber bei höheren wesentlich ausgeprägter. Bei Konzentrationen von 10^{-2} m kam es neben einer starken Enzymausschüttung zu einer bereits optisch nachweisbaren Zellschädigung (Klumpung, Quellung). Größere Meß-Serien zeigten, daß der Enzymaustritt zur Thyroxinkonzentration in gesetzmäßiger Beziehung steht. Durch Änderung der Osmolarität der Lösung konnte die Thyroxinwirkung potenziert werden (Abb. 1).

Bei höheren Thyroxindosen waren bereits makroskopisch Änderungen des Hydratationszustands der Zellen nachweisbar. Durch quantitative Bestimmung des Zellwassergehalts konnten wir zeigen, daß unter Thyroxin eine deutliche Schwellung auftritt. Wir haben diesen Effekt mit einer von LEHNINGER für Mitochondrien angewendete Methode der Lichtabsorptionsmessung weiter geprüft (6). Diese soll eine empfindliche Volumenbestimmung von Erythrocyten (7) und Mitochondrien darstellen (8). PACKER konnte damit auch an Ehrlich-Ascites-Tumorzellen Schwellungsprozesse nachweisen (9). Leukocyten zeigten ebenfalls eine leichte Abnahme der Lichtabsorption bei 520 mμ, die unter Thyroxin wesentlich ausgeprägter wurde. Der Effekt trat bereits bei Konzentrationen von 10^{-6} m auf. Die Ergebnisse der gravimetrischen Analyse sprechen dafür, daß dieser durch einen Schwellungsprozeß bedingt ist (Abb. 2). Laufende Bestimmungen über 1—2 Std zeigten, daß die Abnahme der Lichtabsorption der Zunahme der Enzymaktivität im Suspensionsmedium zeitlich konform geht. Dagegen konnte unter Thyroxin ein vermehrter Austritt von K^+, Na^+ und Phosphat nicht beobachtet werden. Die

Extinktionsabnahme im Lichtabsorptionstest blieb aus, wenn dem Medium ATP
($10^{-3}-10^{-2}$ m) zugesetzt wurde, bei höheren Konzentrationen (10^{-2} m) kam es
sogar einige Male zu einer Zunahme der Absorption. Damit konnte ein weiterer
von Lehninger an Mitochondrien beobachteter Effekt an intakten Zellen reproduziert werden. Ein Einfluß von ATP auf die Enzympermeabilität konnte nicht
geprüft werden, da ATP in diesen Konzentrationen einen direkten Hemmeffekt
auf die Enzyme des Inkubationsmediums ausübt.

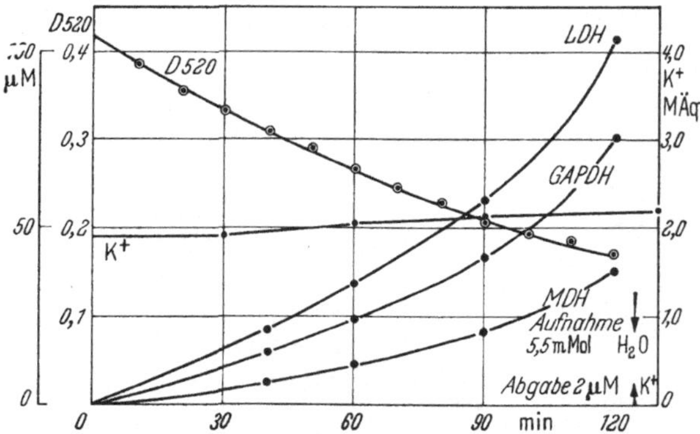

Abb. 2. Enzymaustritt aus weißen Blutzellen. Einfluß von Stoffwechselgiften auf die Permeabilität weißer Blutzellen für Enzymeiweiß. Inkubation in isotoner Salzlösung ph 6.9. Temp. 37 Grad. Abszisse: Zeit in Stunden.
Ordinate: LDH-Aktivitätt in μMol/10⁹ Zellen/h. B: Zusatz der Substanzen zum Medium in der Endkonzentration
von 10^{-3} m

Diskussion

Bereits elektronenoptische Untersuchungen an Leberzellen [Schulz u. Mitarb.
(10)] und an Herzmuskeln [Poche (10, 12)] hatten Wirkungen des Thyroxin nicht
nur an Mitochondrien, sondern auch auf das Zellprotoplasma (Schwellung des
Ergastoplasma bzw. Sarkoplasmareticulum) ergeben. Eigene Untersuchungen
lassen ähnliche Veränderungen auch an intakten isolierten Blutzellen annehmen.
Dabei muß die Frage nach einem Angriffspunkt des Thyroxin an der Zellmembran
in den Vordergrund der Diskussion gestellt werden. Lehninger hat bereits einen
Einfluß des Thyroxin auf die Mitochondrienmembranen diskutiert (6, 13, 14). Er
postuliert, daß die Enzyme der Atemkette Energie nicht nur in energiereiche
Phosphatbindungen, sondern auch in mechanische Energie umwandeln können.
Dieses „Mechanoenzymsystem" soll, in Abhängigkeit vom Oxydo-Reduktions-
zustand der Atemkette, Änderungen an der molekularen Konfiguration oder
Anordnung der Membran hervorrufen können, die eine Änderung der Permeabilität sowie des Volumens herbeiführen können. Diese Hypothese ist wohl für
Mitochondrien, nicht aber für intakte Zellen anwendbar, da die Atemketten-
enzyme in den Strukturen der Mitochondrien lokalisiert sind. Jedoch enthält die
Zellmembran selbst Enzyme, die an Transportmechanismen beteiligt sind (ATP-
asen 15, Phosphatidsäurephosphatase 16). Es ist zu diskutieren, ob solche enzymatisch aktiven Proteine der Membranschichten solche „Mechanoenzym"-
funktionen übernehmen können.

Die Beobachtung des Phänomens des Eiweißdurchtritts durch die für Eiweißmoleküle normalerweise impermeable Zellmembran führt zur Besprechung weiterer

Probleme. Allein ein Vergleich der bekannten Porenradien tierischer Organzellen (3,5—7,1 Å) (*17, 18*) mit dem molekularen Radius des Eiweißmoleküls läßt erkennen, daß eine Zunahme der Porengröße bis zu einer Durchlässigkeit für Eiweißmoleküle (Durchmesser des Aldolasemoleküls 100 Å) (*19*) nicht denkbar ist, auch dann nicht, wenn durch Schwellung eine starke mechanische Dehnung eingetreten ist. Ähnliche Fragen ergaben sich beim Studium der Hämolyse roter Blutzellen. Auch hier ist der Mechanismus des Durchtritts des Hämoglobins unter dem Einfluß der osmotisch bedingten Schwellung ungeklärt (*20*). Direkte Wirkungen des Thyroxin auf die Innenschichten der Mitochondrienmembran im Sinne einer Fragmentierung der Membran wurden vielfach beobachtet (*11, 12, 13*). An intakten Zellen stehen solche Untersuchungen noch aus.

Es ist bekannt, daß sowohl die Phänomene der Schwellung wie des Enzymdurchtritts unspezifisch sind. Die Membranpermeabilität für Enzyme wird nach unseren Beobachtungen auch noch durch Hämolysegifte in niedriger Konzentration, durch Tetrachlorkohlenstoff und starke pH-Verschiebungen gesteigert.

Auch das Phänomen der Schwellung kann durch eine große Zahl von Substanzen hervorgerufen werden, die aber nach LEHNINGER sämtlich in den Zellstoffwechsel eingreifen (*6*). Allein schon daraus geht hervor, daß aus diesen Befunden ein Rückschluß auf biologische Wirkungen des Hormons nicht erlaubt ist. Dies wird weiter bestätigt durch die Tatsache, daß die beschriebenen Effekte nur unter hohen Hormondosen auftreten. Die Untersuchungen zeigen aber, daß die Wirkungsweise der Hormone sowohl mit der Struktur der Zellelemente wie mit der Dynamik des Zellstoffwechsels verknüpft ist.

Literatur

1. BRUNS, F. H., E. BOSSWITZ, H. DENNEMANN, H. D. HORN u. E. NOLTMANN: Klin. Wschr. 7, 342—346 (1961).
2. LÖHR, G. W., u. H. D. WALLER: In: Methoden der enzymatischen Analyse, S. 744 H. U. BERGMEYER. Weinheim, Bergstraße: Verlag Chemie GmbH.
2a. DELBRÜCK, A., E. ZEBE u. TH. BÜCHER: Biochem. Z. **331**, 273 (1959).
3. BECK, W. S., and W. N. VALENTINE: Cancer Res. **12**, 823 (1952).
4. LEHNINGER, A. L.: Physiol. Rev. **42**, 467 (1962).
5. ENGLHARDT, A.: Vortrag 10. Colloquium über die Proteide der menschlichen Körperflüssigkeiten. Brügge 1962.
6. LEHNINGER, A. L.: J. biol. Chem. **234**, 2187 (1959).
7. u. 8. Zit. nach 4.
9. Zit. nach 4.
10. SCHULZ, H., H. LÖW, L. ERNSTER u. F. S. SJÖSTRAND: Elektronenmikroskopy Proc., Stockholm Conf., Stockholm 1957.
11. POCHE, R.: Beitr. path. Anat. 118, 407—420 (1957).
12. —, u. W. LOCHNER: Frankfurt. Z. Path. 72, 34 (1962).
13. LEHNINGER, A. L., and B. L. RAY: Biochim. biophys. Acta **26**, 643 (1957).
14. — J. biol. Chem. **234**, 2465 (1959).
15. POST, R. L., and C. D. ALBRIGHT: In: Membran Transport and Metabolism. S. 219. Prag, August 1960.
16. HOKIN, L. E., and M. R. HOKIN: In: Membran Transport and Metabolism. Prag, August 1960.
17. GORIN, M. H.: J. chem. Phys. **7**, 405 (1939).
18. SOLOMON, A. K.: In: Membran Transport and Metabolism. Prag, August 1960.
19. ZIERLER, K. L.: Amer. J. Physiol. **193**, 3 (1958).
20. LINDEMANN, B.: Naunyn-Schmiedeberg's Arch. exp. Path. Pharm. **206**, 197 (1949).

Aus der II. Medizinischen Klinik der Universität München
(Direktor: Prof. Dr. Dr. G. BODECHTEL)

Der Einfluß von androgenen und oestrogenen Hormonen auf das PBI im Blut des Menschen.[1]

Von

K. KOPETZ, K. VOLKMER und K. SCHWARZ

Wir hatten vor 3 Jahren auf dem Symposion in Homburg Gelegenheit, über Veränderungen der Plasmacorticosteroide unter dem Einfluß von Oestrogenen zu berichten (*1*). Zwischen dem Verhalten der Corticosteroide im Plasma und dem des eiweißgebundenen Jods besteht eine weitgehende Parallelität. Beide Hormone zeigen in der Schwangerschaft (*2—7*) und ebenso nach Zufuhr exogener Oestrogene einen Anstieg, der weit über den physiologischen Bereich hinausgeht, ohne daß sich Zeichen eines Hyperkortizismus oder einer Hyperthyreose einstellen (*8, 9*). Für das eiweißgebundene Jod ist weiterhin gesichert, daß es durch Zufuhr androgener Hormone zu einem Absinken des Plasmaspiegels kommt. Dieser entspricht oft Werten, wie sie beim Myxödem gefunden werden, ohne daß klinische Symptome der Unterfunktion auftreten (*10—12*). Die zu besprechenden Untersuchungen sollten das Verhalten des PBIs unter dem Einfluß einer Oestrogen-Androgen-Kombination klären und die Dosisrelation bestimmen, bei der sich der stimulierende Effekt der Oestrogene (Oe) durch die depressive Wirkung des Androgenzusatzes aufheben läßt. Außerdem sollten Veränderungen des eiweißgebundenen Jods bei Lebercirrhosen nach Gaben von Oestrogenen und Androgenen (A) geprüft werden.

Die Bestimmung des PBI erfolgte nach der Methode von SPITZY, REESE und SKRUBE (*13*). Als Untersuchungsgut dienten 23 Frauen in der Menopause. Bei den Patienten mit Lebercirrhose handelte es sich um 6 Männer. Die Lebercirrhose war jeweils laparoskopisch und bioptisch gesichert.

Zum Vergleich für die folgenden Untersuchungen wurden zunächst die Veränderungen des PBIs bei 5 Patientinnen nach Zufuhr von je 5 mg Oestradiolbenzoat an drei aufeinanderfolgenden Tagen ermittelt (Tab. 1). Die Mittelwerte zeigen unter Oe-Einfluß ein deutliches Ansteigen von 5,6 auf 8,6 und 11,5 γ-% 48 Std nach der ersten Injektion, nach 3 Tagen ist der Wert auf 7,1 γ-% abgesunken, liegt jedoch immer noch deutlich über dem Ausgangswert. Bei einer Patientin mit hohem Ausgangswert handelte es sich um eine Hyperthyreose, auch bei dieser kam es zum Anstieg.

Bei längerdauernder Oe-Medikation, über die von ENGSTROM u. Mitarb. berichtet wurde, zeigte die Kurve innerhalb von 3—4 Wochen einen kontinuier-

---

[1] Mit Unterstützung der Deutschen Forschungsgemeinschaft.

Tabelle 1

Patientin	eiweißgebundenes Jod im Serum in γ %				Patientin	eiweißgebundenes Jod im Serum in γ %			
	Ausgangswert	nach 24 Std	nach 48 Std	nach 72 Std		Ausgangswert	nach 24 Std	nach 48 Std	nach 72 Std
Gruppe I	5 mg Oestradiolbenzoat				Gruppe II	5 mg Testosteronpropionat			
Kl.	5,0	6,0	12,6	6,3	Re.	6,7	3,9	1,4	1,2
Se.	4,2	7,9	11,7	9,3	He.	4,4	1,5	1,2	1,4
Br.	9,4	13,9	10,3	6,8	Li.	5,3	1,5	1,4	1,4
Be.	4,1	8,2	10,0	14,1	Ur.	6,2	2,8	1,6	1,6
Ma.	4,1	7,1	14,0	9,0	Ha.	6,8	4,7	—	—
Mittelwerte	5,6	8,6	11,5	7,1	Mittelwerte	5,9	2,9	1,4	1,4
Gruppe III	5 mg Oestradiolbenzoat + 250 mg Testosteronpropionat				Gruppe IV	5 mg Oestradiolbenzoat + 150 mg Testosteronpropionat			
Be.	3,5	3,1	3,1	—	Ma.	4,7	5,5	3,7	2,3
Ko.	6,5	1,2	2,7	—	Gö.	4,7	5,8	4,4	3,9
Sc.	6,8	6,4	5,6	—	Ke.	4,7	6,3	3,3	2,3
Mittelwerte	5,6	3,6	3,5	—	Ry.	5,8	6,7	4,4	3,6
					Ab.	4,7	5,1	—	—
Gruppe V	5 mg Oestradiolbenzoat + 75 mg Testosteronpropionat				Mittelwerte	4,9	5,9	3,9	3,0
Sc.	4,7	14,1	16,6	12,9	Gruppe VI	Patienten mit Lebercirrhose 5 mg Oestradiolbenzoat			
Pr.	3,9	16,4	20,9	13,9	Wi.	7,3	4,8	5,9	—
Le.	4,3	13,1	15,4	10,7	Kö.	4,8	3,3	1,3	—
Kö.	6,8	21,6	25,3	20,1	Si.	2,3	1,6	5,0	—
St.	3,9	14,8	19,5	12,7	Mittelwerte	4,8	3,2	4,1	—
Mittelwerte	4,7	16,0	19,5	14,1					
Gruppe VII	Patienten mit Lebercirrhose 75 mg Testosteronpropionat								
St.	2,4	1,8	3,4	—					
He.	3,3	6,7	6,4	—					
Wi.	3,0	4,3	3,4	—					
Mittelwerte	2,9	4,3	4,4	—					

lichen Anstieg und verlief dann plateauartig. Ein gelegentliches Absinken einzelner Werte innerhalb dieser 4 Wochen wurde auch von ENGSTROM und MARKHARDT beobachtet. Nach Absetzen des Oe gehen die Werte innerhalb von 4 Wochen wieder zur Norm zurück (*8, 9*).

Ebenfalls als Vergleichsuntersuchung gedacht war die Bestimmung des PBI-Spiegels unter Einwirkung von Testosteronpropionat (Tab. 1). Es fand sich ein übereinstimmender Abfall der Ausgangszahlen bei allen 5 Patientinnen, der nach 48 Std seinen maximalen Wert erreichte und bis 72 Std konstant blieb.

Ähnliche Ergebnisse nach Androgengaben wurden von KEITEL und SHERER sowie von FEDERMAN u. Mitarb. angeführt (*10, 11*). Der hemmende Effekt war bei einzelnen Untersuchungen nicht so ausgesprochen. FELDMAN und CARTER beobachteten nach Testosteronpropionat den niedrigsten Mittelwert mit 4,6 im Vergleich zu 1,4 γ-% bei uns (*16*).

Bei Verabfolgung von 5 mg Oestradiolbenzoat[1] mit dem 50fachen A-Zusatz kommt es zu einer völligen Hemmung des stimulierenden Oe-Effektes (Tab. 1).

Bei geringerer A-Menge und konstanter Oe-Dosis, bei einem Verhältnis von 1:30 zeigt sich nach 24 Std noch ein leichter Anstieg. Erst nach 48 und 72 Std scheint der depressive A-Einfluß zu überwiegen. Überraschend ist das Ergebnis bei Gaben von Oestradiolbenzoat und Testosteronpropionat[1] im Verhältnis von 1:15. Dabei kommt es nicht wie erwartet lediglich zu einer geringeren Bremsung der Oestrogenwirkung, sondern diese wird potenziert. Nach 24 und 48 Std werden erheblich höhere Werte als nach alleiniger Gabe von Oestradiobenzoat erzielt. Ähnlich wie nach Oe allein liegt der 72 Std-Wert etwas tiefer als der vorhergehende. Insgesamt liegt jedoch der Kurvenverlauf deutlich darüber (Tab. 1).

Auf Grund unserer Untersuchungen über Plasmacorticosteroide und Oestrogene lag der Gedanke nahe, PBI-Bestimmungen nach Medikation von Keimdrüsenhormonen auch bei Lebercirrhosen durchzuführen. Wir untersuchten den PBI-Spiegel bei je 3 Patienten nach Oestradiolbenzoat und nach Testosteronpropionat (Tab. 1). Bei Betrachtung der Mittelwerte nach Oestradiol fehlt eine Erhöhung des PBIs entsprechend den Befunden bei Normalpersonen. Es kommt im Gegensatz dazu nach 24 Std zu einem leichten Absinken der Werte.

Ebenso fehlte ein depressiver A-Effekt bei den drei untersuchten Lebercirrhosen. Der geringe Anstieg nach 24 und 48 Std dürfte sich wohl bei einer größeren Anzahl von Untersuchungen als nicht signifikant erweisen. Insgesamt hat man bei Durchsicht der Einzelwerte den Eindruck, daß die Schwankungen unabhängig von der Hormonzufuhr erfolgen.

Diskussion

Die Erhöhung des proteingebundenen Hormonjods nach Oe-Zufuhr ist nach Meinung der meisten Autoren (*12, 14*) verursacht durch eine Steigerung der Thyroxin (T_4)-Bindungskapazität, der wahrscheinlich eine Vermehrung des thyroxinbindenden Globulins (TGB) zugrunde liegt. Die Halbwertszeit des T_4 im Serum wird durch Oe verlängert. Eine Beteiligung der Schilddrüse beim Zustandekommen dieses Mechanismus ist nicht erforderlich, da es auch bei ausreichend behandelten Athyreosen zu dem gleichen Effekt kommt (*12*). Ein meßbarer Effekt der Oe auf die Schilddrüsenspeicherung von I^{131} oder die Konzentration des serumpräcipitablen I^{131} als Ausdruck des intrathyreoidalen Turnovers und auf die renale Clearance konnte nicht nachgewiesen werden (*15*). Von Dowling u. Mitarb. wurde über eine geringe Zunahme des J^{131}-Verteilungsraums berichtet. Die pro Zeiteinheit aus dem T_4-Verteilungsraum entfernte Hormonmenge und periphere Utilisation wird, zumindest bis zur Einstellung eines neuen Gleichgewichts, vermindert. Für die ausschlaggebende Rolle des TBGs sprechen auch Literaturangaben über einzelne Fälle mit kongenitalem Fehlen des TBGs, bei denen nach Oe-Zufuhr keine Verzögerung des peripheren T_4-Turnovers und keine Zunahme der T_4-Bindung des Serums erreicht werden konnte. Andererseits waren bei einem

---

[1] Für die Überlassung von Versuchspräparaten sind wir der Fa. Schering-AG, Berlin, zu besonderem Dank verpflichtet.

Patienten mit einer anscheinend idiopathischen TBG-Vermehrung spontan ähnliche Veränderungen wie bei Normalpersonen nach Oestrogenen festzustellen (*16, 17*). Der Abfall des PBI-Spiegels nach A kommt durch eine herabgesetzte Thyroxinbindungekapazität als Folge einer Verminderung der TBG-Konzentration zustande. Dadurch kommt es zu einer Erhöhung des freien Thyroxins im Serum und des Thyroxinschwundes aus dem Serum und der pro die abgebauten Thyroxinmenge (*11*). Sowohl für die A- als auch die Oe-Wirkung wird der Angelpunkt in Mengenänderungen der Trägerproteine gesehen.

Bei unseren Untersuchungen führte die gleichzeitige Gabe von Oe und A z. T. zu unerwarteten Ergebnissen. Bei hochdosierten A-Zusätzen im Verhältnis von 50:1 zeigte sich ein rein antagonistischer Effekt der durch Oe induzierten Anhebung des PBI-Spiegels. Ganz im Gegensatz dazu kommt es bei einer geringeren A-Dosierung und unveränderter Oestrogenmenge bei einem Verhältnis von 15:1 zu einer synergistischen Wirkung auf das eiweißgebundene Jod. Die in gleicher Dosierung getrennt gegebenen Keimdrüsenhormone hatten eine rein konträre Wirkung gezeigt. Eine Erklärung für das Zustandekommen dieses Effektes kann vorerst nicht angeführt werden. Dieser potenzierende Effekt scheint sich nicht auf den Hormonjodspiegel zu beschränken. Oe führen zu einem Anstieg der Plasmacorticosteroide, als dessen Ursache ebenfalls eine Vermehrung der Trägerproteine angenommen wird. Bei Untersuchung der Plasma-CS und Zufuhr von Oestrogenen und Androgenen zeigte sich in einer früheren Arbeit eine Aufhebung des Oe-Effektes bei einer Dosisrelation von 1:15. Der höchste Anstieg der CS fand sich aber nicht bei dem niedrigsten A-Zusatz, der die geringste Hemmwirkung haben sollte, sondern bei einer mittleren Dosierung (*18*).

Die abnorm geringe Reaktivität von Lebercirrhosen auf Hormongaben und ihre erhöhte Hormontoleranz ist vom Insulin her bekannt. In früheren Untersuchungen stellten wir fest, daß eine Erhöhung der Plasma-CS, wie sie nach Gaben von Insulin und Glucagon bei Normalpersonen zustande kommt, bei Patienten mit Lebercirrhosen ebenso ausbleibt wie der Anstieg der Nebennierenrindensteroide nach Oestrogenzufuhr (*19*).

In den vorliegenden Untersuchungen wurde festgestellt, daß bei Lebercirrhosen sowohl nach Oestradiolbenzoat der übliche PBI-Anstieg als auch der Abfall nach Testosteronpropionat vermißt wird. Dem Einwand, daß bei Lebercirrhosen mit dem schon vorher erhöhten Spiegel endogener Oestrogene eine weitere Stimulierung keinen Effekt mehr haben könne, kann entgegengehalten werden, daß bei einem normalen Verhalten der Lebercirrhosen eben diese erhöhten Oestrogene bereits zu einer Erhöhung der PBI-Werte führen müßten. Diese wurden jedoch von VANNOTTI und BÉRAUD nicht signifikant erhöht, von anderen Untersuchern (*20, 21, 22*), wie auch in unseren Fällen eher niedrig gefunden. Darüber hinaus müßte es nach A-Medikation, insbesondere da es sich bei den Versuchspersonen um Männer handelte, zu einem Absinken der Werte kommen. Der intakten Leberfunktion kommt demnach beim Zustandekommen des Oe- und A-Einflusses auf den PBI-Spiegel eine maßgebliche Rolle zu. Zusammenhänge zwischen Keimdrüsenhormonen und der Leber, insbesondere den Leberproteinen gehen aus Untersuchungen an Ratten hervor. Bei diesen konnten in der Leber geschlechtsspezifische Eiweißkörper nachgewiesen werden, deren Auftreten oder Verschwinden von den Sexualhormonen beeinflußt wird (*23*).

Hinweise auf die Eiweißbindung von Hormonen in der Leber geben die Untersuchungen von Szego und Roberts, sowie von Horwitz u. Mitarb. (*24, 25*). Diese konnten an Rattenleberschnitten und -homogenaten eine Bindung von markiertem Oestron und Oestradiol an Eiweißkörper nachweisen. Eine Störung der Synthese dieser Eiweißkörper und ihrer Bindungsaktivität bei der Dysproteinämie und Hypalbuminämie der Lebercirrhosen wäre vorstellbar. Dem widerspricht allerdings, daß die Thyroxinbindungskapazität bei Lebercirrhosen leicht erhöht gefunden wurde (*26*).

Auffällig bleibt das völlig gleichsinnige Verhalten der Nebennierenrindensteroide und des eiweißgebundenen Jods unter dem Einfluß der Keimdrüsenhormone einschließlich der fehlenden Reaktivität bei Lebercirrhosen.

Literatur

1. Schwarz, K., u. K. Kopetz: 7. Symp. Dtsch. Ges. f. Endokrinologie Homburg/Saar, 263 (1960).
2. Gemzell, C. A.: Acta endocr. (Kbh.) 17, 100 (1954).
3. Doe, R. B., H. H. Zinneman, E. B. Flink and R. A. Ulstrom: J. clin. Endocr. 20, 1484 (1960).
4. Heinemann, M., C. E. Johnson and E. B. Man: J. clin. Invest. 27, 91 (1948).
5. Peters, J. P., E. B. Man and M. Heinemann: Obstet. gynec. Surv. 3, 647 (1948).
6. Robbins, J., and J. H. Nelson: J. clin. Invest. 37, 153 (1958).
7. Dowling, J. T., D. L. Hutchinson, W. R. Hindle and Ch. R. Kleeman: J. clin. Endocr. 21, 779 (1961).
8. Engstrom, W. W., B. Markhardt and A. Liebman: Proc. Soc. exp. Biol. (N. Y.) 81, 582 (1952).
9. — — J. clin. Endocr. 14, 215 (1954).
10. Keitel, H. G., and M. G. Sherer: J. clin. Endocr. 17, 854 (1957).
11. Federman, E. D., J. Robbins and J. E. Rall: J. clin. Invest. 37, 1024 (1958).
12. Engbring, N. H., and W. W. Engstrom: J. clin. Endocr. 19, 783 (1959).
13. Spitzy, H., M. Reese u. H. Skrube: Mikrochim. Acta 4, 488 (1958).
14. Dowling, J. T., N. Freinkel and S. H. Ingbar: J. clin. Invest. 39, 1119 (1960).
15. — S. H. Ingbar and N. Freinkel: J. clin. Endocr. 19, 1245 (1959).
16. Feldman, E. B., and A. C. Carter: J. clin. Endocr. 20, 842 (1960).
17. Beierwaltes, W. H., and J. Robbins: J. clin. Invest. 38, 1683 (1959).
18. Kopetz, K., K. Schwarz u. K. P. Eymer: Klin. Wschr. 40, 1181 (1962).
19. — K. P. Eymer, K. Schwarz u. K. F. Weinges: 8. Symp. d. Dtsch. Ges. f. Endokrinologie, München 1961.
20. Vannotti, A., and T. Béraud: J. clin. Endocr. 19, 466 (1959).
21. Kydd, D. M., and E. B. Man: J. clin. Invest. 30, 874 (1951).
22. Shipley, R. A., and E. B. Chudzik: J. clin. Endocr. 17, 1229 (1957).
23. Bond, H. E.: Nature (Lond.) 196, 242 (1962).
24. Szego, C. M., and S. Roberts: J. biol. chem. 221, 619 (1956).
25. Horwitz, J. P., L. Horn, A. V. Loud and S. C. Brooks: Experientia (Basel) 18, 414 (1962).
26. Tanaka, S., and P. J. Starr: J. clin. Endocr. 19, 84 (1959).

Hypophyse und Schilddrüse

Von

K. Fellinger (Wien)

Mit 5 Abbildungen

Referat

Der Funktionskreis Hypophyse—Schilddrüse ist eines jener Themen, das bei einschlägigen Diskussionen immer wieder zur Sprache kommt, obgleich oder vielleicht gerade deshalb, weil unser Wissen auf diesem Gebiete in den letzten Jahren zweifellos außerordentlich bereichert wurde. Trotz aller Detailkenntnisse stehen aber nicht nur Einzelprobleme, sondern auch grundsätzliche Fragen noch immer zur Diskussion. Vor allem das den Kliniker brennend interessierende Problem der Pathogenese der Hyperthyreose — meist diskutiert in der Fragestellung, ob es sich um eine hypophysär ausgelöste oder um eine primär thyreogene Krankheit handle.

Da diese Fragestellung eine so wesentliche ist, Klinik und Theorie gleichermaßen berührend, gibt sie auch Gelegenheit, die wichtigsten aktuellen Allgemeinfragen im gleichen Rahmen zu besprechen. Ich möchte deshalb meine Ausführungen um diese Fragestellung ausbauen, wobei uns die speziellen Probleme, die sich um das toxische Adenom gruppieren, vielleicht als Ariadnefaden durch das sehr verworrene Labyrinth der sich so vielfach widersprechenden Erkenntnisse werden dienen können. Summative Übersichtsreferate über Hypophysenaktivität, TSH-Verhalten und Nachweis, TSH-Schilddrüsenfunktion usw. sind in den letzten Jahren ja wiederholt und in ausgezeichneter Weise erschienen: Ich weise nur hin auf die einschlägigen Zusammenfassungen von Danowsky (1963), von Purves und Adams (1960) und von Paulsen (1961), um die wichtigsten zu nennen.

Ich brauche wohl auch nicht im einzelnen darauf einzugehen, warum die Fragestellung der Genese der Hyperthyreose nicht schon lange durch quantitative Untersuchungen über Ausschüttung bzw. Blutspiegel des TSH geklärt wurde, was ja zunächst naheliegend erschiene. Die Ursachen sind, einfach genug, sowohl methodischer als auch grundsätzlicher Art: Methodisch, weil der normale Spiegel des TSH im Blut sehr niedrig und die Bestimmungsmethoden recht kompliziert sind, so daß quantitative Bestimmungen (vor allem in klinischer Routinearbeit) technisch sehr schwierig und außerdem mit Fehlerbreiten in und außerhalb der Methodik behaftet sind, die ohne weiteres kleine Differenzen übersehen lassen. Dabei ist zu bedenken, daß ja keineswegs große Differenzen im TSH-Spiegel vorliegen müssen. Zum zweiten auch grundsätzlich, da ja zum Zeitpunkt der bereits entwickelten Hyperthyreose die hochaktive Schilddrüse durch Bindung von TSH einen normalen Blutspiegel trotz erhöhter Produktion vortäuschen könnte. Es hat sich insbesondere Rawson (1955) mit dieser Frage intensiv beschäftigt und in einer Reihe von Untersuchungen experimenteller Natur (in Gewebekulturen) darzutun versucht, daß das TSH im Schilddrüsengewebe inaktiviert wird, wobei er sogar zahlenmäßige Beziehungen zwischen Gewicht des Schilddrüsengewebes und Einheiten des gebundenen thyreotropen Hormons aufzeigen konnte.

Es mag hier auch von Interesse sein, kurz die Untersuchungsergebnisse von Bakke et al. (1962) zu erwähnen, die über die Verschwinderate von zugeführtem TSH beim Menschen berichteten und fanden, daß diese unabhängig vom Vorhandensein einer Schilddrüse weitgehend der Intensität des Stoffwechsels folgt, d. h. beim Hypometabolen verzögert, beim Hypermetabolen beschleunigt ist, letzteres sogar dann, wenn es sich um einen ursprünglich Hypo- oder Athyreoten handelt, der durch medikamentöse Zufuhr von Schilddrüsenpräparaten hypermetabolisch gemacht worden war — ein Verhalten, das die Argumente von Rawson bezüglich des TSH-Mangels infolge Verschwindens des TSH durch Bindung an die Schilddrüse erheblich abschwächt. Die Autoren weisen auch noch sehr nachdrücklich auf die bisher kaum beachtete große Bedeutung des Nierengewebes für Speicherung des TSH (nicht Ausscheidung!) hin, die im Tierversuch bis zu 40% des zugeführten Hormons betragen kann. Die Autoren sehen in der Speicherungsfunktion der Nieren möglicherweise eine eigene, zweite homoiostatische Regulation bzw. Kontrolle für die Thyreoideafunktion.

Ebensowenig haben die Versuche, die TSH-Konzentration im Harn zu bestimmen, weiter geholfen, da die bisher gewonnenen Ergebnisse sehr inkonstant waren. Besonders auffallend war, daß wiederholt bei Hyperthyreoten überhaupt kein TSH im Harn nachgewiesen werden konnte. Rawson erklärt dies wiederum durch die erhöhte Bindung von TSH in der hyperthyreotischen Schilddrüse und erhärtet diese Überlegung dadurch, daß nach Jodgaben bei Hyperthyreotikern TSH im Harn auftritt, weil Jod die Bindung des TSH an die Schilddrüse verhindert, welche Meinung bereits auf ältere einschlägige Auffassungen (Albert 1949) zurückgehen mag.

Es ist begreiflich genug, daß bei untersuchungsmäßig und auch experimentell derartig schwierigen Voraussetzungen nicht nur die Ansichten, sondern auch die Ergebnisse der verschiedenen Untersucher außerordentlich uneinheitlich, ja widersprechend sind, trotz der großen methodischen Fortschritte, die durch die Entwicklung besonders subtiler Methoden der TSH-Bestimmung in den biologischen Flüssigkeiten (durch Bates, 1959) zweifellos heute gegeben sind.

Darf ich vielleicht zunächst ganz konzentriert und kurz die derzeitige Situation bzw. die wichtigsten Argumente skizzieren, wie sie von beiden Seiten für die thyreogene bzw. hypophysäre Genese der Hyperthyreose vorgebracht werden.

Für die Auffassung, daß die Basedowsche Krankheit Folge einer vermehrten Stimulierung der Schilddrüse durch das TSH sei, sprechen, abgesehen von der zunächst an sich naheliegenden Annahme, daß ja bekanntlich durch TSH experimentell und auch klinisch anatomische und funktionelle Veränderungen hervorgerufen werden können, die weitgehend denen bei Hyperthyreose entsprechen, drei weitere Momente:

Erstens und recht schwerwiegend, daß die echte Basedowsche Krankheit, also das Vollbild der Hyperthyreose, meist vom Symptom der Exophthalmie begleitet wird. Dieses wird ja heute in der Regel durch die Einwirkung eines "exophthalmic factor" des HVL erklärt; es wird nun immer wieder darauf hingewiesen, daß öfters — keineswegs stets — der Exophthalmus nach Schilddrüsen-ausschaltung stärker, nach Schilddrüsengaben oder Hypophysenausschaltung geringer wird, was zweifellos zunächst im Sinne einer überfunktionierenden Hypophyse gedeutet werden kann. Daß aber bei der ganzen Exophthalmusfrage vieles, wenn nicht das meiste, noch im Fluß ist, braucht hier nicht betont zu werden.

Zweitens natürlich die positiven Befunde über vermehrt TSH im Blute von Hyperthyreotikern: wir nennen etwa PURVES und GRISBACH (1949), D'ANGELO et al. (1951), GILLILAND und STRUDWICK (1956), kürzlich BAKKE et al. (1962) neben anderen, die vermehrt TSH öfters, keineswegs regelmäßig, im Blute Hyperthyreoter gefunden haben. Dem steht allerdings meist ein Fehlen von TSH im Harn gegenüber.

Drittens werden Kasuistiken vorgestellt wie etwa von ALBEAUX-FERNET et al. (1955), der bei einer 56jährigen Frau mit schwerer Hyperthyreose und Exophthalmus die Hypophysektomie durchführen ließ und anschließend klinische Heilung, Absinken des GU und ein — allerdings nur bescheidenes — Absinken des PBI fand. Ähnlich berichten JAILER und HOLUB (1960) über Heilung eines hyper-thyreotisch Erkrankten bei bestehendem Hypophysentumor nach Hypophysen-bestrahlung, wobei sich auch die Labor-Daten besserten. Überzeugend sind die Einzelfälle aber kaum.

Diesen drei Argumenten für eine hypophysäre Genese der Basedowschen Krank-heit stehen ebenso gewichtige gegenüber, die im entgegengesetzten Sinne sprechen und vor allem von WERNER (1955) und seinem Arbeitskreis vertreten werden. Ich bringe wieder nur die Quintessenz:

Die Befunde von vermehrtem TSH im Serum sind äußerst inkonstant, die Mehrzahl der Untersucher fanden eher keine sichere Vermehrung; im Harn wurde in der Regel keine TSH-Aktivität gefunden.

Histologisch entsprechen die Zellbilder des HVL bei Hyperthyreosen eher jenen bei Thyroxinüberproduktion und nicht bei TSH-Überproduktion, da oft die Basophilie fehlt, worauf schon 1938 WEGELIN hingewiesen hat. Es wurden sogar fibröse Umwandlungen der Hypophyse beschrieben (KRAUS und ANDERSON, 1948). Es sei aber gleich angemerkt, daß doch einige Untersucher auch über aus-gesprochene Basophilie des HVL bei Hyperthyreotikern berichten (ALBEAUX-FERNET et al., 1955, RUSSFIELD, 1955 u. a.).

Das stärkste Argument WERNERs dafür, daß die Hyperthyreose nicht durch eine vermehrte TSH-Aktivität des Hypophysenvorderlappens hervorgerufen werde, ist die Beobachtung, daß sich bei einer unbehandelten Hyperthyreose die Radiojodaufnahme in die Schilddrüse auch durch höchste Dosen Trijodthyronin oder Thyroxin nicht unterdrücken läßt, während nach erfolgreicher Behandlung der Hyperthyreose der „Hemmtest" wieder normale Ergebnisse zeigt. Wir (EGERT und HÖFER, 1961) konnten dieses Verhalten an unserem eigenen Material voll bestätigen und die Argumentation noch etwas weiterführen:

Bei 24 Patienten, die zum Zeitpunkt der Untersuchung nach einer (wegen gesicherter Hyperthyreose durchgeführten) Strumektomie oder Radiojodbehand-lung eindeutig euthyreot waren, konnte durch Schilddrüsenhormongaben die Speicherung unterdrückt werden (Abb. 1, links). Das Ausmaß der Unterdrückung

entsprach durchaus den Verhältnissen bei einer Kontrollgruppe von Normalpersonen (durchschnittlicher Abfall des 24 Std-Speichertests nach Hormongabe
auf 39% des Ausgangswertes).

Bei Patienten, die wegen einer Hyperthyreose strumektomiert oder mit Radiojod
behandelt worden waren, zum Zeitpunkt der Untersuchung aber noch oder wieder
hyperthyreot waren, gelang die Unterdrückung der Radiojodspeicherung durch
Hormongaben nicht (Abb. 1, rechts).

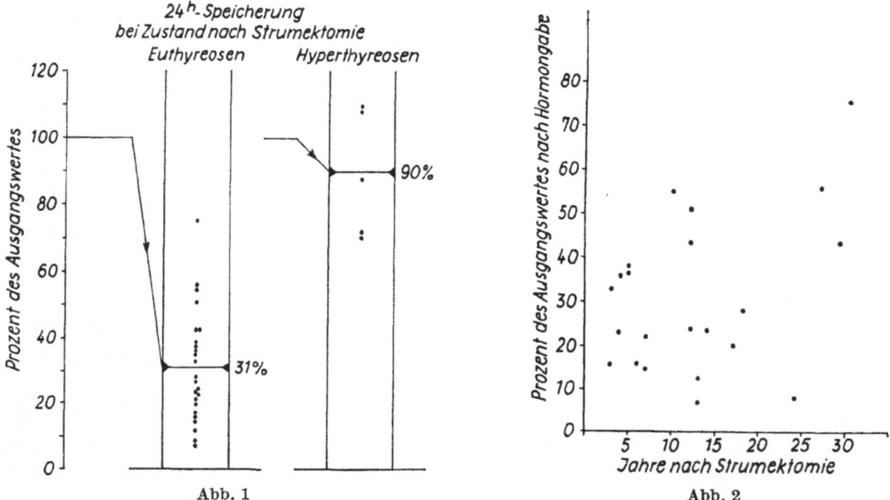

Abb. 1   Abb. 2

Abb. 1. Abfall der 24 Std-Speicherung nach Hormongabe bei 24 euthyreoten und 5 hyperthyreoten Strumektomierten aus: H. Egert und R. Höfer, Der Schilddrüsenhemmtest. Nuklearmedizin 1, 1961, Abb. 3, p. 384

Abb. 2. Verhältnis der Hemmtestwerte zum Intervall nach der Strumektomie aus: H. Egert und R. Höfer, Der
Schilddrüsenhemmtest. Nuklearmedizin 1, 1961, Abb. 6, p. 386

Setzt man das Ergebnis des Hemmtestes bei den euthyreoten Strumektomierten oder Radiojod-Behandelten zum Abstand von der Strumektomie oder Radiojodbehandlung in Beziehung, so zeigt sich keinerlei Abhängigkeit. Dies ist deshalb
von Bedeutung, weil man immer noch argumentieren könnte, daß die Wiederkehr
eines normalen Hemmtestes nach Strumektomie oder Radiojodresektion Ausdruck
der sich nach erfolgreicher Behandlung normalisierenden TSH-Überproduktion
wäre. Dann wäre aber doch zu erwarten, daß die Normalisierung des Hemmtestes
eine Beziehung zum zeitlichen Abstand von der Strumektomie aufwiese, was aber
nicht der Fall ist (Abb. 2).

Diese Untersuchungen scheinen uns ein recht schlüssiger Beweis dafür zu sein,
daß der normale Feedback-Mechanismus zwischen Schilddrüse und Hypophyse
sofort wieder einsetzt, wenn der Blutspiegel an Schilddrüsenhormon bei der
Hyperthyreose durch Reduktion des überfunktionierenden Schilddrüsengewebes
unter die Norm gesenkt wird. Dies kann aber nur dann sein, wenn die Ursache für
die Erkrankung nicht in der Hypophyse gelegen war.

Daß die Senkung des peripheren Schilddrüsen-Hormonspiegels auch beim
Hyperthyreoten einen im wesentlichen normalen Feedback-Mechanismus auslöst,
geht wohl auch daraus hervor, daß bei der durch Thyreostatika hervorgerufenen
Remission einer Hyperthyreose regelmäßig eine Vergrößerung der Schilddrüse zu

beobachten ist, die sich auf zusätzliche orale Hormonmedikation wieder schlagartig rückbildet; ein Verhalten, auf das ja schon PURVES und ADAMS (1960) in diesem Sinne hingewiesen haben.

Schließlich werden auch von WERNER und anderen Kasuistiken vorgestellt, die mir allerdings ebensowenig überzeugend erscheinen, wie die schon zitierten. So z. B. von WERNER und STEWART (1958) ein Fall eines Hypophysentumors mit weitgehender Kompression des Vorderlappens, bei dem eine Hyperthyreose entstand. Deswegen nicht überzeugend, weil der, wenn auch makroskopisch kleine VL-Rest doch funktionell überaktiv hätte sein können. Weiter ist hier der öfters zitierte Fall von McCULLAGH et al. (1960) zu nennen, die bei einer etwa 50 jährigen Frau mit Rezidivhyperthyreose den Hypophysenstiel durchtrennten und isolierten; es traten bei der Patientin dann auch ausgeprägte Zeichen des HVL- und überhaupt Hypophysenausfalls auf. Trotzdem entwickelte sich 1 Jahr später eine zunehmend deutliche Hyperthyreose, die auf die übliche Behandlung gut ansprach. Auch dieser Fall überzeugt deswegen nicht restlos, weil keine Autopsiebefunde vorlagen, die allein das tatsächliche Bestehen einer definitiven und vollkommenen HVL-Atrophie beweisen würden. Das gleiche gilt für einen Fall von FAJANS (1958), der über eine junge Frau referiert, bei der sich nach einem Partus Hypophysenausfallssymptome deutlicher Art entwickelten, die auf Substitution gut ansprachen. Etwa 18 Jahre später, unter weiterlaufender Substitution, entwickelte die Patientin eine ausgeprägte Hyperthyreose, die sich unter thyreostatischer Therapie vorübergehend besserte, schließlich mußte aber doch thyreoidektomiert werden. Auch hier fehlt der Autopsiebefund über den Zustand der Hypophyse. Man wundert sich immer wieder darüber, inwiefern solche in ihrer Beweisführung doch letztlich inkomplette Einzelfälle helfen sollen, ein so schwieriges Problem zu klären.

Es ist hier vielleicht der Platz, auf die Arbeiten von LI et al. (1955) hinzuweisen, die an einem recht großen Material von wegen Neoplasmen Hypophysektomierten zeigen konnten, daß nur die totale Hypophysektomie einen groben Abfall der RJ-Aufnahme in die Schilddrüse und des Serum-PBI bewirkt. Bei subtotaler Hypophysektomie fallen die PBI-Werte und die RJ-Aufnahme entweder überhaupt nicht nennenswert oder nur vorübergehend. LI verlangt daher den Nachweis der Entwicklung einer klinisch und laboratoriumsmäßig eindeutigen Hypothyreose geradezu als Beweis für die Komplettheit einer Hypophysektomie.

Daß aber selbst so grundsätzliche Konzepte einleuchtender Art, wie die zwangsläufige Entwicklung von Hypothyreosen nach totaler Hypophysektomie noch problematisch sind, mögen die sehr genau durchgeführten Arbeiten von PAZIANOS et al. (1960) aus dem Sloan Kettering-Institut bzw. der Cornell-Universität dartun: Die Autoren berichten über 10 euthyreote Frauen, die wegen Mammacarcinom hypophysektomiert wurden. Die komplette Entfernung der Hypophyse wurde dabei in 4 Fällen später durch Autopsie, in 2 Fällen durch Reoperation bestätigt. Die Frauen wurden über 2 Jahre beobachtet. Sie zeigten normales PBI, normale RJ-Speicherung, bei der Autopsie normale bzw. adenomatöse Schilddrüsen, wobei die Adenome sich wie toxische Adenome verhielten. Man braucht wohl nicht zu unterstreichen, wie sehr bei solchen Befunden selbst unsere anscheinend gesicherten Konzepte problematisch werden.

Diese kurzen Excerpte aus dem Feld der Kasuistik mögen hier genügen, um zu zeigen, daß auch mit Fallbeschreibungen die zur Diskussion stehende Frage einer befriedigenden Lösung nicht zugeführt werden kann und durchaus offen bleibt, um so mehr, als ja auch von seiten der Anhänger einer hypophysären Genese der Hyperthyreose Kasuistiken angeboten werden, wie ich schon erwähnte.

Es scheint uns also eine befriedigende, letztlich über Hypothesen hinausgehende Stellungnahme zur nach wie vor offenen Frage der Pathogenese der Basedowschen Krankheit — und damit des klinischen Hauptproblems im Rahmen der Beziehungen Hypophyse-Schilddrüse — weder durch diese Kasuistiken noch durch die bisher erwähnten labormäßigen Untersuchungen über Wirkstoffgehalt von Blut, Harn usw. möglich. Eher käme in Erwägung, daß klinisch-funktionelle Überlegungen weiterhelfen könnten.

Wie schon wiederholt angedeutet, bildet nun ein Hauptargument Werners die Tatsache der fehlenden Hemmung der Schilddrüsenaktivität bei Hyperthyreosen durch zugeführte Thyreoideawirkstoffe, was zunächst auf einen hypophysenunabhängigen Mechanismus schließen läßt. Selbst 2 mg Trijodthyronin — das 20fache der üblichen Tagesdosis — sind nicht imstande, eine nachweisbare Funktionsminderung zu bewirken. Auf unsere eigenen einschlägigen Untersuchungen habe ich ebenfalls hingewiesen, die dartun, daß bei Hyperthyreosen der Feedback-Mechanismus eindeutig ruht, aber durch Reduktion der Thyroxinproduktion wieder aufleben kann, daß also die primäre Störung nicht in der Hypophyse, sondern in der Schilddrüse selbst gelegen zu sein scheint (Egert und Höfer, 1961).

Eine weitere Klärung dieser Fragestellung könnten Untersuchungen über das toxische Schilddrüsenadenom bringen, da hier vielleicht ein analoger Funktionsmechanismus vorliegt, über dessen Art die Untersuchungen der letzten Jahre einigen Aufschluß gegeben haben (Fellinger et al. 1961, 1962, Höfer und Vetter, 1959).

Zunächst, wie verhält sich das toxische Adenom? Es ist autonom, d. h. unabhängig von der TSH-Regulierung. Wir haben in den letzten Jahren rund 120 solcher hyperaktiver Schilddrüsenadenome beobachtet und in allen Fällen war der Feedback-Mechanismus zwischen dem normalen Schilddrüsengewebe und der Hypophyse zwar voll erhalten, nicht jedoch zwischen überfunktionierendem Adenom und Hypophyse. Das läßt sich durch die folgenden Befunde erläutern bzw. aufzeigen:

Es gibt Schilddrüsenadenome (meist im Beginn der Entwicklung), die nach dem Scintigramm eindeutig überaktiv sind, ohne daß klinisch deutliche Hyperthyreose-Zeichen bzw. im Laborversuch (GU, PBI usw.) schon eine vermehrte Hormonproduktion nachweisbar wäre. Es muß daher die Situation offenbar so liegen, daß das autonom gewordene überaktive Adenom die übrige Schilddrüse auf dem Umwege über den Feedback-Mechanismus so unterdrückt, daß sie derart *unter*funktioniert, daß die *Gesamthormonproduktion* von Adenom und gedrosseltem Normalgewebe noch annähernd im Rahmen des Normalen liegt (Abb. 3, a). Führt man solchen Fällen Schilddrüsenwirkstoff zu, so gelingt es, die Speicherung im *gesunden* Gewebe voll zu unterdrücken, im Adenom ändert sich nichts (Abb. 3, b). Der Hemmtest als Gesamttest fällt in diesem Stadium oft noch normal aus.

Bei deutlich werdender klinischer und Labor-Symptomatik stellt sich im Scintigramm eine immer geringere Speicherung im Normalgewebe dar. Steigt nämlich die Hormonproduktion des toxischen Adenoms bis an die Grenzen des

Bedarfes, so kann auch eine völlige Ruhe der Normalschilddrüse die Überproduktion nicht mehr immer völlig kompensieren. Der Hemmtest wird dann allmählich pathologisch ausfallen.

Im Vollbild entsprechen klinische Befunde und Laborbefunde der Hyperthyreose, im Scintigramm findet man *nur* das Adenom abgebildet (Abb. 3,c) und histologische Untersuchungen bei einer Operation zeigen im Normalgewebe sogar Zeichen der Atrophie. Der Hemmtest fällt natürlich negativ aus.

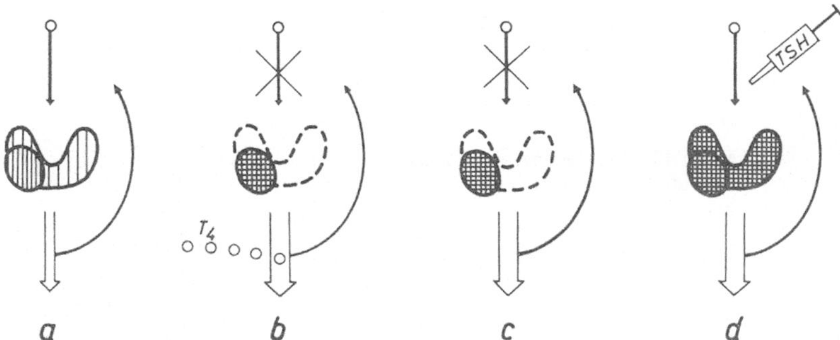

Abb. 3a—d. Schematische Darstellung des feed-back Mechanismus bei einem toxischen Adenom. a) Das hyperaktive Adenom produziert einen Teil des normalen Hormonbedarfs, die übrige, dem feed-back Mechanismus unterworfene Schilddrüse den Rest. b Orale Thyroxinzufuhr unterdrückt die Speicherung im normalen Gewebe, via feed-back. c Das toxische Adenom produziert eine pathologisch hohe Menge Hormon, das Normalgewebe ist via feed-back Mechanismus stillgelegt. d Parenterale TSH-Zufuhr reaktiviert das Normalgewebe

Daß aber auch in diesem Stadium das Normalgewebe noch die *Fähigkeit* des Ansprechens auf TSH zeigt, kann durch Injektion von TSH geprüft werden: Wiederholt man das Scintigramm nach exogener TSH-Zufuhr, so zeigt sich dann auch im Normalgewebe eine deutliche RJ-Aufnahme (Abb. 3,d). Wird andererseits das Adenom selektiv entfernt, so entwickelt sich die Funktion — erkennbar an der RJ-Aufnahme im Scintigramm — im gesunden Schilddrüsenanteil wieder völlig normal.

Ein weiterer Hinweis dafür, daß mit der Entfernung des hyperaktiven Adenoms wirklich auch die „Krankheit" entfernt wurde, liegt in der Tatsache, daß alle einschlägigen Radiojodstoffwechseluntersuchungen nach der Enucleation des Adenoms, gleichgültig wie früh oder wie spät nach der Operation sie durchgeführt werden, völlig normale Ergebnisse zeigen; vor allem konnten wir keineswegs die so typische, und von uns als Strumektomieeffekt bezeichnete (HÖFER, 1961; FELLINGER et al., 1957) irreführende Erhöhung des PBI[131] nach Enucleation eines hyperaktiven Adenoms beobachten.

Aus alldem geht die Autonomie des toxischen Adenoms, also die Unabhängigkeit seiner Aktivität von dem HVL eindeutig hervor und erscheint bewiesen.

Die Frage ist nun die, ob wir aus Vergleichen mit dem Verhalten des toxischen Adenoms auf den Mechanismus der Basedowschen Erkrankung schließen können.

Wir haben zunächst die klinische Symptomatik des toxischen Adenoms mit der Klinik der diffusen Hyperthyreosen verglichen. Tab. 1 zeigt die wichtigsten Symptome gegenübergestellt und man sieht, daß mit wenigen Ausnahmen die Symptomatik identisch ist. Ausnahmen sind höhergradige tachykarde Reaktionen, die beim toxischen Adenom etwas weniger stark auftreten — wohl ohne weiteres durch die quantitativen Hormonverhältnisse allein zu erklären. Der zweite sicherlich wichtige Unterschied ist das Fehlen eines Exophthalmus beim toxischen Adenom. Auf diesen Umstand wurde ja von verschiedenen Seiten immer wieder hingewiesen. Ich kann im Rahmen dieser Diskussion nicht die Exophthalmusprobleme abhandeln, würde auch einem späteren Referat in ungebührlicher Weise vorgreifen. Ich möchte nur zusammenfassen, daß uns das Exophthalmusproblem heute noch weitgehend ungeklärt erscheint.

Tabelle 1. *Vergleich der klinischen Symptomatik*

	150 Hyperthyreosen %	80 Tox. Adenome %
Vergeßlichkeit, Konz. Schwäche	64	79
psychische Labilität	81	95
Schlafstörungen	69	58
Angst	32	42
Hitzeunverträglichkeit	74	63
Hyperhidrosis	84	74
Haarausfall	20	26
Tremor	83	72
Reflexsteigerung	58	42
Muskelschwäche	94	95
Heißhunger	42	37
Schlechter Appetit	36	26
Übelkeit-Erbrechen	28	16
Durst	80	75
Stuhlbeschleunigung	70	58
Gewichtsabnahme	87	90
Herzklopfen (subjektiv)	91	95
Frequenz:		
unter 100/min	28	58
100—120/min	44	21
über 120/min	28	16
Vorhofflimmern	3	10
Dekompensation	12	0
Exophthalmus	36	0
Andere Augensymptome	83	47

Dies demonstriert gut der interessante Fall von Furth et al. (1962), bei dem sich nach Hypophysektomie zunächst der einseitige Exophthalmus völlig zurückbildete und dann nach zweieinhalb Jahren ein schwerer Exophthalmus am anderen Auge auftrat. Allerdings fehlen letztlich auch in diesem Fall wieder der anatomische Beweis der totalen Hypophysektomie, jedoch waren alle Laborproben eindeutig.

Ich glaube jedenfalls nicht, daß man das verschiedene Verhalten hinsichtlich des Exophthalmus allein als sichere Basis nehmen kann, um darauf einen Wesensunterschied in der grundsätzlichen Pathogenese der beiden Zustandsbilder aufzubauen, gebe aber gerne zu, daß hier eine beachtliche und derzeit noch nicht zu klärende Unbekannte vorliegt.

Es mag aber zunächst angezeigt sein, weitere Argumente bezüglich der Vergleichbarkeit der beiden Schilddrüsenstörungen zu diskutieren:

Wir haben in letzter Zeit, wie Höfer (1963) später noch detailliert ausführen wird, die Verteilung einer Tracerdosis Radiojod in den verschiedenen jodierten Verbindungen der Schilddrüse als Funktion der Zeit nach Verabreichung der

Dosis untersucht. Es ließ sich dabei zeigen, daß bei der normalen euthyrecten Schilddrüse die Jodidkonzentration im Schilddrüsenhydrolysat nach 48 Std beträchtlich höher ist als 8 Std nach Verabreichung der Testdosis. Es handelt sich dabei wohl um die Auswirkung der Dejodierungsvorgänge im Laufe der Hormonsynthese.

Untersucht man nun in der gleichen Weise das Hydrolysat einer Schilddrüse, die unter erhöhter TSH-Stimulation steht, so findet man im Gegensatz dazu nach 8 Std die höchste Jodidkonzentration, während sie in weiterem Abstand von der Gabe der Tracerdosis abnimmt (Abb. 4). Es scheint sich bei dieser Abnahme um eine Folge der Ausschüttung von Jodid aus der Schilddrüse unter TSH-Einwirkung, wie sie Rosenberg et al. (1961) und andere beobachtet haben, zu handeln, bzw. um eine vermehrte intrathyreoidale Utilisation des bei der Dejodierung freiwerdenden Jods.

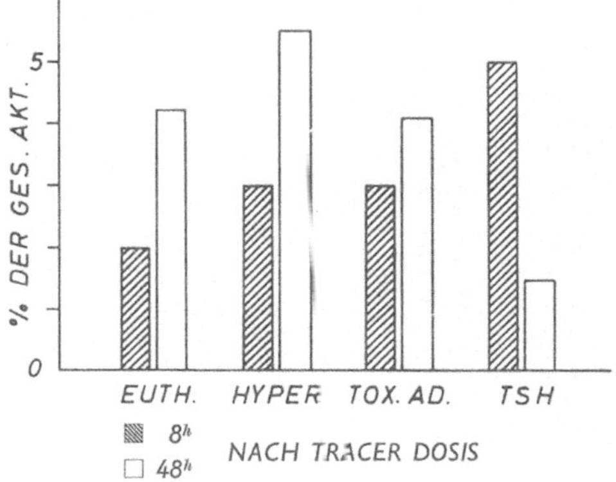

Abb. 4. Erläuterung siehe Text

Sowohl beim toxischen Adenom als auch bei der Hyperthyreose steigt jedoch die Jodidkonzentration mit Abstand vom Zeitpunkt der Gabe der Tracerdosis an, entspricht daher nicht dem Typ der TSH-Stimulation. Es handelt sich hier also um eine Eigenart des intrathyreoidalen Jodstoffwechsels, die im Gewebe einer Hyperthyreose und eines hyperaktiven Adenoms parallel läuft und im Gegensatz zur beobachteten Wirkung einer Stimulation von Schilddrüsengewebe mit TSH steht.

Eine weitere Überlegung: Schon Werner hat als ein Hauptargument gegen die These, daß die Hyperthyreose durch vermehrte Thyreotropinproduktion verursacht werde, die Tatsache angeführt, daß es bei der Hyperthyreose gelingt, durch zusätzliche TSH-Stimulation eine Erhöhung des proteingebundenen Jods im Serum zu erzielen.

Wir konnten den genau gleichen Effekt bei hyperaktiven Adenomen erzielen: Nach Injektion von thyreotropem Hormon kommt es gleichlaufend mit der vermehrten Ausschüttung von im Adenom gespeichertem Radiojod zu einem Anstieg des proteingebundenen stabilen wie auch radioaktiven Jods im Serum.

Schon diese Parallelität des TSH-Effektes beim toxischen Adenom und bei der Hyperthyreose verstärkt die Argumentation Werners. Wir konnten aber auch zusätzlich noch zeigen, daß es zusammen mit dem Anstieg des proteingebundenen Jods im Serum beim toxischen Adenom wie auch bei der Hyperthyreose unter TSH gleichzeitig zu einem Anstieg auch des anorganischen Jodids im Serum kommt (Abb. 5) (Fellinger et al 1961). Dies kann gegen den Einwand zur Beweisführung Werners geltend gemacht werden, daß der von ihm beobachtete TSH-Effekt auf die hyperthyreotische Schilddrüse nur zeigte, daß diese nicht unter maximaler TSH-Stimulation stehe.

Es sei an dieser Stelle der Analog-Untersuchungen Toxisches Adenom — diffuse Hyperthyreose auch eingefügt, daß sich in letzter Zeit Green und Ingbar (1962) mit dem Argument Rawsons (1955), Solomons (1960) u. a. beschäftigt haben, daß

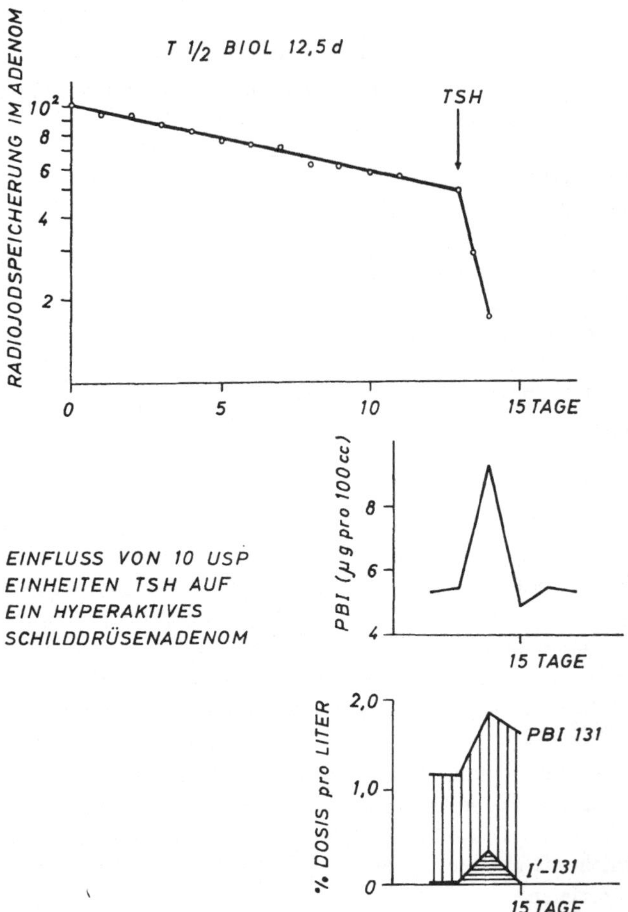

Abb. 5. Einfluß der parenteralen Zufuhr von 10 USP Einheiten TSH auf die biologische Halbwertszeit, PBI[131], anorganisches Jodid[131] im Serum und PBI[127] bei einem Patienten mit toxischem Adenom

nämlich die Hemmung der Hormonsekretion nach Zufuhr von anorganischem Jodid dadurch zu erklären sei, daß das Jodid die Bindung des TSH durch Schilddrüsengewebe verhindert.

Rawson entkräftet damit jene Einwände gegen die hypophysäre Genese der Hyperthyreose, die sich auf das Fehlen von TSH im Harn und Serum von Hyperthyreotikern stützten und er schließt seine Beweiskette damit, daß sich nach Jodidzufuhr auch bei Hyperthyreotikern TSH im Harn und Serum findet.

Green und Ingbar (1962) konnten in sehr schönen Versuchen ebenfalls an einigen Fällen von toxischen Adenomen zeigen, daß die Wirkung von Jodid auf die Verschwinderate von organischem Jod aus der Schilddrüse, also auf die Hormonausschüttung, auch bei völliger Unterdrückung der TSH-Funktion (wie beim toxischen Adenom vorliegend und beweisbar) weiterbesteht. Diese Tatsache, daß Jodid die Ausschüttungsquote des Hormonjods auch bei unterdrücktem TSH ruckartig hemmt, zeigt eindeutig, daß keineswegs ein Jodid-TSH-Antagonismus die Ursache dieses Geschehens sei, daß also die Annahme eines solchen Antagonismus unbegründet ist, womit das oben erwähnte Argument RAWSONs zur Erklärung der mangelnden TSH-Erhöhung bei Hyperthyreosen seine Bedeutung verliert.

Hier ist wohl nun der Platz, darauf hinzuweisen, daß heute überhaupt die ganze Fragestellung in ihrer bisherigen Formulierung (hypophysär bedingt oder primär-thyreogen) revidiert werden muß. Deswegen, weil neben hypophysär entstandenem TSH und der Homoiostase der Schilddrüse selbst ein dritter, vorläufig bezüglich seiner Genese noch nicht klarzustellender Faktor einzuschalten ist, der vielleicht die Diskussion auf eine völlig neue Ebene stellen kann.

Schon das hypophysär gewonnene TSH läßt sich mit chemischen Methoden in mehrere Fraktionen mit TSH-Wirkung zerlegen: nach PIERCE et al. (1956, 1958) in etwa fünf, nach BATES et al. (1959) in drei solche. Auch rein physiologisch kann man etwa drei Arten der Wirkung des hypophysären TSH unterscheiden: eine rasch einsetzende Wirkung bestand in der Ausschüttung präformierten Hormons aus dem Kolloid, beginnend nach meist weniger als 30 min und wenige Stunden andauernd. — Bei wiederholter Injektion folgt die zellstimulierende Wirkung, erkennbar in Hypertrophie und auch mitotischer Vermehrung der Epithelzellen. — Endlich setzt ziemlich verspätet (HALMI et al. 1953) die Stoffwechselwirkung ein: beschleunigte Jodspeicherung und vermehrter Jodeinbau in die Aminosäuren (STANLEY und ASTWOOD, 1949).

1958 haben nun ADAMS sowie McKENZIE, und 1959 MUNRO in einer Reihe sehr interessanter Arbeiten gezeigt, daß die Zufuhr von Serumextrakten Hyperthyreoter eine maximale Erhöhung des PBI^{131} erst nach 10—24 Std bewirkt, während nach Injektion von Standard-TSH bereits nach 2—3 Std das Maximum erreicht ist. Das Halbleben dieses Wirkstoffes war ebenfalls deutlich verschieden vom Halbleben des normalen TSH, und zwar 7,5 Std (ADAMS, 1960) im Gegensatz zu 14 min für das normale thyreotrope Hormon. ADAMS bezeichnete diesen Wirkstoff zunächst als „abnormales TSH", später bürgerte sich der Ausdruck LATS (Long Acting Thyroid Stimulator) ein. LATS unterscheidet sich also vom hypophysären TSH eindeutig:

    a) hat er eine wesentlich längere Halblebenszeit,

    b) läßt er sich mit der Methode von BATES nicht aus Blut extrahieren und

    c) wird er durch Antisera gegen TSH nicht neutralisiert.

Wegen dieser Unterschiede haben ADAMS und seine Mitarbeiter auch die Möglichkeit erwogen, daß es sich hier (da ja LATS besonders bei exophtalmischen Hyperthyreosen gefunden wurde) um eine im exophthalmisch gereizten Orbitalgewebe entstandene Substanz handeln könne. Sie konnten es dort aber nicht nachweisen und so steht der Ort der Produktion des LATS durchaus zur Debatte. Nun haben vor einem Jahre ADAMS und PURVES (1962) noch einen weiteren „abnormalen" thyreoideastimulierenden Wirkstoff im Blut beschrieben, nämlich ein kurzfristig wirkendes TSH (vorläufig bei nur einem Hyperthyreosekranken). Auch dieser Wirkstoff verhält sich ähnlich wie das LATS. Er ist ebenfalls mit der Bates-Methode nicht extrahierbar, mit TSH-Antiserum nicht neutralisierbar, also mit dem hypophysären TSH nicht identisch. Sein Blutspiegel wurde durch Thyreoideagaben nicht unterdrückt, er unterliegt also nicht dem Feedback-Mechanismus. Die Autoren benennen den neuen Faktor als SATS (Short Acting Thyroid Stimulator).

Es liegen bereits eine Reihe von Befunden vor, die darauf hindeuten, daß die positiven Befunde im Serum Hyperthyreoter (positiv im Sinne einer erhöhten TSH-Aktivität) nicht durch vermehrtes hypophysäres TSH, sondern durch „abnormales TSH", also LATS bzw. SATS, bedingt sind. Es wird zweifellos noch eingehender Untersuchungen an größerem Material bedürfen, bis darüber genügend Klarheit geschaffen ist. Eines aber scheint heute schon zwar nicht bewiesen, aber doch rechts wahrscheinlich, daß das LATS bzw. SATS einen neuen thyreostimulierenden Faktor neben dem hypophysären TSH darstellt.

Übersehen wir nun die bisher geschilderte Situation, so kann man etwa wie folgt argumentieren:

1. Die Befunde über das *TSH-Niveau im Blut und Urin* sind widersprechend, aus quantitativen und methodischen Gründen im klinischen Versuch derzeit für letzte pathogenetische Entscheidungen noch kaum verwertbar. Die Annahme, daß ein niederer TSH-Spiegel bei Hyperthyreosen durch eine Bindung der TSH an die Schilddrüsenzelle verursacht würde, scheint nach Bakke (1962) widerlegt. Die Bedeutung des LATS ist noch offen, ebenso seine Entstehung und gesamte Physiopathologie; unklarer noch die Bedeutung des SATS, doch ist anzunehmen, daß sie beide nicht mit dem hypophysären TSH identisch sind.

2. *Kasuistiken* beweisen, soweit vorliegend, kaum etwas Wesentliches. Die meisten Kasuistiken sind irgendwie inkomplett bzw. nicht schlüssig.

3. Es ist als sichergestellt zu betrachten, daß das „toxische Adenom" autonom ist, d. h. nicht von der TSH-Stimulierung abhängt, umgekehrt aber, daß TSH (im Rahmen des Feedback) weitgehend vom Hormonausstoß des toxischen Adenoms unterdrückt wird, was eindeutig aus dem Verhalten des nicht adenomatösen Schilddrüsenanteiles hervorgeht.

4. Es liegt nun nahe, aus dieser Tatsache (der sichergestellten Autonomie des toxischen Adenoms) auf eine parallele Genese der diffusen Basedow-Schilddrüse zu schließen, um so mehr als der klinische Unterschied zwischen den beiden Erscheinungsformen der Überfunktion der Schilddrüse nicht groß ist.

5. Die Annahme eines prinzipiell ähnlichen Mechanismus bei der diffusen Hyperthyreose wird nun, abgesehen von der erwähnten weitgehenden Parallelität des klinischen Geschehens, weiter unterstützt durch andere Argumente:

a) Die diffusen Hyperthyreosen unterliegen ebenfalls nicht dem Schilddrüsenhemmtest: selbst große Mengen Trijodthyronin sind nicht imstande, die Thyreoideafunktion zu unterdrücken, obwohl diese T_3-Mengen an sich genügen, die TSH-Produktion völlig zu hemmen.

b) Sowohl diffuse Hyperthyreosen als auch das toxische Adenom zeigen eine zeitabhängige Verteilung des Radiojod in den verschiedenen Jodverbindungen innerhalb der Schilddrüse, die nicht der Kurve einer TSH stimulierten Schilddrüse entspricht.

c) Durch zusätzliche TSH-Gaben kann sowohl das toxische Adenom als auch die diffuse hyperthyreotische Schilddrüse weiter stimuliert werden: es kommt zu vermehrter Ausschüttung sowohl von anorganischem als auch von organischem Jod.

6. Das eigentlich einzige Argument, das derzeit für eine Rolle der Hypophyse in der Genese der Hyperthyreose spricht, ist das häufige Auftreten eines Exophthalmus bei diffusen Hyperthyreosen, während beim toxischen Adenom nie ein Exophthalmus beobachtet werden konnte. Es muß aber darauf hingewiesen werden, daß die nötigen Voraussetzungen zur Bewertung dieses Befundes, nämlich genaue Kenntnis der Genese des Exophthalmus, noch nicht gegeben sind.

Aus allen diesen Gründen scheinen uns bei der derzeitigen Lage der Forschungsergebnisse mehr Argumente zugunsten der Annahme einer nicht hypophysär-TSH-bedingten Genese der Hyperthyreose zu sprechen, was natürlich nicht ausschließt, daß es vielleicht daneben auch unter Umständen eine hypophysäre Genese der Hyperthyreose gehen *kann*.

Ich darf darauf hinweisen, daß schon vor etwa 40 Jahren JULIUS BAUER hier in Wien die Vermutung ausgesprochen hat, daß im allgemeinen die Hyperthyreosen nicht hypophysär bedingt sind, daß dies aber bei den klimakterischen Hyperthyreosen zutreffen könnte: eine Annahme, die wir seinerzeit (1937) auf Grund unserer damaligen noch mit sicher technisch sehr insuffizienten Methoden durchgeführten Untersuchungen über den TSH-Spiegel im Blute stützen zu können glaubten, während wir schon damals für die jugendlichen und sonstigen nicht dem Klimax angehörigen Hyperthyreosen keine Hinweise auf hypophysäre Aktivität finden konnten.

Wir haben oben ausdrücklich formuliert: „nicht hypophysär-TSH-bedingt" und haben vermieden zu formulieren „primär-thyreogen-bedingt". Dies deswegen, weil die Rolle des LATS, SATS und ähnlicher Faktoren noch weitgehend ungeklärt ist, nicht nur was ihre physio-pathologische Bedeutung, sondern vor allem auch, was den Ort ihrer Entstehung betrifft. Es muß immer wieder betont werden, daß durch den Nachweis dieser Stoffe eine Veränderung der bisherigen Alternative eingetreten ist. Während man bisher formulieren konnte: entweder hypophysär (= TSH) bedingt *oder* autonom-thyreogen, muß man wohl jetzt die Möglichkeit einer Dreieckswahl offen lassen: entweder hypophysär-TSH-bedingt oder primär-thyreogen oder aber durch einen Stimulator noch unbekannter Entstehung provoziert.

Wir persönlich neigen jedenfalls dazu anzunehmen, daß der Regelfall der Hyperthyreose nicht durch eine vermehrte Einsonderung von hypophysärem TSH hervorgerufen ist und glauben, daß dem TSH hypophysärer Genese mehr eine Regulierungsfunktion innerhalb gewisser physiologischer Grenzen zukommt. Ob es daneben, etwa bei Hypophysentumoren oder im Klimakterium, gelegentlich auch hypophysär ausgelöste Hyperthyreosen gibt, steht noch offen.

Wesentliche Aufgabe der Zukunft bzw. der Forschung der nächsten Zeit aber wird es nun sein, aufzuzeigen, „wes Nam' und Art" die sogenannten „abnormalen TSH-Wirkstoffe" sind und welche Rolle *ihnen* in dem Funktionskreis der Schilddrüse zukommt.

Literatur

ADAMS, D. D.: J. clin. Endocr. 18, 699 (1958).
— Endocrinology 66, 658 (1960).
— H. D. PURVES, N. E. SIRETT and D. W. BEAVEN: J. clin. Endocr. 22, 623 (1962).
ALBEAUX-FERNET, M., J. GUIOT, S. BRAUN and J. D. ROMANI: J. clin. Endocr. 15, 1239 (1955).
ALBERT, A.: Ann. N.Y. Acad. Sci. 50, 466 (1949).

BAKKE, J., N. LAWRENCE and S. ROY: J. clin. Endocr. **22**, 352 (1962).

BATES, R. W., M. M. GARRISON and T. B. HOWARD: Endocrinology **65**, 7 (1959).

D'ANGELO, S. A., K. E. PASCHKIS, A. S. GORDON and A. CANTAROW: J. clin. Endocr. **11**, 1237 (1951).

DANOWSKY, T. S.: N. Y. St. J. Med. **1963**, 50.

EGERT, H., u. R. HÖFER: Nuklearmedizin 1, 380 (1961).

FAJANS, ST. S.: J. clin. Endocr. **18**, 271 (1958).

FELLINGER, K.: Wien. Arch. inn. Med. **29**, 375 (1937).

— R. HÖFER and H. VETTER: J. clin. Endocr. **17**, 483 (1957),

— — H. EGERT and H. VETTER: in: Advances of Thyroid Research, S. 347. Pergamon Press, London (1961).

— — — Radiobiol. Radioth. **313**, 291 (1962).

FURTH, E. D., D. V. BECKER, B. S. RAY and S. W. KANE: J. clin. Endocr. **22**, 518 (1962).

GILLILAND, I. C., and J. I. STRUDWICK: Brit. med. J. **1956** I, 378.

GREEN, W., and S. INGBAR: J. clin. Invest. **41**, 173 (1962).

HALMI, N. S., B. N. SPIRTOS, E. M. BOGDANOVE and H. J. LIPNER: Endocrinology **52**, 19 (1953).

HÖFER, R.: in: Fortschritte der Schilddrüsenforschung. S. 70. Herausgeg. von K. OBERDISSE u. E. KLEIN. Stuttgart, G. Thieme, 1962.

—, u. H. VETTER: in: Medical Isotope Scanning, Seminar IAEA and WHO, 1959, 213.

JAILER, J. W., and D. A. HOLUB: Amer. J. Med. **28**, 497 (1960).

KRAUS, J. E., and W. A. D. ANDERSON: in Anderson: Pathology 1948, 1019.

LEPP, A., and P. STARR: J. clin. Endocr. **22**, 800 (1962).

LI, M. C., J. E. RALL, J. B. MACLEAN, M. B. LIPSETT, B. S. RAY and O. H. PEARSON: J. clin. Endocr. **15**, 1228 (1955).

MACCULLAGH, E. P., S. W. REYNOLDS and J. M. MACKENZIE: J. clin. Endocr. **20**, 1029 (1960).

MCKENZIE: Endocrinology **62**, 865 (1958).

—, Endocrinology **63**, 372 (1958).

MUNRO, D. S.: J. clin. Endocr. **19**, 64 (1959).

PAULSEN, F.: in: Fortschritte der Schilddrüsenforschung, S. 102. Herausgeg. von K. OBERDISSE u. E. KLEIN. Stuttgart, G. Thieme, 1962.

PAZIANOS, A. G., R. BENUA, B. S. RAY and O. H. PEARSON: J. clin. Endocr. **20**, 1051 (1960).

PIERCE, J. G., and J. F. NYC: J. biol. Chem. **222**, 777 (1956).

— L. K. WYNSTON and M. E. CARSTEN: Biochim. biophys. Acta 28 434 (1958).

PURVES, H. D., and D. D. ADAMS: Brit. med. Bull. **16**/2, 128 (1960).

—, and W. E. GRIESBACH: Brit. J. ex. Path. **30**, 23 (1949).

RAWSON, R. W.: In: S. C. WERNER, The Thyroid, S. 441, 1955.

ROSENBERG, I. N., J. C. ATHANS, A. BEHAR and C. S. AHN: In: Advanves of Thyroid Research, S. 194, 1961.

RUSSFIELD, A. B.: J. clin. Endocr. **15**, 1393 (1955).

SOLOMON, D. H., and J. TH. DOWLING: Ann. Rev. Physiol. **22**, 615 (1960).

STANLEY, M. M., and E. B. ASTWOOD: Endocrinology **44**, 49 (1949).

WEGELIN, C.: Arch. Anat. path. **15**, 703 (1938).

WERNER, S. C.: The Thyroid, 1955.

—, and W. B. STEWART: J. clin. Endocr. **18**, 266 (1958).

Diskussion

F. HOFF (Frankfurt):

Herr FELLINGER sieht die Ursache der Thyreotoxikose vorwiegend in der Schilddrüse selbst. Er stützt sich dabei auf das toxische Adenom, das zweifellos eine lokale Schilddrüsenerkrankung ist und das er in der Pathogenese der Thyreotoxikose ziemlich gleichsetzt. Zu berücksichtigen sind aber für die Pathogenese der Thyreotoxikose, wie ich schon in meinem Schilddrüsenreferat auf dem Internistenkongreß 1937 darlegte, als Glieder eines Funktionskreises Schilddrüse, Hypophyse und Hypothalamus. An jedem dieser Glieder kann primär eine Störung einsetzen, stets ist dann der ganze Funktionskreis in Mitleidenschaft gezogen. Ich stimme Herrn FELLINGER zu: Das toxische Adenom stellt eine lokale Erkrankung der

Schilddrüse dar, es kann ähnlich wie eine örtliche Thyreoiditis eine Thyreotoxikose hervorrufen. Wenn das Adenom entfernt wird oder die Thyreoiditis ausheilt, ist die Krankheit geheilt. Das Regulationssystem Hypophyse-Zwischenhirn ist an sich in Ordnung. Deshalb sehen wir ja beim toxischen Adenom über den Funktionskreis eine Stillstellung der Schilddrüse außerhalb des Adenoms durch Herabsetzung des thyreotropen Hormons. Bei der Thyreotoxikose ist das aber grundsätzlich anders. Trotz des erhöhten Spiegels von Schilddrüsenhormon kommt keine Hemmung der Bildung von thyreotropem Hormon zustande. Es liegt eine Störung der übergeordneten Regulationen vor. Deshalb kann auch nach Strumektomie ein Rezidiv eintreten. Nun gibt es auch Fälle, in denen eine Thyreotoxikose primär von der Hypophyse oder vom Zwischenhirn ausgeht. Hierfür werden eigene kasuistische Beobachtungen angeführt, z. B. Thyreotoxikose nach Virusencephalitis, nach Fleckfieberencephalitis, Myxödem bei Hypophysentumor, aber auch nach Herderkrankungen im Hypothalamus. Während das toxische Adenom eine lokale Schilddrüsenerkrankung ist, dürften in der Pathogenese der Thyreotoxikose Störungen der übergeordneten Regulationen, der Hypophyse und des Hypothalamus mitwirken. Diese Störungen des Regulationssystems sind wohl oft erblich oder konstitutionell angelegt.

E. KLEIN (Düsseldorf):

Es kommt bei der Beurteilung von klinischen Hinweisen auf zentrale Faktoren sehr darauf an, in welcher Phase ihres Verlaufs eine Hyperthyreose erstmals untersucht wird, weil subcorticale Komponenten ebenso Folge wie Ursache der überschießenden Hormonsynthese der Schilddrüse sein können. So gehen die zweifellos hypophysär bedingten echten endokrinen Augensymptome gelegentlich und nachweisbar dem Ausbruch der Hyperthyreose lange voran, während sie sich in anderen Fällen, auch ohne daß iatrogene Maßnahmen im Spiel sind, erst auffallend spät hinzugesellen. Abgesehen vielleicht von den Verhältnissen beim toxischen Adenom gibt es bei voll entwickeltem Krankheitsbild mit oder ohne endokrine Ophthalmopathie weder ein klinisches noch trotz aller spezieller Verfahren ein laboratoriumstechnisches Kriterium dafür, ob eine Hyperthyreose primär oder sekundär thyreogen ist.

K. OBERDISSE (Düsseldorf):

Bei allen Betrachtungen über die Pathogenese der Hyperthyreose muß der negative Suppressionstest im Vordergrund stehen. Die erhöhte Aktivität der Schilddrüse, gemessen an der Radiojodaufnahme, läßt sich durch Zufuhr von Schilddrüsenhormon nicht unterdrücken, ganz im Gegensatz zur euthyreoten Struma. Bei dem toxischen Adenom ist der Reglermechanismus nicht gestört, was auch aus der Inaktivierung des umgebenden Schilddrüsengewebes bei Autonomie des Adenoms hervorgeht. Der negative Suppressionstest ist ein so konstantes Phänomen, daß man ihn geradezu bei der Differentialdiagnose der euthyreoten und hyperthyreoten Struma zur Entscheidung als letzte Instanz heranziehen kann. Man kann dieses Phänomen nicht als Argument gegen die hypophysäre Bedingtheit der Hyperthyreose anführen. Es läßt sich nur daraus schließen, daß bei der Hyperthyreose das suprathyreoidale System, das Hypophyse und Hypothalamus einschließt, nicht auf Schilddrüsenhormon anspricht und daß es infolgedessen zu einer Entzügelung dieses Systems mit der übermäßigen Abgabe von Schilddrüsen-stimulierenden Stoffen kommt. Hier ergeben sich durchaus Parallelen zu anderen Überfunktionszuständen, z. B. Cushing-Syndrom mit bilateraler Rindenhypertrophie. Auch hier haben wir bei einer Reihe von Fällen die Überproduktion von Cortisol nicht durch Dexamethason bremsen können. Der negative Suppressionstest im Falle der Hyperthyreose sagt allerdings nichts darüber aus, ob es sich bei der Stimulierung um Thyreotropin oder einen anderen ähnlichen Faktor handelt, der von der Hypophyse oder vielleicht auch von suprathyreoidalen Gebilden abgegeben wird. Es ist richtig, daß der Suppressionstest nach Strumektomie wieder positiv wird, aber eben doch erst dann, wenn die Euthyreose wieder eingetreten ist.

K. FELLINGER:

Selbstverständlich hat Herr HOFF recht, wenn er darauf hinweist, daß das Problem mit der Besprechung der Beziehung Hypophyse-Schilddrüse nicht erschöpft ist, sondern weiter noch durch den Einfluß des Hypothalamus auf die Hypophyse kompliziert wird. Es war aber nicht möglich, in diesem Rahmen auf diesen höheren Regulationsmechanismus einzugehen, sondern die Fragestellung wurde ganz bewußt auf die Beziehung Hypophyse-Schilddrüse allein eingeschränkt, nicht zuletzt auch deswegen, weil diese Seite der Problematik ja auch von Herrn Greer gesondert behandelt wird. Es ist auch nicht einzusehen, wieso durch eine Erwägung der Beziehungen zwischen Hypothalamus und Hypophyse die engere Fragestellung (autochtone oder hypophysäre Genese der Hyperthyreose) wesentlich geklärt werden soll. Was die Behauptungen Herrn Hoffs betrifft, daß bei der Thyreotoxikose „keine Hemmung der Bildung von thyreotropem Hormon" zustande komme, so kann ich nur darauf hinweisen, daß das ja gerade das zu diskutierende Problem ist, und ich habe mit meinen Ausführungen mich bemüht darzulegen, daß bisher überhaupt noch keine endgültige Klärung des Verhaltens des thyreotropen Hormons bei der Hyperthyreose möglich war.

Ich weise diesbezüglich auch auf die Diskussionsbemerkung von Herrn Klein hin, der mit Recht gesagt hat, daß wir bisher noch kein sicheres labor-technisches Kriterium dafür haben, ob eine Hyperthyreose primär oder sekundär thyreogen sei, welche Situation ja die Basis für meine Ausführungen abgab.

Herrn Oberdisse kann ich nur nochmals darauf hinweisen, daß ein wesentlicher Punkt meiner Ausführungen die Tatsache war, daß der Schilddrüsenhemmtest automatisch mit dem Absinken des Hormonspiegels im Blute, nach durchgeführter Operation oder dergleichen wieder einsetzt und daß das Wiedereinsetzen des Hemmtestes — was ich besonders hervorgehoben habe — keinerlei Beziehung zum Abstand von der Strumektomie zeigte. Im gleichen Sinne spricht auch das Auftreten einer Strumaentwicklung mit Unterdrückung der Hyperthyreose durch Schilddrüsenhemmstoffe.

Zum dritten endlich möchte ich nochmals unterstreichen, daß ich meine Überlegungen nicht auf ein einzelnes Argument allein aufgebaut haben, sondern auf die Summe einer Anzahl von Argumenten, die klinisch und labormäßig in ähnlicher Richtung deuten. Ich gebe gerne zu, daß, und das war wohl auch der Tenor meiner Ausführungen, das Problem noch in keiner Weise restlos geklärt ist. Zweck der Darlegung war, meine persönliche Meinung auf Grund einer Zusammenschau einer Reihe von alten und neuen Tatsachen und Überlegungen vorzutragen.

Aus der 2. Medizinischen Universitätsklinik Wien (Prof. Dr. K. Fellinger)

Zur Dynamik der Jodierungsvorgänge in der Schilddrüse

Von

R. Höfer und G. Pfeiffer

Mit 6 Abbildungen

Einleitung

Die bisherigen Ergebnisse der Erforschung der Biosynthese der Schilddrüsenhormone wurden in umfassender Weise von Pitt-Rivers in ihrer Monographie „Thyroid Hormones" dargestellt, und sie führten zur Aufstellung des wohlbekannten Schemas, daß in der Schilddrüse Jodid aus der Zirkulation konzentriert und nach Oxydation in ein Tyrosinmolekül zu Monojodtyrosin eingebaut wird; dann erfolgt die weitere Jodierung zu Dijodtyrosin und schließlich die Kopplung von Dijodtyrosin zu Thyroxin.

Eine typische Versuchsanordnung, wie sie zur Aufstellung dieses Schemas führte, stellt ein in vivo Tierexperiment dar, bei dem der zeitliche Ablauf der Verteilung einer Tracerdosis Radiojod in den verschiedenen jodierten Verbindungen in der Schilddrüse untersucht wurde. Abb. 1 (Pitt-Rivers, unveröffentlicht), z. B. zeigt, daß nach Verabreichung einer Tracerdosis Radiojod dieses zunächst in der Monojodtyrosinfraktion (MIT) erscheint, später dann in der Dijodtyrosinfraktion (DIT) und als letztes in der Thyroxinfraktion (T_4), womit bewiesen erscheint, daß MIT der Vorläufer von DIT und DIT der Vorläufer von Thyroxin ist, wie es in klassischer Weise von Harington (1926) vorausgesagt worden war.

Es wäre nun von Interesse, ähnliche Untersuchungen über den zeitlichen Ablauf der Verteilung einer Tracerdosis beim Menschen unter verschiedenen physiologischen und pathologischen Bedingungen zu machen. Dies stößt aber auf beträchtliche methodische Schwierigkeiten. Bei einem Tierversuch, wie er auch der Abb. 1 zugrunde liegt, wird einer Serie von Versuchstieren Radiojod verabreicht. Die Schilddrüsen von kleineren Gruppen werden nun zu verschiedenen Abständen nach Gabe der Tracerdosis hydrolysiert, die interessierenden Verbindungen abgetrennt und die Aktivität jeder einzelnen Fraktion bestimmt. Die so erhaltenen Werte werden als Funktion der Zeit graphisch dargestellt und zeigen somit, wie das Radiojod in den Tyrosinen und Thyroninen im Laufe der Hormonsynthese auftritt.

Um den gleichen Versuch beim Menschen durchzuführen, müßte man nach Gabe einer Tracerdosis zu verschiedenen Zeiten mehrfach biopsieren. Gegen ein solches Vorgehen spricht von vornherein, daß es kaum möglich ist, bei einem Patienten mehrmals in kurzen Abständen hintereinander Biopsien durchzuführen.

Weiterhin ist bekannt, daß die Verteilung einer Dosis Radiojod innerhalb der Schilddrüse durchaus nicht gleichförmig ist und daß somit auch der Ablauf des intrathyreoidalen Jodumsatzes von Gewebsbezirk zu Gewebsbezirk unterschiedlich sein muß. Es werden daher verschiedene Gewebsproben nicht ideal miteinander vergleichbar sein.

Nicht zuletzt muß man auch noch bedenken, daß alle Methoden zur Auftrennung eines Schilddrüsenhydrolysates in seine verschiedenen jodierten Komponenten schwierig sind, und auch nur geringe Veränderungen der Arbeitsbedingungen können daher zu recht

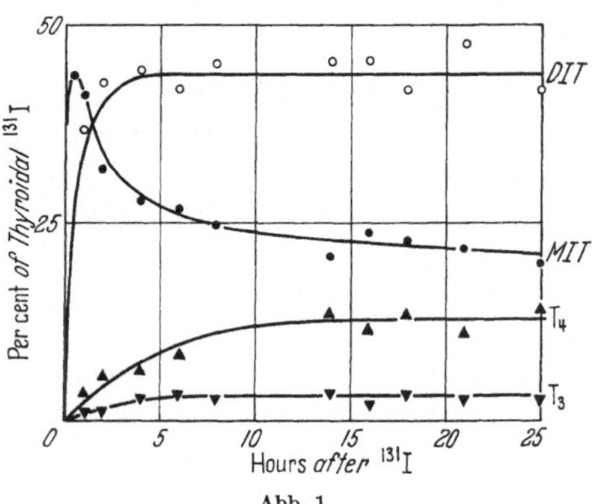

Abb. 1
Lt. R. Pitt-Rivers (unveröffentlicht)

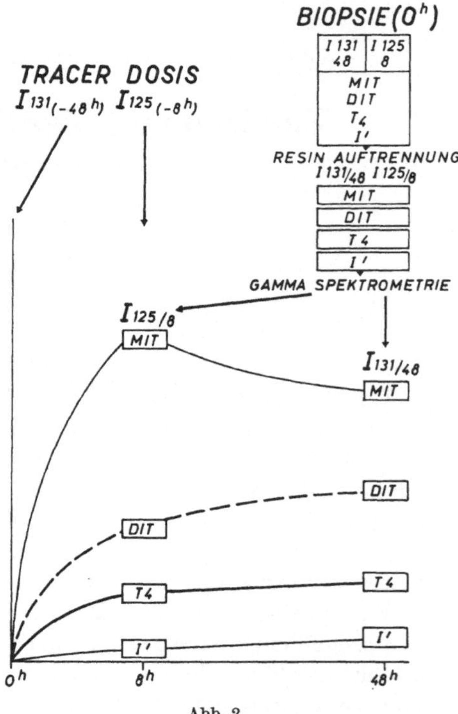

Abb. 2.
Schema des Arbeitsgangs mit Doppelmarkierung

beträchtlichen Divergenzen der Ergebnisse führen, wodurch der Vergleich verschiedener Gewebsproben weiterhin kompliziert wird.

Wir haben deshalb eine Methode entwickelt, die diese Fehlermöglichkeiten bei Untersuchungen zur Dynamik des intrathyreoidalen Jodtransportes vermeidet. Im Prinzip besteht diese Methode darin, daß wir, anstatt nach einer einmaligen Tracerdosis mehrmals Gewebsproben zu gewinnen, nur eine einzige Gewebsprobe entnehmen und untersuchen, und dafür zu verschiedenen Zeitpunkten vorher verschiedene Jodisotope verabreichen.

Methodik

Abb. 2 zeigt schematisch unseren Arbeitsvorgang. Es wird 48 Std vor der Biopsie eine Testdosis von Jod-131 gegeben und 8 Std vor der Biopsie eine zweite Testdosis, diesmal Jod-125. In der nun entnommenen Gewebsprobe wird daher die Verteilung des Jod-125 in den einzelnen Verbindungen repräsentativ für die Verhältnisse 8 Std nach Verabreichung einer Testdosis sein, während die Verteilung des Jod-131 die Verhältnisse 48 Std nach Verabreichung der Dosis wiedergibt. Es ist jetzt nur noch notwendig, die eine gewonnene Probe aufzuarbeiten, die einzelnen Fraktionen zu separieren und dann in jeder einzelnen Fraktion mit Hilfe eines

Gamma-Spektrometers einerseits den Jod-125-Gehalt und andererseits den Jod-131-Gehalt zu messen.

Im einzelnen gehen wir in folgender Weise vor. Nach Applikation von je etwa 50 μC der beiden Isotope wird in dem entsprechenden Zeitabstand im Rahmen der Strumektomie eine Probe entnommen und ein etwa 300 mg schweres Gewebsstück aufgearbeitet. Im wesentlichen folgen wir dabei den Angaben von R. PITT-RIVERS und B. I. SACKS (1963).

Möglichst sofort nach der Biopsie wird das Gewebsstück in einem Veronalpuffer bei einem p_H von 8,4 im Eisbad homogenisiert. Um Rejodierungsvorgänge zu vermeiden, wird außerdem eine kleine Menge Thioharnstoff zugesetzt. Das Homogenat wird mit etwas Pankreatin versetzt und 24 Std lang in einem rotierenden Brutschrank bei 37° hydrolysiert. Die hydrolysierte Probe wird bei 3000 UpM 30 min zentrifugiert. Die aus ihrer Peptidbindung freigesetzten Aminosäuren befinden sich nun in der überstehenden Flüssigkeit. Es hat sich gezeigt, daß bei diesem Vorgehen die Hydrolyse bis zu 95% komplett war.

Die Auftrennung in die einzelnen Komponenten erfolgt an einer Anionenaustauschersäule. Aus einem Dowex 1-Anionenaustauscher von der Korngröße 200—400 mesh, der in den Biorad-Laboratorien speziell hergestellt wird, wird eine Säule von 30 mm Höhe und 11 mm Durchmesser bereitet. Der Austauscher wird nun mit gesättigtem Natriumacetat in die Acetatform gebracht und durch Waschen mit einem Acetatpuffer auf ein p_H von 5,6 eingestellt. Die überstehende Flüssigkeit der zentrifugierten Probe wird aufgesetzt und etwa 1—2 Std gewartet, damit sich das Gleichgewicht einstellen kann. Vor Elution der einzelnen Fraktionen wird die Säule eiweißfrei gewaschen, wobei streng darauf zu achten ist, daß das p_H des dazu verwendeten destillierten Wassers nicht unter 6 liegt. Die Elution der einzelnen jodierten Verbindungen erfolgt mit Essigsäure in ansteigender Konzentration, und zwar wird das MIT mit 0,025%, das DIT mit 1% und das Thyroxin zusammen mit dem Trijodthyronin (T_3) mit 50% Essigsäure aus der Säule eluiert. Das anorganische Jodid wird anschließend mit 3n-Natriumbromidlösung ausgewaschen. Wir enden also mit 4 reinen Fraktionen eines bestimmten Volumens.

Ein aliquoter Teil jeder einzelnen Fraktion wird nun in einem Bohrlochkristall unter Verwendung eines Ein-Kanal-Impulshöhenanalysators gemessen. Die Bestimmung der Jod-131-Aktivität erfolgt im 0,364 MeV-Bereich, die der Jod-125-Aktivität im Summenpeak (26 + 35,4 keV). Alle Jod-125-Messungen müssen für die mitgemessenen Jod-131-Aktivitäten korrigiert werden. Durch Multiplikation mit dem Verdünnungsfaktor erhält man die Aktivität der einzelnen Fraktionen, die schließlich in Prozenten der Gesamtaktivität als Funktion der Zeit dargestellt werden.

Ergebnisse

Da die Methode doch recht kompliziert und zeitraubend ist, haben wir erst über einige Resultate zu berichten. In Abb. 3 ist das Ergebnis der Bearbeitung einer Gewebsprobe von einem euthyreoten Patienten dargestellt. Es wurde in diesem, wie in allen folgenden Fällen, die erste Dosis 48 Std und die zweite 8 Std vor der Strumektomie gegeben. Abb. 3 zeigt ein fast identisches Kurvenbild mit Abb. 1: Es kommt zunächst zur Bildung von MIT, mit dessen Abfall steigt das DIT an, als letztes zeigt die Thyroxinkurve einen Anstieg. Auch hier sehen wir also wieder einen Beweis dafür, daß MIT der Vorläufer von DIT und DIT die Vorstufe von T_4 ist. Hinzuweisen wäre auch noch auf das Verhalten des ungebundenen Jodids, das mit zunehmendem Abstand vom Zeitpunkt der Gabe der Tracerdosis an ansteigt, ein Hinweis darauf, daß ungebundenes Jodid in der Schilddrüse vorwiegend durch Dejodierungsprozesse entsteht.

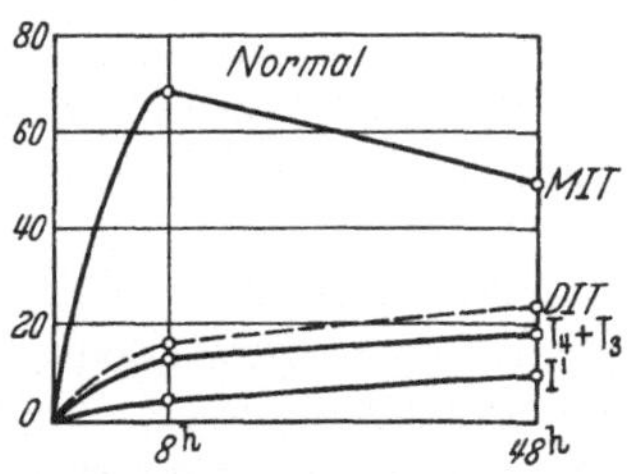

Abb. 3. Gewebsprobe aus einer euthyreoten Struma: auf der Ordinate sind die Zeitpunkte nach Gabe der Tracerdosis aufgetragen, auf der Abszisse die Aktivität der einzelnen Fraktionen in Prozent der Gesamtaktivität

Als Beispiel dafür, wie die Verhältnisse bei fehlender, bzw. stark herabgesetzter TSH-Stimulation liegen, kann das Ergebnis einer Untersuchung gelten, die bei einem Patienten mit einem hyperaktiven Schilddrüsenadenom durchgeführt wurde (Abb. 4). Das Nicht-Adenomgewebe steht bei einem toxischen Adenom kaum unter TSH-Stimulation (K. Fellinger et al., 1961) und wir erhalten daher ein ähnliches Bild, wie Taurog (1958) es im Rattenversuch mit hypophysektomierten Tieren gezeigt hat: Die Überführung von MIT in DIT ist stark vermindert, und die Thyroxinsynthese sehr stark gehemmt. Auffallend ist hier außerdem, daß zwischen den 8 Std- und den 48 Std-Werten kaum Unterschiede bestehen, also offenbar sehr frühzeitig ein Gleichgewicht eintritt, eine Beobachtung, die ebenfalls schon Taurog (1958) im Tierversuch gemacht hatte.

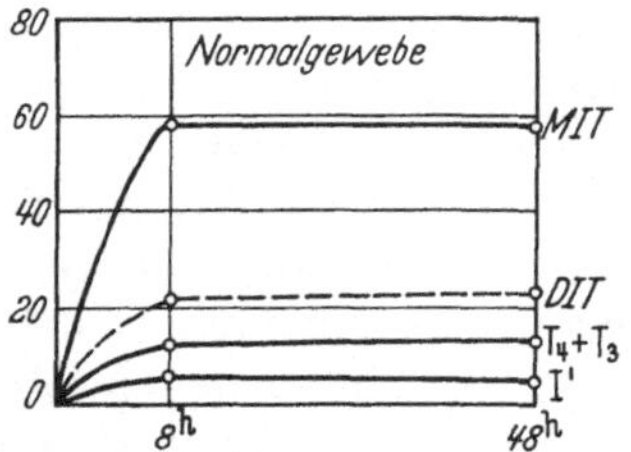

Abb. 4. Gewebsprobe aus der Schilddrüse eines Patienten mit einem hyperaktiven Adenom. Die Probe selbst wurde dem „Nicht-Adenomgewebe" entnommen. Wie bei Abb. 3 sind wieder die Prozentanteile an der Gesamtaktivität gegen die Zeit aufgetragen

Abb. 5 und Abb. 6 zeigen Patienten, deren Schilddrüse unter erhöhter TSH-Stimulation stand. In einem Fall (Abb. 5) wurde TSH parenteral zugeführt, im anderen Fall (Abb. 6) handelt es sich um eine mehrmals strumektomierte Patientin. In beiden Fällen liegt der hervorstechendste Unterschied gegenüber den bisher gezeigten Fällen im deutlichen Absinken der Jodidkonzentration nach 48 Std im Vergleich zum 8 Std-Wert. Es dürfte sich hier wahrscheinlich um eine vermehrte Jodidausschüttung durch die

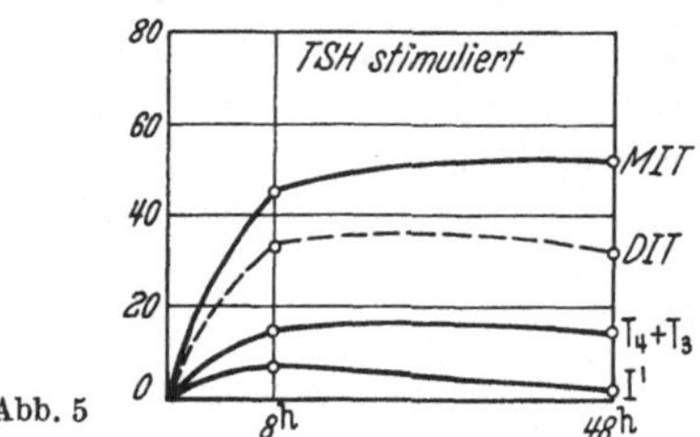

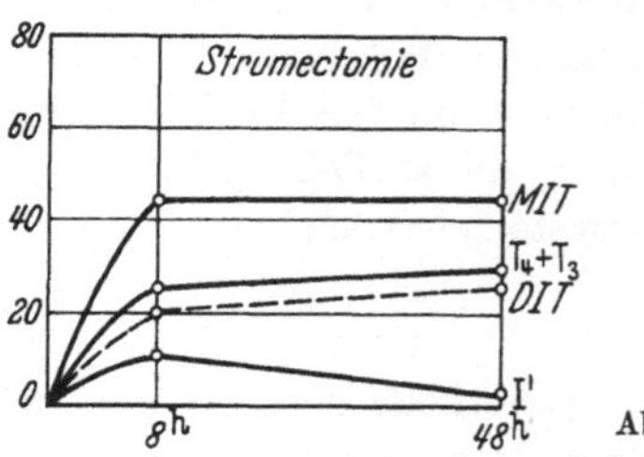

Abb. 5. Gewebsprobe aus einer Struma nach exogener Stimulierung mit TSH. Beschriftung wie in Abb. 3
Abb. 6. Gewebsprobe aus der Schilddrüse einer mehrmals strumektomierten Patientin. Beschriftung wie in Abb. 3

TSH-Stimulation, bzw. um eine vermehrte Reutilisation des aus Dejodierungsvorgängen freigewordenen Jods handeln. In letzter Zeit haben Rosenberg et al. ähnliche Befunde erhalten können.

Es ist zweifellos verfrüht, aus den bisherigen Ergebnissen weitreichende Schlüsse zu ziehen, aber wir glauben, daß es mit dieser Methode möglich sein wird, weitere Aufschlüsse über die intrathyreoidalen Jodierungsvorgänge zu gewinnen.

Literatur

FELLINGER K., R. HÖFER, H. EGERT and H. VETTER: Advances in Thyroid Research p. 347 (1961).
HARINGTON, C. R.: Biochem. J. 20, 300 (1926).
PITT-RIVERS, R., and B. I. SACKS: Biochem. J. 82, 111 (1963).
TAUROG, A., W. TONG and I. L. CHAIKOFF: Endocrinology 62, 664 (1958).
ROSENBERG, I. N., J. C. ATHANS. A. BEHAR and C. S. AHN: Advances in Thyroid Research p. 194 (1961).

Aus der 2. Med. Klinik und Poliklinik der Med. Akademie Düsseldorf
(Direktor: Prof. Dr. OBERDISSE)

Über den EPF-Gehalt im Serum endokriner Ophthalmopathien

Von

F. A. HORSTER und E. KLEIN

Mit 2 Abbildungen

Der Exophthalmus produzierende Faktor (EPF) wurde noch nicht identifiziert. Gesichert erscheint, daß er in allen Hypophysenvorderlappenextrakten enthalten und dem TSH verwandt, aber nicht mit ihm identisch ist (*4, 5, 18*). So unterscheiden sich TSH und EPF z. B. in Sedimentationskonstante und Molekulargewicht (*2*). Differente thyreogene und exophthalmogene Vorderlappenanteile konnten auch in Tierversuchen nachgewiesen werden (*3, 5, 6*). TSH ist stets auch in Seren nachweisbar, die EPF enthalten, während sich EPF nicht in allen TSH-haltigen Seren findet (*16*). Ebensowenig wie TSH ist wahrscheinlich der sog. lang wirkende Schilddrüsen-Stimulator, kurz LATS (Long Acting Thyroid Stimulator) mit dem EPF identisch (*15*). LATS ist zwar bei hyperthyreotischen endokrinen Ophthalmopathien häufiger als bei Hyperthyreosen ohne Augenbeteiligung anzutreffen, findet sich aber auch im Serum von Normalpersonen und hypophysektomierten Tieren (*15, 19*). EPF verschwindet nach Hypophysektomie stets aus dem Serum und ist nur bei endokrinen Ophthalmopathien regelmäßig nachzuweisen (*14*).

Der TSH-Gehalt des Serums und die Schilddrüsenfunktion stehen in keiner festen Beziehung zu den klinischen Symptomen einer endokrinen Ophthalmopathie (*8, 9, 12, 17*). Es stellte sich daher die Frage, ob bei endokrinen Ophthalmopathien eine Korrelation zwischen dem EPF-Gehalt des Serums, der Stärke des Exophthalmus und der Höhe des intrathyreoidalen Jodumsatzes nachweisbar ist. Der intrathyreoidale Jodumsatz wird als sog. PBI^{131} im Trichloressigsäuresediment des Serums bestimmt und in Prozent der Dosis/Liter Serum ausgedrückt; der intrathyreoidale Jodumsatz ist bei endokrinen Ophthalmopathien pathognomonisch beschleunigt (*8, 12*). Wenn auch zu den klinischen Symptomen einer endokrinen Ophthalmopathie Lidschwellungen, peri-, intra- und extraoculäre Ödeme, Bindehaut und Hornhautaffektionen und Augenmuskellähmungen zählen, so ist das einzige meßbare und daher auch statistisch erfaßbare Symptom der Exophthalmus. Deshalb dienten hier die Hertelwerte als klinisches Signum einer endokrinen Ophthalmopathie, wobei wir Werte über 19 mm dann als pathologisch ansehen, wenn sie von anderen soeben geschilderten Symptomen begleitet werden.

Als Beleg für die Schilddrüsenfunktion wird das chemisch analysierte Hormonjod im Blut, das sog. PBI angegeben (*12*).

Den EPF-Gehalt des Serums bestimmen wir wie vielerorts (*1, 5, 10, 11, 20*) im biologischen Test an Fischen: Das Blut wird eine Stunde nach Entnahme zentrifugiert und sofort verwendet oder tiefgefroren. Untersucht wird das Testserum zugleich mit einem Kontrollserum, einer Kaltblüter NaCl-Lösung und einer TSH-Lösung bekannter Konzentration. Je sieben Karpfen von 4—10 g Gewicht bilden eine Versuchsgruppe. Ein Volumen von 5% des Körpergewichtes wird dreimal in zwölfstündigen Abständen injiziert. Während des Versuches werden die Fische in

	n	*PBI* [γ %]	*PBI*[131] [% Dosis/l]	*ICD* [% Änderung]
Ohne endokrine Ophthalmopathie				
Euthyreosen	*26*	*6,2*	*0,02*	*± 3 %*
Hyperthyreosen	*24*	*11,1*	*1,05*	*± 3 %*
HVL Adenome	*3*	*6,8*	*0,08*	*± 4 %*
SD Malignome	*3*	*6,1*	*0,10*	*± 4 %*
Endokrine Ophthalmopathie				
euthyreot	*14*	*6,3*	*1,55*	*+ 18 %*
hyperthyreot	*32*	*11,0*	*1,35*	*+ 19 %*

Abb. 1. Mittelwerte von Hormonjodgehalt (PBI) und intrathyreoidalem Jodumsatz (PBI[131]) sowie prozentualer Änderung der Intercornealdistanz (ICD) bei den einzelnen Krankheitsgruppen.

150 l-Aquarien bei konstanten Licht- und Temperaturverhältnissen gehalten. Das einzige Kriterium bei der Bestimmung des EPF im biologischen Test am Fisch ist die Änderung des Abstandes von einem Corneascheitel des Fischauges zum anderen, der sog. Inter-Corneal-Distanz (ICD). Wir bestimmen diese Distanz vor und während des Versuches lichtmikroskopisch mit einer Genauigkeit von $^1/_{100}$ mm. Die physiologische Schwankungsbreite der ICD beträgt, wie wir in mehreren hundert Messungen feststellen konnten, 3%. Erst bei einer prozentualen Zunahme der ICD von 5% und mehr, erscheint uns der Nachweis eines EPF gesichert.

Wie aus Abb. 1 ersichtlich ist, unterschieden wir Gruppen mit und ohne endokrine Ophthalmopathie. Angegeben sind die Anzahl der untersuchten Seren (*n*), die Mittelwerte des PBI, des PBI[131] und der prozentualen Änderung der ICD. Signifikante Differenzen ergaben sich in den Gruppen ohne endokrine Ophthalmopathien insofern, als bei den Hyperthyreosen das PBI mit 11,1 (Schwankungsbreite 7,5—18,0 γ-%, mittlere Streuung $\pm$ 3,2 γ-%) und das PBI[131] mit 1,09 (Schwankungsbreite 0,36—3,70, mittlere Streuung $\pm$ 0,48) %/Dosis/Liter erhöht war gegenüber den normalen Werten bei Euthyreosen, HVL-Adenomen und SD-Malignomen. Die bei den endokrinen Ophthalmopathien angegebenen Daten zeigen, daß das PBI[131] bei euthyreoten (1,55 $\pm$ 0,5) und bei hyperthyreoten

Augenveränderungen (1,3 ± 0,45) im Vergleich zu Euthyreosen ohne endokrine Ophthalmopathie (0,09 ± 0,05) signifikant erhöht war.

Abb. 2 gibt vergleichend die Daten für die prozentuale ICD-Änderung, das PBI[131] und die Hertelwerte wieder. Es handelt sich in der Abbildung ausschließlich um endokrine Ophthalmopathien. Jede Säule repräsentiert den an sieben Fischen getesteten EPF-Gehalt eines Serums, ausgedrückt als prozentuale ICD-Zunahme.

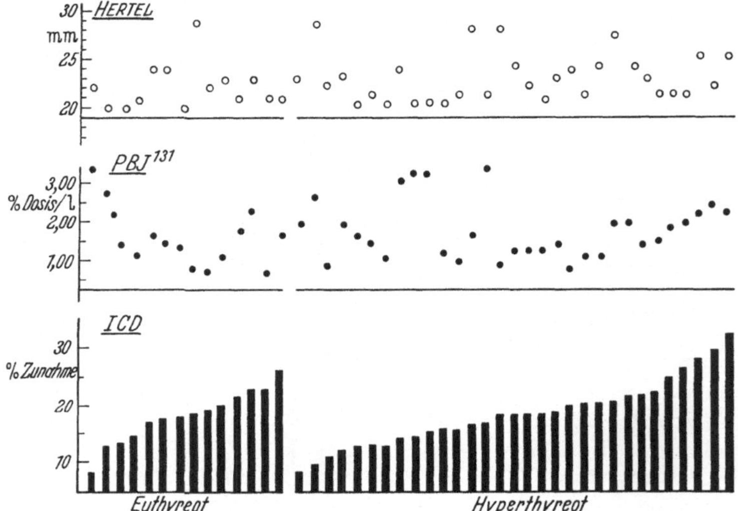

Abb. 2. Endokrine Ophthalmopathien: Höhe der Säulen = prozentuale ICD-Zunahme. Schwarze Punkte = der jeder Säule entsprechende PBI[131]-Wert. Kreise = zugehöriger Hertelwert.

Darüber sind als schwarzer Punkt der PBI[131]-Wert und in der oberen Reihe als Kreis der entsprechende Hertelwert angegeben. Der Normalbereich liegt stets unterhalb der waagerecht ausgezogenen Linien. Die Abbildung mag erkennen lassen, daß einem zunehmenden EPF-Gehalt des Serums weder ein ansteigender PBI[131]-Wert des Serums noch ein zunehmender Exophthalmus entsprechen, d. h. daß offenbar kein Zusammenhang zwischen den angeführten Parametern besteht.

Zusammenfassung

1. Im biologischen Test am Karpfen konnte bestätigt werden, daß im Serum endokriner Ophthalmopathien immer der biochemisch noch nicht identifizierte EPF nachzuweisen ist.

2. Es besteht kein Zusammenhang zwischen der Aktivität dieses Faktors einerseits und dem Ausmaß von Hormonproduktion und intrathyreoidalem Jodumsatz sowie dem Grad des Exophthalmus andererseits.

Literatur

1. Börner, R.: Berichte 59. Zusammenkunft Dtsch. Ophthalm. Ges. 1956, S. 255.
2. Brunish, R., Hayashi K. and J. Hayashi: Arch. Biochem. 98, 135 (1962).
3. Canadell, J., y J. Barraquer: Exoftalmia endocyrina. Publicaciones monograficas del Instituto Barraquer, Madrid, 1958.

4. Condliffe, P. G., u. R. W. Bates: I. Internat. Kongr. Endokrinol. Copenhagen 1960, Abstract 132.
5. Dobyns, B. M., and S. L. Steelman: Endocrinology **52**, 705 (1953).
6. —, and L. A. Wilson: J. clin. Endocr. **14**, 1393 (1954).
7. Haynie, T. B., R. J. Winzler, J. Matovinovic, E. A. Carr and W. H. Beierwaltes: Endocrinology **71**, 782 (1962).
8. Horst,W., u. K. Ullerich: Hypophysen-Schilddrüsen-Erkrankungen und endokrine Ophthalmopathie. Stuttgart: F. Enke Verlag 1958.
9. El Kabir, D. J.: In: Advances in Thyroid Research. London: Pergamon Press 1961.
10. Kemper, F., u. A. Loeser: Acta endocr. (Kbh.) **38**, 200 (1961).
11. Der Kinderen, P. J., Maria Houstra-Lanz, u. F. Schwarz: J. clin. Endocr. **20**, 712 (1960).
12. Klein, E.: Der endogene Jodhaushalt des Menschen und seine Störungen. Stuttgart: G. Thieme Verlag 1960.
13. — H. Zimmermann u. H. Lins: Endokrinologie **39**, 44 (1960).
14. McGill, D. A.: Quart. J. med. **29**, 423 (1960).
15. McKenzie, J. M.: In: Advances in Thyroid Research. London: Pergamon Press 1961.
16. Pimstone, B.: S. Afr. med. J. **36**, 579 (1962).
17. Querido, A., and I. D. F. Lameijer: Proc. roy. Soc. Med. **49**, 209 (1956).
18. Wegelius, O.: Acta endocr. (Kbh.) **22**, 157 (1960).
19. Werner, S. C.: J. Amer. med. Ass. **177**, 551 (1961).
20. Wernze, H., u. K. Wernze: Klin. Wschr. **40**, 262 (1962).

Diskussion

D. Emrich (Freiburg):

Wurde der EPF bei Fällen von endokriner Ophthalmopathie bestimmt, die keine Umsatzbeschleunigung im J^{131}-Test zeigten und welche Ergebnisse wurden dabei gewonnen?

E. Klein:

Wir haben unter 210 hyperthyreoten und 38 euthyreoten endokrinen Ophthalmopathien nur bei 3 der letzteren nicht die an sich obligatorische Beschleunigung des thyreoidalen Jodumsatzes gefunden, obgleich kein Anhalt für eine andere als endokrine Genese festzustellen war. Nur in einem dieser Fälle wurde der EPF bestimmt und seine Aktivität erhöht gefunden.

Aus der Medizinischen Klinik (Dir.: Prof. Dr. E. WOLLHEIM) und dem Pathologischen Institut
der Universität Würzburg (Dir.: Prof. Dr. H. W. ALTMANN)

Vergleichsuntersuchungen über Exophthalmus-Reaktion und Schilddrüsenaktivierung unter Thyreotropin beim Goldfisch

Von

H. WERNZE und G. DHOM

Mit 2 Abbildungen

Seit der Veröffentlichung von ALBERT 1945 über die Erzeugung eines Exophthalmus durch Hypophysenvorderlappen-Präparate an dem Meeresfisch Fundulus heteroclitus ist die Messung der Exophthalmusreaktion an Fischen zu einem einfach zu handhabenden biologischen Test entwickelt worden. Neben den von amerikanischen Autoren verwendeten Fundulus-Arten (*4, 7, 8, 9, 10, 15, 20*) wurden außerdem mit Erfolg Karpfen (*3, 11, 12, 14, 21*) und Goldfische (*5, 18, 23*) herangezogen.

Zwischen der Höhe der Dosis EPS- (= exophthalmus producing substance) -reicher Hypophysenvorderlappenextrakte und dem Grad des Exophthalmus soll nach DOBYNS u. Mitarb. (*9*) beim Fundulus heteroclitus eine grobe Beziehung bestehen. Der KINDEREN u. Mitarb. (*14*) haben bei Karpfen sogar reproduzierbare Dosis-Wirkungs-Kurven als Grundlage für die quantitative Vergleichstestung des Exophthalmus-Producing-Factors im Serum von Patienten mit endokrinem Exophthalmus herausgearbeitet.

Andererseits ist aber bereits ALBERT bei seinen Untersuchungen aufgefallen, daß bei Verwendung verschiedener Dosen eines Hypophysenvorderlappenextraktes immer nur eine bestimmte Quote der Testfische mit einem Exophthalmus reagieren. DOBYNS (*8*) hat in seiner ersten Mitteilung 1954 über den Nachweis des Exophthalmus-Producing-Factors im Serum ebenfalls die große individuelle Streuung innerhalb der Fischkollektive hervorgehoben. Einzelne Tiere bleiben gänzlich ohne Reaktion.

Wir haben diese Angaben mit verschiedenen Thyreotropin (TSH)-Präparaten und mit Seren von Patienten mit endokriner Ophthalmopathie ebenso wie McGILL (*18*) an Goldfischen bestätigen können. KEMPER (*13*) hat bei Versuchen an Karpfen, die 5mal in Abständen von 12 Std mit Thyreotropin behandelt wurden, ebenfalls eine Versagerquote festgestellt.

Unsere Versuchsergebnisse aus insgesamt 10 Testserien bei einmaliger Gabe von 0,5 mg TSH (= 1,25 IE) pro 5 g Fisch zeigten zunächst, daß die Häufigkeit, mit der die Fische einen Exophthalmus produzieren wie auch die Stärke der Reaktion beträchtlich voneinander abwichen. Das galt auch für die Versuche, die in gleichen Monaten durchgeführt wurden. Vergleicht man die Mittelwerte der Exophthalmus-Reaktion bei verschiedener Dosierung von Hypophysenvorderlappen-Extrakt in der zusammenfassenden Arbeit von DOBYNS u. Mitarb. 1961, so ergeben sich auch bezüglich der Dosis-Wirkungs-Beziehungen Überschneidungen. Wodurch diese stark unterschiedliche Reaktionsweise zu erklären ist, konnte von den Autoren, die nunmehr über 10jährige Erfahrung mit dem Fischtest verfügen, für den Fundulus heteroclitus nicht eindeutig bestimmt werden.

Grundsätzlich dürften als Erklärung 2 Faktoren in Betracht kommen:

1. Eine fehlerhafte Injektion, wobei wir als fehlerhaft nicht den während oder sofort nach der Injektion erkennbaren Verlust an Injektionsmaterial verstehen, sondern einen nach Wiedereinbringen der Fische ins Bassin eventuell unkontrollierbar bleibenden Rückfluß aus der Injektionsstelle, begünstigt durch die Schwimmaktivität der Tiere.

2. Eine stark schwankende biologische Ansprechbarkeit der Testfische, die sich nicht allein auf jahreszeitliche Einflüsse erstreckt.

Da die Schilddrüse zahlreicher bislang untersuchter Fische auf TSH-Gabe mit einer Aktivitätssteigerung reagiert (*6, 16*), erschien es uns aus den erwähnten methodischen Gründen aufschlußreich, die Exophthalmus-Reaktion mit der histologischen Schilddrüsen-Reaktion am Einzeltier zu vergleichen. Der Nachweis einer thyreotropen Stimulierung wird dadurch erleichtert, daß beim Goldfisch normalerweise eine ausgesprochene Ruheschilddrüse mit fast endothelartigem Follikelepithel vorliegt (*6*).

Wir haben hierzu Versuche an insgesamt 58 Goldfischen[1] im Gewicht zwischen 4,2 und 6,1 g durchgeführt. Die Fische erhielten in verschiedenen Gruppen einmalig jeweils 0,25 — 2,0 mg/5 g Fisch (entsprechend 0,63—5,0 IE) thyreotropes Hormon mit Exophthalmus-Aktivität[2] über den After in die Cölomhöhle injiziert, 10 Kontrollfische zum Vergleich lediglich das Lösungsmittel 0,7%ige Kochsalzlösung. Das Injektionsvolumen betrug 0,25 ml/5 g Fisch.

Die Messung der Intercornealdistanz mit einer Plastikschublehre erfolgte nach 3, 6, 12 und 24 Std, anschließend die Tötung der Tiere in Urethannarkose. Sodann wurde der Unterkiefer herauspräpariert, in Formalin fixiert, in Serie geschnitten und nach H.E. gefärbt. Das Schilddrüsengewebe der meisten Knochenfische ist kein Organ mit abgegrenzter Kapsel, sondern zeigt in der Nachbarschaft der größeren Kiemengefäße verstreut gelegene Einzelfollikel wechselnder Größe. Die Auswertung der Epithelzellhöhe erfolgte anhand von Mikrofotogrammen. Die Errechnung des mittleren Epithelhöhendurchmessers bezieht sich auf durchschnittlich 110 Einzelmessungen pro Fisch.

In Abb. 1 haben wir die zytometrischen Ergebnisse den jeweiligen Maximalwerten der Exophthalmus-Reaktion innerhalb des Versuchszeitraumes gegenübergestellt. Es zeigt sich, daß es in jeder Versuchsgruppe auch bei der sehr hohen Dosis von 2 mg TSH Fische gibt, die keinen Exophthalmus entwickeln. Der Prozentsatz der Nichtreagenten liegt zwischen 33 und 44%. In den gesamten Versuchsgruppen gibt es demgegenüber nur 4 Tiere, das entspricht rund 8%, die nicht mit einer Schilddrüsenaktivierung reagieren. Zu erwähnen ist, daß sich bei diesen 4 Fischen auch kein Exophthalmus entwickelt hatte. Wir glauben, daß man

---

[1] Zierfischzucht W. GRASSL, Dachau/München.

[2] Charge 494 E 18, PARKE, DAVIS u. Co., Detroit.

diese Gruppe als Injektionsversager ansehen muß. Das schließt nicht aus, daß auch bei den restlichen 44 Fischen mit Schilddrüsenaktivierung teilweise ein Verlust an Injektionsmaterial erfolgt sein kann.

Das Ausmaß der Schilddrüsen-Reaktion ist auch im hohen Dosenbereich von 2 mg TSH nicht von der kleinsten TSH-Dosis unterschieden. Das erklären wir damit, daß offenbar die von uns gewählte kleinste TSH-Dosis von 0,25 mg im 24 Std-Zeitraum bereits eine maximale Stimulierung bewirkt.

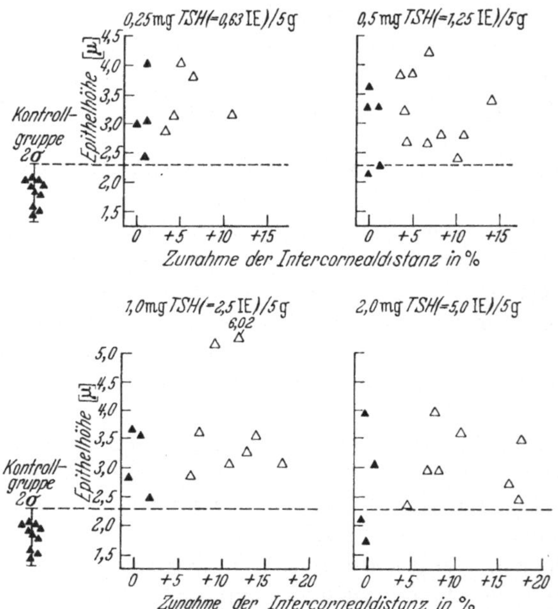

Abb. 1. „Schilddrüsenaktivierung" und Exophthalmusreaktion nach 0,25—2,0 mg TSH beim Goldfisch (△ = sichere, ▲ = fehlende Exophthalmus-Reaktion). Am linken Rand Einzelwerte mit 2 σ Streubereich für den mittleren Epitheldurchmesser der Kontrollgruppe (Mittelwert 1,82 μ)

Bezogen auf die mittlere Epithelhöhe der Kontrollgruppe beträgt die Zunahme des Epitheldurchmessers im Durchschnitt in den Versuchsgruppen 68% bis 95%. Die Exophthalmusreaktion ist im Durchschnitt bei höherer TSH- und dementsprechend höherer EPS-Dosis verstärkt.

Wird die gleiche TSH-Menge nicht einmalig, sondern wiederholt injiziert, so sprechen anfängliche Versager auch später nur äußerst selten mit einem Exophthalmus an. Daß solche Fische dennoch im allgemeinen eine gleichkräftige Schilddrüsenaktivierung entwickeln, ist in Abb. 2 dargestellt.

Inwieweit bei den Fischen mit aktivierter Schilddrüse, aber fehlender Exophthalmus-Reaktion besondere Lokalfaktoren des Retrobulbärraumes oder spezielle Plasma-Inhibitoren der EPS eine Rolle spielen, ist nicht zu beantworten. Für das Zustandekommen der Protrusio bei Fischen ist bekanntlich ebenfalls eine Anhäufung saurer Mucopolysaccharide und parallel damit eine Zunahme des Wassergehaltes im Retrobulbärgewebe maßgeblich (4).

Als synergistische oder potenzierende Faktoren, zumindest beim experimentellen Exophthalmus, sind wiederholt ACTH oder Nebennierenrindenhormone herausgestellt worden. CANADELL und BARRAQUER haben den exophthalmus-verstärkenden Effekt von ACTH bei Injektion eines ACTH-TSH-Gemisches an Goldfischen nachweisen können. Dabei wurde angenommen, daß ACTH und damit

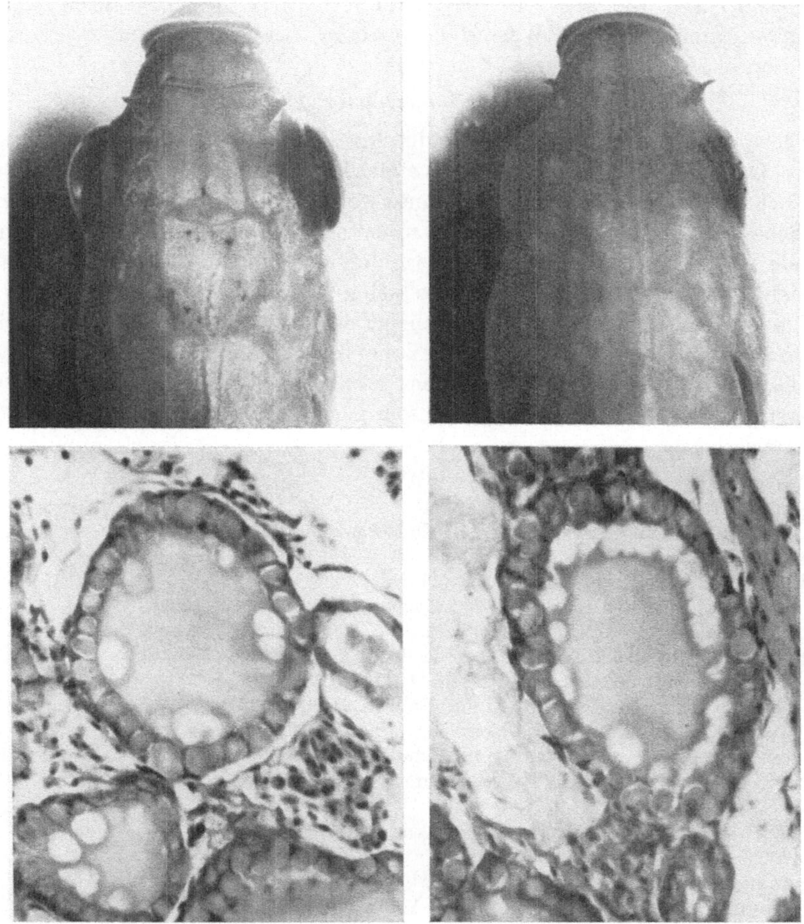

Abb. 2. Behandlung beider Fische mit 2 mal 0,5 mg TSH/5 g Gew. im Abstand von 24 Std. Tötung nach 48 Std. Beachte den Exophthalmus links (Zunahme der ICD + 17%), rechts das Fehlen der Reaktion, bei beiden Fischen die deutlichen Zeichen der „Schilddrüsenaktivierung"

die Aktivität der Nebennierenrinde das Retrobulbärgewebe gegenüber dem Exophthalmuseffekt des TSH-Präparates sensibilisiere. Eigene Versuche haben gezeigt, daß es bei Fischen mit vorhergehender Injektion von ACTH und nachfolgender Gabe von TSH nicht gelingt, die Exophthalmus-Versagerquote auszuschalten.

Die Bedeutung noch unbekannter biologischer und vermutlich äußerer Milieu-Faktoren geht auch aus den paradoxen Versuchsergebnissen von LANGFORD (15) und DOBYNS (10) hervor. Danach entwickelt der Fundulus heteroclitus aus den Gewässern der Bermuda-Inseln nicht auf Hypophysenvorderlappenextrakt, wohl aber auf Schilddrüsenhormone einen Exophthalmus, während die gleichen Fische von den Ost- und Südküsten der USA ein gegensätzliches Verhalten zeigen[1]. Ebenso bemerkenswert ist, daß es offenbar bei den Bermuda-Inseln Fische gibt, die auf Zufuhr von Methyltestosteron und Testosteronphenylacetat einen Exophthalmus entwickeln (*17*). Die äußeren Temperaturverhältnisse scheinen nach unseren Befunden, zumindest bei Wassertemperaturen zwischen 15 und 23° auf die Reaktion ohne Einfluß zu sein.

Zusammenfassung

Die Exophthalmusreaktion an Goldfischen nach einmaliger oder auch wiederholter Gabe von Thyreotropin ist, vergleichbar den Befunden am Fundulus heteroclitus, größeren Schwankungen unterworfen. Als Gründe, beurteilt an Hand der Schilddrüsenaktivierung, kommen in erster Linie biologisch bedingte Unterschiede der Ansprechbarkeit, selten eine fehlerhafte Injektionstechnik in Betracht. Bei der Testung der Exophthalmus-Producing-Aktivität im Serum von Patienten mit endokriner Ophthalmopathie erscheint es vor allem bei der quantitativen Wertbestimmung zweckmäßig, nur Fische mit annähernd vergleichbarer Exophthalmusreaktion zu berücksichtigen. Nichtreagenten innerhalb kleiner Versuchsgruppen schließen das Vorhandensein einer EPS-Aktivität im Testmaterial nicht aus.

Literatur

1. Albert, A.: Endocrinology **37**, 389 (1945).
2. Aterman, K., and S. M. Greenberg: Endocrinology **52**, 510 (1953).
3. Börner, R.: Ber. 59. Zus. dtsch. Ophthalm. Ges. **1956**, 255.
4. Brunish, R.: Endocrinology **62**, 437 (1958).
5. Canadell, I. M., and I. Barraquer: Endocrinology **64**, 1017 (1959).
6. Chavin, W.: J. exp. Zool. **133**, 1 (1956).
7. Dobyns, B. M., and S. L. Steelman: Endocrinology **52**, 705 (1953).
8. —, and L. A. Wilson: J. clin. Endocr. **14**, 1393 (1954).
9. — A. Wright and L. Wilson: J. clin. Endocr. **21**, 648 (1961).
10. —, — and M. A. Sanders: Endocrinology **70**, 864 (1962).
11. Horster, F. A., u. E. Klein: 10. Symposium Dtsch. Ges. Endokrinol. Wien, 1963.
12. Kemper, F., u. A. Loeser: 9. Symposium Dtsch. Ges. Endokrin. Mainz, 1962.
13. — persönl. Mitteilung.
14. Der Kinderen, P. J., M. Houtstra-Lanz and F. Schwarz: J. clin. Endocr. **20**, 712 (1960).
15. Langford, H. G.: Endocrinology **60**, 390 (1957).
16. Leloup, J., and M. Fontaine: Ann. N. Y. Acad. Sci. **86**, 316 (1956).
17. Matty, A. J. D. Menzel and J. E. Bardach: J. Endocr. **17**, 314 (1958).
18. McGill, D. A.: Quart. J. Med. **29**, 423 (1960).
19. —, and S. P. Asper: New. Engl. J. Med. **267**, 133, 188 (1962).
20. Schultz, R. O., A. E. Braley and H. E. Hamilton: Amer. J. Ophthal. **50**, 783 (1960).
21. Schwarz, F., P. J. Der Kinderen and M. Houtstra-Lanz: J. clin. Endocr. **22**, 718 (1962).
22. Smelser, G. K., and V. Ozanics: Amer. J. Ophthal. **39**, 146 (1955).
23. Wernze, H., u. K. Wernze: Klin. Wschr. **40**, 262 (1962).

Diskussion

F. Kemper (Münster):

Auch bei der Verwendung von Karpfen (Cyprinus carpio) zum Nachweis einer EPF-Aktivität reagierten nicht alle eingesetzten Tiere. Im Gegensatz zum Goldfisch fallen hier

---

[1] Vgl. auch Fußnote in (*19*).

jedoch nur 15 bis max. 20% aus. Wie eigene Untersuchungen mit Farbstoffinjektionen ergaben, dürfte ein Teil dieser Versager mit den schon von Herrn WERNZE erwähnten Schwierigkeiten bei der Injektion zusammenhängen. Daneben gibt es sicherlich auch echte Versager, die im Wesen der biologischen Methodik liegen. Bei strenger Beachtung der methodischen Bedingungen und unter der Voraussetzung einer genügend großen Anzahl von Fischen je Kontroll- und Versuchsgruppe ist der Karpfen zum Nachweis des EPF gut geeignet.

E. KLEIN (Düsseldorf):

Nach allen bisherigen Erfahrungen ist offenbar der Goldfisch für den Nachweis des EPF ungeeignet und sollte man, zum mindesten hierzulande, besser junge Karpfen benutzen. Die Provokation eines Exophthalmus am Südsee-Fundulus durch Schilddrüsenhormone (LANGFORD) ließ sich von DOBYNS (4. Int. Kropfkonferenz London 1960) und wohl auch von LANGFORD selber später nicht reproduzieren.

H. WERNZE:

Betreffs Erzeugung eines Exophthalmus an Fischen durch Schilddrüsenhormone ist zu sagen, daß nicht nur am Fundulus heteroclitus, sondern auch an einer Papageienfischart (Sparisoma squalidum) von MATTY, MENZEL u. BARDACH unter Thyroxin und Trijodthyronin ein Exophthalmus erzeugt werden konnte. Zu dem Widerruf der Befunde von LANGFORD erscheint die Fußnote in einer Arbeit von McGILL u. ASPER [New Engl. J. Med. **267**, 133 und 188 (1962)] beachtenswert.

Aus der I. Medizinischen Universitätsklinik in Wien
(Suppl. Leiter: Prof. Dr. H. Jesserer)

Über den Einfluß der hypophysären Regulation auf die Verteilung der jodierten Aminosäuren im Serum

Von

N. Honetz und R. Kotzaurek

Mit 2 Abbildungen

Seit der Entdeckung von Trijodthyronin als zweitem Schilddrüsenhormon durch J. Gross und R. Pitt-Rivers (6) gewann die Auftrennung der Schilddrüseninkrete praktische Bedeutung, zumal dem Trijodthyronin eine rund fünffache Stoffwechselwirksamkeit gegenüber Thyroxin zugeschrieben und schon sehr frühzeitig die Möglichkeit einer Verschiebung des physiologischen Verhältnisses beider Inkrete diskutiert wurde. Zur Trennung dieser beiden Hormone und einer Reihe ihrer Metaboliten aus Schilddrüsengewebe bzw. Serum bediente man sich anfänglich fast ausschließlich der Butanolextraktion mit nachfolgenden komplizierten Waschungen. Die eigentliche Trennnung der einzelnen jodhaltigen Aminosäuren erfolgte allerdings erst mit Hilfe der Papierchromatographie. Um den Schwierigkeiten des chemischen Nachweises der einzelnen Substanzen am Papier zu entgehen, bediente man sich größtenteils Aktivitätsmessungen in Chromatogrammen nach Gabe von ^{131}J. Mit dieser Technik gelang es zwar, noch kleinere Mengen zu erfassen, doch ließ sie keine quantitativen Aussagen zu. Erst die Einführung der Absorption des Untersuchungsmaterials an einen Ionenaustauscher an Stelle der Butanolextraktion gestattete es, durch Verminderung der methodischen Fehlerquellen eine brauchbare Arbeitsvorschrift zur getrennten quantitativen Bestimmung von Thyroxin und Trijodthyronin auszuarbeiten. In der Entwicklung dieses speziellen Arbeitsgebietes verdienen folgende Autoren besonders erwähnt zu werden: R. Pitt-Rivers (13), J. Gross (5), J. Roche u. Mitarb. (14), R. H. Mandl u. R. J. Block (11), N. F. Maclagan u. Mitarb. (10), G. Feuer (3), J. Wynn (16), T. Béraud (1), E. Klein (9), R. Höfer (7) sowie H. Spitzy u. Mitarb. (12).

An der I. Medizinischen Universitätsklinik in Wien wurden seit vier Jahren einschlägige Untersuchungen durchgeführt, so daß die Schwierigkeiten der verschiedenen Verfahren wohl bekannt waren, ehe vor einem halben Jahr eine neue Methodik eingeführt wurde, die eine Fortentwicklung der Jodbestimmungsmethode nach Spitzy, Reese und Skrube (15) darstellt. Ihre relative Einfachheit gestattet es, die Fehler sehr klein zu halten und somit auch kleinste Mengen von Schilddrüsenhormonen noch exakt zu erfassen. 2,0 ml Serum läßt man durch eine geeichte Sephadex-G 25[1]-Säule laufen und der Eiweißanteil wird direkt in einem

---

[1] Sephadex der Firma Pharmacia, Uppsala, Schweden.

mit 80%iger Ameisensäure und 80%iger Essigsäure vorbehandelten Dowex[1] (1 × 2, 10 mesh) beschickten Glaszylinder einer auseinandernehmbaren Fritte aufgefangen. Anschließend wird 1 Std geschüttelt, die Fritte zusammengesetzt und das denaturierte Eiweiß mit isotoner Kochsalzlösung, dann mit bidestilliertem Wasser und schließlich seine Reste mit verdünnter Essigsäure (pH 3,0) entfernt. Die Elution der Schilddrüsenhormone erfolgt mit einem Gemisch von konzentrierter Ameisensäure und konzentrierter Essigsäure in einem Verhältnis von 2:1. Das Elutionsmittel wird schließlich in einem Oberflächenverdampfer ent-

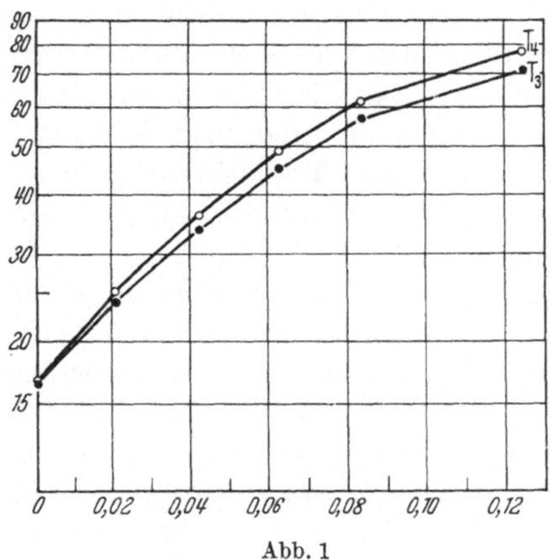

Abb. 1

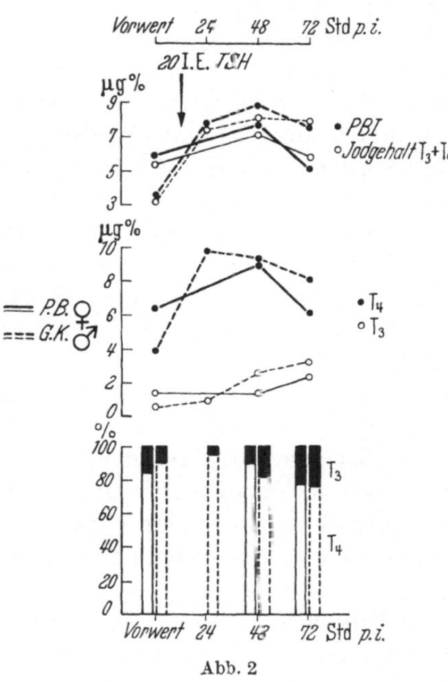

Abb. 2

fernt und der Rückstand in 0,4 ml ammoniakgesättigtem Methanol gelöst und davon zweimal 0,1 ml an den Startpunkten der Chromatographiestreifen (Schleicher-Schüll 2043) getrennt aufgetragen. Es wurde mit einem n-Butanol-Dioxan-Ammoniak-Gemisch (5:1:4 Vol-%) als Lösungsmittel in absteigender Form gearbeitet und damit regelmäßig eine brauchbare Trennung von Thyroxin und Trijodthyronin erzielt. Als Vergleichssubstanzen wurden kleinste Mengen (etwa 0,1 µg) chromatographiereiner, jodierter Aminosäuren und radioaktives Trijodthyronin verwendet, die beiderseits des zu untersuchenden Eluats aufgetragen und mit der modifizierten „Berlinerblaureaktion" nach GMELIN und VIRTANEN (4) färberisch dargestellt bzw. aktivitätsmäßig analysiert wurden. Entsprechend den Positionen der Vergleichssubstanzen wurden an den Untersuchungsstreifen Papierscheibchen im Durchmesser von 25 mm ausgeschnitten und eluiert. In einer eigens zu diesem Zwecke entwickelten Apparatur werden die Substanzen mit Hilfe von 2,0 ml ammoniakgesättigtem Methanol aus dem Papier eluiert und direkt in die Bestimmungskölbchen nach SPITZY, REESE und SKRUBE übergeführt, das Elutionsmittel anschließend im Vakuum abgedampft, der Rückstand der katalytischen Jodreaktion unterworfen, colorimetriert und die Mengen von Thyroxin und Trijodthyronin mit Hilfe von getrennten Eichkurven ermittelt (Abb. 1).

---

[1] Dowex der Firma Fluka A. G., Buchs SG., Schweiz.

Um die erhaltenen Resultate mit gleichzeitig ermittelten PBI-Werten zu korrelieren, müssen erstere auf ihren Jodgehalt bezogen werden.

Um die Verteilung der Schilddrüsenhormone vor und nach Stimulierung mit thyreotropem Hormon zu erfassen, wurde die angegebene Methodik an zwei Patienten klinisch erprobt. Es wurden in jedem Falle 20 IE TSH (Ambinon[1]) einmalig intramuskulär verabfolgt. Die dabei erhaltenen Ergebnisse sind aus Abb. 2 ersichtlich.

Hier ist oben mit stark ausgezogenen bzw. unterbrochenen Linien das Verhalten des eiweißgebundenen Serumjod (PBI) vor und nach der Verabreichung von thyreotropem Hormon wiedergegeben. In beiden Fällen war der 48 Std-Wert am höchsten, wobei das PBI einmal von 5,9 auf 7,7 μg-% und das anderemal von 3,5 auf 8,8 μg-% angestiegen war. Nur in einem Fall war der Ausgangsspiegel nach 72 Std wieder erreicht worden. Im anderen Fall, bei dem es zu einem 150%igen PBI-Anstieg gekommen war, stellte sich bei dem Patienten auch ein länger anhaltendes Druckgefühl in der Schilddrüsengegend ein. Die dünn ausgezogenen bzw. unterbrochenen Linien geben das Verhalten der auf den Jodgehalt bezogenen Summen der gleichzeitig bestimmten Thyroxin- und Trijodthyroninmengen wieder. Bei ihrer Gegenüberstellung zu den PBI-Werten wurde zu keinem Zeitpunkt eine Abweichung von mehr als 10% festgestellt.

Bei der getrennten Bestimmung von Thyroxin und Trijodthyronin im Serum zeigte sich nach der Stimulierung mit TSH ein unterschiedliches Verhalten beider Schilddrüsenhormone. Das Thyroxin erreichte bei beiden Patienten frühzeitig sein Maximum, was auch im PBI-Anstieg seinen Ausdruck fand, um nach 72 Std deutlich abzusinken. Im Gegensatz dazu wies der Trijodthyroninspiegel in dem einen Fall nach 48 Std und in dem anderen erst nach 72 Std einen Anstieg auf, zu Zeitpunkten also, in denen die Thyroxin- bzw. PBI-Maxima schon deutlich überschritten waren. Nach 72 Std betrug die Trijodthyroninerhöhung das Doppelte bzw. das Sechsfache des Ausgangswertes. Um das gegensätzliche Verhalten beider Schilddrüsenhormone nach Stimulierung mit thyreotropem Hormon noch deutlicher zum Ausdruck zu bringen, wurde im unteren Anteil des Diagrammes ihr prozentuales Verhältnis zueinander zu den angegebenen Zeitpunkten graphisch festgehalten. Die Verhältnisse der Vorwerte betrugen 85:15 sowie 91:9 und die nach 72 Std 77:23 und 76:24. Das bedeutet, daß sich das Verhältnis zu diesem Zeitpunkt zugunsten von Trijodthyronin deutlich verschoben hat. Ein gleichgerichtetes Ergebnis haben Hydovitz und Arons (8) durch Aktivitätsbestimmungen in Chromatogrammen erhalten. Ob die aus dem Diagramm nach 24 Std bzw. auch teilweise noch nach 48 Std ersichtliche geringgradige Verschiebung zugunsten vonThyroxin echt ist, kann einerseits wegen Ausfalles einerBestimmungsserie, andererseits deshalb nicht entschieden werden, weil so kleine noch in die Fehlerbreite der Methodik fallende Änderungen des absoluten Trijodthyroninspiegels schon deutliche Verschiebungen des Hormonverhältnisses bei variabler Gesamtsumme bedingen.

Besprechung

Die hier angewendete Methodik bietet den Vorteil, daß nur kleine Serummengen zur Verarbeitung notwendig sind und sie, ein geschultes Personal voraus-

---

[1] Ambinon der Firma Organon-OSS (Holland).

gesetzt, relativ einfach zu handhaben ist. Ihre Fehlerbreite ist so gering, daß deutlichere Hormonverschiebungen erfaßt und damit reproduzierbar werden. Eine Steigerung der Genauigkeit der Methodik ist nur durch getrennte Elution von Thyroxin und Trijodthyronin vom Ionenaustauscher mit nachfolgender quantitativer Bestimmung unter Weglassung der Papierchromatographie möglich.

Bezüglich der Ergebnisse erscheint es derzeit nicht berechtigt, weitere Hypothesen über die TSH-Wirkung abzuleiten. Die Resultate sind lediglich in bisher erworbene Erkenntnisse einzubauen. So sind die Thyroxinerhöhungen im Serum 24 und 48 Std nach der TSH-Stimulierung mit den bisher bekannten Untersuchungsergebnissen von eiweißgebundenem Serumjod durchaus in Einklang zu bringen [BOWERS u. Mitarb. (2)]. Für die Erfassung des zeitlich nachfolgenden, im Vergleich dazu geringgradigen Trijodthyroninanstieges ist die PBI-Bestimmung überfordert, doch müßte letztere eher in der Hormonwirksamkeit am Erfolgsorgan zum Ausdruck kommen. Ferner ergibt sich aus den Resultaten die Folgerung, daß die Stimulierung der Schilddrüse mit Rückkehr des PBI zum Ausgangswert keineswegs als abgeschlossen gelten kann, sondern daß die Untersuchungen zeitlich solange fortzusetzen sind, bis auch der Ausgangswert des Trijodthyronins erreicht ist. Zum besseren Verständnis der Wirksamkeit von TSH auf die Schilddrüse erscheint eine mehrmalige Verabfolgung von thyreotropem Hormon bei gleicher Versuchsanordnung erforderlich.

Zusammenfassung

Es wurden erstmals mittels einer neu ausgearbeiteten Methode die einzelnen Schilddrüsenhormone quantitativ erfaßt und ihr Verhalten auf eine einmalige Injektion von 20 IE TSH (Ambinon) geprüft. Dabei ergab sich bei den beiden untersuchten Fällen eine gute Übereinstimmung der Werte untereinander wie auch mit dem gleichzeitig bestimmten eiweißgebundenem Serumjod. Die getrennte Bestimmung der beiden Hormone erfolgte 24, 48 und 72 Std nach der TSH-Verabreichung und zeigte bei beiden Patienten ein Verhältnis Thyroxin:Trijodthyronin von rund 9:1 als Ausgangswert, wobei sich dieses bei dem einen Patienten 72 Std und bei dem anderen bereits 48 Std nach der TSH-Gabe deutlich zugunsten des Trijodthyronin verschob.

Literatur

1. BÉRAUD, T.: Répartition de l'iode organique plasmatique en physiopathologie thyroïdienne. Schweiz. med. J. **90, 1340** (1960).
2. BOWERS, C. Y., P. J. MURISON, D. L. GORDON and W. LOCKE: Effect of thyrotropin on the serum protein-bound iodine level in various thyroid states (TSH-PBI-test).
3. FEUER, G.: Papierchromatographische Bestimmung der Schilddrüsenhormone. Acta physiol. Acad. Sci. hung. **12,** 19 (1957).
4. GMELIN, R., and A. I. VIRTANEN: A sensitive colour reaction for the paperchromatographic detection of iodide, iodinated thyronines, and thyronines. Acta chem. scand. **13,** 1469 (1959).
5. GROSS, J.: Thyroid hormones. Brit. med. Bull. **10,** 218 (1954).
6. —, and R. PITT-RIVERS: II. Thyroid hormone physiology and biochemistry. Triiodothyronine in relation to thyroid physiology. Recent Progr. Hormone Res. **10,** 109 (1954).
7. HÖFER, R.: Der Jodstoffwechsel nach Strumektomie. Fortschritte der Schilddrüsenforschung. S. 70. Herausgeg. von K. OBERDISSE u. E. KLEIN. Stuttgart, G. Thieme, 1961.
8. HYDOVITZ, J. D., and W. L. ARONS: Effect of thyrotropin on the pattern of thyroid hormones in plasma. J. Endocr. **17,** 1332 (1957).

9. Klein, E.: Der endogene Jodhaushalt des Menschen und seine Störungen. Stuttgart: G. Thieme, 1960.
10. Maclagan, N. F., C. H. Bowden and J. H. Wilkinson: The metabolism of thyroid hormones. II. Detection of thyroxine and triiodothyronine in human plasma. Biochem. J. **67**, 5 (1957).
11. Mandl, R. H., and R. J. Block: Methods for the qualitative, semiquantitative and quantitative determination of iodoamino acids and of inorganic iodide in iodoprotein digests and in human serum. Arch. Biochem. **81**, 25 (1959).
12. Müller, K., H. Skrube u. H. Spitzy: Zur Isolierung der Schilddrüsenhormone aus dem Blutserum mit DOWEX 1 $\times$ 2. Mikrochim. Acta **1962**, 1144.
13. Pitt-Rivers, R., and J. R. Tata: The thyroid hormones. Pergamon Press 1959.
14. Roche, J., and R. Michel: On the peripheral metabolism of thyroid hormones. Ann. N. Y. Acad. Sci. **86**, 454 (1960).
15. Spitzy, H., M. Reese u. H. Skrube: Eine neue, einfache Jodbestimmung im Blutserum unter Anwendung der Isothermdiffusion. Mikrochim. Acta **4**, 488 (1958).
16. Wynn, J.: Organic iodine constituents in human serum. Arch. Biochem. **87**, 120 (1960).

Division of Endocrinology, Department of Medicine, University of Oregon Medical School,
Portland, Oregon

Hypothalamus und Schilddrüse

Von

Monte A. Greer

Referat

Man hat lange vermutet, daß die Schilddrüse in einem bestimmten Maße unter
der Kontrolle des Zentralnervensystems steht. Gewisse Merkmale der Hyperthyreose, zum Beispiel Tremor, Schweißausbrüche, Hyperaktivität und Tachykardie
können durch einen rein nervösen Mechanismus entstehen. Weiter stellten viele
Beobachter fest, daß einer klinischen Hyperthyreose oft hochgradige emotionale
Störungen vorausgehen. Man hat daher immer wieder die Frage aufgeworfen, ob
nicht die Basedowsche Krankheit psychosomatischer Natur sei.

Bei der Entwicklung der wissenschaftlichen Endokrinologie in der ersten
Hälfte dieses Jahrhunderts ergaben sich nur wenig experimentelle Befunde, die
eine solche Hypothese stützten. Als dann die Rolle der Hypophyse bei der Steuerung der Schilddrüsenfunktion nach und nach aufgedeckt wurde, schien es, als ob
die Hypophyse zu der Schilddrüse die gleiche Beziehung habe wie zu den anderen
untergeordneten Drüsen. Die Hypophyse war die Steuerdrüse, welche die untergeordneten Drüsen über einen Rückkopplungseffekt kontrollierte. Die Adenohypophyse sezerniert Thyrotropin in variierenden Mengen, um im zirkulierenden
Blut einen konstanten Thyroxinspiegel zu unterhalten. In dieser Beziehung verhielt sich die Hypophyse wie ein Thermostat, die Schilddrüse wie ein Ofen. Man
nahm an, daß Schilddrüse und Hypophyse nur voneinander abhängig seien, daß
sie im wesentlichen unabhängig von nervösen Kontrollen seien. Man dachte sich
eine rein humorale Beziehung. Im letzten Jahrzehnt trat nun ein merklicher Wan-
del in den Anschauungen über die Hypophysenfunktion ein. Man arbeitete die
Bedeutung des Pfortadersystems der Hypophyse heraus, das von der eminentia
mediana des Hypothalamus zu der Adenohypophyse zieht, und verlegte die Betonung auf ein neues, höher gelegenes Steuergebiet. Man glaubt heute allgemein,
daß dieses Steuerzentrum der Hypothalamus sei. Viele und ganz unterschiedliche Experimente zeigten, daß die Hypophyse nur dann normal arbeitet, wenn
sie in direkter Verbindung mit dem Hypothalamus steht und ein offenes und
funktionierendes Pfortadersystem hat. Andererseits können, wenn das Pfortadersystem unversehrt bleibt, bestimmte, lokalisierte Läsionen des Hypothalamus
definierte Alterationen der Hypophysensekretion hervorrufen.

Die Bedeutung des Zentralnervensystems für die Schilddrüsenfunktion war
erstmalig eindeutig nachgewiesen, als gefunden wurde, daß elektrolytische
Läsionen im vorderen Hypothalamus die Schilddrüsenhypertrophie verhindern

konnten, die gewöhnlich aus einer chronischen Propylthiourazil-Fütterung resultiert. Tiere mit solchen Läsionen bilden aber nach TSH-Injektionen Kröpfe. Dies zeigt, daß Läsionen im Hypothalamus die TSH-Sekretion blockieren.

Schließlich fand man, daß das Gebiet des Nucleus paraventricularis von größter Bedeutung für die Steuerung der Schilddrüsenfunktion zu sein scheint. Verhältnismäßig kleine Läsionen in diesem Gebiet vermindern die TSH-Sekretion, während wirksame Läsionen in anderen Gebieten des Hypothalamus nahezu ausnahmslos mit einer Atrophie der Nuclei paraventriculares verbunden sind.

Eine elektrische Reizung des Hypothalamus hat den entgegengesetzten Effekt, nämlich einen Anstieg der Schilddrüsen-Sekretion. Dies wurde von Harris u. Mitarb. beim Kaninchen und von Matsuda u. Mitarb. beim Hund nachgewiesen. Die größte Wirkung scheint man zu erhalten, wenn man den vorderen Hypothalamus in dem Gebiet reizt, in dem Läsionen eine Verminderung der TSH-Sekretion verursachen. Wenn auch die Bedeutung des vorderen Hypothalamus für die Steuerung der Schilddrüsenfunktion klar bewiesen ist, so ist es doch noch unbekannt, ob Hypothalamus, Adenohypophyse und Schilddrüse ein verhältnismäßig autonomes System bilden, oder ob noch andere Teile des Zentralnervensystems über eine Modifizierung der Hypothalamus-Aktivität an der Steuerung der Schilddrüsenfunktion wesentlich beteiligt sind. Der Hypothalamus ist ein ungemein komplexes System und ist reich versehen mit Nervenverbindungen zu anderen Gebieten, besonders zum Limbus-System.

Angesichts der Tatsache, daß die Schilddrüse auf Änderungen der Umgebung reagieren kann, würde man erwarten, daß einige dieser Verbindungsfasern die Thyrotropinsteuerung des Hypothalamus modulieren. Jedoch mindert die Entfernung großer Gebiete im Vorderhirn die Fähigkeit der Adenohypophyse, TSH in maximalen Mengen zu produzieren, nur ganz unwesentlich.

Es erscheint nun außer Frage, daß für die Erzeugung einer Schilddrüsen-Hypertrophie größere TSH-Mengen nötig sind als für eine Steigerung der Synthese oder der Abgabe von Schilddrüsenhormon. Wenn daher in Versuchstieren nach einer langdauernden Verabreichung einer schilddrüsenhemmenden Substanz ein Kropf entsteht, der jenem von Kontrolltieren vergleichbar ist, so kann man ziemlich sicher sein, daß die TSH-Sekretion der Adenohypophyse nicht wesentlich gebremst ist. Diese Technik wurde bei Ratten angewandt, und es wurde gefunden, daß die Entfernung der Neokortex, der Corpora Amygdala oder des Epithalamus die Fähigkeit zur maximalen TSH-Sekretion nicht vermindert. Mess berichtete, daß die Zerstörung der Nuclei habenulares die TSH-Sekretion etwas bremst. Diese Ergebnisse konnten aber in unserem Laboratorium von Yamada und Matsuda nicht reproduziert werden. Wie ich hörte, hat auch Mess selbst diesen Gedanken weitgehend aufgegeben.

Matsuda hat kürzlich in unserem Laboratorium eine Technik ausgearbeitet welche in der Ratte die Entfernung des ganzen Vorderhirnes von dem Colliculus superior bis zu dem Diaphragma sellae erlaubt.

Unter diesen Bedingungen, wo das Vorderhirn bis hinunter zu dem Hypothalamus entfernt war, und wo der Hypothalamus infolge der Durchschneidung der hinteren Nervenverbindungen isoliert war, entwickelten die Ratten Kröpfe, die genau so groß waren wie jene der unversehrten Kontrolltiere. Wenn dagegen nur die Eminentia mediana, der Hypophysenstiel und die Hypophyse selbst erhalten blieben, entwickelte sich kein Kropf. Dies weist darauf hin, daß es der Hypothalamus ist, der einen maximalen Anstieg der TSH-Sekretion verursacht oder erlaubt, und zwar ohne irgendwelche Beteiligung des restlichen Nervensystems, da ja die hinteren Nervenverbindungen durchschnitten waren. Wenn auch die Zahl der Versuchstiere sehr klein ist, so zeigen doch die Ergebnisse, daß der Hypothalamus selbst für den Anstieg der TSH-Sekretion von wesentlicher Bedeutung ist, da bei Ratten, in denen die Eminentia mediana sozusagen als isolierte Insel übrig gelassen wurde, sich keine Kröpfe entwickeln. Diese Ergebnisse stimmen mit früheren überein, welche zeigten, daß Läsionen im vorderen Hypothalamus die kropfbildende Wirkung von Schilddrüsenhemmern aufhebt.

Nun kommen aber wichtige, modifizierende Einflüsse auf das TSH-Zentrum aus dem Hypothalamus selbst, wie verschiedene Experimente zeigen. Ganz kürzlich wies Andersson eine intrahypothalamische Kopplung bei der TSH-Abgabe nach. Viele Untersucher zeigten, daß Änderungen der Umgebungstemperatur Änderungen der Schilddrüsenfunktion verursachen. Wenn man Tiere der Kälte aussetzt, wird die Schilddrüsen-Sekretion erhöht, während bei einer Erhöhung der Körpertemperatur sich die Schilddrüsen-Sekretion vermindert. Andersson entwickelte nun eine Technik zur lokalen Kühlung des „Kühlzentrums" mittels eines stereotaxisch implantierten Kältefingers bei Ziegen. Dieser Eingriff verursachte einen erheblichen Anstieg der allgemeinen Körpertemperatur. Die Schilddrüsensekretion stieg höher an, als wenn das Tier der Kälte ausgesetzt worden wäre. Da normalerweise ein Anstieg der Körpertemperatur einen Abfall der Schilddrüsenaktivität verursacht, kann man aus diesem Experiment der lokalisierten Kühlung entnehmen, daß auf lokale Kälte hin die TSH-Sekretion direkt im Hypothalamus aktiviert wird.

Weitere Beweise für einen intrahypothalamischen Mechanismus bei der Steuerung der TSH-Abgabe wurden durch folgende Experimente geliefert. Thyroxin wurde in den Hypothalamus in Mengen injiziert, welche zu klein waren, um bei intraperitonealer Applikation irgendwelche Änderungen der Schilddrüsen-Funktion zu verursachen. Solche Untersuchungen haben zuerst von Euler und Holmgren bei Kaninchen durchgeführt. Diese Autoren fanden, daß Injektionen von Thyroxin in die Hypophyse die Schilddrüsen-Funktion unverzüglich unterdrückten, daß aber ähnliche Injektionen in den Hypothalamus wirkungslos waren. Diese Untersuchungen wurden von Yamada in unserem Laboratorium bei der Ratte wiederholt. Die Wirksamkeit von Thyroxininjektionen in die Hypophyse war schnell bestätigt. Es ergab sich aber, daß in der Ratte intrahypothalamische Injektionen von gleichem Volumen und gleichem Thyroxin-Gehalt gleicherweise wirksam waren. Andere Untersucher, z. B. Daume und Hohlweg und Kovacs, haben im Folgenden den hemmenden Effekt intrahypothalamischer Thyroxininjektionen bestätigt. Der Grund für von Eulers negatives Versuchsergebnis ist möglicherweise darin zu suchen, daß das injizierte Flüssigkeitsvolumen sehr klein war im Verhältnis zu jenem, das Yamada in die Ratte injizierte. Das Thyrotropin-Zentrum im Hypothalamus ist offensichtlich ziemlich groß. So mag das von von Euler injizierte Volumen so klein gewesen sein, daß es nicht auf genügend Zellen des Zentrums einwirkte und sie zur TSH-Abgabe-Hemmung veranlaßte. In Yamadas Experimenten andererseits wurde ein so großes Volumen injiziert, daß eine genügende Durchtränkung des gesamten Thyrotropin-Zentrums garantiert war.

BROWN-GRANT und PURVES stellten die Theorie auf, daß der grundlegende Mechanismus bei der Steuerung der TSH-Sekretion durch den Hypothalamus ein Filter-System im Hypothalamus oder in der Eminentia mediana sei. Nach diesem Konzept wird die Thyroxin-Menge, welche die Adenohypophyse erreicht, durch einen verstellbaren Filter in Hypothalamus reguliert. Wenn dieser Filter durch eine Läsion im Hypothalamus zerstört ist oder durch eine Transplantation der Hypophyse ausgeschaltet ist, erreichen größere Thyroxinmengen aus dem zirkulierenden Blut die Adenohypophyse, so daß bei einem bestimmen Thyroxinspiegel im Blut eine stärkere Hemmung der THS-Produktion eintritt als in den normalen Kontrolltieren. Für diese Theorie spricht, daß die Adenohypophyse, wie festgestellt wurde, Receptoren besitzt, an denen das Thyroxin angreifen und die TSH-Produktion hemmen kann. Zu Gunsten dieser Theorie spricht weiter, daß in Tieren mit transplantierten Hypophysen oder mit Läsionen im Hypothalamus, in welchen der Filtermechanismus nicht wirksam sein kann, geringere Thyroxin-Mengen für die Hemmung der TSH-Produktion notwendig sind als in Normaltieren. Diese Hypothese kann aber nicht erklären, warum in Tieren mit Läsionen im Hypothalamus oder mit Hypophysentransplantaten keine maximale TSH-Sekretion eintritt, wenn das Schilddrüsenhormon, etwa nach langzeitiger Verabreichung von Propylthiourazil, nahezu vollständig aus dem Körper entfernt wird. Wenn es sich um einen Filtermechanismus handeln würde, müßte man erwarten, daß Abwesenheit von Schilddrüsenhormon im Körper zu einer maximalen Thyrotropin-Ausschüttung führt, gleichgültig wo die Hypophyse sich befindet und ob der Hypothalamus zerstört ist oder nicht. Da dies aber nicht der Fall ist, müssen wir offensichtlich positive Einflüsse des Hypothalamus postulieren, die die Thyrotropin-Abgabe stimulieren.

Die Natur dieses Einflusses des Hypothalamus ist zur Zeit noch nicht aufgeklärt. Da die Adenohypophyse kaum mit Nerven versorgt ist, und da, wie nachgewiesen wurde, das Pfortadersystem von ganz besonderer Bedeutung für das normale Funktionieren der Adenohypophyse ist, nimmt man heute allgemein an, daß über das portale System gewisse Substanzen von Hypothalamus zu der Hypophyse transportiert werden. Für die Existenz einer solchen neurohumoralen Kontrolle wurden im Falle der ACTH- und LH-Sekretion ziemlich starke Beweise geliefert. Die Beweisgründe für ein TRF, einen „Thyrotropin Releasing Factor" analog dem „Corticotropin Releasing Factor", CRF, sind bestenfalls fragmentarisch und verwirrend. Verschiedene Untersucher berichten über Experimente zum Nachweis und zur Isolation von TRF. Diese Experimente sind aber nicht voll überzeugend. Zu diesem Zeitpunkt muß die neurohumorale Kontrolle der Thyrotropin-Abgabe als wahrscheinliche, aber unbewiesene Hypothese angesehen werden. Überblickt man das Gebiet, so erscheint es außer Frage, daß unsere einfache und so präzise Thermostat- und -Ofen-Anschauung der Steuerung der Schilddrüsenfunktion, die bis vor 10 Jahren allgemein akzeptiert war, falsch sein muß. Anstatt dessen sind wir mit einer rasch wachsenden Masse von Informationen konfrontiert, die uns klar zeigen, daß der Hypothalamus ein integraler Teil des Steuersystems der Schilddrüse ist, welches die Homoeostase durch einen konstanten Thyroxinspiegel im zirkulierenden Blut aufrechterhält. Welche Strukturen und welche Mechanismen die Aktivität des Hypothalamus modifizieren und wie nun genau der Hypothalamus auf die Thyrotropin-Sekretion der Hypophyse einwirkt, das sind Probleme, die gegenwärtig in einer ganzen Anzahl von Laboratorien intensiv studiert werden. Wir wollen hoffen, daß sie bald klarer erscheinen.

Literatur

1. HARRIS, G. W., and J. W. WOODS: J. Physiol. (Lond). **143**, 246 (1958).
2. SHIZUME, K., K. MATSUDA, M. IRIE, S. IINO, J. ISHII, S. NAGATAKI, F. MATSUZAKI and S. OKINAKA: Endocrinology **70**, 298 (1962).
3. MESS, B.: Endokrinologie **35**, 196 (1958).
4. YAMADA, T.: Endocrinology **69**, 706 (1961).
5. MATSUDA, K.: Endocrinology **72**, 972 (1963).
6. —, J. W. KENDALL, jr., C. DUYCK and M. A. GREER: Endocrinology **72**, 845 (1963).
7. ANDERSSON, B., L. EKMAN, G. G. GALE and J. W. SUNDSTEN: Life Sciences **1**, 1 (1962).
8. EULER, C. von, and B. HOLMGREN. J. Physiol. (Lond.) **131**, 125 (1956).
9. YAMADA, T., and M. A. GREER. Endocrinology **64**, 559 (1959).
10. — Endocrinology **65**, 216 (1959).
11. — Endocrinology **65**, 920 (1959).
12. DAUME, E., and W. HOHLWEG: Endokrinologie **38**, 51 (1959).
13. KOVACS, S., and M. VERTES: Endokrinologie **40**, 159 (1961).
14. BROWN-GRANT, K.: Ciba Foundation Colloquia on Endocrinology **10**, 97 (1957).
15. AVERILL, R. L. W., H. D. PURVES and N. E. SIRETT: Endocrinology **69**, 735 (1961).

Diskussion

A. STURM (Wuppertal):

Nachdem ich 1926 mikrojodanalytisch einen von der Schilddrüsenfunktion abhängigen physiologischen Blutjodspiegel in Höhe von 8%γ-Jodeiweiß nachweisen konnte, bestimmte ich 1932 zusammen mit R. SCHNEEBERG den Jodgehalt einzelner Hirnteile. Ich konnte feststellen, daß bei Mensch, Hund und Kaninchen vor allem nach Thyroxininjektion bzw. Thyreoidingaben das Tuber cinereum und die benachbarten basalen Hirnformationen in der Umgebung des 3. Ventrikels jodhaltiger waren als andere Hirnteile und daß nach Hypophysektomie das Tuber cinereum diesen Jodreichtum verliert. 1955 habe ich diese Versuche zusammen mit W. WERNITZ mit radiojodtechnischen Methoden wieder aufgenommen, konnte die alten Versuche bestätigen und erweitern:

Injizierte man 1 mC J^{131} bei Meerschweinchen intraperitoneal, so zeigte sich 2 Std später, in der sog. Jodidphase, eine einheitliche Jodverteilung im Gehirn. In der Hormonphase, d. h. 24 Stunden nach intraperitonealer Jodinjektion, war eine starke Anreicherung von Hormonjod im Hypophysenhinterlappen und im Tuber cinereum nachweisbar. Führte man den gleichen Versuch beim hypophysektomierten Tier mit sekundärer Schilddrüsenatrophie durch, so fehlte die Hormonjodanreicherung. Gab man zusätzlich TSH zur Aktivierung der ruhiggestellten Schilddrüse, so trat der Jodreichtum der vorgenannten Hirnteile wieder deutlich in Erscheinung. Spritzte man beim Normaltier Thyroxin mit radioaktiv markiertem J^{131}, so war dieselbe Hormonjodanreicherung nachzuweisen wie in der Hormonphase des Radiojodtestes. Die an Trockenorganen gewonnenen Meßergebnisse der Strahlungsintensitäten wurden mittels Autoradiographie kontrolliert und voll bestätigt.

Damit erscheint hinreichend bewiesen, daß eine bestimmte Affinität des basalen Hypothalamus zum Schilddrüsenhormon besteht — in Übereinstimmung mit den Tierexperimenten von COURRIER, JENSEN, CLARK, BROLIN, UOTILA und vor allem GREER. Der Hypothalamus ist wahrscheinlich der Receptor für Schilddrüsenhormon in dem Reglerkreis Schilddrüse — Hypothalamus — Hypophyse, in dem der Schilddrüsenhormonspiegel des Blutes die Reglergröße, die Schilddrüse das Regelglied darstellt.

Aus der Medizinischen Poliklinik der Universität Würzburg (Direktor: Prof. Dr. H. Franke)

Die Beurteilung der peripheren Hormon-jodversorgung mit Hilfe eines J^{132}- Kurztests

Von

W. Börner

Mit 1 Abbildung

Seit einigen Jahren ist es möglich, den peripheren Umsatz an Schilddrüsen-hormonen mit Hilfe von radioaktiv markiertem Thyroxin und Trijodthyronin sowie durch chromatographische Trennung der einzelnen Schilddrüsenhormone und ihrer Metaboliten zu beurteilen [Hamolsky et al. (1953) (6), Sterling et al. (1954) (12), Ingbar and Freinkel (1955) (7), Friis (1958) (4), Klein (1960) (8)]. E. Klein hat kürzlich über die ersten derartigen systematischen Untersuchungen an einem größeren Krankengut berichtet (9). Verständlicherweise erfordern diese Untersuchungen für jeden Patienten einen recht erheblichen Aufwand und sind u. a. auch mit einer relativ hohen Strahlenbelastung verbunden, so daß sie für die Anwendung in der klinischen *Routine* nicht in Frage kommen können.

Auf der anderen Seite gestatten die bisher aus der Literatur bekannt gewordenen zahlreichen Schilddrüsenfunktionsproben mit Radiojod jedoch kaum eine Aussage über die periphere Hormonjodversorgung.

Der von uns eingeführte J^{132}-Kurztest, welcher an anderer Stelle bereits aus-führlich beschrieben wurde (3), erlaubt dagegen außer einer gleichzeitigen Messung der Radiojodaufnahme durch die Schilddrüse und der Kreislaufzeit Cubitalvene — Oberschenkel (10 cm proximal vom oberen Rand der Patella) auch eine Be-urteilung der peripheren Versorgung mit wirksamen Schilddrüsenhormonen.

Mit Hilfe zweier Strahlungsmeßapparaturen, bestehend aus Szintillations-zähler FH 451 (NaJ-Kristall ⌀ 30 mm, Tiefe 20 mm) mit Bleikollimator (27 mm), Strahlungsmeßgerät FH 49 und Linienschreiber PC 120[1] werden die Impulsraten über Halsregion und Oberschenkel kontinuierlich aufgezeichnet. Die Anordnung über dem Oberschenkel dient dabei zur individuellen Korrektur der extrathyr-eoidalen Gewebsaktivität. Durch eine einfache Kompensationsschaltung ist es möglich, die Differenz der Impulsraten beider Strahlungsmeßgeräte mit einem dritten Linienschreiber gleichzeitig zu registrieren. Nach i. v.-Injektion der Test-dosis von 10 μC J^{132} (in 4 ml physiol. NaCl-Lösung) wird der Abstand des Detektors vom Oberschenkel durch Variation des Rückzugs im Kollimator so geändert, daß die mit Hilfe des Differenzschreibers registrierte Kurve bei Extrapolation auf den Injektionszeitpunkt durch den Nullpunkt verläuft.

---

[1] Die Strahlungsmeßgeräte, Szintillationszähler, Kollimatoren und Metrawatt-Linien-schreiber wurden von der Firma Frieseke & Hoepfner, GmbH, Erlangen-Bruck, bezogen.

Somit registrieren wir bei unserem Kurztest gleichzeitig drei Kurven: die Halskurve, die Oberschenkelkurve und die Differenzkurve aus beiden. Die letztere stellt die eigentliche Radiojodaufnahme durch die Schilddrüse dar (Abb. 1). Als Beobachtungszeitraum haben sich 20 min als ausreichend, aber auch als notwendig erwiesen. In Fällen sehr niedriger Speicherung wird nach 2 Std eine weitere Messung von etwa 5 min Dauer in gleicher Meßanordnung angeschlossen, um eine nicht thyreogen bedingte verlangsamte Verteilung des Radiojods im Gewebe von einer Hypothyreose unterscheiden zu können.

Bei geringer oder fehlender Jodspeicherung der Schilddrüse erlaubt die Beurteilung der Oberschenkelkurve *allein* eine Aussage über die Versorgung der Körperperipherie mit wirksamen Schilddrüsenhormonen. Hierzu bilden wir das um den radioaktiven Abfall von J¹³² korrigierte Verhältnis der Oberschenkel-Impulsraten bei 20 min und 5 min p. i. Diesen Quotienten bezeichnen wir als „Gewebewert". Bei einem Mangel an Schilddrüsenhormonen in der Peripherie kommt es zu einem charakteristischen Anstieg der Oberschenkelkurve. Der Gewebewert wird deutlich größer als 1. Dagegen kommt es bei normaler hormoneller Versorgung spätestens nach 2 min zu einem Abstrom des Radiojods aus dem Gewebe, d. h. der Gewebewert ist gleich oder kleiner als 1. Vorbedingung für die meßtechnische Erfassung des Gewebewertes ist ein relativ geringer Abstand (0—10 cm) des Strahlungsdetektors vom Oberschenkel. Wegen der Gültigkeit des 1/r²-Abstand-Gesetzes für die einzelnen vom Detektor erfaßten Volumenelemente des Oberschenkelgewebes muß sich eine Verschiebung der Aktivität von den zentral gelegenen Gefäßen zur Peripherie hin in einer Erhöhung der Impulsrate äußern.

Wir beschäftigten uns mit der Frage, ob der Gewebewert durch die verschiedene Dicke und den unterschiedlichen Fettanteil des Oberschenkels beeinflußt werden kann. Zu diesem Zweck wurden die Gewebewerte der einzelnen Schilddrüsenfunktionsklassen sowohl gegen das Körpergewicht als auch gegen das relative Gewicht (wirkliches Gewicht in Prozent des Sollgewichts der jeweiligen Körperlänge) als Maß des Körperfettgehaltes aufgetragen. Für beide Bezugsgrößen konnte eine Korrelation nicht gefunden werden. Wir glauben damit nachgewiesen zu haben, daß eine möglicherweise vorhandene Beziehung zwischen Oberschenkeldicke und Gewebewert nicht von ausschlaggebendem Einfluß sein dürfte.

Nur bedingt zu verwerten ist der Gewebewert bei Patienten mit konsumierenden Erkrankungen, dekompensierten Herzfehlern und auch bei Patienten, die Pharmaka erhalten haben, von welchen bekannt ist, daß sie den Radiojodtest stören.

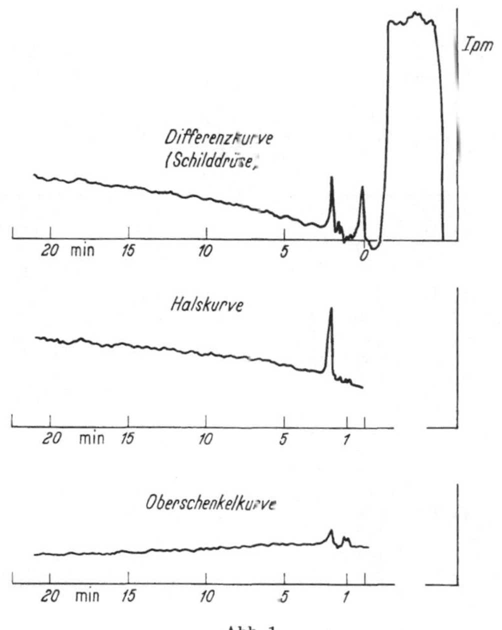

Abb. 1

Die Auswertung der Oberschenkelkurve ergibt einen umso höheren Gewebewert, je schwerer das klinische Bild der Unterfunktion ist und je länger dieses schon in unbehandeltem Zustand vorgelegen hat. Durch Verabreichung von Schilddrüsenhormonen gelingt es, den Gewebewert auf normale Werte zu senken. In Tab. 1 soll gezeigt werden, wie bei athyreoten Patienten der Gewebewert nach Einleitung einer Substitutionsbehandlung auf Werte um 1 zurückgeht.

Tabelle 1

Patient	Test Nr.	Tag der Untersuchung	20 min-Speicherwert der Schilddrüse (%)	Gewebewert	Kreislaufzeit (sec^{-1})	Körpergewicht (kg)	Körperlänge (cm)	Substitution mit Schilddrüsenhormonen pro Tag
R. R. ♀	6	1. 12.	0	1,72	—	109	168	ab 11. 12. 100 γ Thybon
	17	15. 12.	0	1,08	26,0	106		ab 15. 12. 100 γ Thybon
	25	21. 12.	0	1,00	29,0	101		dann 0,1—0,2 g Thyreoidin
E. W. ♀	245	16. 5.	0	1,22	25,0	65,8	157	ab 19. 5. 100 γ Thybon
	269	24. 5.	0	0,94	20,0	64,5		ab 24. 5. 100 γ Thybon
	279	31. 5.	0	0,95	19,2	64,0		ab 31. 5. 100 γ Thybon
	287	22. 6.	0	0,92	13,0	59,2		dann 0,1—0,2 g Thyreoidin
W. S. ♂	110	1. 3.	0	1,28	20,6	63,0	163	ab 1. 3. 0,1 g Thyreoidin + 80 γ Thybon
	129	8. 3.	0	1,14	22,0	60,0		ab 8. 3. 0,1 g Thyreoidin + 80 γ Thybon
	371	10. 10.	0	1,02	13,0	58,0		ab 10. 10. 0,15 g Thyreoidin
	395	8. 11.	0	1,03	14,4	59,0		dann 0,15 g Thyreoidin
O. H. ♀	408	22. 11.	0	1,26	29,2	88,0	163	ab 22. 11. 100 γ Thybon
	419	29. 11.	0	1,05	30,2	87,0		ab 29. 11. 80 γ Thybon
	427	6. 12.	0	1,00	24,0	85,0		ab 6. 12. 80 γ Thybon
	432	14. 12.	0	1,03	26,0	83,5		ab 14. 12. 0,2 g Thyreoidin + 40 γ Thybon
	436	19. 12.	0	1,00	18,0	83,0		ab 19. 12. 0,2 g Thyreoidin + 20 γ Thybon
I. H. ♀	954	16. 1.	0	1,23	28,8	72,3	163	ab 2. 2. 40 γ Thybon
	1000	14. 2.	0	1,11	21,8	67,2		ab 9. 2. 50 γ Thybon

Der Gewebewert hat sich noch bei einer zweiten Patientengruppe als nützliches diagnostisches Kriterium bewährt. Bei Strumektomierten mit Verdacht auf Hypothyreose ergibt sich häufig eine Diskrepanz zwischen dem klinischen Bild und dem Ergebnis des Radiojod-Langtests. Die Radiojodspeicherung der Schilddrüse liegt bei diesen Patienten im Normbereich, während die J^{131}-Serumwerte meist leicht erhöht sind. Durch die Verkleinerung des Jodpools ist bei normaler oder verminderter täglicher Hormonproduktion und -sekretion das Verhältnis J^{131}/J^{127} zwangsläufig erhöht. Mit anderen Worten, es findet sich ein normaler oder verminderter PBI^{127}-Spiegel bei einem („relativ") erhöhten PBI^{131}-Spiegel. Auf die Problematik dieser möglichen Fehlinterpretation von Radiojodtestergebnissen bei verkleinertem Jodpool wurde von GERBAULET c. s. (5), KOUTRAS c. s. (10) und SILVER (11) bereits ausführlich hingewiesen. Unter der bereits erwähnten Voraussetzung einer nicht zu hohen, aber noch im Normbereich liegenden Radiojodspeicherung der Schilddrüse ist der Gewebewert solcher Patienten entsprechend der mangelhaften Hormonversorgung des Organismus meist erhöht (vgl. Tab. 2).

Auch bei Mangel an wirksamen Schilddrüsenhormonen im Gefolge einer sekundären hypophysär bedingten Hypothyreose (Hypophysentumoren, Zustand nach Y^{90}- oder Au^{198}-Implantation der Hypophyse), einer Jodfehlverwertung oder einer Dystopie von Schilddrüsengewebe kann sich die Bestimmung des Gewebewertes, insbesondere im Hinblick auf eventuell erforderliche therapeutische Maßnahmen, als aufschlußreich erweisen.

Tabelle 2

| Patient | Test Nr. | Struma-opera-tion | Gewebe-wert | 20 min-Speicher-wert der Schild-drüse (%) | Langtest | | | | | | Kreis-laufzeit (sec⁻¹) |
					2 Std (%)	8 Std (%)	24 Std (%)	48 Std (%)	Ges. Se-rum J^{131} (%/1)	PBI¹³¹ (%/1)	
V. S. ♀	27	1937 1947	1,07	4,4	10	14	24	23	0,2	0,1	19,0
M. H. ♀	214	1934 1958	1,45	3,6	28	46	56	51	0,7	0,6	23,6
A. K. ♀	234	1947	1,14	1,6	13	22	34	34	0,6	0,6	24,8
P. C. ♂	407	1920 1952	1,29	0	15	25	32	30	0,9	0,8	24,2
M. H. ♂	718	1961	1,12	0	10	23	29	22	1,5	1,4	19,0

Wenn wir abschließend versuchen, den Zusammenhang zwischen Versorgung der Peripherie mit wirksamen Schilddrüsenhormonen und dem Verlauf der Oberschenkelkurve zu deuten, müssen wir zunächst feststellen, daß bei normaler und erhöhter Jodidaufnahme der Schilddrüse der Kurvenverlauf im Gewebe im wesentlichen nur ein indirektes Maß für die Schilddrüsenspeicherung darstellt. Je nach dem Grad der Speicherung fällt die Oberschenkelkurve durch die Verminderung der Gewebsaktivität mehr oder weniger stark ab und der Gewebewert ist kleiner als 1. In solchen Fällen kommt dieser Größe wenig Bedeutung zu. Dagegen finden wir bei unbehandelten Hypothyreosen stets einen Anstieg der Oberschenkelkurve im Beobachtungszeitraum und somit einen Gewebewert, der deutlich über 1 liegt. Hormonell ausreichend substituierte Unterfunktionen haben andererseits einen Gewebewert um 1. Die Radiojodausscheidung durch die Niere beeinflußt den Verlauf der Registrierkurven im Beobachtungszeitraum von 20 min nicht, da sie selbst bei Unterfunktionen im Mittel nur 1,7% der Testdosis beträgt (3).

Worauf führen wir nun den erhöhten Gewebewert bei Mangel an wirksamen Schilddrüsenhormonen zurück ? Mit großer Wahrscheinlichkeit ist der Anstieg der Oberschenkelkurve durch die sekundären funktionellen und anatomischen Veränderungen bedingt, wie sie bei der Hypothyreose vorgefunden werden (1, 2, 13):

Bei erniedrigtem Schlag- und Minutenvolumen ist die Strömungsgeschwindigkeit des Blutes verlangsamt, während der periphere Widerstand erhöht ist. Pathologisch-anatomisch finden wir Anreicherungen von chondroitinhaltigen Mucoproteiden in den Extracellularräumen, fadenförmig verengte Capillaren und letztlich auch ausgedehnte atheromatöse Gefäßveränderungen. Darüber hinaus kommt es zu Permeabilitätsstörungen der Zellen mit Elektrolytverschiebungen. In allen diesen sekundären Veränderungen sehen wir die Ursache für die verzögerte Verteilung des Radiojods im Gewebe, die in einem Anstieg der Oberschenkelkurve zum Ausdruck kommt.

Die vorliegenden Untersuchungen wurden mit dankenswerter Unterstützung des Bundesministeriums für wissenschaftliche Forschung durchgeführt.

Literatur

1. Bansi, H. W.: Pathophysiologie, Klinik und Therapie der Hypothyreosen. Internist 1, 397 (1960).
2. — Krankheiten der Schilddrüse. In: Handbuch der inneren Medizin, 4. Auflage, Bd. VII/1 Berlin-Göttingen-Heidelberg: Springer 1955.
3. Börner, W.: Ein neuer Radiojodkurztest zur Schilddrüsenfunktionsprüfung mit gleichzeitiger Beurteilung der peripheren Hormonjodversorgung. Klin. Wschr. 39, 990 (1961).
4. Friis, T.: Thyroxine metabolism in man estimated by means of I^{131}-labeled l-thyroxine. Acta endocr. (Kbh.) 29, 587 (1958).
5. Gerbaulet, K., W. Fitting u. W. Maurer: Über Messungen der quantitativen Jodid-Aufnahme der Schilddrüse und der Konzentration des Serum-Jodids. I. Experimentell-theoretischer Teil: Grundsätzliche Zusammenhänge und Deutung des klinischen Radio-Jod-Tests. Klin. Wschr. 38, 474 (1960).
6. Hamolsky, M. W., A. St. Freedberg, G. S. Kurland and L. Wolksky: The exchangeable thyroid hormone pool. J. clin. Invest. 32, 453 (1953).
7. Ingbar, S. H., and N. Freinkel: Simultanous estimation of rates of thyroxine degradation and thyroid hormone synthesis. J. clin. Invest. 34, 808 (1955).
8. Klein, E.: Der endogene Jodhaushalt des Menschen und seine Störungen. Stuttgart: Georg Thieme 1960.
9. — Der normale und pathologische Umsatz von Schilddrüsenhormonen in der Körperperipherie. Klin. Wschr. 40, 3 (1962).
10. Koutras, D. A., W. D. Alexander, W. W. Buchanan, J. Crooks and E. J. Wayne: Studies of stable iodine metabolism as a guide to the interpretation of radioiodine tests. Acta endocr. (Kbh.) 37, 597 (1961).
11. Silver, S.: Radioactive Isotopes in Medicine and Biology. Second Edition, Philadelphia: Lea & Febiger 1962.
12. Sterling, K., J. C. Lashof and E. B. Man: Disappearance from serum of I^{131}-labeled l-thyroxine and l-triiodothyronine in euthyroid subjects. J. clin. Invest. 33, 1031 (1954).
13. Wezler, K., u. A. Böger: Der Blutdruck und seine maßgebenden Komponenten bei einigen pathologischen Zuständen. Ergebn. Physiol. 41, 569 (1939).

Diskussion

E. Klein (Düsseldorf):

Seinem Aufbau und Ablauf nach erfaßt der geschilderte Kurztest keineswegs die Versorgung der Körperperipherie mit Hormonjod, sondern lediglich das Verhalten von Jodid in ihr. Dieses hängt natürlich weitgehend von der durch Schilddrüsenhormone gesteuerten Stoffwechselsituation der Gewebsverbände ab, ist aber ein grundsätzlich ebenso unspezifisches Maß dafür wie etwa ihr Sauerstoffverbrauch oder Enzymmuster. Damit vermehrt der Kurztest die Zahl indirekter Untersuchungsmethoden der Schilddrüsenfunktion, die wir durch direkte Verfahren zu ersetzen trachten. Die Hormonversorgung der Gewebe kann z. Z. nur durch die von Ihnen auch angeführten komplizierten Verfahren erfaßt und allenfalls durch den in vitro-Test mit radioaktivem Trijodthyronin, dessen Aussagefähigkeit aber durch mancherlei Faktoren eingeschränkt ist, einigermaßen abgeschätzt werden.

R. Höfer (Wien):

Ich finde auch, daß der Kurztest nicht die Hormonversorgung mißt.

V. Lachnit (Wien):

Ich bezweifele die Spezifität des angegebenen Kurztestes, weil die damit erhaltenen Gewebewerte nicht nur von der Speicherung über der Schilddrüse, sondern vorzüglich von dem Blutminutenvolumen abhängen, wie Sie auch angedeutet haben. Haben Sie auch bei euthyreoten Kreislaufkranken mit erhöhtem oder vermindertem Minutenvolumen derartige Untersuchungen vorgenommen?

F. Petersen (Hamburg):

Wenn der Gewebewert des J^{132} nach 20 min noch von anderen Faktoren abhängt als von der Jodid-Clearance, müßte er different sein bei Hypothyreosen und bei für die Jodaufnahme blockierten Schilddrüsen. Haben Sie ensprechende Untersuchungen durchgeführt?

W. Börner:

In Tab. 1 wird an Hand einer Reihe athyreoter Patienten die Abhängigkeit des Gewebewertes von der ausreichenden Substitution mit Schilddrüsenhormonen veranschaulicht. Es ist damit nachgewiesen, daß der Gewebewert eine Aussage über die Versorgung der Peripherie mit wirksamen Schilddrüsenhormonen erlaubt. Die Korrelation ist eindeutig. Ich möchte darauf hinweisen, daß der Gewebewert sicher auch mit anderen markierten Ionen als Jodid bestimmt werden kann. In unserem Test ergibt sich der Gewebewert jedoch ohne jeden zusätzlichen Aufwand zusammen mit der Radiojodspeicherung und der Kreislaufzeit.

Wie bereits erwähnt, hat der Gewebewert nur dann einen Aussagewert, wenn die Jodidclearance vernachlässigt werden kann, also bei keiner oder geringer 20 min-Speicherung der Schilddrüse. Zwischen Hypothyreosen (Gewebewert deutlich > 1) und Euthyreosen, deren Schilddrüsenfunktion durch Medikamente blockiert ist (Gewebewert ungefähr 1), bestehen deutliche Unterschiede. Bei cardial dekompensierten Patienten konnten wir in einzelnen Fällen mit niedriger Radiojodspeicherung eine Erhöhung des Gewebewertes feststellen. Differentialdiagnostisch ist der Gewebewert jedoch für diese Patientengruppe ohne Bedeutung, weil meist eine normale 20 min- bzw. 2 Std-Speicherung der Schilddrüse vorliegt.

Aus der II. Medizinischen Universitätsklinik München (Direktor: Prof. Dr. Dr. G. BODECHTEL)

Änderungen der Schilddrüsen- hormonkonzentration im Liquor cerebrospinalis bei Schilddrüsenerkrankungen

Von

K. VOLKMER, K. SCHWARZ UND K. KOPETZ

Mit 1 Abbildung

Zahlreiche Untersuchungen haben gezeigt, daß die meisten anorganischen und organischen Substanzen im Liquor cerebrospinalis zu den entsprechenden Bestandteilen des Blutes in einem bestimmten Verhältnis stehen (DEMME, LÜTHY, MEYER u. a.). Der jeweilige Blut-Liquorquotient ist unter physiologischen Bedingungen recht konstant, mit Ausnahme der freien Aminosäuren (KNAUFF u. Mitarb.). Bei den bereits von LACHNIT und WEIS sowie SCHWARZ nachgewiesenen Hormonen der Hypophyse und der Nebennierenrinde im Liquor lagen jedoch die Konzentrationen niedriger als im Blut. Untersuchungen von SCHRADER und WEINGES zeigten, daß sowohl unter phsyiologischen als auch unter pathologischen Bedingungen kein Insulin bzw. keine insulinähnliche Aktivität im Liquor cerebrospinalis sich nachweisen ließ.

STURM u. Mitarb. haben in den Jahren 1933 und 1934 den Jodgehalt im Gehirn von Menschen, Hunden, Katzen und Kaninchen untersucht und gefunden, daß im Tuber cinereum, im Pallidum, vor allem aber in der Hypophyse und hier im Hypophysenhinterlappen der Jodgehalt um vieles höher ist als im Blut. Diese Befunde wurden 20 Jahre später von amerikanischen Arbeitsgruppen aufgegriffen, die sich mehr und mehr der außerordentlich empfindlichen und exakten Radiojodmethoden bedienten, und in allen wesentlichen Punkten bestätigt. JENSEN und CLARK zeigten, daß der Jodreichtum der Hypophyse in erster Linie auf einer Thyroxinanreicherung im HHL beruht. FORD und GROSS haben den Stoffwechsel markierter Schilddrüsenhormone in der Hypophyse und im Gehirn bei Kaninchen untersucht und auch hier eine sehr hohe Anreicherung im HHL gefunden.

Wir haben uns von klinischer Seite deshalb die Frage gestellt, ob den so regelmäßig zu beobachtenden Symptomen des ZNS bei Schilddrüsenerkrankungen nicht Änderungen des PBI im Liquor zugrunde liegen und wie das Verhältnis zwischen Blutjodspiegel und Liquorjodspiegel unter physiologischen und pathologischen Bedingungen ist.

Die Untersuchung des proteingebundenen Jods im Liquor wurde nach der Jodbestimmungsmethode von SPITZY, REESE und SKRUBE durchgeführt, mit der einen Abweichung, daß zur Fällung mit Trichloressigsäure 5 cm³ Liquor pro Untersuchung verwendet wurden. Der Liquor wurde mittels Lumbalpunktion gewonnen. Wir haben bei allen Untersuchungen Doppelbestimmungen gemacht und dafür entsprechend 10 cm³ Liquor entnommen. Den Liquorverlust haben wir mit stets frischer steriler physiologischer Kochzalzlösung wieder aufgefüllt.

In der ersten Gruppe wurden bei 15 euthyreoten Patienten gleichzeitig Liquor und Blut entnommen und das eiweißgebundene Jod bestimmt. Wir fanden eine Serumeiweißjodkonzentration um 6,1 γ-% und eine Liquoreiweißjodkonzentration um 1,6 γ-%.

Bei der zweiten Gruppe handelte es sich um 9 Patienten mit nachgewiesener Hyperthyreose. Bei diesen Probanden lag der Spiegel des proteingebundenen Jods im Blutserum bei 10,5 γ-%, während der PBI-Spiegel im Liquor gegenüber der ersten Gruppe deutlich höher bei 4,9 γ-% lag (Abb. 1).

Diese Befunde zeigen, daß auch beim Menschen im Liquor cerebrospinalis erhöhte Konzentrationen der Schilddrüsenhormone nachzuweisen sind, die wahrscheinlich eine Folge der erhöhten Blutkonzentration sind und weniger ein Permeabilitätsproblem darstellen. Die Untersuchungen lassen die Frage offen, ob auch bei Hyperthyreosen größere Mengen von PBI die Blut-Gehirn-Schranke passieren. Immerhin ist es von klinischer Seite interessant, zu diskutieren, ob nicht die so markanten psychischen Änderungen der menschlichen Persönlichkeit beim Myxödem, bzw. beim

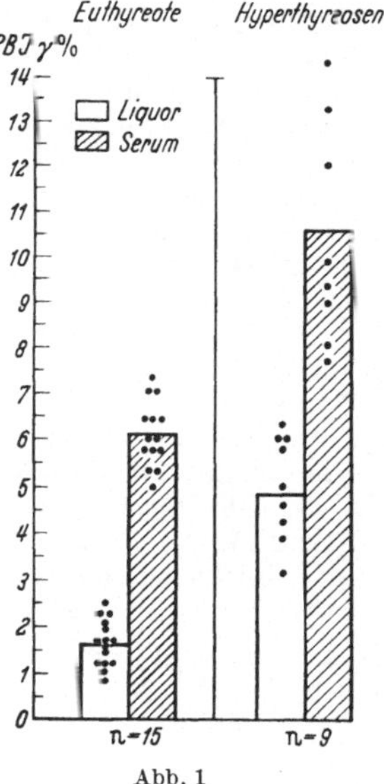

Abb. 1

Basedow-Kranken eine Folge des zu geringen oder stark erhöhten Schilddrüsenhormongehalts im Gehirn sind. Dafür sprechen ebenfalls die tierexperimentell erhobenen Befunde mit markiertem Thyroxin bzw. nach Thyreoidektomie.

In der letzten Gruppe waren Patienten mit dem Verdacht auf einen intracerebralen Prozeß. Vor der Durchführung der notwendigen Carotisangiographie wurde bei diesen Patienten ebenfalls Liquor und Blut entnommen. Die zweite Entnahme des Liquors erfolgte während der Luftencephalographie. Die Untersuchungswerte vor der parenteralen Jodgabe (Urografin) sind in der ersten Gruppe mit enthalten. Der Liquorjodspiegel nach Urografingabe schwankte zwischen 15,2 und 21,6 γ-%. Die höchsten Werte fanden sich bei zwei Patienten, bei denen 2 Tage nach einer Carotisangiographie eine Luftencephalographie durchgeführt wurde. Der niedrigere Wert von 15,2 γ-% fand sich bei 2 Patienten, bei welchen erst nach 8 Tagen eine Pneumencephalographie vorgenommen wurde. Diese auffälligen Befunde erheben die Frage, ob nicht im Liquor das parenteral verabreichte Jod schneller ausgeschieden wird als im Blut, wo bekanntlich das Jod über Monate noch einen sehr hohen bis in die Hunderte von γ-% gehenden Spiegel aufweist.

Es sollte bei diesen Untersuchungen gezeigt werden, daß auch im Liquor cerebrospinalis proteingebundenes Jod nachzuweisen ist. Das Verhältnis zum Serumjodspiegel ist ähnlich wie bei den bereits nachgewiesenen Hormonen der Hypophyse und der Nebennierenrinde. Die Konzentrationen sind hier wesentlich niedriger. Bei den 9 Hyperthyreosen ist der Liquorjodspiegel gegenüber dem der ersten Gruppe ebenfalls erhöht, wie dies auch im Blutserum der Fall ist. Ob das parenteral verabreichte Jod aus dem Liquor schneller ausgeschieden wird als aus Blut, kann anhand der wenigen Fälle noch nicht ausgesagt werden.

Literatur

Demme, H.: Die Liquordiagnostik in Klinik und Praxis, 2. Aufl. München und Berlin: Urban & Schwarzenberg 1950.

Ford, D. H., and J. Gross: Endocrinology 62, 4, 416 (1958).

Jensen, J. M., and D. E. Clark: J. Lab. clin. Med. 38, 663 (1951).

Knauff, H. G., P. Schabert u. H. Zickgraf: Die Konzentration der freien Aminosäuren im Liquor cerebrospinalis und ihre Beziehungen zur Konzentration der freien Plasmaaminosäuren. Klin. Wschr. 1961 I, 778.

Lachnit, V., u. J. Weis: ACTH-Aktivität des Liquors bei hypophysären und interrenalen Erkrankungen. Dtsch. Arch. klin. Med. 202, 275 (1955).

Lüthy, F.: Liquor cerebrospinalis. In: Handbuch der inn. Med., 4. Aufl., Bd. 5/I. Berlin-Göttingen-Heidelberg: Springer 1953.

Meyer, H.: Der Liquor. Berlin-Göttingen-Heidelberg: Springer 1949.

Schrader, A., u. K. F. Weinges: Vergleichende Bestimmungen der insulinähnlichen Aktivität im Blut und Liquor cerebrospinalis. Klin. Wschr. 7, 344 (1962).

Schwarz, K.: Über den Nachweis und die Bedeutung der Steroidhormone im Liquor cerebrospinalis. Dtsch. Z. Nervenheilk. 177, 464 (1958).

Sturm, A.: Münch. med. Wschr. 97, 35, 1125 (1955).

— CIBA-Foundation: The cerebrospinal fluid. London: J. & A. Churchill, 1958.

Aus der Chirurgischen Universitätsklinik Hamburg-Eppendorf (Direktor: Prof. Dr. L. ZUK-SCHWERDT) und dem Pathologischen Institut der Universität Hamburg (Direktor: Prof. Dr. Dr. h. c. C. KRAUSPE)

Experimentelle Untersuchungen am Lymphgefäßsystem der Schilddrüse

Von

H. KIRSCHNER, J. KRACHT und V. BAY

Mit 2 Abbildungen

In experimentellen Untersuchungen am Hund gelang EICKHOFF, KRACHT u. HORST, KRACHT, HORST u. EICKHOFF sowie DOBYNS u. HIRSCH der Nachweis, daß die Schilddrüse Hormonjod nicht nur in die Blutbahn, sondern auch in das Lymphgefäßsystem sezerniert. Bei dieser Species wird die Schilddrüsenlymphe über perifollikuläre und perilobuläre Klappen enthaltende Lymphgefäße an die Kapsel herangeführt, von dort über makroskopisch nicht präparierbare, aber durch intrathyreoidale Kontrastmittelgabe in vivo darstellbare perithyreoidale Bahnen beiderseits in einen cervicalen Sammellymphknoten abgeleitet, um von dort über den Truncus lymphaticus cervicalis beiderseits getrennt in den Venenwinkel einzumünden. Durch Unterbindung der ableitenden cervicalen Lymphbahnen entfalten sich die intrathyreoidalen Lymphgefäße nach dem Prinzip der Rückstauung. Mit dieser Methode prüften wir an 12 Hunden das Verhalten von cervicalem Sammellymphknoten und Schilddrüse bei akuter und chronischer Lymphstauung und modifizierten wie folgt:

1. akute Lymphstauung durch Resektion des Truncus cervicalis bzw. durch Exstirpation des cervicalen Sammellymphknotens a) einseitig, b) beidseitig, c) durch zusätzliche Resektion einer oder beider Venae jugulares externae, d) durch einseitige Venenresektion ohne Manipulation am ableitenden Lymphgefäßsystem. Tötung nach 4 Tagen.

2. Versuch einer chronischen Lymphstauung durch Eingriffe wie bei 1 a—d. Tötung zwischen dem 28. und 41. Tag nach dem jeweiligen Eingriff. Die Befunde wurden durch intraoperative Messung des Gewebsdrucks in der Schilddrüse ergänzt.

Bereits wenige Minuten nach Abklemmung, Unterbindung oder Resektion des Truncus lymphaticus cervicalis schwillt der in seinem Abfluß behinderte cervicale Lymphknoten an und gewinnt an Konsistenz. Innerhalb von Stunden ist er auf das Mehrfache der Norm vergrößert und verhärtet. Dem entspricht histologisch das Bild des akuten Lymphödems. Unter Schwund des lymphatischen Gewebes reichert sich gestaute Lymphe innerhalb und außerhalb der erweiterten Sinus an. In den Randpartien bleiben die lymphatischen Strukturen am längsten erhalten. Die Stauung setzt sich auf den Hals und Schlundbereich fort und führt innerhalb

von Tagen zu einem großen submandibulären subcutanen Ödemsack. In diesem
Stadium finden sich ohne wesentliche Organvergrößerung in der Schilddrüse perifollikuläre Lymphangiektasien, die gelegentlich zur Aufsplitterung des Follikel-

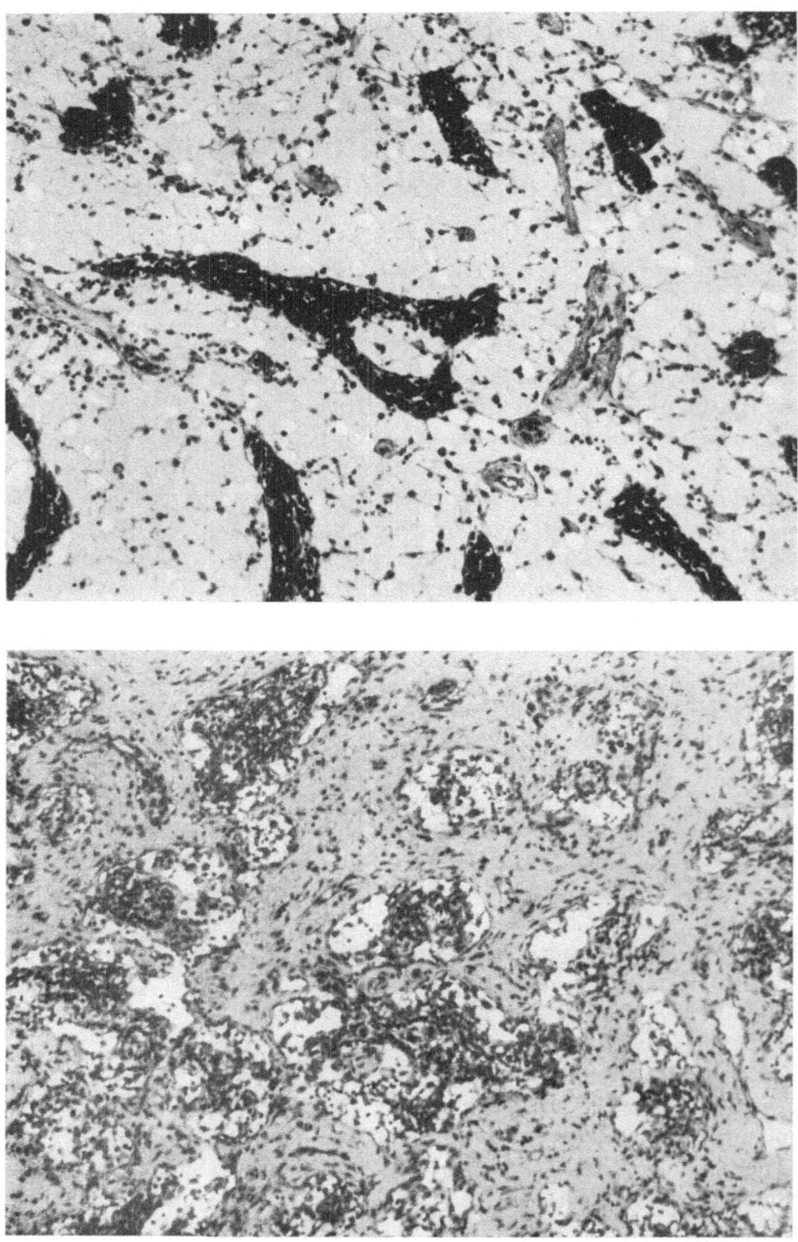

Abb. 1. Cervicaler Sammellymphknoten des Hundes. *Oben:* Akutes Lymphödem, 3 Tage nach Durchtrennung und
Unterbindung des Truncus cervicalis. *Unten:* Ödemsklerose, 36 Tage nach Durchtrennung und Unterbindung des
Truncus cervicalis. Goldner, Vergr. 130fach

verbandes und zum Phänomen sog. schwimmender Follikel führen. Durch zusätzliche Resektion der Vena jugularis werden diese Veränderungen quantitativ potenziert, wobei zusätzlich eine venöse Hyperämie kennzeichnend ist. Die alleinige

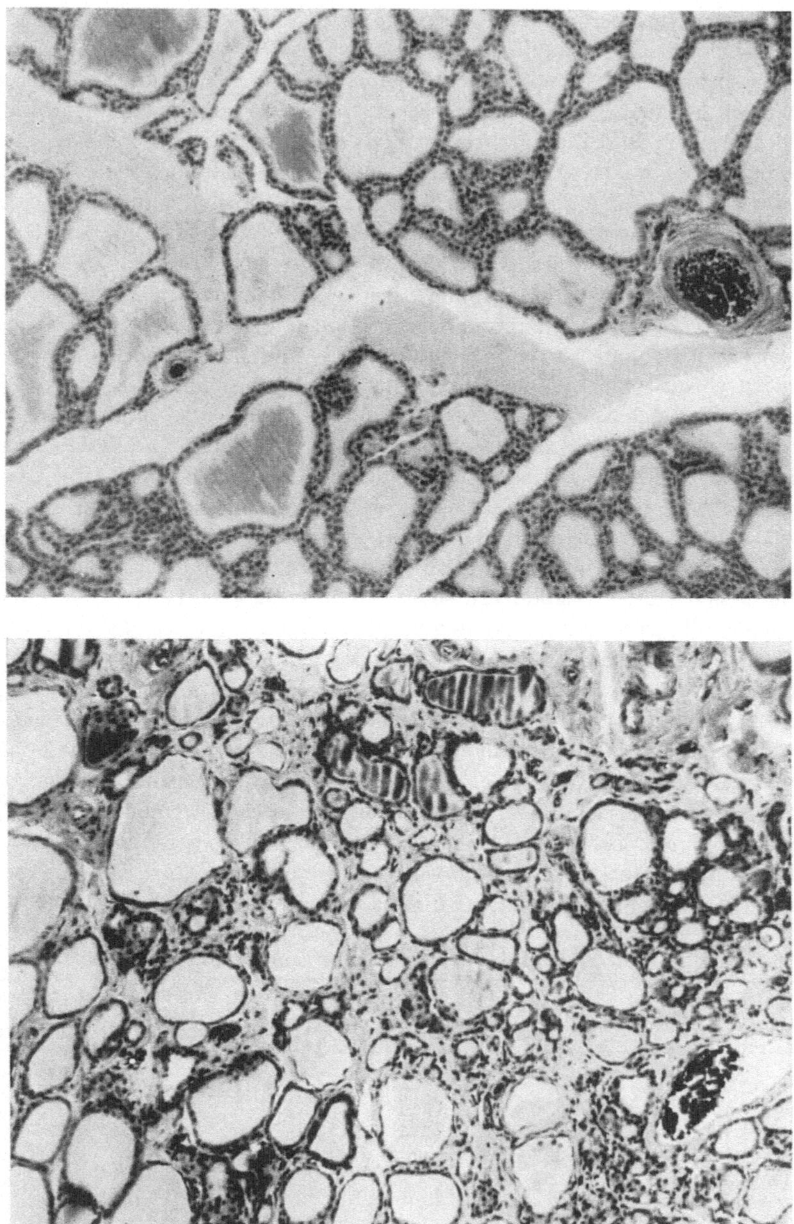

Abb. 2. Schilddrüse des Hundes. *Oben:* Lymphangiektasien mit kolloidähnlichem Inhalt, 3 Tage nach Durchtrennung und Unterbindung des zugehörigen Sammellymphknotens. *Unten:* Sklerose des Zwischengewebes, verkleinerte Follikel und Abflachung des Follikelepithels sowie venöse Hyperämie, 41 Tage nach Exstirpation des zugehörigen Sammellymphknotens und Unterbindung der V. jugularis. Goldner, Vergrößerung 130fach.

venöse Stauung bewirkt dagegen keine sicheren Veränderungen am Lymphgefäßsystem der Schilddrüse. Unter längerer Lymphstauung erfolgt eine zunehmende
Sklerosierung des cervicalen Lymphknotens nach Art der Ödemsklerose (Abb. 1).
Dies bedeutet, daß kompensatorische Abflußwege hier nicht oder nicht ausreichend beschritten werden. Im Gegensatz zum cervicalen Sammellymphknoten
fehlen bei chronischer Lymphstauung vergleichbare Veränderungen in der Schilddrüse. Das Ausmaß der Lymphangiektasien übersteigt nicht nur die Veränderungen
des akuten Stadiums, sondern hat sich in der Regel sogar weitgehend zurückgebildet. Werden jedoch zusätzlich die Vena jugularis externa und vom unteren
Schilddrüsenpol caudalwärts ziehende Venen ausgeschaltet, treten auch in der
Schilddrüse nach längerer Versuchsdauer örtlich degenerative Veränderungen in
Form von Sklerosierung des Zwischengewebes und Follikelatrophie auf. Die Fol-
likelgröße nimmt dabei durchschnittlich ab, die Follikelepithelhöhe reduziert sich
bis zur endothelartigen Form (Abb. 2). Diese Veränderungen entsprechen den in
menschlichen Strumen bekannten Degenerationen. Zur Deutung der Diskrepanz
histologischer Befunde am cervicalen Sammellymphknoten und Schilddrüse bei
alleiniger chronischer Lymphstauung einerseits und Schilddrüsensklerose nach
zusätzlicher Ausschaltung des venösen Abflusses andererseits muß davon ausgegangen werden, daß die Schilddrüse offensichtlich längerdauernde Behinderungen
des Lymphabflusses zu kompensieren vermag. Es liegt nahe, hierfür die Existenz
lymphatico-venöser Kommunikationen zu fordern, wie sie von Threefoot u.
Mitarb. anhand von Korrosionspräparaten bei der Ratte und durch Lymphangio-
graphie beim Menschen nachgewiesen worden sind. Für die Existenz derartiger
Verbindungen in der Schilddrüse selbst, in ihrer Kapsel bzw. extrathyreoidal
zwischen Schilddrüse und Sammellymphknoten beim Hund spricht die Tatsache,
daß erst durch Lymph- und Venenstauung eine maximale Abflußbehinderung
geschaffen wird, die zwangsläufig degenerative Veränderungen nach sich zieht.
In funktioneller Hinsicht ist der Schluß naheliegend, daß ähnliche Kompensations-
vorgänge auch bei einseitig behindertem Hormontransport existieren und daß ein
System vikariierend für das andere eintreten kann. In diesem Zusammenhang sei
auf die Schwierigkeiten zur Erzeugung eines chronischen Lymphödems im Tierexperiment durch isolierte Lymphgefäßausschaltung auch in anderen Körperregionen hingewiesen. Lymphatico-venöse Verbindungen dürften auch hierbei
den entscheidenden kompensierenden Faktor darstellen (Kirschner).

Tabelle 1. *Mittlere Druckwerte in Hundeschilddrüsen nach Stauung in mm Hg*

Nach Ligatur von:	30 min nach Ligatur		48 Std nach Ligatur	
	rechts	links	rechts	links
1. V. jugul. links	4	9	—	—
2. Trunc. cerv. links	3	14	—	—
3. V. jugul. und Trunc. cerv. links.	3	25	3	10
4. V. jugul. und Trunc. cerv. links und V. jugul. rechts . .	10	25	—	—
5. V. jugul. bds.	8	9	—	—
6. Trunc. cerv. bds.	15	15	—	—
7. V. jugul. und Trunc. cerv. bds.	23	24	9	10

Die morphologischen Befunde an der Schilddrüse und ihre Deutung werden
durch Gewebsdruckmessungen sinnvoll ergänzt (Tab. 1). Wir stellten fest, daß die

Druckwerte der Schilddrüse 30 min nach Ligatur des Truncus lymphaticus cervicalis stärker anstiegen, als nach Ausschaltung der Venal jugularis. Nach kombinierter Eliminierung beider Systeme auf beiden Seiten resultiert ein maximaler Druckanstieg in beiden Schilddrüsenlappen, während nach nur einseitiger Ausschaltung kontralateral im intakten lymphogen-venösen Abfluß der Norm entsprechende Werte gefunden werden. Es muß jedoch berücksichtigt werden, daß die jeweiligen Drucksteigerungen lediglich im kurzfristigen Versuch erzielbar sind, da sich bereits 48 Std nach dem Eingriff eine Tendenz zur Normalisierung der Druckwerte abzeichnet.

Zusammengefaßt geht aus unseren Untersuchungen am Beispiel der Schilddrüse einerseits die kompensierende Wirkung lymphatico-venöser Verbindungen bei alleiniger Lymphabflußbehinderung und andererseits die Bedeutung einer kombinierten lymphogen-venösen Stauung für die Erzeugung eines chronischen Lymphödems und damit verbundener degenerativer Veränderungen im parenchymatösen Organ hervor. Die experimentellen Befunde lassen sich nicht ohne weiteres auf die menschliche Schilddrüse transformieren, obwohl sich Ansatzpunkte für die Bearbeitung der Genese degenerativer Veränderungen in Strumen andeuten.

Literatur

DOBYNS, B. M., and E. Z. HIRSCH: J. clin. Endocr. 16, 153 (1956).
EICKHOFF, W., J. KRACHT u. W. HORST: Verh. dtsch. Ges. Path. 40, 265 (1956).
KIRSCHNER, H.: Bruns' Beitr. klin. Chir. 205, 1 (1962).
KRACHT, J., W. HORST u. W. EICKHOFF: Verh. dtsch. Ges. inn. Med. 66, 374 (1960).
THREEFOOT, S. A., W. T. KENT and B. F. HATCHETT: J. Lab. clin. Med. 61, 9 (1963).

Aus dem Pathologischen Institut Bezirksprosektur Duisburg
(Direktor: Prof. Dr. med. W. EICKHOFF)

Das Lymphbahnsystem
der menschlichen Schilddrüse

Von

W. EICKHOFF

Mit 2 Abbildungen

Unter Anwendung einer verfeinerten Methode konnte durch Injektion gewöhnlicher Tuschelösung das Lymphbahnsystem der menschlichen Schilddrüse in seinem gesamten Aufbau dargestellt und mit histologischen bzw. photographischen Abbildungen wiedergegeben werden. Anatomische Eigenheiten in der histologischen Struktur der Schilddrüse ermöglichen den gewünschten Erfolg der parenchymatösen Injektionen, wenn sie in der Injektionstechnik durch besondere Kautelen ausgenutzt werden. Entscheidend wichtig ist nämlich, daß die Endothelien der Lymphcapillaren im Gegensatz zu denen von Blutcapillaren nicht von einer Basalmembran umschlossen werden, sondern unmittelbare Verbindungen zum umgebenden Bindegewebe besitzen (SHDANOW). Das bedeutet, daß eine interstitiell injizierte Flüssigkeit eine Volumenvermehrung des Bindegewebes auf umschriebenem Raum bedingt, die die Faserverbindungen zwischen Lymphcapillarendothelien und Bindegewebe unter Spannung setzen, so daß die Lymphcapillaren durch diese radiär angreifenden Zugwirkungen erweitert werden. Die Verankerung der Blutcapillaren zu ihrer Umgebung ist dagegen durch den Einbau einer Basalmembran und weit reichender Faserzüge bedeutend lockerer, so daß sie nach der interstitiellen Injektion infolge der Druckvermehrung zusammengepreßt werden.

Die injizierte Tuschelösung gelangt zunächst in die Lymphbahnanfänge, in die interfollikulären Lymphcapillaren, die korbartig die Schilddrüsenfollikel umgeben. Diese Anfänge des intrathyreoidalen Lymphbahnnetzes sind die Quellorte der Schilddrüsenlymphe und geben ihren Inhalt an die nächst größeren Straßen weiter. Der Fluß der Injektionsmasse von der Capillare am Follikel bis zur Organperipherie wird in unseren Versuchen augenfällig durch Schlierenbildungen und Strömungsbilder in den Lymphwegen demonstriert (Abb. 1). Die elektive Lymphbahnfüllung geht auch daraus noch hervor, daß einmal in den Blutgefäßen keine Tusche zu finden ist und andererseits die Injektionsmasse in geschlossenen Kanälen an der Kapsel das Organ verläßt.

Die Verhältnisse an der Follikelbasis konnten folgendermaßen erkannt werden. Dem Follikelepithelsaum, der außen von einer Basalmembran (WISSIG, WALLER, ROOS) umhüllt wird, liegt unmittelbar das Netz der Blutcapillaren an. Die Blutcapillaren sind in der übermäßigen Mehrzahl als mit Erythrocyten gefüllte Querschnitte mit ovalen, massig imponierenden Endothelkernen zu erkennen und führen nirgends Tuschepartikel. Jenseits vom Blutcapillarnetz, im interfollikulären Bindegewebe, verlaufen die Lymphcapillaren, die als flächen- bis seenhafte Gebilde zu denken sind. Sie sind einzig von zarten Endothelien mit schlanken,

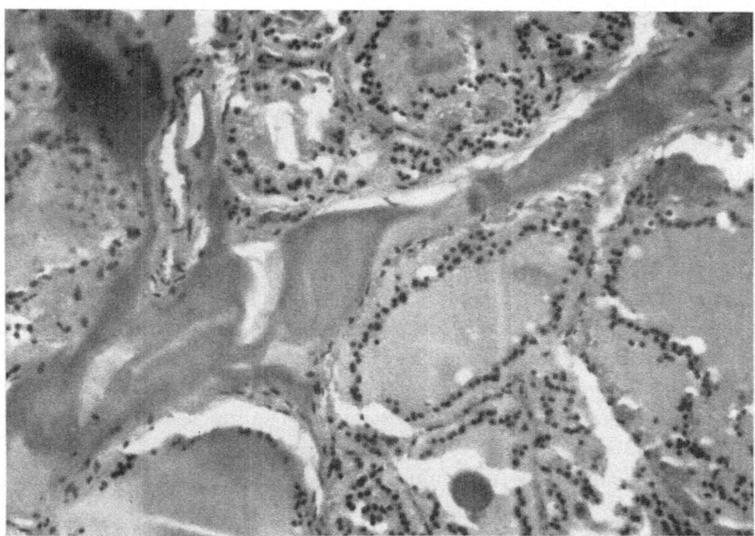

Abb. 1. Strömungsbilder der injizierten Tusche in perifollikulären und perilobulären Lymphbahnen. (Leitz Phot. Mikr. Obj. Plan 10, Ok. 8, Paraffin, HE)

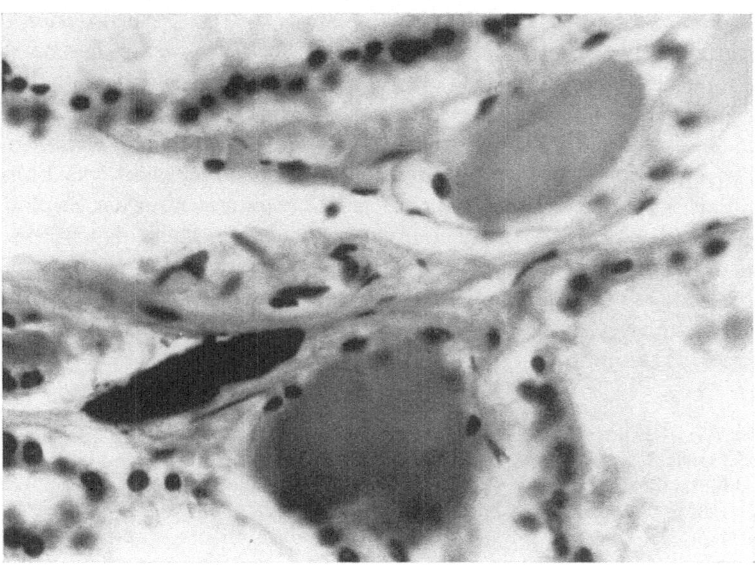

Abb. 2. Diagonal verlaufende, teils erweiterte (injizierte), teils kollabierte perifollikuläre Lymphbahn. (Leitz Phot. Mikr. Obj. Pl. 40, Ok. 8, Paraffin, HE)

spindelförmigen Kernen umsäumt und passen sich in ihrer Lichtungsgröße völlig der Umgebung an. So kommt es, daß interfollikuläre Lymphcapillaren in den Zwickeln zwischen benachbarten Follikeln weit eröffnet und von Tuschemassen gefüllt sind. Im weiteren Verlauf können sie sich wieder verengern oder direkt zwischen zwei Nachbarfollikeln kollabieren. Sie sind dann nur noch an der charakteristischen Doppelreihe ihrer Endothelkerne weiter zu verfolgen (Abb. 2).

Aus den perifollikulären Lymphcapillaren dringt die Tusche in die perilobulären Lymphwege vor. Diese besitzen den gleichen Wandbau wie die vorgeschalteten Capillaren, verlaufen aber in Bindegewebszügen, die mehrere Follikel zu Lobuli zusammenfassen. Infolgedessen erhalten sie in ihrem Bild bereits einen individuellen Charakter und sind nicht mehr so unmittelbar von der Umgebung abhängig. An den Schnittpunkten mehrerer solcher perilobulärer Lymphbahnen entstehen kleine „Lymphtümpel", in die typischerweise Blutgefäßbündel eingebettet sind.

In den massiven Bindegewebstrabekeln, die von der Kaspel aus die Schilddrüse durchziehen, verlaufen die trabekulären Lymphbahnen zur Organoberfläche und ergießen ihren Inhalt in die Kapsellymphgefäße. Die Trabekelbahnen zeigen vereinzelte muskuläre Elemente in ihrer Wand und besitzen besonders in Kapselnähe erstmalig Klappen. Blutgefäße werden von ihnen umspült.

Zwischen den beiden Blättern der Organkapsel sammelt sich die Schilddrüsenlymphe in dem äußerst dichten und engmaschigen Netz der Kapselgefäße. Muskulatur, kollagene und elastische Fasern bilden die Wandung, Klappen unterteilen in regelmäßigen Abständen das Gefäßrohr und geben ihm ein perlschnurartiges Aussehen.

An bestimmten, regelmäßig lokalisierbaren Orten der Organoberfläche verdichten sich die Kapsellymphbahnen und gehen in die ableitenden thyreoidalen Lymphgefäße über, die den tiefen Lymphknoten des Halses mehr oder weniger verzweigt zustreben. Dabei konnten je nach ihrem Verhalten zu den Blutbahnen zwei Lymphgefäßtypen unterschieden werden, die „Trabantenbahnen", die bereits in der Kapsel die Nähe der Blutbahnen suchen und auch außerhalb des Organs enge Nachbarschaft zu ihnen behalten, und die „selbständigen oder Kantengefäße", die an Lymphsammelstellen allein, d. h. ohne eng nachbarschaftliche Blutgefäße die Schilddrüse verlassen. Die Trabantengefäße lagern sich an der Schilddrüsenvorderfläche überwiegend den Arterien an, an der Hinterfläche den Venen.

Über weitere Einzelheiten, insbesondere der erstmaligen photographischen Wiedergabe dieser Lymphbahnverhältnisse an der menschlichen Schilddrüse und am Lymphbahnsystem des Halses, wurde schon an anderer Stelle berichtet (Eickhoff; Herberhold).

Literatur

Eickhoff, W.: Die intrathyreoidalen Lymphbahnen des Menschen. Verh. dtsch. Ges. Path. **46**, 293 (1962).
— Die abführenden thyreoidalen und cervikalen Lymphgefäße des Menschen. Endokrinologie **43**, 1 (1962).
Herberhold, K.: Über die intrathyreoidalen Lymphbahnen des erwachsenen Menschen. Inaug. Diss. Tübingen 1962.
Roos, B.: The submicroscopic structure of the rat thyroid gland. Path. et Microbiol. (Basel) **23**, 129 (1960).
Shdanow, D. A.: Über das Lymphsystem. Leningrader med. Z. **1952**.
Waller, U.: Zur submikroskopischen Struktur der Rattenschilddrüse. Acta endocr. (Kbh.) **35**, 334 (1960).
Wissig, S. L.: The anatomy of secretion in the follicular cells of the thyroid gland. J. biophys. biochem. Cytol. **7**, 419 (1960).

Aus der 2. Medizinischen Klinik und Poliklinik der Medizinischen Akademie Düsseldorf
(Direktor: Prof. Dr. K. OBERDISSE)

Untersuchungen über Enzyme des Energiestoffwechsels in menschlichen Schilddrüsen

Von

D. REINWEIN und A. ENGLHARDT

Mit 1 Abbildung

Aus tierexperimentellen Befunden von WEISS (1951) und LINDSAY u. JENKS (1960) ist bekannt, daß die Schilddrüse außer der Hormonbildung eine Reihe von Synthesen im Intermediärstoffwechsel leisten kann. Über die menschliche Schilddrüse liegen nur die Ergebnisse von DUMONT (1960) und TELKKÄA et al. (1960) über Enzyme des Tricarbonsäure-Cyclus vor. Um einen weiteren Einblick in die energetischen Leistungen der Schilddrüse zu gewinnen, haben wir 20 Enzyme in operierten Schilddrüsen von 37 Patienten mit normaler und pathologischer Drüse biochemisch untersucht.

Untersuchungsgut und Methoden

Wir untersuchten 5 Patienten mit normaler Schilddrüse (Kehlkopf-Carcinom), 18 mit blander diffuser Struma und 14 mit hyperthyreoter Struma. Der Operation gingen außer den üblichen klinischen Untersuchungen mit Grundumsatzbestimmung Messungen des Jodstoffwechsels mit Jod[131] und die chemische Analyse des Hormonjodes im Blut (PBI) nach KLEIN (1952) voraus. 10 Patienten mit hyperthyreoter Struma hatten präoperativ Lugolsche Lösung und Favistan bzw. Propycil, 4 nur Lugolsche Lösung erhalten. 3 Patienten mit blander Struma waren ebenfalls kombiniert und 3 nur mit Lugolscher Lösung vorbehandelt worden. Laut Grundumsatz und klinischem Befund war die Stoffwechsellage in allen Fällen zum Zeitpunkt der Operation euthyreot.

Sogleich nach Resektion der Schilddrüse erfolgte die Aufarbeitung des Gewebes. Wir homogenisierten es im Verhältnis 1:5 mit 0,2 m Phosphatpuffer, p_H 7,2, im Starmix. Im Überstand des bei 20000 × g in der Kühlzentrifuge sedimentierten Homogenates erfolgten die Bestimmung des Proteins (BEISENHERZ et al. 1953) und der Enzyme. Die Aktivitäten folgender Fermente wurden gemessen: 1. Glucose-6-Phosphat-Dehydrogenase (ZF, G6-PD). 2. Aldolase. 3. 3-Phosphoglyceratkinase (PGK). 4. Lactat-Dehydrogenase (LDH). 5. Glycerinaldeyhd-phosphat-Dehydrogenase (GAPDH). 6. Malat-Dehydrogenase (MDH). 7. Isocitrico-Dehydrogenase (ICDH). 8. β-Ketoacylthiolase. 9. β-Oxacyl-Dehydrogenase. 10. Acyl-Dehydrogenase. 11. Cytochrom-c-Oxydase (Cyt. ox.). 12. Cytochrom c-Reduktase (Cyt. red.). 13. Bernsteinsäure-Deyhdrogenase (BSDH). 14. Glutamat-Dehydrogenase (GSDH). 15. Glutamat-Oxalacetat-Transaminase (GOT). 16. Glutamat-Pyruvat-Transaminase (GPT). 17. TPN-Glutathion-Reduktase (GSSD-T). 18. Glutathion-DPN-Reduktase (GSSD-D). 19. Alkalische Phosphatase (AP). 20. Saure Phosphatase (SP). Die Bestimmungen der Enzyme 2, 4, 15 und 16 erfolgten nach den Vorschriften der „Biochemika Test Boehringer", diejenigen der Enzyme 1, 3, 5 bis 7 und 14 in einer Modifikation der Originalmethode von DELBRÜCK et al. (1959). Die Fermente 8 bis 10 wurden nach WIELAND et al. (1955), 11 bis 13 in einer Modifikation nach KERPPOLA u.

164   D. Reinwein und A. Englhardt:

Pitkänen (1960), 17 und 18 nach Horn u. Bruns (1958), 19 und 20 nach Gutman u. Gutman (1938) bestimmt. Bei den im optischen Test gemessenen Enzymen betrug das p_H 7,40 und die Temperatur 25° C, bei den Phosphatasen 4,0 bzw. 11,0 und 37° C.

Die Enzymaktivitäten sind in IE (1 IE = 1 μMol Substratumsatz pro Minute bei 25° C) pro g Gewebe (Feuchtgewicht) bzw. 100 mg Extraktprotein (Spez. A.) ausgedrückt.

Ergebnisse

In Abb. 1 sind die mittleren spezifischen Enzymaktivitäten von 5 normalen Schilddrüsen, 18 blanden und 14 hyperthyreoten Strumen wiedergegeben. Die

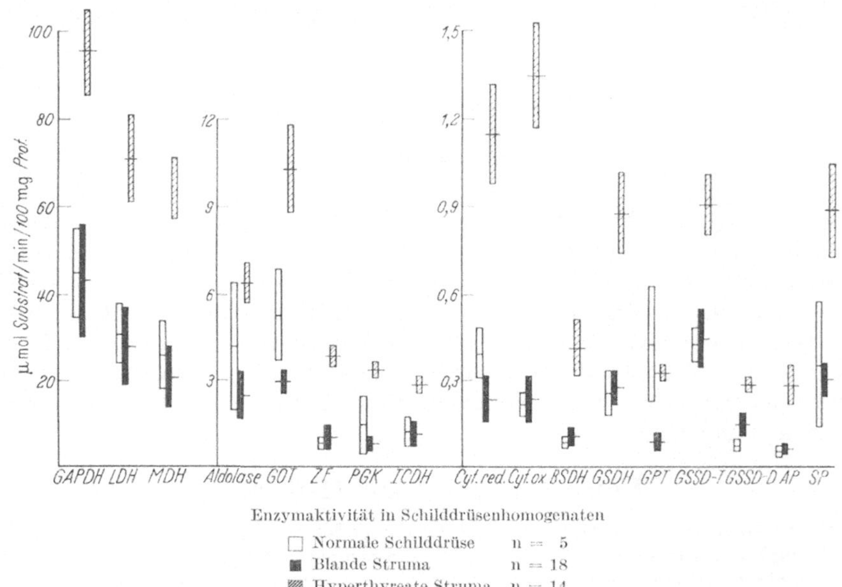

Abb. 1

höchsten Aktivitäten mit einem Substratumsatz über 20 μMol finden wir bei der GAPDH, LDH und MDH, einen Umsatz zwischen 1 bis 6 μMol weisen die GOT, Aldolase, G6-PD, PGK und ICDH auf; Werte unter 1 μMol zeigen die Cyt. red., Cyt. ox., BSDH, GSDH, GPT, GSSD-T, GSSD-D, AP und SP. Enzyme des Fettsäure-Cyclus, die β-Ketoacylthiolase, β-Oxacyl-Dehydrogenase und Acyl-Dehydrogenase, ließen sich nicht nachweisen; Inhibitoren wurden andererseits ausgeschlossen.

Blande Strumen zeigen gegenüber normalen Schilddrüsen eine geringere Enzymaktivität. Ausnahmen machen die G6-PD, GSSD und AP mit etwas höheren Werten. Keiner dieser Unterschiede ist signifikant. Auch in Strumen von Patienten, die mit Propycil oder Lugolscher Lösung oder kombiniert vorbehandelt worden sind, ergibt sich grundsätzlich das gleiche Enzymspektrum wie bei nicht vorbehandelten Strumen.

In hyperthyreoten Strumen finden wir eine deutliche Aktivitätszunahme aller Enzyme außer der GPT, die unabhängig von der Art der medikamentösen Vorbehandlung ist. Die Unterschiede sind mit einem $p < 0,001$ signifikant. Im Serum war dagegen kein Enzymzuwachs gegenüber Kontrollen festzustellen. Stellt man die spezifische Aktivität hyperthyreoter denjenigen euthyreoter Strumen gegenüber, ergeben sich für die am Elektronentransport beteiligten Enzyme sowie AP, G6-PD, PGK, GOT und GPT die höchsten Werte. Sie betragen das 3,5 bis 6fache der Vergleichsdaten. Ähnliche Unterschiede finden wir, wenn das Feuchtgewicht der Gewebe als Bezugsgröße gewählt wird. Zwischen dem Schweregrad des klinischen Bildes und den Daten des Jodstoffwechsels einerseits und den Aktivitätsänderungen in der Drüse andererseits bestehen keine derartigen Beziehungen, wie sie bei den Schilddrüsen-Proteasen festgestellt wurden (REINWEIN 1962).

Besprechung der Ergebnisse

Unsere Untersuchungen beim Menschen zeigen übereinstimmend mit tierexperimentellen Ergebnissen, daß die Schilddrüse zu einer Reihe von Stoffwechselleistungen fähig ist. Typisch scheint für die Drüse eine relativ hohe Aktivität der G6-PD und eine niedrige Aktivität der Enzyme des Tricarbonsäure-Cyclus und des Aminosäurestoffwechsels sowie die fehlende Enzymausstattung zur Oxydation von Fettsäuren zu sein. Im Vergleich zur Leber, dessen Enzymmuster SCHMITT u. SCHMITT (1960) unter gleichen Testbedingungen gemessen haben, beträgt die Enzymausrüstung der Schilddrüse für die Glykolyse 20 bis 50%, den Krebs-Cyclus 5 bis 20% und den Aminosäurestoffwechsel 1 bis 10%. Möglicherweise deuten diese Veränderungen darauf hin, daß hier die Energie zu einem großen Teil durch den Glucoseabbau auf dem Wege des Pentose-Shunts bereitgestellt werden kann, worauf DUMONT (1960b) schon hingewiesen hatte.

Blande Strumen unterscheiden sich kaum von normalen Schilddrüsen. Allerdings ist hier eine weitere Aktivitätszunahme der G6-PD nachzuweisen, während die glykolytischen Enzyme abnehmen. Wieweit die in hyperthyreoten Strumen gefundenen Veränderungen iatrogen oder drüsenspezifisch sind, kann nicht eindeutig geklärt werden, weil alle Patienten präoperativ vorbehandelt worden sind. Folgende Befunde lassen aber darauf schließen, daß der medikamentöse Einfluß nur gering sein kann. In 2 hyperthyreoten Strumen, die nur mit Lugolscher Lösung vorbehandelt worden sind, ist die Aktivitätssteigerung genau so groß wie in den übrigen Strumen (Lugol + Favistan). Kein Zuwachs an Aktivität zeigen dagegen 6 euthyreote Strumen, von denen jeweils 3 mit Lugolscher Lösung und 3 kombiniert vorbehandelt worden sind. Auch in vitro fanden wir bei keinem der 17 Enzyme durch 10^{-3} bis 10^{-5} m Jodid, Propycil oder Favistan Änderungen der Aktivität. Die Aktivitätszunahme scheint spezifisch für die Schilddrüse zu sein, weil der Gesamtstoffwechsel zum Zeitpunkt der Operation laut Sauerstoffverbrauch normal gewesen ist.

Zusammenfassend ist festzustellen, daß die Enzymausstattung der menschlichen Schilddrüse im Vergleich zur Leber eine geringere Glykolyse ermöglicht und die Energiebildung zu einem relativ größeren Teil über den Pentose-Shunt erfolgt. Gering ist der Substratumsatz durch den Krebs-Cyclus, noch geringer der Umsatz im Aminosäurestoffwechsel, während die Enzyme zur Oxydation der Fettsäuren fehlen. Blande Strumen unterscheiden sich kaum von normalen Drüsen. Dahingegen zeigen hyperthyreote Strumen eine signifikant erhöhte Aktivität von 16 Enzymen. Die Veränderungen sind eher drüsenspezifisch als iatrogen bedingt; sie lassen darauf schließen, daß die klinische Besserung nicht mit der Regulation aller Stoffwechselvorgänge in der Drüse parallel geht.

Literatur

Beisenherz, G., H. J. Boltze, Th. Bücher, R. Czok, K. H. Garbade, E. Meyer-Arendt u. G. Pfleiderer: Z. Naturforsch. 8b, 555 (1953).

Delbrück, A., E. Zebe u. Th. Bücher: Biochem. Z. 331, 273 (1959).

Dumont, I. E.: J. clin. Endocr. 20, 1246 (1960a).

— Biochim. biophys. Acta 40, 354 (1960b).

Gutman, A. B. and E. B. Gutman: J. clin. Invest. 17, 473 (1938).

Horn, H. D., u. F. H. Bruns: Biochem. Z. 331, 58 (1958).

Kerppola, W., and E. Pitkänen: Endocrinology 67, 162 (1960).

Klein, E.: Biochem. Z. 322, 388 (1952).

Lindsay, S., and P. R. Jenks: Internat. Congr. Series No. 26, 42 (1960).

Reinwein, D.: Acta endocr. (Kbh.) Suppl. 67, 156 (1962).

Schmitt, E., u. F. W. Schmitt: Klin. Wschr. 38, 957 (1960).

Telkkää, A., K. J. Heikkilea and V. K. Hopsu: Acta endocr. (Kbh.) 35, 135 (1960).

Weiss, B.: J. biol. Chem. 193, 509 (1951).

Wieland, O., D. Reinwein and F. Lynen: In: Biochemical Problems of Lipids, S. 155, ed. by G. Popjak and E. I. Breton. London: Butterworth Sci. Publ. 1955.

Aus der Chirurgischen Universitätsklinik Hamburg
(Direktor: Prof. Dr. ZUKSCHWERDT)

Das toxische Adenom der Schilddrüse

(Klinische und histologische Befunde bei 45 operierten Fällen)

Von

V. BAY

Mit 1 Abbildung

Der ersten Beschreibung des toxischen Adenoms durch PLUMMER folgten für lange Zeit nur spärliche Mitteilungen.

Erst das Lokalisations-, Funktions- und Regulationsstudium mit Radiojod ermöglichte eine schnelle zuverlässige Diagnose. Die Unabhängigkeit der Funktion des Adenoms von der Hypophysenregulation konnte nachgewiesen werden.

Nach HORST unterscheiden wir kompensierte und dekompensierte Adenome.

Unsere Hamburger Arbeitsgruppe beobachtete in 10 Jahren 151 toxische Adenome, von denen 106 radiologisch und 45 operativ behandelt wurden. Die Zahl der operierten Fälle nahm in den letzten Jahren fortlaufend zu (Tab. 1). Teils ist dieses begründet durch die Steigerung des gesamten Materials, teils durch Einschränkung der radiologischen Indikationsstellung, um Material für die histologische Grundlage des toxischen Adenoms zu gewinnen.

Langzeitbeobachtungen zeigten den Übergang vom kompensierten toxischen Adenom in das dekompensierte unter Zunahme der Größe, wie dieses auch FELLINGER beschrieb.

Tabelle 1.

Gesamtmaterial der operierten Strumen der Chirurgischen Universitätsklinik Hamburg von 1952—1962.

	Gesamtzahl der op. Sturmen	Hyperthyr.	Struma uni + multinodosa				
			kalte[1] Knoten	warme[1] Knoten	toxische Adenome		
					dekomp.	komp.	nicht auton.
1952	30	3	26	3	0	1	0
1953	37	2	35	2	0	0	0
1954	32	1	30	2	1	0	0
1955	30	5	20	12	3	1	1
1956	52	9	41	12	1	1	0
1957	50	10	40	8	0	0	0
1958	56	8	42	10	1	1	0
1959	56	9	44	15	0	1	0
1960	51	6	34	16	0	5	0
1961	102	10	74	19	8	4	1
1962	148	16	106	19	9	8	6
Insgesamt	644	79	492	118	23	22	8

[1] In einer Struma vorkommende kalte und warme Knoten wurden extra aufgeführt

Große Adenome weisen oft kalte Bereiche auf, die histologisch als ausgedehnte degenerative Bezirke geklärt werden. Die Weiterentwicklung führt meist zu Cysten, die nur noch einen Randsaum aktiven Gewebes enthalten.

Es lag nahe, zunehmende Drucksteigerungen für die regressiven Veränderungen verantwortlich zu machen. Tatsächlich fanden wir bei prä- und intraoperativer systematischer Druckmessung in Adenomen mit cystischer Umwandlung Werte bis 75 mm Hg, während gleichmäßige parenchymatöse Adenome nur 8–10 mm Hg aufwiesen. Die degenerativen Veränderungen sind also Folge der Drucksteigerung im Adenom durch sein schnelles Wachstum mit Beeinträchtigung zunächst des venösen Abflusses (bedingt durch obliterierende Venenveränderungen nach Hamperl und Ratzenhofer), später der arteriellen Zufuhr.

Tabelle 2. *Klinische Symptome des toxischen Adenoms*

	%
1. *Kardiovasculär:*	
Herzklopfen, Tachykardie .	56
Atemnot bei Belastung . .	24
2. *Nervös:*	
Allgemeine Nervosität . . .	60
Schlafstörungen	28
Tremor.	27
Schwindel	24
Schwitzen	35

Die kompensierten toxischen Adenome verliefen euthyreotisch, die dekompensierten meist hyperthyreotisch, aber ohne Exophthalmus. Die nächste Tabelle (Tab. 2) zeigt die klinischen Symptome. Im Vordergrund stehen kardiovasculäre und nervöse Zeichen. Nicht selten wurde auch über psychische Veränderungen, insbesondere depressive Stimmungsschwankungen sowie Menstruationsstörungen und Verlust der Libido berichtet. Häufig wurden von den Patienten als „Ursachen" des Erkrankungsbeginns Geburten, Operationen oder Phasen innersekretorischer Unruhe wie Menarche und Klimakterium angegeben.

Bei 39 Patienten fand sich das toxische Adenom in einer uninodösen Struma, 6 hatten mehrere Knoten, von denen einer der aktive war. Einmal stellten wir 2 toxische Adenome in einer Struma multinodosa fest.

Der Durchmesser der dekompensierten Adenome war 4,5 cm und damit deutlich größer als bei den kompensierten mit 2,4 cm. Die Herzfrequenz war bei den kompensierten nicht, bei den dekompensierten deutlich erhöht. Blutdruck und EKG zeigten keine wesentlich von der Norm abweichenden Werte, dagegen war die Kreislaufzeit (mit Magnorbin bestimmt) mit 9,3 sec auffallend beschleunigt gegenüber 19 sec bei Gesunden. Ähnliche Befunde konnte Jores beim Morbus Basedow erheben. Als Ursache der Beschleunigung der Kreislaufzeit vermuten wir eine vermehrte Öffnung arterio-venöser Anastomosen, ohne sie bis jetzt sicher durch capillarmikroskopische Untersuchungen beweisen zu können. Die arterio-venöse Relation von normal 1 : 3 fanden wir allerdings im Mittel auf 1 : 6 verändert, außerdem beobachteten wir erhebliche Kaliberschwankungen der Endschlingen. Über die Bedeutung dieser Befunde läßt sich noch nichts Endgültiges sagen (Franke).

In der Behandlung des toxischen Adenoms stehen sich Operation und Radiojodelimination gleichwertig gegenüber. Finden sich „kalte" Bezirke im toxischen Adenom, so verdient die Operation den Vorzug. Sie muß den anatomischen und funktionellen Besonderheiten Rechnung tragen. Die typische Resektion nach Enderlen-Hotz führt durch Reduktion des normalen Schilddrüsengewebes zumindest zu vorübergehender Hypothyreose. Wir empfehlen die sorgfältige totale Enucleation des toxischen Adenoms ohne Ligatur der Schilddrüsenarterien (ZUKSCHWERDT). Das ruhende Schilddrüsengewebe muß geschont werden. Die histologische Untersuchung unserer toxischen Adenome verdanken wir Herrn Prof. KRAUSPE.

Makroskopisch waren alle gut abgekapselt, größenmäßig zwischen einer Erbse und einer Männerfaust. Die Schnittfläche zeigte häufig degenerative Veränderungen mit Erweichungscysten, Nekrosen und alten Blutungsherden oder Cysten, die lediglich am Rande aktives Gewebe enthielten.

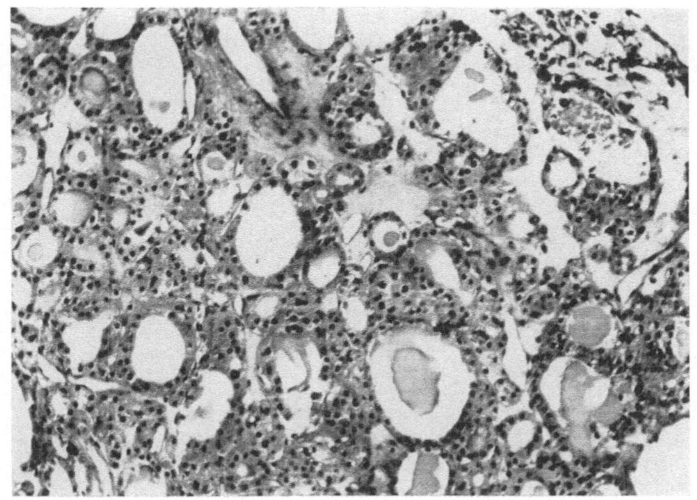

Abb. 1. Toxisches Adenom mit verschiedenen Funktionszuständen der Follikel neben degenerativen Veränderungen

Die *mikroskopische* Untersuchung ergab 38mal ein folliculäres Adenom, wobei das trabeculäre, embryonale und fetale Adenom unter dieser Bezeichnung eingereiht wurde, entsprechend der Einteilung von WARREN und MEISSNER. 7 Adenome waren von papillärem Bau. Neben sekretorisch aktiven Epithelien und Speicherfollikeln sahen wir in nahezu allen Fällen degenerative Veränderungen (Abb. 1). *Anzeichen für maligne Entartung fanden sich bei keinem unserer toxischen Adenome.* Die bei einigen trabeculären Adenomen vorhandene Polymorphie der Zellen mahnt allerdings zur Vorsicht in der Beurteilung. Die Nachuntersuchung aller Patienten mit operierten toxischen Adenomen, deren Operationen z. T. 10 Jahre zurückliegt, ergab bis jetzt kein Rezidiv. Alle berichteten über anhaltende Beschwerdefreiheit.

Literatur

FELLINGER, K., R. HÖFER and H. VETTER: J. clin. Endocr. 17, 483 (1957).
— — H. EGERT and H. VETTER: In: Advances in Thyroid Research, p. 347. Oxford. London, New York, Paris: Pergamon Press, 1961.

Franke, J.: Dtsch. Zahnärztl. Z. **16**, 1475 (1961).

Hamperl, H.: Upsala Läk. -Fören.Förh. **1/2** 99 (1949).

Horst, W.: Klinische Radiojoddiagnostik der Schilddrüsenerkrankungen. In: Strahlenbiologie, Strahlentherapie, Nuklearmedizin und Krebsforschung. S. 785—930. Stuttgart 1959.

— C. Schneider u. Kl. J. Thiemann: Verh. dtsch. Ges. inn. Med. **66**, 356 (1960).

— I. Petersen, Kl. J. Thiemann u. L. Zukschwerdt: Dtsch. med. Wschr. **85**, 711 (1960).

Jores, A.: Zit. nach Bürger, M., u. K. Seidel: Münch. med. Wschr. **102**, 609 (1960).

Plummer, H. S.: Amer. J. med. Sci. **146**, 790 (1913).

—, and W. M. Boothby: Amer. J. Physiol. **63**, 406 (1923).

— Trans. Ass. Amer. Phycans **43**,. 159 (1928).

Ratzenhofer, M.: III. Österr. Ärztetag, Salzburg, S. 214, Wien 1950.

Warren, S., and W. A. Meissner: Atlas of Tumor Pathology, Section IV,: Tumors of the Thyroid gland. Armed Forces Institute of Pathology. Washington 1953.

Zukschwerdt, L.: Strahlentherapie (Sonderband) **49** 1929 (1961).

—, u. W. Horst: Langenbeks Arch. klin. Chir. **301**, 486 (1962).

—, u. V. Bay: Vortrag Schilddrüsensymposion, Innsbruck 1962. Wien. med. Wschr. **113**, 823 (1963).

Aus der Chirurgischen Universitätsklinik und Poliklinik Hamburg
(Direktor: Prof. Dr. L. Zukschwerdt)

Das Adenylsäuresystem
nach Eingriffen an der Schilddrüse[1]

Von

O. Scheibe

Mit 2 Abbildungen

Nach großen chirurgischen Eingriffen kommt es im Rahmen kataboler Stoffwechselveränderungen zu einer negativen Energielage in den Erythrocyten; wir sehen einen Abfall des Adenosintriphosphats (ATP), des Quotienten ATP/ADP und statistisch gesichert des Quotienten ATP/AMP. Durch Zufuhr von Zuckern, am besten der Fructose, kann dieser Abfall verhindert und in eine positive Energielage mit einem Ansteigen dieser Werte verwandelt werden (1).

Einen postoperativen Anstieg von ATP, ATP/ADP und auch des Quotienten aus Pyruvat/Lactat (BTS/MS) ohne Zufuhr energieliefernder Substanzen finden wir nur nach Schilddrüsenresektionen und nur bei subtotaler oder totaler Entfernung. Den Grund für dieses Verhalten können wir in der Stoffwechselwirkung des Schilddrüsenhormons finden. Kleine Thyroxinkonzentrationen steigern in geringem Umfang die Größe der Atmungskettenphosphorylierung, große Dosen dagegen hemmen sie bis zur vollständigen Entkopplung (2, 3, 4) und setzen den Ausnutzungsgrad physiologischer Energielieferanten herab; damit fallen die ATP-Werte, der Quotient ATP/ADP und ATP/AMP im Blut ab. Fällt durch die operative Entfernung des Schilddrüsengewebes dieser entkoppelnde Effekt weg, steigen die Werte wieder an (Abb. 1 u. 2).

Aber auch nach subtotaler Resektion *euthyreoter* Strumen (10 Fälle), die weder im Radiojodstoffwechsel-Studium noch im Grundumsatz eine faßbare Überfunktion zeigen, fanden wir postoperativ diese positive Energielage. Der postoperative Stoffwechsel verhält sich also ebenso wie der nach subtotaler Resektion einer *hyperthyreoten* Struma oder heißer Knoten.

Der entkoppelnde Einfluß des Schilddrüsenhormons muß sich aber auch in den Werten vor der Operation bemerkbar machen. Tatsächlich fanden wir einen tieferen Ausgangswert für ATP, geringer auch für ATP/ADP und ATP/AMP. Das gleiche postoperative Verhalten und der erniedrigte Ausgangswert deuten an, daß sich beide Schilddrüsenerkrankungen – die euthyreote *und* die hyperthyreote Struma – im Stoffwechselverhalten nicht unterscheiden, daß also auch die sog. euthyreote Struma Schilddrüsenhormon in klinisch unterschwelliger, aber stoffwechselaktiver Menge *vermehrt* ausschüttet.

---

[1] Die Untersuchungen wurden mit Mitteln der Deutschen Forschungsgemeinschaft durchgeführt.

Die positive Energielage nach subtotaler oder totaler Schilddrüsenentfernung
ist aber nicht eine Eigenheit der Schilddrüsenoperation: andersartige Eingriffe
an diesem Organ, die wenig Gewebe entfernen, verändern postoperativ den Stoffwechsel gegensätzlich; sie zeigen die negative Energielage wie nach anderen großen

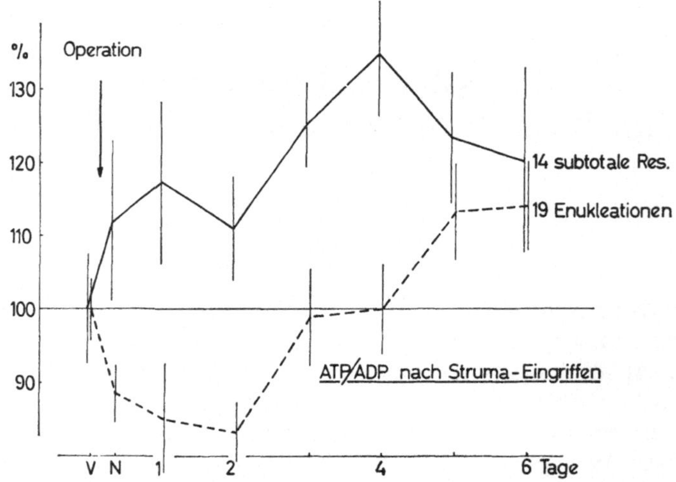

Abb. 1. ATP/ADP-Quotient nach 14 subtotalen Strumaresektionen und 19 Enucleationen

Eingriffen und einen leicht angehobenen präoperativen ATP-Ausgangswert (vgl.
Abb. 1), der an die stimulierende Wirkung kleiner Thyroxindosen erinnert. Mit
den vorliegenden Stoffwechseluntersuchungen übersehen wir mehr dieser wenig

Blut-ATP nach Struma-Eingriffen

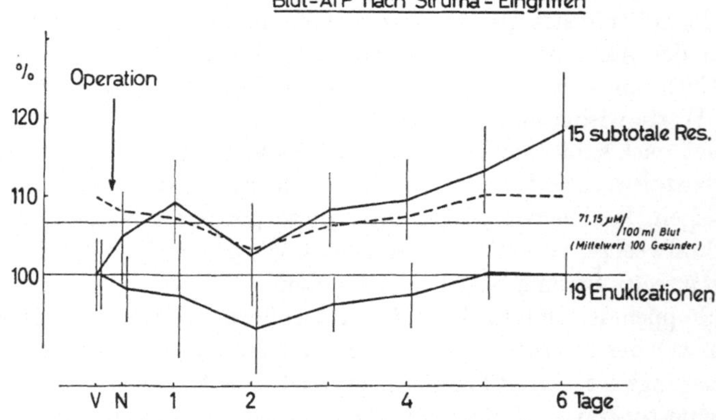

Abb. 2. Blut-ATP-Werte nach 15 subtotalen Strumaresektionen und nach 19 Enucleationen (gestrichelte Linie),
bezogen auf den Mittelwert aus 100 Stoffwechselgesunden

Gewebe entfernenden Eingriffe, insgesamt 19 Enucleationen eines oder mehrerer
Knoten bzw. Teilresektionen eines multinodulären Schilddrüsenlappens, da etwa
vier Fünftel unserer Kranken im Raum Hamburg an meist uninodösen Knoten-
kröpfen leiden.

Viel seltener sehen wir die Hyperthyreose oder sog. heiße Knoten (5 Fälle). Mit anorg. Jod wird die Thyroxinabgabe gebremst (5, 6, 7, 8); entsprechend findet sich auch die Energielage im Erythrocyten angehoben. Während bei der Hyperthyreose der Blut-ATP-Wert und der Quotient ATP/ADP nach subtotaler Resektion auf Werte um 160% des präoperativen Wertes ansteigt, fallen diese unter Jodeinfluß ab; es entsteht also ein Stoffwechselbild wie nach Operationen in anderen Körperregionen. Der Einfluß des anorganischen Jods zeigt sich auch während der Operationsvorbereitung: durch Hemmung der Thyroxinausschüttung hört die Entkopplung der oxydativen Phosphorylierung auf und der ATP-Wert im Erythrocyten steigt an. Beispielsweise fand sich bei einer 47jährigen „Basedow"-Kranken am Aufnahmetag, also vor Beginn der Jodmedikation, ein ATP-Wert von 60,7 μM/100 ml Blut. Der Wert vor der Operation im Höhepunkt der Jodwirkung betrug 77,9 μM/100 ml. Die täglich gemessenen postoperativen Werte lagen zwischen 50 und 60 μM/100 ml Blut, also bis 15% unter dem Ausgangswert. Ähnliche Werte zeigt der ATP/ADP-Quotient, der Anstieg des BTS/MS-Quotienten fehlt.

Aus unseren Untersuchungen läßt sich folgendes sagen:

1. Die sog. euthyreote Struma hat ebenfalls hyperthyreote Eigenschaften und schüttet Schilddrüsenhormon in klinisch allerdings unterschwelliger, aber stoffwechselaktiver Menge aus; die Folge ist ein erniedrigter Ausgangswert des energiereichen Phosphats ATP und der Quotienten ATP/ADP und ATP/AMP.

2. Die subtotale Entfernung großer euthyreoter Strumen führt ebenso wie die subtotale Resektion von hyperthyreoten Strumen und die Totalentfernung der Struma maligna in den ersten 6 Tagen nach dem Eingriff zu einem Anstieg der energiereichen Phosphate; der entkoppelnde Effekt des Schilddrüsenhormons auf endogene Atmung und Phosphorylierung fällt weg; dieser Einfluß ist wahrscheinlich abhängig von der Menge resezierten Strumagewebes und nicht von der präoperativen Funktion.

3. Die Knotenentfernung dagegen führt zu einer postoperativen Senkung des Blutenergiespiegels und ähnelt damit der Veränderung nach anderen Eingriffen.

4. Die Gabe anorganischen Jods bei der Hyperthyreose normalisiert den Stoffwechsel, d. h. der postoperative Energiespiegel im Blut zeigt wie nach allen großen Operationen fallende Tendenz.

Literatur

1. SCHEIBE, O.: Postoperative Veränderungen des Adenylsäuresystems. Klin. Wschr. **40**, 303—312 (1962).
2. MARTIUS, C., u. B. HESS: Über den Wirkungsmechanismus des Schilddrüsenhormons: Naunyn-Schmiedeberg's Arch. exp. Path. Pharmak. **216**, 45—46 (1952).
3. — Über den Wirkungsmechanismus des Schilddrüsenhormons. Biochem. Z. **326**, 191—198 (1955).
4. — Die oxydative Phosphorylierung und ihre hormonelle Steuerung. Klin. Wschr. **35**, 223—225 (1957).
5. KÜHNAU, J.: Biochemie der Schilddrüse. Naunyn-Schmiedeberg's Arch. exp. Path. Pharmak. **216**, 4—16 (1952).
6. VOSS, R., H. L'ALLEMAND u. F. X. EISENREICH: Hypothermie dei pharmakologischer Drosselung der Schilddrüse. Langenbecks Arch. klin. Chir. **289**, 319—321 (1958).
7. BECKER, W. H., u. R. VOSS: Die Wirkung von parateral verabreichtem Jod auf den Glykogengehalt von Herzmuskel-, Gehirn- und Lebergewebe. Klin. Wschr. **38**, 949—950 (1960).

8. Staib, I., u. W. Niepmann: Zur Bedeutung hoher Joddosen in der prä-und postoperativen Behandlung hyperthyreoter Strumen. Chirurg **32**, 513—516 (1961).

Diskussion

D. Reinwein (Düsseldorf):

Haben Sie den Einfluß der Zellmembran-ATP-ase berücksichtigt?

O. Scheibe:

Da keine Gewebsuntersuchungen mit Homogenisierung im physiologischen Milieu sondern Blutuntersuchungen mit $HClO_4$-Extraktion durchgeführt wurden, spielt die ATP-ase keine Rolle.

D. Reinwein:

War bei den Patienten mit positiver postoperativer Energielage eine Jodvorbereitung durchgeführt worden?

O. Sceibe:

Nein.

Aus dem Therapeutischen Strahleninstitut (Chefarzt: Prof. Dr. Gauwerky) und der I. Med.
Abtlg. (Chefarzt: Prof. Dr. Bansi) des Allgemeinen Krankenhauses St. Georg, Hamburg

Iatrogene Strumen

Von

F. Petersen und H. W. Bansi

Mit 1 Abbildung

Als iatrogene Strumen werden jene Schilddrüsenvergrößerungen aufgefaßt, die bei euthyreoten Patienten durch eine nicht indizierte Verabreichung von schilddrüsenwirksamen Präparaten erzeugt werden, oder die als Nebenwirkung gewisser Medikamente auftreten, wobei die Indikation zur Behandlung ein von der Schilddrüse unabhängiges Leiden darstellt.

Als Ursache für die Entstehung iatrogener Strumen kommen drei Gruppen von Pharmaka in Frage:

a) Anorganische und organische Jodverbindungen (mit Ausnahme von Schilddrüsenhormonen bzw. -hormonanalogen.)

b) Antithyreoidale Substanzen (Thiourazile, Mercaptoimicazole und Perchlorate).

c) Medikamente mit antithyreoidalem Nebeneffekt. Thiocyanat (*8, 9, 11, 19, 63*), PAS (*16, 28, 36, 50*), Butazolidin (*14, 30, 67*), Kobalt (*12, 43, 61, 65*), gelegentlich auch Sulfonamide (*6, 48, 59*), Sulfanylharnstoffe (*49*), Hydantoinderivate (*25*) und BAL (*17*).

Von 1953—1962 waren unter 5567 euthyreoten Patienten, die zum Radiojodstoffwechselstudium überwiesen wurden, 3326 Strumenträger. 158 dieser Strumen, d. i. 4,8%, waren iatrogen entstanden oder verschlimmert. In 148 Fällen war eine nicht indizierte thyreostatische Prämedikation die Ursache, 5 Strumen entstanden nach Gabe von Irgapyrin®, 3 nach jodhaltigen Medikamenten, 2 nach PAS. Nicht enthalten sind in der Auswertung Patienten mit „heißem" Adenom, endokriner Ophthalmopathie sowie Thyreoiditis; ferner Patienten, die mit der Fragestellung einer Schilddrüsenunterfunktion, einer hypophysären Insuffizienz oder einer Jodfehlverwertung überwiesen wurden und Fälle, in denen ein Schilddrüsenmalignom vorlag.

1. Einfluß von Jod auf die Schilddrüse

Es ist gleichgültig, in welcher Form bzw. Verbindung das Jod verabreicht wird, die Dejodasen des Organismus spalten jeweils Jodid ab (*1, 13, 37, 70*) und lassen es schilddrüsenwirksam werden. Je nach der Dosierung, der Dauer der Jodapplikation und der Reaktionsbereitschaft der Schilddrüse kann die Wirkung grundsätzlich verschieden sein. Jod kann eine Struma reduzieren oder induzieren, es kann die Schilddrüsenfunktion hemmen oder auch stimulieren, in Einzelfällen wird sogar eine Unterfunktion hervorgerufen oder eine Stoffwechselentgleisung im Sinne einer Hyperthyreose ausgelöst. Bansi (5) hat daher vom Janus-Gesicht des Jods gesprochen.

Während niedrige Joddosen die Schilddrüse stimulieren, tritt eine Hemmung der Jodaufnahme der Schilddrüse ein, sobald der Jodidspiegel im Blut bei Schilddrüsengesunden 20—35 γ-% überschreitet (21, 62, 72, 79, 80). Nach der heutigen Anschauung, die auf experimentellen und tierexperimentellen Untersuchungen basiert, greift ein Überangebot von Jod an drei Punkten in den Schilddrüsenstoffwechsel ein.

1. Durch den homöostatischen Effekt wird die Ausschüttung des TSH vermindert, ferner wird das TSH in der Schilddrüsenzelle inaktiviert (2, 24, 60, 77, 79).

2. Bei vermehrter Jodzufuhr verringert sich die Jodidmenge, die nach dem Durchlaufen einer hypothetischen Reaktionsform in die Hormonsynthese eintreten kann (3, 20, 58).

3. Die Hormonsynthese ist bei der Kopplung der Tyrosine zu den Thyroninen blockiert (18, 79, 80).

Bei längerer Verabreichung von Jod vermögen im allgemeinen die Schilddrüse und die Hypophyse sich der erhöhten Zufuhr anzupassen, so daß die Hemmung nur vorübergehend ist. Gelegentlich bleibt dieser Effekt jedoch bestehen, so daß bei langhaltenden Jodapplikationen Strumen und sogar Unterfunktionen entstehen können. Der erste Fall eines Jod-Myxödems wurde von Haines 1928 (26) beschrieben, inzwischen sind etwas über 50 Fälle publiziert worden (10, 18, 22, 23, 31, 40, 46, 22, 53, 54, 56, 57, 66, 68, 75, 76, 78). Der folgende Fall demonstriert die Stoffwechselbeeinflussung:

Die 65jährige Pat. W. Z. erhielt wegen eines Asthma bronchiale seit 7 Jahren Felsol®, das pro Pulver 10 mg Phenyldimethyljodpyrazolon enthält. Seit 6 Jahren hat sich die Schilddrüse langsam vergrößert. Klinisch deuteten eine etwas rauhe Haut, ein leichtes Frieren und eine Obstipation auf eine geringe Unterfunktion. Das Cholesterin i. S. war auf 370 mg-% erhöht.

Das Radiojodstoffwechselstudium ergab eine Jodaufnahme von 52, 35, 24% nach 2, 24, 48 Std. Die effektive HWZ war auf 1,2 Tage verkürzt. Die Gesamt-Serumaktivität nach 48 Std betrug 0,20%/1, das PBJ[131] war nur 0,02%/l. Nach einer raschen Jodaufnahme verließ das Jod die Schilddrüse wieder mit einer sehr kurzen Halbwertzeit, größtenteils ohne in die Hormonsynthese einzutreten, so daß nach 48 Std vorwiegend anorganisches Jod im Serum enthalten war. Das Radiochromatogramm zeigte folgende Aufteilung der Jodfraktionen:

	DJT in %	MJT in %	J in %	T4 in %	T3 in %	Unbekannt in %
nach 8 Std . . .	9	9	50	4	9	19
nach 24 Std . . .	6	9	36	11	6	32
nach 48 Std . . .	1,5	8,5	50	3	9	28

Während die Tyrosine (MJT, DJT) im oberen Bereich der Norm lagen, war der Prozentsatz der Thyronine (T3, T4) sehr stark vermindert, die Hormonsynthese stagnierte somit im Bereich der Tyrosine.

Das nicht in die Hormonsynthese eingetretene Jod ließ sich bei analogen Fällen durch den KSCN-Test aus der Schilddrüse verdrängen (47, 56, 57). 12 Tage nach Absetzen des Felsols führten wir den KSCN-Test durch, zu dieser Zeit ließ sich bereits kein freies Jod mehr aus der Schilddrüse eliminieren. Die Jodaufnahme der Schilddrüse betrug jetzt 71, 69, 67% nach 2, 24,

48 Std, die effektive HWZ war 7,1 d. Der Schilddrüsenstoffwechsel war nicht mehr blockiert und zeigte einen Nachholbedarf im Sinne eines Reboundphänomens. Das Reboundphänomen ist vorwiegend durch das TSH bedingt (73); es weist darauf hin, daß nach der Depression unter der Jodwirkung eine kurze Periode mit vermehrter Ausschüttung von TSH folgt. Die Jod-Struma entsteht unter verminderter Einwirkung von TSH durch Kolloidstauung und Hyperplasie zur Kompensation der Stoffwechselstörung. Die Rückbildung der Struma erfolgte nach Absetzen der Jodmedikation sehr rasch, bereits nach 3 Wochen war bei der Pat. der Halsumfang um 2 cm kleiner geworden.

Die Entwicklung einer Struma mit nachfolgender Basedowifizierung durch langdauernde Gaben kleiner Jodmengen ist ein relativ seltenes Ereignis (5, 51), Von den 5567 Pat. waren 120 mit Jod vorbehandelt; in nur einem Fall beobachteten wir eine Basedowifizierung. Zur Auslösung ist daher außer der Jodnoxe eine besondere Bereitschaft der Schilddrüse zur Stoffwechselautonomie erforderlich, wobei es noch offen ist, ob der Schilddrüse, der Hypophyse oder einem übergeordneten Zwischenhirnzentrum pathogenetisch die größere Bedeutung zukommt.

Der 57 jährige Pat. O. T. erhielt wegen einer Lues im Stadium III mit Aortitis luica seit 4 Jahren Josikol, 3×5 Tropfen täglich, das 10% Kalium jodatum (KJ) enthält. Die Überweisung erfolgte, weil sich unter der Behandlung eine kleine Struma von 70 g gebildet hatte. Bei der Erstuntersuchung bot der Patient klinisch keine hyperthyreotischen Zeichen. G. U. + 26%. Cholesterin 230 mg-%.

Das Radiojodstoffwechselstudium ergab eine Jodaufnahme der Schilddrüse von 34, 61, 58% nach 2, 24, 48 Std, das PBJ[131] betrug 0,28%/l, die effektive HWZ war 6,5 d. Da es sich bei dem PBJ[131] um einen Grenzwert handelte, führten wir einen Suppressionstest mit Trijodthyronin durch. Die Jodaufnahme war mit den Werten 58, 65, 62 nach 2, 24, 48 Std nicht hemmbar, was für eine autonome Schilddrüsenfunktion sprach. Wegen des unauffälligen klinischen Bildes konnten wir uns zunächst zu einerSchilddrüsenbehandlung nicht entschließen.

Nach 2 Monaten trat plötzlich ein linksseitiger Exophthalmus auf, bei dem die Hertel-Werte 19,5 — 100 — 20,5 gemessen wurden. Das anschließende Radiojodstoffwechselstudium zeigte jetzt eine Veränderung im Sinne einer Hyperthyreose: Jodaufnahme 62, 80, 69% nach 2, 24, 48 Std, PBJ[131] 0,72%/l, effektive HWZ 4,8 d. Zwischenzeitlich waren eine innere Unruhe, ein Fingertremor und eine Gewichtsabnahme von 3,5 kg eingetreten.

Zur Limitierung der Schilddrüsenfunktion wurde eine Radiojodtherapie durchgeführt. Spätere Kontrollen ergaben normale Werte für die Jodaufnahme der Schilddrüse und eine hohe Plasmaaktivität nach 2 Std von über 2%/l, was für eine niedrige Jodidclearance der Schilddrüse bei Euthyreose spricht. Auch klinisch waren keine Überfunktionszeichen mehr nachzuweisen. Der Exophthalmus bildete sich günsigerweise vollständig zurück.

2. Strumigene Wirkung antithyreoidaler Substanzen

Die Entdeckung des Thioharnstoffes als Thyreostaticum beruht letztlich auf der Beobachtung des strumigenen Effektes, den eine einseitige Kohlernährung beim Kaninchen hervorruft (4, 15, 37). Die Hemmung der Schilddrüsenfunktion und die Bildung einer Struma sind durch die hypophysäre Regulation eng miteinander verbunden. Der erniedrigte Hormonjodspiegel bedingt eine vermehrte Ausschüttung von TSH, wodurch die Schilddrüse zur Hyperplasie angeregt wird. So können durch eine antithyreoidale Behandlung nicht nur eine Unterfunktion und eine Struma, sondern auch ein Exophthalmus hervorgerufen werden.

Wie Tab. 1 zeigt, wurden 12% der euthyreoten Patienten thyreostatisch vorbehandelt. Von den 659 Vorbehandelten entwickelten 23% eine Struma. Die thyreostatischen Vorbehandlungen sind in den letzten Jahren zurückgegangen, wobei jedoch berücksichtigt werden muß, daß im Anfang mehr stationäre Schwerkranke zur Untersuchung kamen und später vorwiegend leichtkranke Patienten

Tabelle 1. *Häufigkeit von iatrogenen Schäden bei euthyreoten Patienten nach thyreostatischer Vorbehandlung*

Jahre	Euthyreote Patienten	davon thyreostatisch vorbehandelt		Iatrogene Schäden		
				Struma-wachstum	Myxödem	Exophthalmus
1953—1955	325	59	[18%]	13	1	—
1956	304	50	[16%]	12	—	1
1957	387	57	[15%]	12	1	1
1958	423	62	[14%]	15	1	—
1959	640	95	[15%]	25	6	3
1960	984	118	[12%]	35	4	2
1961	1196	123	[10%]	21	2	2
1962	1289	95	[7%]	15	2	—
Insgesamt	5557	659	[12%]	148 [2,7%]	17 [0,3%]	9 [0,16%]

ambulant überwiesen wurden. Bei den 9 Fällen mit Exophthalmus hat sich in 4 Fällen die Ophthalmopathie wieder zurückgebildet, in 5 Fällen ist sie unverändert geblieben. In keinem Fall lagen die Hertel-Werte über 22, Augenmuskelparesen wurden nicht beobachtet.

Die Tab. 2 gibt die Art der Medikamente an, mit denen die Patienten in den letzten 2 Jahren vor der Untersuchung behandelt wurden; wenn ein Thyreostaticum gewechselt wurde, ist das zuletzt gegebene vermerkt.

Tabelle 2. *Zahl und Art der Vorbehandlung mit schilddrüsenwirksamen Präparaten bei euthyreoten Patienten*

Jahre	vorbehandelt mit			vorbehandelt mit Thyreostatika		
	jodhaltigen Präparaten		Lycopus	Thiour-azile	Mer-captoimi-dazole	Per-chlorate
	Jod	Tyrosine				
1953—1957 1016 Patienten	19	7	35	95	68	3
1958—1960 2056 Patienten	42	6	118	88	72	115
1961—1962 2485 Patienten	35	12	122	67	71	80
Insgesamt 5557 Patienten	96	25	275	250	211	198

Im Angriffspunkt auf den Schilddrüsenstoffwechsel unterscheiden sich die Thioharnstoffe und Mercaptoimidazole von den Perchloraten. Die Perchlorate hemmen kompetitiv die Jodaufnahme der Schilddrüse (*42, 71, 81*). Die Thiourazile und Mercaptoimidazole blockieren durch Fermentschädigung den Einbau des Jods in das Tyrosin, so daß die Bildung von Monojodtyrosin und vor allem von Dijodtyrosin behindert wird und die Hormonsynthese stagniert (*6, 32, 64, 69*). Der folgende Fall weist darauf hin, daß die Stoffwechselbeeinflussung bei den Perchloraten langfristig sein kann.

Dem 51jährigen Patienten H. I. wurden von Januar — Mai 1961 wegen eines Verdachtes auf eine Schilddrüsenüberfunktion 2 × 15 Tropfen Irenat® (600 mg) täglich verabreicht. Eine

Grundumsatzbestimmung war vor der antithyreoidalen Behandlung nicht vorgenommen worden. Unter der Therapie trat Anfang Mai ein Exophthalmus auf, die Struma vergrößerte sich, Gesicht und Hände schwollen an. Mitte Juni, 4 Wochen nach Absetzen des Medikamentes kam der Patient zu uns zur Untersuchung. Es bestand noch das Vollbild eines Myxödems. Im Halsbereich war eine kleinfaustgroße Struma von relativ derber Konsistenz zu tasten. Für den Exophthalmus wurden die Hertel-Werte 22 — 100 — 22 gemessen. Unter einer substituierenden dreiwöchigen Behandlung mit 50 γ Trijodthyronin täglich trat eine rasche Befundbesserung ein. Die Ödeme schwemmten aus, der Patient nahm 10 kg an Gewicht ab, der Halsumfang wurde um 3 cm kleiner. Nachdem klinisch eine euthyreote Stoffwechsellage erreicht war, wurde auf eine weitere Substitution verzichtet. Der Exophthalmus ist bisher unverändert geblieben. Im Radiojodstoffwechselstudium waren noch sehr lange Veränderungen nachzuweisen:

Datum der Untersuchung	Grund- umsatz in %	Cholest. i. S. mg-%	PBJ¹³¹ %/l	BEI¹³¹ %/l	Jodaufnahme in %			effekt. HWZ in d
					2 Std	24 Std	48 Std	
Juni 1961. . . .	—11	334	4,46	2,92	43	23	17	1,6
September 1961 .	+ 3	267	2,05	1,80	38	54	47	2,9
Dezember 1961 .	+ 5	—	0,98	0,85	22	51	44	3,4
Juli 1962	+ 3	291	0,53	0,46	28	52	48	4,4

Die Werte zeigen ein sogenanntes partielles Reboundphänomen in der Hormonphase (*39*) mit beschleunigtem Jodumsatz. Das PBJ¹³¹ war nach 14 Monaten noch nicht vollständig normalisiert. Auffällig ist ferner die Differenz zwischen dem PBJ¹³¹ und dem BEI¹³¹ bei der ersten Untersuchung. Da leider damals eine Radiochromatographie nicht durchgeführt wurde, kann nicht mit Sicherheit gesagt werden, ob es sich um eine vermehrte Bildung von Tyrosinen im Sinne einer Jodfehlverwertung handelte, oder ob andere nicht alkalisch eluierbare organische Jodverbindungen vorlagen.

Die Abb. 1 zeigt den zeitlichen Verlauf des Reboundphänomens in der Hormonphase bei 5 Fällen. Die beiden Fälle mit langanhaltender Erhöhung des PBJ¹³¹ sind mit Perchlorat vorbehandelt worden. Der Abfall der Kurven verläuft hier in der halblogarithmischen Darstellung in zwei Exponentialfunktionen. Wir möchten daher annehmen, daß bei diesen Fällen an der Erhöhung des PBJ¹³¹ zwei Komponenten ur-

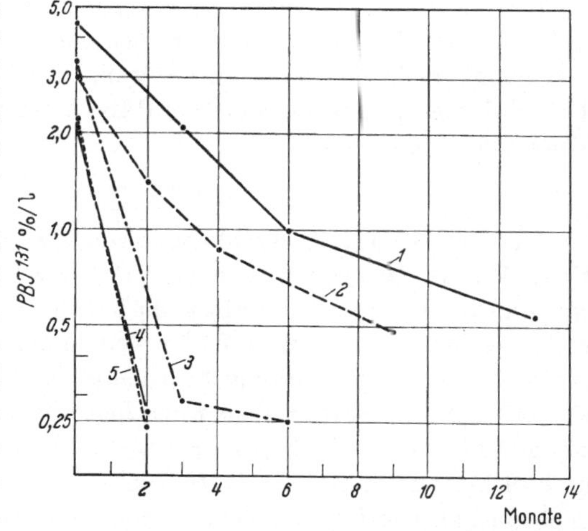

Abb. 1. Zeitlicher Verlauf des Reboundphänomens in der Hormonphase nach thyreostatischer Vorbehandlung euthyreoter Patienten. Vorbehandelt wurden Fall 1 u. 2 mit Perchlorat, Fall 3 mit Mercaptoimidazol, Fall 4 mit Propylthiourazil und Fall 5 mit Methylthiourazil.

sächlich wirksam sind, die wir als Nachholbedarf (schnelle Komponente) und Pooleinengung des Hormonjodraumes (langsame Komponente) auffassen möchten. Die Perchlorate haben eine sehr lange Haftfähigkeit in der Schilddrüse, da sie sich stoffwechselindifferent verhalten (*27*, *41*, *45*), sie blockieren somit für lange Zeit einen Teil der Zellfunktion und engen den Hormonjodraum ein.

3. Medikamente mit antithyreoidalem Nebeneffekt

Von den 5 Strumen, die nach Gabe von Butazolidin auftraten, wiesen 2 Fälle eine erhöhte PBJ^{131}-Ausscheidung mit beschleunigtem Jodumsatz bei niedriger Jodaufnahme auf. Wahrscheinlich wurde hier die Hormonsynthese so eingeschränkt, daß eine Einengung des Hormonjodraumes resultierte. Experimentell konnte ein Hemmeffekt auf die Jodaufnahme der Schilddrüse nachgewiesen werden (44), diese Wirkung kann durch Injektion von thyreotropem Hormon aufgehoben werden (47). Da jede Senkung des Hormonjodspiegels mit einer vermehrten Ausscheidung von thyreotropem Hormon beantwortet wird, ist es verständlich, daß die Hemmung mit Butazolidin im Experiment nur vorübergehend erzielt werden kann (38). Es wäre somit zu prüfen, ob in den wenigen Fällen, bei denen durch Butazolidin eine Struma hervorgerufen wird, eine Störung in der Regulation Hypophyse—Thyroidea besteht oder unter Umständen die TSH-Reserve vermindert ist. Ferner muß berücksichtigt werden, daß als Grundleiden bei den Patienten eine chronische Polyarthritis vorlag. Manche Hinweise (34) sprechen für ein koexistierendes thyreohypophysäres Syndrom bei rheumatischen Arthritiden. Rheumatische Syndrome und eine Arthritis rheumatica werden wesentlich häufiger bei Patienten mit Strumen als bei solchen ohne Struma gefunden (33). Tierexperimentell ließ sich eine Arthritis durch Desoxycorticosteronacetat nur erzeugen, wenn vorher eine Thyreoidektomie durchgeführt wurde (29). Das Problem der Butazolidin-Struma erscheint somit vielschichtiger.

Bei den beiden Patienten, die unter Gabe von PAS eine Struma entwickelten, ließ sich zum Zeitpunkt der Untersuchung, als die Medikamente schon mehrere Monate abgesetzt waren, keine Störung der Schilddrüsenfunktion nachweisen. Der Wirkungsmechanismus der bei PAS zur Bildung von Strumen führt, soll dem Thiourazil ähnlich sein.

Zusammenfassung

An einem selektiven Krankengut von 5567 euthyreoten Patienten betrug die Häufigkeit der iatrogenen Strumen 2,7%. Der größte Teil der iatrogenen Strumen entsteht durch länger dauernde, nicht indizierte Verabreichung von Thyreostatica und ist somit vermeidbar. Falls bei Medikamenten mit antithyreoidalem Nebeneffekt eine strumige Wirkung beobachtet wird und eine Fortsetzung der Medikation wegen des Grundleidens wünschenswert ist, kann dem Effekt durch gleichzeitige Gabe von Trijodthyronin entgegengewirkt werden. Bei Jod-Strumen tritt nach Absetzen der Jodapplikation eine rasche Verkleinerung des Kropfes ein, in einem Fall von Jod-Myxödem normalisierte sich die Stoffwechsellage innerhalb weniger Tage nach Beendigung der medikamentösen Jodzufuhr.

Literatur

1. Albert, A., and F. R. Keating: J. clin. Endocr. 11, 996 (1951).
2. — and R. W. Rawson: J. clin. Invest. 25, 916 (1948).
3. Alexander, N. M.: Endocrinology 68, 671 (1961).
4. Astwood, E. B.,T. Sullivan, A. Biselli and R. Tyslowitz: Endocrinology 32, 210(1943).
5. Bansi, H.W.: Handbuch der inneren Medizin, Bd. VII/1. Berlin, Göttingengen,Heidelberg: Springer-Verlag 1955.
6. — Thyreotoxikose und antithyreoidale Substanzen. Stuttgart: G. Thieme-Verlag 1951.

7. — Jod. Schilddrüsendiagnostik mit Radiojod. In: H. SCHWIEGK u. F. TURBA: Künstliehe radioaktive Isotope in Physiologie, Diagnostik und Therapie. Berlin, Göttingen, Heidelberg: Springer-Verlag 1961

8. BARKER, H. H., H. A. LINDBERG and M. H. WALD: J. Amer. med. Ass. 117, 1591 (1941).

9. BEAMISH, R. E., W. F. PERRY and V. M. STORRIE: Amer. Heart J. 48, 433 (1954).

10. BELL, G. O.: Trans. Amer. Goiter Ass. 1952, 28

11. BLACKBURN, C. M., F. R. KEATING and S. F. HAINES: J. clin. Endocr. 11, 1503 (1951).

12. BREIDAHL, H., and R. FRASER: Proc. roy. Soc. Med. 48, 1026 (1955).

13. BROWNSTONE, S., and R. PITT-RIVERS: Lancet 1959/II, 376

14. CASTENFORS, H., O. LÖVGREN and A. M. ALLGOTH: Acta rheum. scand. 2, 244 (1957).

15. CHESNY, A. M., T. A. CLAWSON and B. WEBSTER: Bull. Johns Hopk. Hosp. 43, 261 (1928).

16. COULAND, E.: Rev. Tuberc. (Paris), 18, 261 (1954).

17. CURRENT, J. V., J. B. HALES and B. M. DOBYNS: J. clin. Endocr. 20, 13 (1960).

18. DIMITRIADOU, A., and R. FRASER: Proc. roy. Soc. Med. 54, 345 (1961).

19. DONIACH, I. R., and R. FRASER: Lancet 1950/I, 855.

20. FAWCETT, D. M., and S. KIRKWOOD: J. biol. Chem. 204, 787 (1953); 205, 795 (1953).

21. FEINBERG, W. D., D. L. HOFFMANN and CH. A. OWEN: J. clin. Endocr. 19, 576 (1959).

22. GOLD, E.: Surgery 45, 424 (1959).

23. GOLDNER, M. G.: Metabolism 4, 545 (1955).

24. GREER, M. A., and L. J. DEGROOT: Metabolism 5, 682 (1956).

25. GUINET, P., et M. BERGER: Ann. Endocr. (Paris) 12, 544 (1951).

26. HAINES, F. S.: Endocrinology 12, 55 (1928).

27. HALMI, N. S., R. STUELKE and M. D. SCHNELL: Endocrinology 58, 634 (1956).

28. HAMILTON, R. R.: Brit. med. J. 1953/I, 29.

29. HARRISON, R. G., and T. J. BARNETT: Ann. rheum. Dis. 12, 275 (1953).

30. HULLIGER, L., A. WALSER u. H. LÜTHY: Schweiz. med. Wschr. 90, 1348 (1960).

31. HURXTHAL, L. M.: Lahey Clin. Bull. 4, 73 (1945).

32. IINO, S., T. YAMADA and M. A. GREER: Endocrinology 68, 582 (1961).

33. KALLIOLA, H., J. L. KALLIOMÄKI and A. RINTALE: Ann. Med. intern. Fenn. 46, 97 (1957).

34. KALLIOMÄKI, J. L., and T. E. HOLOPAINEN: Acta rheum. sand. 2, 213 (1956).

35. KENNEDY, T. H., and H. D. PURVES: Brit. J. exp. Path. 22, 241 (1941).

36. KJERULF-JENSEN, K., and G. WOLFFBRANDT: Acta pharmacol. (Kbh.) 7, 376 (1951).

37. KLEIN, E.: Klin. Wschr. 30, 462 (1952).

38. — Arzneimittel Forsch. 6, 726 (1956).

39. — Der endogene Jodhaushalt und seine Störungen. Stuttgart: G. Thieme-Verlag 1960.

40. — Internist 3, 481 (1962).

41. — In: Fortschritte der Schilddrüsenforschung, 81. Stuttgart: G. Thieme-Verlag 1962.

42. KLEINSORG, H., u. H. L. KRÜSKEMPER: Dtsch. med Wschr. 1955, 578.

43. KRISS, J. P., W. H. CARNES and R. T. GROSS: J. Amer. med. Ass. 157, 117 (1955).

44. KRÜSKEMPER, H. L., u. A. MARSCH: Klin. Wschr. 33, 285 (1955).

45. —. and H. REILICH: Acta endocr. (Kbh.) 32, 579 (1959).

46. LAROCHE, G., et M. HIRSCH: Presse méd. 68, 2119 (1960).

47. LINSK, A. J., B. C. PATON, M. PERSKY, M. ISAACS and H. S. KUPPERMANN: J. clin. Endocr. 17, 416 (1957).

48. MCGAVACK, TH. H.: N. Y. St. J. Med. 51, 1729 (1951).

49. — W. SEEGERS, H. HAAR and V. ERK: Diabetes 6, 80 (1957).

50. MCGREGOR, A. G., and A. G. SOMNER: Lancet 1954, II, 931

51. MEANS, J. H.: The Thyroid and its Diseases. Philadelphia: J. B. Lippincott Comp. 1948.

52. MORGANS, M. E., and W. R. TROTTER: Lancet 1959, II, 374.

53. MORNEX, R., J. O. PEYRIN, E. POMMATAU, M. BERGER et G. RIFFAT: Ann. Endocr. (Paris) 21, 704 (1960).

54. NIXON, P. G. F.: Brit. med. J. 5021, 748 (1957).

55. OPPENHEIMRE, J. H., and H. T. MCPHERSON: Amer. J. Med. 30, 281 (1961).

56. PALEY, K. R., E. SOBEL and R. S. YALOW: J. clin. Endocr. 18, 850 (1958).

57. PARIS, J., W. M. MCCONAHEY, C. A. OWEN JR., L. B. WOOLNER and R. C. BAHN: J. clin. Endocr. 20, 57 (1960).

58. PITT-RIVERS, R.: Physiol. Rev. 30, 194 (1950).

59. Pitt-Rivers, R.: Ann. N. Y. Acad. Sci. **86**, 362 (1960).
60. Rawson, R. W.: Ann. N. Y. Acad. Sci. **50**, 491 (1949).
61. Reimold, E.: Arch. Kinderheilk. **156**, 265 (1958).
62. Reinwein, D., and E. Klein: Acta endocr. (Kbh.) **35**, 485 (1960).
63. Richards, C. E., R. J. Brockhurst and T. H. Coleman: J. clin. Endocr. **9**, 446 (1949).
64. Richards, J. B., and S. H. Ingbar: Endocrinology **65**, 198 (1959).
65. Robey, J. S., P. M. Veazy and J. D. Crawford: New Engl. J. Med. **255** 955 (1956).
66. Rubinstein H. M., and L. Oliner: New Engl. J. Med., **256**, 47 (1957).
67. Scott K. G., J. B. Freriks and W. A. Reilly: Proc. Soc. exp. Biol. (N. Y.) **2** (150 (1953).
68. Skaggs J. T., and R. A. Cooke: J. Allergy **17**, 377 (1956).
69. Slingerland D. W., D. E. Graham, R. K. Josephs, P. F. Mulvey, A. P. Trakas and E. Yamazaki: Endocrinology **65**, 178 (1956).
70. Stanbury, J. B., A. A. H. Hassenaar and J. W. A. Meijer: J. clin. Endocr. **16**, 735 (1956).
71. —, and J. B. Wyngaarden: Metabolism **1**, 533 (1952).
72. Stanley, M. M.: J. clin. Endocr. **12**, 191 (1952).
73. Studer, H., u. F. Wyss: Schweiz. med. Wschr. **50**, 1536 (1961).
74. Talmas, V., F. Dossin et H. J. Ernould: Ann. d'Endocr. **19**, 884 (1958).
75. Turner, H. H., and R. B. Howard: J. clin. Endocr. **16**, 141 (1956).
76. Van der Laan, W. P.: Metabolism **5**, 640 (1956).
77. Van der Laan, J. E., W. P. Van der Laan and M. A. Logan: Endocrinology **29**, 93 (1941).
78. Wilfingseder, P.: Wien. klin. Wschr. **74**, 648 (1962).
79. Wolff, J., and I. L. Chaikoff: J. biol. Chem. **172**, 855 (1948); **174**, 555 (1948).
80. —, — Endocrinology **42**, 468 (1948); **43**, 174 (1948).
81. Wyngaarden, J. B., B. M. Wright and P. Ways: Endocrinology **50**, 537 (1952).

Laboratoire de Pathologie Générale, Université de Louvain, Louvain, Belgium

Intrathyroid Disturbances
in Endemic and Sporadic non Toxic Goitre[1]

by

C. BECKERS and M. DE VISSCHER

On the pathogenesis of the non toxic goitre very little is still known. Numerous factors have been considered, particularly iodine deficiency, goitrogenic factors in the diet, and congenital or acquired abnormalities of the hormonosynthesis. Since a few years, our group has been involved in detailed studies on the physiopathology of endemic goitre in the Uele, in the former Belgian Congo[2]. Similar investigations have been performed on sporadic cases of non toxic goitre in Belgium. The purpose of this communication is to present some of the main results we obtained in the study of the intrathyroid disturbances which characterize both endemic and sporadic non toxic goitre.

Material and Methods

Specimens of goitrous thyroid glands were obtained from 20 patients living in the endemic goitre area of the Uele, which is situated in the northern part of the Republic of Congo.

Similar specimens were obtained in 9 euthyroid goitrous patients living in Belgium. Subtotal thyroidectomy was performed because of local compressions. No cases of thyroiditis or thyroid cancer have been included in the present study.

For comparison purpose, "normal" thyroid tissue was also investigated. Specimens were obtained from five patients totaly thyroidectomized for localized carcinoma. Specimens called "normal" are portions of histologicaly normal structure, located outside of the tumor.

All the patients were given a dose of 300—500 μc carrier-free ^{131}I, 2 to 5 days before the surgical procedure. After thyroidectomy, every gland was carefully dissected. Samples were taken for homogenization or extraction of the soluble proteins. Informations regarding the procedures of these investigations have been presented previously (1—7).

Results

a) Soluble thyroid proteins

Such a study involves the determination of the whole amount in proteins of the colloid (i.e. thyroid extract), and also the content in iodinated proteins, particularly thyroglobulin. These investigations are based on the use of well-known

---

[1] This work was supported in part by a grant from the "Fonds de la Recherche Scientifique Médicale", Belgium.

[2] "Groupement pour l'Etude du Goitre dans les Uélés", Universities of Louvain and Brussels.

technics, as electrophoresis, analytical ultracentrifugation, "salting-out" curves and paper chromatography (*4, 7*). In endemic as well as in sporadic goitre, the general characteristics of thyroglobulin appear to be normal. Although thyroglobulin is the main component of the colloid, another compound was regularily found, called prethyroglobulin for its electrophoretic properties. Except in one case of endemic cretinism, prethyroglobulin is not iodinated. After hydrolysis of thyroglobulin by pancreatin, the MIT/DIT ratio is 2,70 $\pm$ 0,35 (s.e.) and the iodothyronine content is very low (chromatography in butanol-acetic acid-water solvent).

b) Studies on enzyme activity of the goitrous tissue

The results can be summarized as follows:

1. the capacity of the goitrous tissue to organify iodine is normal in endemic as well as in sporadic non toxic goitre (*4, 7, 8*);

2. the activity of the iodotyrosine-deiodinating system is reduced, at least in endemic goitre (*5, 7*);

3. the efficiency of the proteolytic system of the goitrous gland is reduced, as compared with normal tissue (*6, 7*).

Discussion

Here below, we comment shortly some particular points which we consider as being important for the understanding of the pathogenesis of the non toxic goitre.

1. The general characteristics of thyroglobulin as a protein appear to be normal at least by the methods used here.

2. The level of iodinated amino-acids has undergone a considerable change: a higher proportion of MIT than of DIT, and a low concentration of T_4 and T_3 were observed. The circumstances which provoke disturbances of this nature in man are not yet very well understood. It is known that the hormone synthesis in the thyroid occurs in several stages and is for the greatest part under enzymatic control. As proposed by Pitt-Rivers et al. (*9*), we believe that the high MIT/DIT ratio can be the result of a disturbance of the iodination of MIT. In "normal" thyroid gland and in hyperactive hyperthyroid tissue, the ratio MIT/DIT is less than 1. All these observations therefore suggest that thyroid hormone synthesis is slowed down in non-toxic goitre. The thyroid changes might be the consequence of some extrinsic factors such as antithyroid substances or iodine deficiency. As we have shown, iodine deficiency could be particularly evoked in the case of the endemic goitre of the Uele. However, it must be kept in mind that in endemic as well as in sporadic goitre, the total thyroid iodine pool is unexpectedly high in all the goitrous glands.

3. The proteolytic system of the goitrous gland is slowed down. The high MIT/DIT ratio can be the result of a trouble of iodination of MIT into DIT.

4. Our investigations have brought to light another abnormality of the intrathyroid content, confirming similar observations by de Groot and Carvalho (*10*). An abnormal iodinated protein called prethyroglobulin, is always found. This compound is present in much larger quantities in those parts of the goitre that have

undergone more pronounced alterations. This point has teen confirmed by analytical ultracentrifugation. This prethyroglobulin may be of the same type of protein or peptide as those observed in the blood or in the thyroid tissue of certain goitrous patients (*11*).

If we accept a pathogenic schema common to endemic and sporadic goitres, we must ask ourselves what is the aetiological factor responsible for the disturbance in hormonogenesis. In the endemic goitre of the Uele Region, hormone synthesis is at first impeded by a severe lack of iodine. In Belgium, where strictly speaking there is no endemic, metabolic studies have shown that goitrous subjects are also affected by iodine deficiency, although much less severely than in Congo. This unexpected result fits in with similar observations made recently in Scotland by ALEXANDER, KOUTRAS and coworkers (*12*). Does this mean that in endemic and sporadic goitre alike iodine deficiency is the sole aetiological factor ? For the endemic goitre of the Uele, we were not able to demonstrate the existence of another mechanism impeding the hormonogenesis. Combined aetiological factors seem more likely in sporadic goitre. Evidence of this is the unequal distribution of goitre in the same environment. Personally, we have in mind particular subthreshold deficits of one or the other intrathyroid enzymatic mechanisms. These metabolic deficiencies — of an hereditary character — would impede hormonogenesis, as soon as there is a slight iodine lack in the body.

In our opinion, those investigations suggest that the goitre disease, once set in, is a process which tends to maintain itself. In other words, a vicious circle is set up: a primary disturbance in hormone production leads to thyroid hyperplasia while the goitre degeneration which eventually ensues, causes disturbances in intrathyroid metabolism (cascade effect). The biochemical abnormalities which we found in nearly all goitres whatever their origin, reflect the deterioration of the main intrathyroid systems, resulting in reduced efficiency of thyroid hormone synthesis.

References

1. DE VISSCHER, M., et M. DE SMET: Acta clin. belg. **14**, 329 (1959).
2. DE SMET, M., et M. DE VISSCHER: Ann. Soc. belge Méd. trop. **40**, 601 (1960).
3. DE VISSCHER, M., C. BECKERS, H. G. VAN DEN SCHRIECK, M. DE SMET, A. M. ERMANS, H. GALPERIN and P. A. BASTENIE: J. clin. Endocr. **21**, 175 (1961).
4. BECKERS, C., and M. DE VISSCHER: Metabolism **10**, 695 (1961).
5. —, — Rev. franç. Étud. clin. biol. **4**, 281 (1961).
6. —, — J. clin. Endocr. **22**, 711 (1962).
7. — L'hormonogenèse dans les goitres endémiques et sporadiques. Ed. Arscia Bruxelles. 1963.
8. —, and M. DE VISSCHER: J. clin. Endocr. **23**, 149 (1963).
9. PITT-RIVERS, R., D. HUBBLE, and W. H. HOATHER: J. clin. Endocr. **17**, 1313 (1957).
10. DE GROOT, L. J., and E. CARVALHO: J. clin. Endocr. **20**, 21 (1960).
11. DOWLING, J. T., S. H. INGBAR and N. FREINKEL: J. clin. Endocr. **21**, 1390 (1961).
12. ALEXANDER, N. D., D. A. KOUTRAS, J. CROOKS, W. W. BUCHANAN, E. M. MacDONALD, M. H. RICHMOND and E. J. WAYNE: Quart. J. Med. **31**, 281 (1962).

Aus der Medizinischen Universitätsklinik mit Poliklinik der Universität Erlangen
(Direktor: Professor Dr. N. HENNING)

Autoradiographischer perinucleärer Jodnachweis in cytologischen Punktaten menschlicher Strumen

H. J. SCHMIDT, N. HENNING, F. SCHEIFFARTH, S. WITTE,
G. KLEYENSTEIBER, F. WOLF und L. ZICHA

Mit 2 Abbildungen

Verabreichtes Radiojod des Isotops J^{131} wurde autoradiographisch bisher als "ring-reaction" über dem apikalen Anteil der Schilddrüsenepithelzellen und im Follikellumen nachgewiesen (*1, 2, 14, 15, 19, 20, 21, 22, 25, 26, 28, 29, 31, 32, 35, 36, 37, 41, 42, 48*). In Autoradiogrammen menschlicher Schilddrüsenpunktate wiesen SCHMIDT, HENNING und WITTE (*46*) das Jod je nach Zeitintervall der Punktionen nach Jodapplikation in Granulaform nach. Der Jodnachweis beschränkte sich dabei nicht nur auf einen dem apikalen Zellanteil zugehörigen Zellrandsaum, sondern gelang im überwiegenden Anteil des Cytoplasmas. Die Thyreocyten erzeugten dabei im Gegensatz zum Kolloid nie eine homogene,

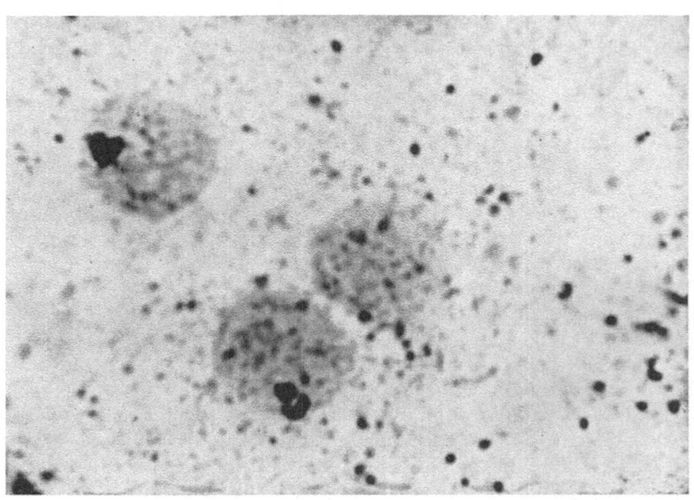

Abb. 1. Kernständige cytoplasmatische solitäre Jodgranula. Punktion einer diffusen Struma bei mäßiger Hyperthyreose 1 Std. nach Applikation von 50 μ C J^{131}. 800 ×

diffuse Schwärzung, sondern markierten eine granulaförmige cytoplasmatische Jodlokalisation. Dabei stellte sich in Punktionsausstrichen mit nur noch spärlichem cytoplasmatischem Jodnachweis in einem oft hohen Prozentsatz in den

Thyreocyten ein perinucleärer Schwärzungspunkt wechselnder Größe dar (Abb. 1 u. 2). Die bisherigen elektronenoptischen Untersuchungen der Zellen, insbesondere der Drüsenzellen, erbrachten nun den Nachweis der cytoplasmatischen Ergastoplasma-Membranen (α-Cytomembranen nach SJÖSTRAND), die nach BRAUNSTEINER, BRAUNSTEINER, FELLINGER und PAKESCH (3, 4, 5, 6, 7), DEMPSEY (12), DEMPSEY und PETERSON (13), EKHOLM und SJÖSTRAND (16), GABE und ARVY (23),

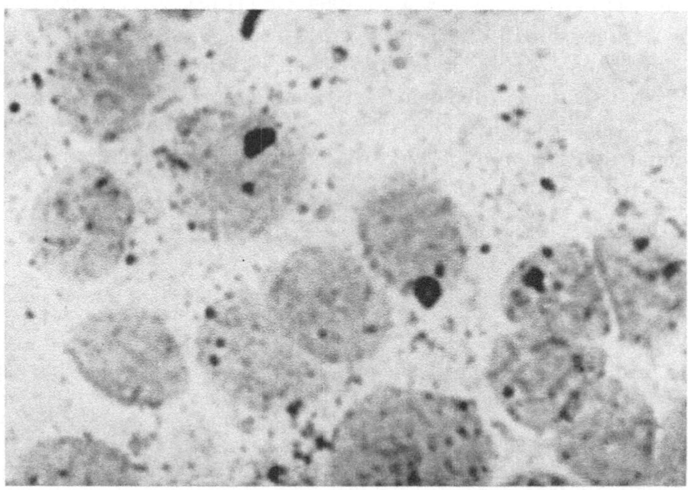

Abb. 2. Kernständige cytoplasmatische solitäre große Jodgranula. Punktion einer Struma bei Morbus Basedow 80 min nach Applikation von 5 μ C J¹³¹. 780 ×

HAGUENAU (27), MONROE (34), PALAY (40), PORTER (43) und WISSIG (51, 52) in Schilddrüsenzellen besonders ausgebildet sind. Dieses das Cytoplasma ausfüllende Lamellensystem hypertrophiert bei gleichzeitiger Zellvergrößerung nach Thyreotrophingabe, bei Kälteexposition und nach Thiouracil-Applikation, während es nach Hypophysektomie wieder verschwindet. Außerdem wies die Elektronenmikroskopie eine gut ausgebildete, aus Membranen und Bläschen bestehende Golgi-Region nach, der aber die 1955 von PALADE beschriebenen Ribosomen entlang der Ergastoplasma-Membran fehlen. Der Nachweis des Golgi-Apparates mit besonderer Betonung seiner perinucleären Lokalisation wurde unter anderem im exokrinen Pankreas, Duodenum und Epididymis der Maus, wie in Melanom-Zellkulturen (9, 10, 11, 23, 30, 43, 45, 47) unter Hinweis seines ubiquitären Charakters vor allem in den Schilddrüsenzellen beschrieben (12, 13, 16, 18, 23, 27, 34, 40, 43, 50, 51, 52). Auf Grund dieser Untersuchungen wird angenommen, daß das Ergastoplasma und sein synthetisiertes Protein mit dem perinucleären Raum und dem Golgi-System in Verbindung stehen (Prozymogenbildung, Melaninvorstufen).

Die von uns nachgewiesenen perinucleären Schwärzungspunkte (Abb. 1 u. 2) von teilweise auffallender Größe nach Jod¹³¹-Verabreichung wurden fast nur in Punktionen hyperthyreoter Strumen gefunden. Als möglicher Ausdruck einer bestimmten Sekretionsphase sind sie nicht regelmäßig in allen Thyreocyten vorhanden. Teilweise gelangen sie auf Grund ihrer perinucleären Lage nach der

Fixation über dem Kernbereich zur Abbildung. Bei einer Zugehörigkeit zu Kernstrukturen wäre jedoch zu fordern, daß regelmäßig eine cytoplasmatische perinucleäre Lokalisation fehlt. Tonutti und Wissig (*50, 51, 52*) sowie weitere Autoren vertreten die Ansicht, daß das Schilddrüsenprotein in der Golgi-Region gebildet wird, wogegen allerdings das Fehlen der Paladeschen Granula sprechen würde. Ob Ergastoplasma-Protein in Intervallen in den Golgi-Apparat gelangt (*9, 10, 11, 39, 43*) und dort jodiert wird, oder die festgestellten perinucleären Jodgranula die Wirkungslokalisation eines vom Nucleus oder Nucleolus abgegebenen, für Jod adaptiven Enzymproteins darstellen, konnte bisher nicht aufgeklärt werden. Wir halten daher zugleich wegen der mangelnden Kenntnisse über die Funktion des Golgi-Systems, des intrathyreoidalen Jodstoffwechsels und der intrathyreoidalen Protein-Jodierung diese autoradiographischen Befunde für erwähnenswert.

Literatur

1. Basser, A. R.: The uptake of radioiodine by the thyroid cells using nuclear emulsion. Med. Austr. 1, 1003 (1956).
2. Bogoroch, R.-B., M. Israelovitsch and C. P. Leblond: The chemical nature of the materials retained in radioautographic preparation of thyroid glands of rats after radioiodine administration. J. Nat. Cancer Inst. 12, 225 (1951).
3. Braunsteiner, H., K. Fellinger and F. Pakesch: Electron microscopic observations on the thyroid. Endocrinology 53, 123 (1953).
4. — — — Ergebnisse und Probleme histologischer Untersuchungen im Elektronenmikroskop. Klin. Wschr. 1953, 357.
5. — — — Demonstration of a cytoplasmic structure in plasma cells. Blood 8, 916 (1963).
6. — — — Probleme elektronenmikroskopischer Gewebsuntersuchungen für Fragen der internen Medizin. Z. wiss. Mikr. 62, 173 (1955).
7. — Elektronenmikroskopische Befunde an Zellen. In: Henning, R., u. Witte S.: Internationales Symposion über klinische Cytodiagnostik, 5. Stuttgart: Thieme 1958.
8. Cottier, H.: Cytologische Aspekte der Plasmaproteinsynthese. In: Symposion über Biochemie und Klinik der menschlichen Bluteiweiße. Bull. schweiz. Akad. med. Wiss. 17, 50 (1961).
9. Dalton, A. J., and M. D. Felix: Studies on the Golgi substance of the epithelial cells of the epididymis and duodenum of the mouse. Amer. J. Anat. 92, 277 (1953).
10. — — Electron microscopy of mitochondria and the Golgi complex. In: Symposium of the Society for experimental biology, number X.,: Mitochondria and other cytoplasmic inclusions, 152. Cambridge: University Press 1957.
11. — GOLGI apparatus and secretion granules. In: Brachet, J., and A. E. Mirsky. The Cell, Vol. II.: Cells and their component parts., 607. New York: Academic Press 1961.
12. Dempsey, W. E.: Comparative and microscopic anatomy of the thyroid. In.: Werner, S. C. The Thyroid, 109. New York: P. B. Hoeber, Inc. 1955.
13. —, and R. R. Peterson: Electron microscopic observations on the thyroid gland of normal, hypophysectomized, cold- exposed and thiouracil treated rats. Endocrinology 56, 46 (1955).
14. Doniach, J., and S. R. Pelc: Autoradiographs with radio-active iodine. Proc. roy. Soc. Med. 42, 957 (1949).
15. —, and J. H. Logothetopoulos: Radioautography of inorganic iodine in the thyroid. J. Endocronology 13, 65 (1956).
16. Ekholm, R., and F. S. Sjöstrand: The ultrastructure of the thyroid gland of the mouse. In: Electron microscopy proceedings of the Stockholm Conference, 171 (1957).
17. Esser, H. O.: Die ultrastrukturelle Organisation der Zelle. Behringwerk-Mitt. 38, 127 (1960).

18. FELDMAN, J. D.: Fine structure and metabolism of the iodinedeficient thyroid. In: PITT-RIVERS, R.: Advances in thyroid research, 318. London: Pergamon Press 1961.

19. FITZGERALD, P. J.: The use of the radioautographic technique in pathology. Bull. N. Y. Acad. Med. 28, 680 (1952).

20. — E. SIMMEL, J. WEINSTEIN and C. MARTIN: Radio-autography: Theory, technic, and applications. Lab. Inv. 2, 211 (1953).

21. — J^{131} concentration and thyroid morphology. In: The Thyroid, Brookhaven Symposia, Nr. 7, Brookhaven National Laboratory Upton N. Y., 220 (1955).

22. — Autoradiography in cytology. In: MELLORS. R. C.: Analytical cytology, 410. New York: Blakist. Div., Inc. 1959.

23. GABE, M., and L. ARVY: Gland cells. In: BRACHET, J., and A. E. MIRSKY: The Cell, Vol. II. 1 New York: Academic Press 1961.

24. GERSH J., and T. CASPERSSON: Total protein and organic iodine in the colloid and cells of single follicles of the thyroid gland. Anat. Rec. 78, 303 (1940).

25. GROSS, J., and C. P. LEBLOND: The presence of free iodinated compounds in the thyroid and their passage into the circulation. Endocrinology 48, 714 (1951).

26. — The dynamic cytology of the thyroid gland. In: Internat. Rev. Cytolog. VI, 265. New York: Academic Press, Inc. 1957.

27. HAGUENAU, F.: The Ergastoplasm. In: Internat. Rev. Cytolog. VII, 468. New York: Academic Press, Inc. 1958.

28. HAMILTON, J. G., M. N. SOLEY and K. B. EICHHORN: Deposition of radioactive iodine in human thyroid tissue. Univ. Californ. Publ. Pharmacol. Vol. 1, 339 (1940).

29. HARBERS, E.: Autoradiographie als histochemisches Untersuchungsverfahren. In: GRAU-MANN, W. und K. H. NEUMANN: Handbuch der Histochemie, Bd. I, 436. Stuttgart: Fischer 1958.

30. LACY, D., and C. E. CHALLICE: The structure of the Golgi apparatus in vertebrate cells examined by light and electron microscopy. In: Symposium of mitochondria and other cytoplasmic inclusions, 62. Cambridge: University Press 1957.

31. LEBLOND, C. P., and J. GROSS: Thyreoglobulin formation in the thyroid follicle visualized by the "coated" autographic technique. Endocrinology 43, 306 (1948).

32. — — The mechanism of the secretion of thyroid hormone. J. clin. Endocr. 9, 149 (1949).

33. — Fate of iodine in the body. J. Amer. pharm. Ass. 40, 595 (1951).

34. MONROE, B. G.: Electron microscopy of the thyroid. Anat. Rec. 116, 345 (1953).

35. NADLER, N. J.. and C. P. LEBLOND: The site and rate of formation of thyroid hormone. In: The Thyroid, Brookhaven Symposia, Nr. 7, Brookhaven National Laboratory, Upton, 40 (1955).

36. — The role of epithelial cell and colloid in the formation of thyroid hormone in the thyroid follicle. I. Internat. Congr. Endocrinology, Session XIIIc, 609, Copenhagen 1960.

37. — J. CARNEIRO and C. P. LEBLOND: The rate of synthesis, secretion and breakdown of thyroglobulin in the mouse thyroid follicle. Excerpt. Med. Internat. Congr., Series, Nr. 26, 43 (1960).

38. PALADE, G. E.: A small particulate component of the cytoplasm. J. biophys. biochem. Cytol. 1, 59 (1955).

39. — In: Symposium on electron microscopy, 170. Brit. An. Ass. London: Arnold Press 1960.

40. PALAY, S. H.: Frontiers in cytology 13, 332. New Haven: Yale Univ. Press. Inc. 1958.

41. PITT-RIVERS, R., and W. R. TROTTER: The site of accumulation of iodine in the thyroid of rats treated with thiouracil. Lancet. 265, 918 (1953).

42. — Biosynthesis of the thyroid hormones. Brit. med. Bull. 16, 118 (1960).

43. PORTER, K. R.: The ground substance. Observations from electron microscopy. In: BRACHET, J., and A. E. MIRSKY. The cell, Volume II. Cells and their component parts, 664. New York: Academic Press, 1961.

44. ROOS, B.: Die submikroskopische Struktur der Rattenschilddrüse. Path. et Microbiol. (Basel) 23, 129 (1960).

45. ROSE, G. G., and J. S. STEHLIN: The Golgi complex and melanin elaboration of human melanomas in tissue culture. Cancer. Res. 21, 1455 (1961).

46. Schmidt, H. J., N. Henning u. S. Witte: Autoradiographische Untersuchungen des menschlichen intrathyreoidalen Jodstoffwechsels. Dtsch. Arch. klin. Med. **208**, 505 (1963).
47. Sjöstrand, F. S., and V. Hanzon: Ultrastructure of Golgi apparatus of exocrine cells of mouse pankreas. Exp. cell Res. **7**, 415 (1954).
48. — The ultrastructure of cells as revealed by the electron microscope. Int. Rev. Cytol. **5**, 456 (1956).
49. Taylor, S.: Genesis of the thyroid nodule. Brit. med. Bull. **16**, 102 (1960).
50. Tonutti, E.: Die Schilddrüse. Abschn. II.: Histophysiologie. In: Staemmler, M., u. E. Kaufmann: Lehrbuch der speziellen pathologischen Anatomie, 11. und 12. Auflage, I. Band, 2. Hälfte, 1292. Berlin: W. de Gruyter 1956.
51. Wissig, S. L.: The anatomy of secretion in the follicular cell of thyroid gland. Thesis, Yale Univ., New Haven, Conn. (1956).
52. — The anatomy of secretion in the follicular cells of the thyroid gland. J. biophys. biochem. Cytol. **7**, 423 (1960).

Aus der Medizinischen Univ.-Poliklinik Heidelberg
(Direktor: Prof. Dr. H. PLÜGGE)

Das Schilddrüsenphonogramm der Hyperthyreose und seine Bedeutung für die Hämodynamik und Therapie dieser Erkrankung

Von

G. SCHWARZ, H. SCHÖNTHAL und F. BAHNER

Mit 1 Abbildung

Durch ihre oberflächliche Lage ist die Schilddrüse der Palpation und Auskultation direkt zugänglich. Bei Hyperthyreosen findet man mit großer Regelmäßigkeit eine Volumenzunahme der Drüse, die zu einem Teil Folge der starken Durchblutung des Organs ist. Die Schilddrüsendurchblutung kann bei Hyperthyreosen um mehr als das 10fache gegenüber der Norm gesteigert sein. Die intensive Durchblutung der hyperthyreotischen Schilddrüse führt zur Bildung eines charakteristischen Strömungsgeräusches dadurch, daß sich zwischen Hals- und Schilddrüsengefäßen eine relative Stenose bildet. In älteren Darstellungen der Klinik der Hyperthyreose ist diesem Strömungsgeräusch große diagnostische Bedeutung beigemessen worden. Das Interesse moderner Autoren konzentriert sich dagegen mehr auf die Ergebnisse von Laboruntersuchungen.

Wir haben bei allen unseren Hyperthyreosefällen ein Strömungs- oder Gefäßgeräusch über der Schilddrüse feststellen können, es phonographisch registriert und seinen Verlauf unter der thyreostatischen Therapie verfolgt. Alle phonographischen Ableitungen erfolgten über dem punctum maximum des Geräusches, am liegenden Patienten, bei verschiedenen Frequenzabstimmungen und unter Standardbedingungen der Verstärkung.

Die Abb. 1 zeigt ein typisches Hyperthyreosegeräusch. Es ist spindelförmig, erstreckt sich über Systole und Diastole, hat im diastolischen Anteil Decrescendo-Charakter und liegt im mittleren Frequenzbereich. Rechts auf der Abb. 1 ist zum Vergleich das Geräusch einer arteriovenösen Fistel abgebildet, das in seiner Form völlig mit dem Strömungsgeräusch der Hyperthyreose übereinstimmt. Das Gefäßgeräusch der hyperthyreotischen Schilddrüse ist leicht von lokalen Gefäßgeräuschen, wie sie gelegentlich im Verlauf der Carotis entstehen, abzugrenzen, denn die funktionellen Carotisgeräusche füllen nur einen kleinen Teil der Systole aus. Das Strömungsgeräusch der hyperthyreotischen Schilddrüse ist ein Shuntgeräusch. Die Form des systolischen Geräuschanteils entspricht den Systolika, die bei Shuntvitien mit relativer Stenose gefunden werden. Die kontinuierliche Abnahme des Geräusches in der Diastole entsteht durch die Abnahme des Druckgradienten zwischen Schilddrüsenarterien und -venen, denn die Durchblutungsgröße und die

Intensität des Strömungsgeräusches hängen vom Druckgradienten zwischen
Arterien und Venen und vom Gefäßquerschnitt ab. Der Shuntcharakter des
Geräusches geht auch aus seinem hämodynamischen Verhalten hervor. Beim Pressen — im Valsalva-Versuch — verschwindet es fast vollständig, um nach Ende des
Preßversuches an Intensität zuzunehmen. Durch das Pressen wird das Schlag-
volumen vermindert und der venöse Druck erhöht. Beide Effekte führen zur Verminderung des arteriovenösen Druckgradienten, zur Unterbrechung des arteriovenösen

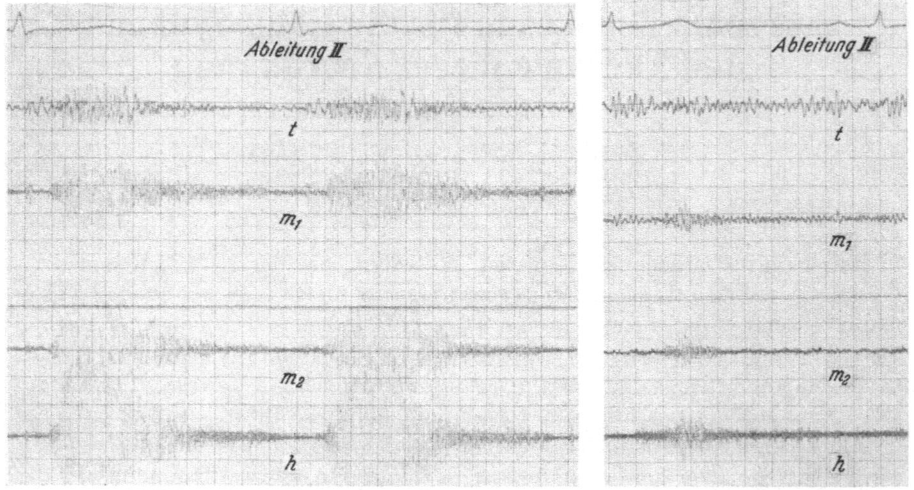

Schilddrüsen-Phonogramm einer Hyperthyreose   Phonogramm einer a-v-Fistel

Abb. 1

Schilddrüsen-Shuntes und zu einer Rückbildung des Geräusches.

Auch durch Lagewechsel ändert sich das Strömungsgeräusch der Hyperthyreose. Die nächste Abbildung zeigt die Lageeinflüsse auf die Geräuschform, die
vermutlich über eine Änderung des Blutdruckes hervorgerufen werden. Nicht nur
die Geräuschform ändert sich, auch die geräuscharme Brücke zwischen zwei
Systolen wird im Liegen und Stehen länger.

Die Dauer und Intensität des Strömungsgeräusches der hyperthyreotischen
Schilddrüse ist von der diastolischen Füllung des Herzens abhängig. Bei absoluter
Arrhythmie führt die bessere diastolische Füllung des Herzens — bei langem
R-R-Abstand der vorhergehenden Systole — zu einer Verlängerung und Verstärkung des Strömungsgeräusches und umgekehrt. Das gleiche Phänomen wird
bei einer Extrasystole deutlich. Das Verhältnis von R-R-Abstand und Geräusch-
dauer kann auch graphisch dargestellt werden. In einem bestimmten Bereich ist
die Dauer des Strömungsgeräusches dem vorhergehenden R-R-Abstand proportional.

Quantitative Aussagen über die Größe des arteriovenösen Schilddrüsenshunts
sind durch das Schilddrüsenphonogramm nur mit Vorbehalt möglich, weil extrathyreoidale Schallfilter zu einer von Fall zu Fall wechselnden Dämpfung des
Geräusches führen können. Beim gleichen Patienten lassen sich bei Einhaltung

Tabelle 1

| Name | Alter Ge-schlecht | Diagnose | Therapie | Dauer von | | Rezidiv (Nachbeobachtungzeit)Bemerkungen |
				Behand-lung Mon.	Ge-räusch Mon.	
H. K.	48 W	Struma basedowi-fikata	Perchlorat (Irenat)	12	12	∅ (1 Jahr)
O. St.	47 W			18	18	∅ (2 Jahre)
J. K.	23 M			5	5	∅ (1 Jahr) Exophthalmus blieb stationär
E. F.	25 M			15	15	∅ (2 Jahre)
A. A.	40 W			12	12	Rezidiv 1 Jahr nach Abschluß der Behandlung, Adenomknoten ging völlig zurück
M. G.	47 M	tox. Adenom		15	15	∅ (2,5 Jahre)
E. Pf.	23 W	diff. toxische Struma		6	6	∅ (1,5 Jahre)
H. H.	33 W			13	13	∅ (0,5 Jahre)
A. G.	24 W			11	11	∅ (3 Jahre)
E. Sch.	35 W			10	10	3 Jahre nach Ende der 1. Behandlung Hyperthyreoserezidiv
O. Sch.	24 M			8	8	2 Jahre nach Ende der 1. Behandlung Hyperthyreoserezidiv
L. A.	31 W			12	12	1 Jahr nach Ende der 1. Behandlung Hyperthyreoserezidiv
E. E.	47 W			18	18	∅ (1 Jahr)
H. B.	55 W			6	6	2,5 Jahre nach Ende der 1. Behandlung Rezidiv
K. H.[1]	34 W			10	10	∅ (6 Monate)
B. H.	49 M			6	6	∅ (5 Monate)
Z. Z.	37 W			13	13	∅ (3 Jahre)
A. S.	27 W			11	11	6 Mon. nach Abschluß der 1. Behandlung Rezidiv; 2. Behandlung seit 3 Mon. abgeschlossen
				6	6	
A. A.	41 W			11	11	Rezidiv unmittelbar nach vorzeitigem Absetzen der Behandlung. Geräusch war noch vorhanden
B. E.	24 W			13	13	

Zahl der Fälle: 20; Rezidive: 5; Rezidive durch vorzeitiges Absetzen der Therapie: 2; Behandlungsdauer: 5—18 Monate, alle Rezidive ließen sich erneut mit Perchlorat behandeln.

[1] Irenatallergie, Weiterbehandlung mit Methylmercaptoimidazol.

von Standardbedingungen der Ableitung aus Form und Dauer des Geräusches aber doch quantitative Aussagen über die Größe des arteriovenösen Schilddrüsenshunts machen.

Unter der thyreostatischen Therapie nehmen Dauer und Intensität des Strömungsgeräusches der hyperthyreotischen Schilddrüse kontinuierlich ab, um schließlich nach erfolgreicher Behandlung ganz zu verschwinden.

Da es schwierig ist, die Dauer einer thyreostatischen Behandlung bei der Hyperthyreose festzulegen, weil die Behandlungszeit von Fall zu Fall erheblich schwankt, haben wir uns daran gewöhnt, so lange zu behandeln, bis das Strömungsgeräusch verschwunden ist. Die Therapie der Hyperthyreose soll solange fortgesetzt werden, wie die gesteigerte Aktivität der Schilddrüse fortbesteht. Solange ein Strömungsgeräusch über der Schilddrüse festzustellen ist, besteht nach unseren Erfahrungen noch eine gesteigerte Schilddrüsenaktivität.

Zu Beginn der Behandlung geben wir 1200—1600 mg Perchlorat pro Tag und gehen mit der Dosis zurück, wenn die peripheren Symptome der Hyperthyreose (das beste Zeichen ist die Normalisierung der Pulsfrequenz) verschwunden sind. Die Erhaltungsdosis [2—3 mal 5 Tropfen Perchlorat[1]] geben wir so lange, wie das Gefäßgeräusch fortbesteht.

In Tab. 1 sind bei 20 unausgewählten Patienten mit Hyperthyreose Behandlungsdauer, Dauer der Nachweisbarkeit des Strömungsgeräusches und Rezidiv-Quote zusammengestellt. In 5 Fällen beobachteten wir echte Rezidive, die erst längere Zeit nach Abschluß der Behandlung auftraten. Bei 2 Patienten wurde die Perchlorat-Therapie vorzeitig abgesetzt, d. h. bevor das Strömungsgeräusch verschwunden war. In beiden Fällen kam es unmittelbar nach Unterbrechnug zu einer akuten Verschlechterung mit Wiederauftreten von Hyperthyreose-Symptomen.

Schließlich hat die Feststellung des Strömungsgeräusches der Schilddrüse noch eine Bedeutung in der Erkennung anbehandelter Hyperthyreosen. Bei richtig dosierter thyreostatischer Behandlung verschwinden die Hyperthyreose-Symptome der Peripherie oder des gesteigerten Stoffwechsels meist nach 3 bis 4 Wochen. Diese anbehandelten Hyperthyreosen sind nur schwer als solche zu erkennen, denn alle Laboruntersuchungen sind nicht zu verwerten. In diesem Fall erlaubt das Strömungsgeräusch nachträglich die Diagnose, denn es besteht so lange, wie die vermehrte Aktivität der Schilddrüse besteht.

---

[1] Irenat® Troponwerke

Aus der II. Med. Univ.-Klinik und Poliklinik Hamburg-Eppendorf
(Direktor: Prof. Dr. A. JORES)

Kasuistischer Beitrag
zur Frage der Entstehung einer Panmyelopathie
und fraglichen Leukose nach Radiojodtherapie
einer Hyperthyreose

Von

H. FRAHM und U. PETERSEN

Über die Entwicklung von Leukämien nach Anwendung von Röntgenstrahlen sowie natürlicher und künstlicher radioaktiver Stoffe liegen eindeutige Befunde vor. Naturgemäß wird von dieser Problematik auch die Therapie von Schilddrüsenerkrankungen mit J^{131} berührt. Die beobachtete Entstehung von Leukosen nach Behandlung von Schilddrüsen-Carcinomen mit J^{131} wird übereinstimmend mit der erforderlichen hohen Dosierung des radioaktiven Jod in Zusammenhang gebracht (*2, 8, 15*). Ungeklärt ist jedoch die seit 1955 diskutierte Beziehung zwischen Leukämieentwicklung und vorausgegangener Radiojodtherapie von Hyperthyreosen. In der Literatur fanden wir Mitteilungen über 23 Fälle, bei denen diese Frage erörtert wird (*1, 3, 5, 6, 7, 8, 9, 10, 12, 13, 14, 15, 16, 17*). Wir beobachteten nunmehr ebenfalls einen Fall, bei dem sich nach zweimaliger Radiojodtherapie einer Hyperthyreose eine Panmyelopathie und später mit großer Wahrscheinlichkeit eine Leukose entwickelten.

Es handelte sich um eine Patientin, die 1957 im Alter von 41 Jahren erstmalig in unsere Klinik zur Diagnostik und Behandlung kam. 1944 hatte sich bei ihr im Anschluß an einen Partus eine Hyperthyreose entwickelt. Bis 1954 erhielt sie in unregelmäßigen Abständen verschiedene antithyreoidale Substanzen in sehr niedriger Dosierung. Nach einem Krankenhausaufenthalt 1955 nahm sie regelmäßig täglich 25—50 mg Mercaptoimidazol bis zum Jahre 1957. Wir stellten 1957 das typische klinische Bild einer Hyperthyreose mit Struma, Tremor, Tachykardie, positiven Augensymptomen usw. fest. Das Radiojodstoffwechselstudium bestätigte die klinische Diagnose. Wegen einer zweifellos toxisch bedingten leukopenischen Anämie sahen wir zunächst von einer Radiojodbehandlung ab. Nach einem erneuten Radiojod-Test im April 1958 veranlaßten wir sofort die Radiojodtherapie, da sich die Blutbildverhältnisse als unauffällig erwiesen. Wegen einer Resthyperthyreose mit Entwicklung einer doppelseitigen benignen Exophthalmopathie war im Nov. 1958 eine zweite Radiojodbehandlung erforderlich. Im April 1958 hatte die Pat. 18 mC und im Nov. 1958 6 mC J^{131} erhalten. Radiojoddiagnostik und -therapie waren im Isotopeninstitut (Leiter: Prof. Dr. HORST) der Radiologischen Klinik des Universitätskrankenhauses Hamburg-Eppendorf (Direktor: Prof. Dr. PRÉVÔT) vorgenommen worden.

Anhand der uns vom behandelnden Hausarzt zur Verfügung gestellten Befunde konnten wir feststellen, daß die hämatologische Situation bei der Pat. bis 1954 unauffällig gewesen war. Ab 1955 unter Dauerbehandlung mit antithyreoidalen Substanzen bestand eine Anämie wechselnden Ausmaßes, gelegentlich trat eine Tendenz zur Leukopenie auf. Nach Absetzen der Thyreostatika normalisierte sich das Blutbild für länger als zwei Jahre. Die Thrombocytenzahl war bis Anfang 1959 immer normal gewesen. Im Sternalmark hatte sich bis Mitte 1960 kein pathologischer Befund gezeigt. Ab Mitte 1959 entwickelten sich eine zunehmende Anämie mit Erythrocytopenie und ab 1960/61 konstant eine schwere Leukopenie mit ausgeprägter Lymphocytose (80 bis 95%). Das Sternalmark bot Mitte 1960 erstmalig das Bild einer schweren toxischen Markhemmung. 1961 traten im peripheren Blut atypische weiße Zellen auf, die einer lymphatischen Leukämie zuzuordnen waren. Klinisch bestand das Vollbild einer schweren hämorrhagischen Diathese bei Panmyelopathie und lymphatischer Leukämie. Infolge massiver unstillbarer Blutungen kam die Pat. am 12. 10. 1961 unter den Zeichen eines Kreis-Herzlaufversagens ad exitum.

Die Histologie der Lymphknoten zeigte eine beträchtliche Aufhebung der normalen Struktur, eine Hyperplasie von Reticulumzellen, eine plasmacelluläre Transformation lymphatischen Gewebes und Vermehrung kleiner cytoplasmaarmer Lymphocyten. Im Knochenmark fanden sich eine Reifungshemmung der myelopoetischen Vorstufen mit vermehrt unreifen und atypischen Elementen im Sinne einer Neoplasie. Teilweise waren die Zellelemente sehr unreifen Plasmazellen ähnlich. Die histologische Untersuchung und Beurteilung erfolgte im Pathologischen Institut des Universitätskrankenhauses Hamburg-Eppendorf (Direktor: Prof. Dr. Krauspe).

Diskussion

Bei epikritischer Betrachtung des Krankheitsverlaufes unserer Patienten kann kein Zweifel daran bestehen, daß die mehrjährige Behandlung mit antithyreoidalen Substanzen zu einer vorübergehenden leukopenischen Anämie bei sonst unauffälligen Blutbildverhältnissen geführt hat. Nach Absetzen der Medikamente kam es zur Normalisierung des Blutbildes. Die ersten Anzeichen einer Panmyelopathie machten sich nach einem länger als 2jährigem Intervall bemerkbar. Der Zeitraum zwischen der ersten Radiojodtherapie mit 18 mC und der zweiten mit 6 mC J^{131} und klinischem Beginn der Panmyelopathie betrug dagegen nur 1 bzw. $^1/_2$ Jahr. Der klinische Verdacht auf eine Leukose entstand mit dem Auftreten atypischer Zellen im peripheren Blutbild 3 bzw. $2^1/_2$ Jahre nach Radiojodbehandlung. Wenn auch der pathologisch-anatomische Befund nicht absolut beweisend für eine Leukämie ist, so spricht er unter Würdigung der Klinik eher dafür als dagegen. In jedem Fall besteht unseres Erachtens Anlaß genug, die Frage des Kausalzusammenhangs zwischen Therapie der Hyperthyreose und der späteren Panmyelopathie und wahrscheinlichen Leukose zu diskutieren. In unserem Falle sind folgende Möglichkeiten in Betracht zu ziehen: 1. Die vorausgegangene Therapie mit antithyreoidalen Substanzen ist die Ursache. 2. Die zweimalige Radiojodbehandlung im Abstand von 7 Monaten mit einer Gesamtdosis von 24 mC J^{131} stellt eine ursächliche Noxe dar. 3. Nach Vorbehandlung mit Thyreostatika bestand eine latente Schädigung; das J^{131} hatte einen auslösenden Effekt. 4. Es handelt sich um ein rein zufälliges Zusammentreffen.

Schon aus zeitlichen Gründen kommen als mögliche alleinige Ursache unter Berücksichtigung des länger als zweijährigen Intervalls die Thyreostatika weniger in Betracht als das J^{131}. Auch wäre die lange symptomlose Latenzzeit ungewöhnlich. Unter der Vorstellung, daß dem J^{131} eine schädigende Bedeutung zukommt, ließe sich dagegen der von uns beobachtete Fall zwanglos in die Kasuistik einreihen, die unter dieser Fragestellung anhand von 23 Fällen in der Literatur diskutiert wird. Das Alter der veröffentlichten Fälle liegt zwischen 28 und 73 Jahren mit der größten Dichte im 5. und 6. Dezennium. Die Höhe der zugeführten J^{131}-Dosis bewegt sich zwischen 2,1—28 mC, am häufigsten wurde zwischen 6—10 mC J^{131} verabfolgt. Das Intervall zwischen Radiojodtherapie und Auftreten

einer Leukämie erstreckt sich von 6 Monaten bis zu 7 Jahren in zwei Extrem-
fällen, die Mehrzahl aller Fälle liegt bei $1^1/_2-2$ Jahren. Gegen den möglichen
Zusammenhang zwischen Knochenmarkschädigung bzw. Leukoseentstehung und
Radiojodtherapie sprechen gewichtige Argumente der Strahlenbiologie. Die Dosen
des verabfolgten J^{131} sind zu niedrig, die Intervalle zu kurz, um die wesentlichen
zu nennen. Der beobachtete Zeitraum zwischen Leukämieentstehung und Strah-
leneinwirkung wird durchschnittlich mit 4—6 Jahren angegeben. Andererseits
sind aber gerade in jüngerer Zeit Untersuchungen bekannt geworden, nach denen
es zu Veränderungen an den Chromosomen der Leukocyten im zirkulierenden
Blut umittelbar nach Zufuhr von J^{131} kommt. BOYD u. Mitarb. berichteten 1961
über einen Abfall der Zellen mit normalen Chromosomen von 90 auf 62—55%
nach Dosen von 100—150 mC J^{131} (4). Chromosomen mit strukturellen Anomalien
waren zahlreich. Änderungen der Chromosomen nach Form und Zahl fanden
auch MACINTYRE und DOBYNS (1962) 12 Std nach J^{131}-Zufuhr bei einer Serum-
aktivität von 4,1 mC (11).

Bei einer Zahl von 23 Fällen, die in der Literatur mit der Frage der Leukoseentstehung nach Radiojodbehandlung wegen Hyperthyreose erörtert werden,
kann ein zufälliges Zusammentreffen weder bejaht noch verneint werden. Die
Schlußfolgerung des unmöglichen Kausalzusammenhangs ist nicht mehr zulässig.
Zu berücksichtigen ist weiter die mögliche größere Fallzahl, da kaum anzunehmen
ist, daß mit den beschriebenen 23 Fällen das gesamte Krankengut ausgeschöpft
ist. Erforderlich wären daher nicht nur die systematischen Verlaufsbeobachtungen
und die Erfassung aller radiojodbehandelter Patienten, sondern insbesondere
exakte Erhebungen darüber, wie groß der Anteil der an Leukämie erkrankten
Personen ist, der in der Vorgeschichte eine Radiojodtherapie aufweist. Es besteht
daher auch in der Literatur die Forderung nach Mitteilung entsprechender
Kasuistik, um die Voraussetzungen für eine statistische Beurteilung zu schaffen.
Unter diesem Aspekt erschien es uns gerechtfertigt, über unsere Beobachtung
zu berichten.

Literatur

1. ABBATT, J. D., H. E. A. FARAN and R. GREEN: Lancet **1956** I, 782.
2. BLOM, P. S., A. QUERIDO and C. H. W. LEEKSMA: Brit. J. Radiol. **28**, 165 (1955).
3. BLOMFIELD, G. W., H. ECKERT, M. FISHER, H. MILLER, D. S. MUNRO and G. M. WILSON: Brit. med. J. **1959** I, 63.
4. BOYD, L., W. W. BUCHANAN and B. LENNOX: Lancet **1961** I, 977.
5. BURNS, TH. W., R. VICKERS and J. F. LOWNEY: Arch. int. Med. **106**, 97 (1960).
6. CHAPMAN, E. M.: Proc. of Conference on Radioiodine, Argonne Cancer Research Hospital. 1956, p. 33.
7. CHILDS, D.: In Proc. of the Conference on Radio-Iofine, Nov. 5 and 6, 1956, Chicago.
8. DELARUE, J., M. TUBIANA and J. DUTREIX: Bull. Ass. franç. Cancer **40**, 263 (1953).
9. GREEN, M., M. FISHER, H. MILLER and G. M. WILSON: Brit. med. J. **5246**, 210 (1961).
10. KENNEDY, W. M., and R. G. FISH: New Engl. J. Med. **260**, 76 (1959).
11. MACINTYRE, M. N., and B. M. DOBYNS: J. clin. Endocr. **22**, 1171 (1962).
12. POCHIN, E.: Brit. J. Radiol. **29**, 31 (1956).
11. — Brit. med. J. **1960** II, 1545.
14. SALOMON, S., and S. RÜBENFELD: Arch. int. Med. **106**, 178 (1960).
15. SEIDLIN, S. M., E. SIEGEL, S. MELAMED and A. A. YALOW: Bull. N. Y. Acad. Med. **31**, 410 (1955).
16. VETTER, H., and R. HÖFER: Brit. J. Radiol. **32**, 263 (1959).
17. WERNER, S. C., and E. H. QUIMBY: J. Amer. med. Ass. **165**, 1558 (1957).

Aus der I. Medizinischen Klinik der Universität München
(Direktor: Prof. Dr. H. Schwiegk)

Untersuchungen über Sekretion und Abbau von Cortisol bei Patienten mit Hypo- und Hyperthyreose

Von

H. J. Karl und W. Decker

Mit 1 Abbildung

Untersuchungen von Percoff (*1*), Levin (*2*), Peterson (*3*) und Schwarz (*4*) zeigten, daß bei Patienten mit Hypo- und Hyperthyreose die Konzentration der 17-Hydroxycorticosteroide im Blut innerhalb des Normbereichs ist. Die sog. biologische Halbwertzeit von Cortisol, berechnet aus der Schwundrate des Hormons nach i.v. Verabreichung war jedoch bei Hyperthyreosen im Vergleich zu Normalpersonen verkürzt, bei Hypothyreosen verlängert [Brown (*5*), Peterson (*3*)]. Dabei war die Ausscheidung von Hormongruppen von Nebennierenrindensteroiden — der 17-Hydroxycorticosteroide und der 17-Ketosteroide — bei Schilddrüsenüberfunktion normal oder leicht erhöht [Peterson (*3*), Schwarz (*4*), Goldenberg (*6*)], bei Schilddrüsenunterfunktion meist vermindert [Levin (*2*), Talbot (*7*), Felber (*8*)].

Die Bestimmung von Hormongruppen läßt jedoch keine genauere Aussage über die Cortisolproduktion und den Cortisolabbau zu. Wir haben deshalb mit neuen und verfeinerten Methoden zum Nachweis einzelner Steroidhormone und zur Bestimmung der Sekretionsrate von Cortisol untersucht, ob bei Patienten mit Hyper- und Hypothyreose die Ausscheidung einzelner Cortisolmetaboliten und die Cortisolsekretionsrate verändert ist.

Der Nachweis der einzelnen Steroide Tetrahydrocortisol (THF), Allotetrahydrocortisol (AlloTHF) und Tetrahydrocortison (THE) erfolgte, nach Hydrolyse des Urins mit β-Glucuronidase, Extraktion mit Chloroform und papierchromatographischer Trennung des Neutralextrakts in den Systemen Bush BL 1 und B 5, mit der Reaktion nach Porter und Silber (*9*). Als Vergleichssubstanzen dienten bei der Chromatographie und bei der quantitativen Auswertung die Reinsubstanzen der einzelnen Steroide[1]. Die Sekretionsrate von Cortisol wurde nach i.v. Verabreichung von 0,1 μC 4-^{14}C-Cortisol (Spez. Aktivität 7,83 mC/mmol[1]) nach dem Verdünnungsprinzip durch Messung der spez. Aktivität der beiden im Urin ausgeschiedenen Cortisolmetaboliten Tetrahydrocortisol und Tetrahydrocortison mit der von uns angegebenen Methode [Karl und Raith (*10*)] bestimmt.

---

[1] Tetrahydrocortisol und Tetrahydrocortison wurde uns entgegenkommenderweise von Prof. Dr. W. Klyne, London, 4-^{14}C-Cortisol von der Endocrinology Study Section, National Institutes of Health zur Verfügung gestellt.

Die Ausscheidung der Summe der Hauptmetaboliten von Cortisol, THF, AlloTHF und THE bei 41 Patienten mit klinisch gesicherter Hyperthyreose zeigt die Abb. 1. Je nach Schwere der Erkrankung wurden die Patienten in 3 Gruppen mit leicht, mittel und stark erhöhtem Grundumsatz unterteilt und außerdem die Steroidhormonausscheidung zur Erkrankungsdauer nach anamnestischen Angaben der Kranken in Beziehung gesetzt. Der „Normalbereich" der Ausscheidung der Cortisolmetaboliten war bei 15 gesunden Versuchspersonen 2,5—9,0 mg/Tag.

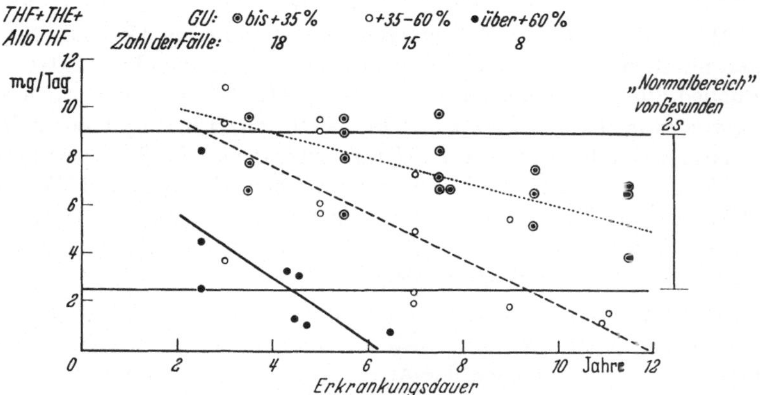

Abb. 1. Die Ausscheidung der Summe der Hauptmetaboliten von Cortisol (Tetrahydrocortisol, Allotetrahydrocortisol und Tetrahydrocortison) bei Patienten mit Schilddrüsenüberfunktion, bezogen auf Dauer und Schwere der Erkrankung

Die *2s*-Grenze ist in der Abbildung angegeben. Bei den Hyperthyreosen war in 60% der Fälle (24 Patienten) die Ausscheidung der Cortisolmetaboliten innerhalb des Normalbereichs. Nur bei 8 Patienten war in den ersten Jahren der Erkrankung die Ausscheidung leicht vermehrt, bei 4 schweren und 5 leichteren Fällen mit länger dauernder Erkrankung dagegen vermindert. Die Regression für jede Gruppe der Patienten ist verschieden, die Differenz des Steigungsmaßes war jedoch nur zwischen den leichten und den schweren Fällen signifikant (P < 0,05).

Offenbar nimmt bei Patienten mit Schilddrüsenüberfunktion im Verlauf und abhängig von der Schwere der Erkrankung die Ausscheidung der Cortisolmetaboliten immer mehr ab, ein Befund, der für eine verminderte Cortisolsekretion der Nebennierenrinde dieser Patienten spricht. Dies stimmt auch mit der klinischen Beobachtung überein, daß schwere Hyperthyreosen häufig Symptome einer Nebennierenrindeinsuffizienz zeigen.

Wenn auch eine verminderte oder vermehrte Ausscheidung von Cortisolmetaboliten auf eine entsprechend veränderte Cortisolproduktion der Nebennierenrinde hinweist, so sind genauere Aussagen über die Größe der Cortisolsekretion nur durch Bestimmung der Sekretionsrate möglich.

Der „Normalbereich" (*2s*) der Cortisolsekretionsrate ist nach unseren Untersuchungen an 18 gesunden Versuchspersonen 7—23 mg/Tag, im Mittel 15 mg/Tag. Bei 9 Patienten mit Hyperthyreose betrug die Cortisolsekretionsrate im Mittel 19,9 mg/Tag. Nur in 2 Fällen, bei denen auch die Ausscheidung der Cortisolmetaboliten im Urin vermehrt war, lag die Sekretionsrate mit 24,6 und 32,0 mg/Tag

über dem *2s*-Bereich von Normalen. Alle übrigen Patienten hatten Cortisol-
sekretionsraten innerhalb des Normalbereichs. 3 Kranke aus dieser Gruppe
wurden strumektomiert und 14 Tage nach der Operation wurde die Sekretionsrate erneut bestimmt. Im Vergleich zu den Werten vor der Operation (im Mittel
19,3 mg/Tag) war die Sekretionsrate nach der Strumektomie im Mittel um 33%
geringer (im Mittel 13,0 mg/Tag).

Dieser Befund weist darauf hin, daß die Cortisolproduktion der Nebennierenrinde direkt oder indirekt vom Schilddrüsenhormonspiegel beeinflußt wird.

Der Abbau des von der Nebennierenrinde sezernierten Cortisols führt bei
Patienten mit Hyperthyreose zu den gleichen Stoffwechselendprodukten wie sie
bei Normalen durch Untersuchungen von GOLD (*11*) bekannt sind. Nach Verabreichung von radioaktivem Cortisol an Patienten mit Hyperthyreose fanden wir
im chromatographisch aufgetrennten Neutralextrakt nach Radiopapierchromatographie die gleichen aktiven Zonen, entsprechend Cortolen und Cortolonen,
THF, AlloTHF und THE, wie bei gesunden Versuchspersonen. Der Anteil von
THE an der Gesamtausscheidung von Cortisolmetaboliten war jedoch bei den
Hyperthyreosen größer als bei Normalen.

Nach Untersuchungen von ROMANOFF (*12*) und HELLMAN (*13*) ist bei Hyperthyreosen neben einem vermehrten Abbau von Steroiden mit 19-C-Atomen zu
5α-Metaboliten vermutlich auch der Abbau von Steroiden mit 21-C-Atomen zu
11-Ketoverbindungen bevorzugt. Wir haben deshalb untersucht, ob das Verhältnis
der Ausscheidung von THF/THE abhängig von der Funktion der Schilddrüse
verändert ist. Die Ergebnisse unserer Untersuchungen sind in Tab. 1 zusammengefaßt. Bei 15 gesunden Versuchspersonen ist der Quotient THF/THE im Mittel
0,55 mit einer Streuung $s = 0,15$. Dieser Wert stimmt weitgehend mit den Ergebnissen der Untersuchungen von GOLD (*11*) bei Normalen überein. Im Vergleich
dazu betrug der Quotient bei 5 Patienten mit Hypothyreose im Mittel 0,85 und bei

Tabelle 1: *Mittlerer Quotient* THF/THE *bei Patienten mit normaler,
verminderter und gesteigerter Schilddrüsenfunktion*

Untersuchte Personengruppen (Zahl der Fälle)	Mittlerer Quotient: Tetrahydrocortisol (mg/Tag im Urin) / Tetrahydrocortison (mg/Tag im Urin)		
Normalpersonen (15)	0,55	*s* 0,15	0,1 > P > 0,2
Patienten mit Hypothyreose (5)	0,85	*s* 0,45	
Patienten mit Hyperthyreose (22)	0,36	*s* 0,44	0,01 > P > 0,01
Patienten mit Hyperthyreose (7)			
14 Tage *vor*/*nach* Strumektomie . .	0,39 / 0,83		0,01 > P > 0,001

22 Patienten mit Hyperthyreose im Mittel 0,36. Bei beiden Patientengruppen
war jedoch die Streuung mit $s = 0,45$ wesentlich größer als bei Normalpersonen.
Die Differenz der Mittelwerte der Quotienten zwischen Patienten mit Hypo- und
Hyperthyreose sowie die Differenz der Mittelwerte der Quotienten zwischen
Patienten mit Hyperthyreose vor und nach Strumektomie war sigifikant (0,01
> P > 0,001). Patienten mit Schilddrüsenüberfunktion scheiden somit relativ
mehr Tetrahydrocortison (THE) aus als solche mit Schilddrüsenunterfunktion
oder Strumektomierte.

Cortisol wird bekanntlich im Prinzip sowohl über seine Dihydro- und Tetrahydroderivate und Cortole als auch nach Reduktion zu Cortison zu den entsprechenden Metaboliten, also Tetrahydrocortison (THE) und Cortolonen abgebaut. Veränderungen der sog. biologischen Halbwertzeit von Cortisol scheinen von der Aktivität und Menge spezifischer Enzymsysteme in der Leber abhängig zu sein. Offenbar werden diese auch durch Schilddrüsenhormone beeinflußt, denn nach Untersuchungen von YATES (*14*) und McGUIRE (*15*) führt im Tierversuch die Verabreichung von Trijodthyronin zu einer Vermehrung der 5α-Δ^4-Steroidhydrogenase und gesteigerter Aktivität des Coenzyms TPNH, wodurch die Reduktion des Ring A des Steroidskelets und damit der Abbau von Cortisol beschleunigt wird.

Die relativ vermehrte Ausscheidung von THE bei Hyperthyreosen ist allein damit nicht zu erklären. THE stammt fast ausschließlich von Cortison und der Anteil aus dem Abbau von Cortisol über THF zu THE beträgt nach Untersuchungen von RAPAPORT (*16*) nur etwa 1%. Bei Hyperthyreosen muß also das Gleichgewicht Cortisol $\leftrightharpoons$ Cortison zugunsten von Cortison verschoben sein und es kann angenommen werden, daß ein erhöhter Schilddrüsenhormonspiegel neben der Δ^4-Steroidhydrogenase auch die 11β-Dehydrogenase mit den entsprechenden Coenzymen aktiviert. Welche Bedeutung diesem Befund in der Wechselwirkung zwischen Nebennierenrinde, Hypophysenvorderlappen und Schilddrüse zukommt, ist noch nicht geklärt.

Zusammenfassend läßt sich sagen, daß bei Patienten mit Hyperthyreose die Ausscheidung der Hauptmetaboliten von Cortisol, Tetrahydrocortisol, Allotetrahydrocortisol und Tetrahydrocortison im Verlauf und offenbar abhängig von der Schwere der Erkrankung abnimmt. Die Bestimmung der Cortisolsekretionsrate ergab Hinweise, daß die Cortisolproduktion der Nebennierenrinde vom Schilddrüsenhormonspiegel beeinflußt wird. Der Abbau von Cortisol erfolgt bei Patienten mit Schilddrüsenüberfunktion vorwiegend über Cortison und dessen Metaboliten und die Ausscheidung von Tetrahydrocortison ist im Vergleich zu Normalen und Patienten mit Hypothyreosen relativ vermehrt.

Literatur

1. PERCOFF, G. T., A. A. SANDBERG, D. H. NELSON and F. H. TYLER: Arch. intern. Med. **93**, 1 (1954).
2. LEVIN, M. E., and W. H. DAUGHADAY: J. clin. Endocr. **15**, 1499 (1955).
3. PETERSON, R. E.: J. clin. Invest. **37**, 736 (1958).
4. SCHWARZ, K.: Klin. Wschr. **37**, 654 (1959).
5. BROWN, H., E. ENGLERT and S. WALLACH: J. clin. Endocr. **18**, 167 (1958).
6. TALBOT, M. B., N. S. WOOD, J. WORCESTER, E. CHRISTO, A. M. CAMBELL and A. S. ZYG-MUNTOWICZ: J. clin. Endocr. **11**, 1224 (1951).
7. FELBER, J. P., W. J. REDDY, H. A. SEDENKOW and G. W. THORN: J. clin. Endocr. **19**, 895 (1959).
8. GOLDENBERG, I. S., L. LUTWAK, P. J. ROSENBAUM and M. A. HAYES: J. clin. Endocr. **15**, 227 (1955).
9. PORTER, C. C., and R. H. SILBER: J. biol. Chem. **210**, 923 (1954).
10. KARL, H. J., L. RAITH u. W. DECKER: 9. Symp. dtsch. Ges. Endocrinol. Berlin-Göttingen-Heidelberg: Springer-Verlag 1962.
11. GOLD, N. I., E. SINGLETON, D. A. McFARLANE and F. D. MOORE: J. clin. Invest. **37**, 813 (1958).
12. ROMANOFF, L. P., R. M. RODRIGUEZ, J. M. SEELYE and G. PINCUS: J. clin. Endocr. **17**, 777 (1957).

13. Hellman, L. H., L. Bradlow, B. Zumoff and T. F. Gallagher: J. clin. Endocr. 21, 1231 (1962).
14. Yates, F. E., J. Urquhart and A. L. Herbst: Amer. J. Physiol. 195, 373 (1938).
15. McGuire, J. S., and G. M. Tomkins: J. biol. Chem. 234, 794 (1959).
16. Rappaport, R., and C. J. Migeon: J. clin. Endocr. 22, 1065 (1962).

Diskussion

W. Teller (Marburg):

Es ist Ihnen in Ihren Untersuchungen gelungen, allo-Tetrahydrocortisol (allo-THF) papierchromatographisch sauber von Tetrahydrocortisol (THF) und Tetrahydrocortison (THE) abzutrennen. In der abschließenden Besprechung Ihrer Ergebnisse wird das allo-THF jedoch nicht mehr erwähnt. Wurde es bei der Bestimmung des Quotienten THF/THE dem Nenner oder dem Zähler zugerechnet oder absichtlich ganz aus den Kalkulationen weggelassen? Hellman et al.: [J. clin. Endocr. 21, 1231 (1961)], sowie Gold and Crigler [J. clin. Endocr. (1963) im Druck] haben gezeigt, daß unter T_3 eine Verschiebung der Steroidmetaboliten im Harn zugunsten der 5 α Verbindungen eintritt. Dies gilt sowohl für die C_{19} als auch für die C_{21} Metaboliten, was die genannten Autoren mit einer Stimulierung der 5 α-Reduktase in der Leber durch das Schilddrüsenhormon erklären [McGuire and Tomkins: Nature 182, 261 (1958)].

Es wäre in diesem Zusammenhang von Interesse, auch bei Ihren Untersuchungen zu prüfen, ob unter T_3 oder T_4 ebenfalls eine absolut vermehrte Ausscheidung von allo-THF im Harn sowie ein Ansteigen des Quotienten allo-THF/THF erfolgt ist.

Haben Sie in Wiederfindungsversuchen mit markierten Steroiden feststellen können, wie hoch Ihre Verluste an Steroidmaterial während des Aufarbeitungsganges waren?

H. J. Karl:

Die Ausscheidung von allo-THF wurde bei der Berechnung des Quotienten THF/THE von uns weder in den Nenner noch in den Zähler miteinbezogen, sondern nicht berücksichtigt. Im Gegensatz zu den Ergebnissen der Belastungsversuche mit Trijodthyronin (T_3) der bereits im Vortrag erwähnten Autoren fanden wir, daß bei Hyperthyreosen die Ausscheidung von allo-THF nur in einzelnen Fällen erhöht war, im Mittel jedoch der von Normalen entsprach. Es ist aber zu bedenken, daß theoretisch beim Abbau von Cortisol und Cortison für jedes der beiden Corticosteroide je 4 Tetrahydrometaboliten, sowohl aus der Pregnan- als auch aus der Allopregnanreihe zu erwarten wären, aber bisher nur THF, allo-THF und THE erfaßt werden.

Da wir die Ausscheidung einzelner Cortisolmetaboliten nach Verabreichung von T_3 oder T_4 nicht untersucht haben, können wir auch keine Angaben über den Quotienten allo-THF/THF unter Belastung mit Schilddrüsenhormonen machen.

Radioaktive Glucuronsäureester von Cortisolmetaboliten stehen bisher nicht zur Verfügung, so daß Wiederauffindungsversuche bei der Bestimmung von THF oder THE, die den gesammten Arbeitsgang einschließlich Hydrolyse erfassen, mit radioaktiven Steroiden nicht möglich sind. Wir haben aus dem Urin von Patienten, denen 4-^{14}C-Cortisol verabreicht worden war ^{14}C-Tetrahydrocortison isoliert und diesen radioaktiven Metaboliten von Cortisol benützt, um den Verlust des Arbeitsgangs nach der Hydrolyse mit β-Glucuronidase zu bestimmen. Er betrug im Mittel 30%.

Aus der Frauenklinik der Medizinischen Akademie Düsseldorf
(Direktor: Professor Dr. med. R. ELERT)

Über den Einfluß von thyreotropem Hormon und Thyroxin auf die Gonaden der Ratte

Von

R. BUCHHOLZ und H. SCHMIDT-ELMENDORFF

Mit 2 Abbildungen

In den letzten 20 Jahren haben zahlreiche Autoren in tierexperimentellen und klinischen Untersuchungen zu zeigen versucht, daß ein funktioneller Zusammenhang zwischen Schilddrüse und Ovar besteht.

So stellten GRUMBRECHT und LÖSER schon im Jahre 1939 fest, daß bei Hypothyreose die Eireifungsvorgänge unvollkommen ablaufen. Als Ursache für die verzögerte Eireifung nahmen diese Autoren an, daß bei Hypothyreose die von der Schilddrüse ausgehende Sensibilisierung der Ovarien für gonadotrope Wirkstoffe der Hypophyse ungenügend sei. Umgekehrt soll nach Meinung von GRUMBRECHT bei Hypothyreose die Eireifung durch thyreogene Sensibilisierung des Ovars beschleunigt werden.

Die Gonaden der Ratte erscheinen als Erfolgsorgane für Gonadotropine in besonderer Weise geeignet, evtl. bestehende Zusammenhänge zwischen Thyroxin und thyreotropem Hormon und der gonadotropinabhängigen Gonadenfunktion zu erhellen.

In den folgenden Untersuchungen soll über den Einfluß von Thyroxin und thyreotropem Hormon auf eine Anzahl von gonadotropen Erfolgsorganen berichtet werden. Einige dieser Erfolgsorgane gelten als hochspezifische Indicatoren für follikelstimulierendes bzw. luteinisierendes Hormon.

Tab. 1 zeigt die untersuchten Erfolgsorgane für Gonadotropine.

Tabelle 1

1. *Augmentation-Reaktion.* Zunahme des Ovargewichtes von intakten, infantilen Ratten, die mit HCG behandelt werden (STEELMAN und POHLEY 1953).
2. *Ascorbinsäuresenkung.* Senkung der Ascorbinsäure in Ovarien von intakten, infantilen Ratten, die mit PMS und HCG vorbehandelt wurden (PALOW 1961).
3. *Prostatagewichtszunahme* bei hypophysektomierten infantilen Ratten.
4. *Testisgewichtszunahme* bei hypophysektomierten infantilen Ratten.
5. *Uterusgewichtszunahme* bei hypophysektomierten infantilen Ratten.
6. *Ovargewichtszunahme* bei hypophysektomierten infantilen Ratten.

Test 1 gilt als Nachweis für FSH-Aktivität, während Test 2 und 3 hochspezifische Indicatoren für LH-Aktivität sind. Die drei letzten Teste sind weder spezifisch für FSH noch für LH, sondern sprechen auf beide Hormone an. Sie können deshalb als Nachweis für gesamtgonadotrope Aktivität gelten.

Folgende Hormone wurden verwandt:

1. *Thyreotropes Hormon (TSH)*. Internationales Standardpräparat.
2. *Thyreotropes Hormon*. Pretiron (Schering).
3. *Thyroxin*. (Roche).
4. *Follikelstimulierendes Hormon. (NIH-FSH-S1)*.
5. *Luteinisierendes Hormon (NIH-LH-S1)*.
6. *Menschliches Menopause Gonadotropin (HMG)* Laborstandard.

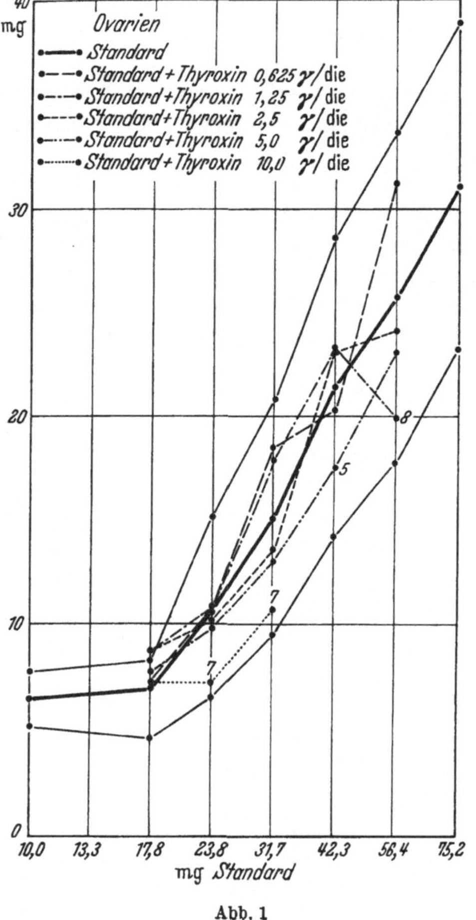

Abb. 1

Die erste Abbildung zeigt die Untersuchung des Einflusses von Thyroxin auf die Ovarien von hypophysektomierten infantilen Ratten.

300 hypophysektomierte, weibliche Ratten wurde in 5 Gruppen zu je 60 Ratten aufgeteilt, die je Gruppe 17,8, 23,8, 31,7, 42,3 und 54,4 mg des Gonadotropinstandards erhielten.

Jede Gruppe von Ratten wurde noch einmal unterteilt in 6 Untergruppen zu je 10 Tieren.

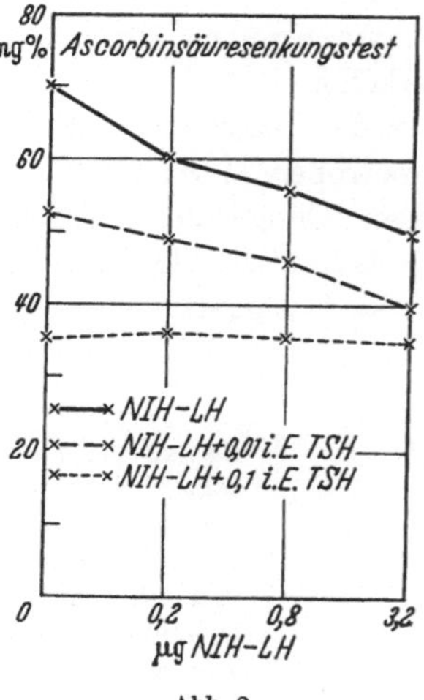

Abb. 2

Die erste Untergruppe erhielt zusätzlich zum Gonadotropin noch 0 μg Thyroxin, die zweite 2,5 μg, die dritte 5,0 μg, die vierte 10,0 μg, die fünfte 20,0 μg und die sechste 40,0 μg Thyroxin.

Während die ausgezogene Linie die Dosenwirkungskurve der Ratten darstellt, die nur Gonadotropin erhielten, repräsentieren die unterbrochenen Linien die Wirkungskurven von solchen Ratten, denen zusätzlich Thyroxin verabreicht wurde.

Offensichtlich hat Thyroxin weder eine hemmende noch eine fördernde Wirkung auf die Gewichtszunahme der Ovarien. Die Werte für eine Kombination von Gonadotropin und Thyroxin befinden sich alle innerhalb der Vertrauensgrenze der Werte für Gonadotropin allein.

Auch die gleichzeitig in diesem Versuch registrierte Uterusgewichtszunahme und damit die Oestrogenproduktion der hypophpsektomierten Ratte zeigt *keine* Beeinflussung durch Thyroxin.

In einem weiteren Experiment wurden 300 hypophysektomierten, männlichen Ratten in gleicher Weise wie in dem vorhergehenden Versuch Gonadotropin und Thyroxin injiziert.

Auch hier fand sich *kein* Einfluß des Schilddrüsenhormons Thyroxin auf das Hodengewicht.

Die gleichzeitig gemessene Gewichtszunahme der Prostata und damit die Androgenproduktion wurde ebenfalls nicht durch Thyroxin beeinflußt.

Schließlich wurde in einem weiteren Versuch der Einfluß von Thyroxin auf den Augmentations-Test bei intakten, weiblichen Ratten untersucht, ein Test, von dem man annimmt, daß er spezifisch für follikelstimulierende Aktivität ist. Aber auch in diesem Versuch zeigte sich *keinerlei* Einfluß des Thyroxin auf die follikelstimulierende Aktivität von Gonadotropinen.

Es erhebt sich nun die Frage, ob das *thyreotrope Hormon oder TSH* einen Einfluß auf die gonadotropen Erfolgsorgane der Ratten hat.

Zu diesem Zweck wurde in einer weiteren Serie von Experimenten die Wirkung der TSH-Präparate „Pretiron" von SCHERING und des Internationalen Standards für TSH auf den Augmentations-Test bei intakten, infantilen Ratten getestet.

Es zeigte sich, daß schon der Zusatz von 10 Meerschweinchen-Einheiten Pretiron pro Ratte einen signifikanten Einfluß auf die Augmentation-Reaktion hatte.

Als dieser Versuch mit dem TSH-Standard anstelle des Pretirons wiederholt wurde, ließ sich selbst mit einer Dosierung von 100 μg-Einheiten TSH pro Ratte kein Einfluß auf den Augmentations-Test erzeugen.

Es darf daher angenommen werden, daß Pretiron seinen Effekt auf den Augmentations-Test durch Kontaminierung mit FSH-Aktivität ausgeübt hat.

Schließlich untersuchten wir den Einfluß des Internationalen Standards für TSH auf die LH-spezifische Ascorbinsäuresenkung.

Abb. 2 zeigt, daß dieses Präparat eine signifikante Wirkung auf die Ascorbinsäuresenkung hat.

Die Frage, ob dieser Effekt des Internationalen Standards für TSH auf den ICSH-spezifischen Test auf einer Kontaminierung mit LH-Aktivität beruht, läßt sich z. Z. nicht sicher beantworten.

Es erscheint außerordentlich schwierig, thyreotropes Hormon von Luteinisierungshormon zu trennen. So enthalten nach KIRKHAM auch hochgereinigte LH-Präparate, wie des NIH-LH, das die 2000fache LH-Aktivität des HMG-Standards besitzt, noch 30 mal 10 Einheiten TSH pro mg LH.

Zum Schluß seien folgende Punkte noch einmal hervorgehoben:

1. Thyroxin zeigte keinen Einfluß auf die gonadotropen Endorgane von hypophysektomierten, männlichen und weiblichen Ratten, wie den Gewichtsanstieg von Ovar, Uterus, Hoden und Prostata. Auch die Augmentation-Reaktion bei intakten, weiblichen Ratten blieb von Thyroxin unbeeinflußt.

2. Die Wirkung des TSH-Präparates Pretiron auf den Augmentation-Test wird auf FSH-Kontaminierung dieses Präparates zurückgeführt. Das Standardpräparat für TSH besitzt diese Wirkung auf den Augmentation-Test nicht.

3. Der Einfluß des Internationalen Standards für TSH auf die ICSH-spezifische Ascorbinsäuresenkung könnte ebenfalls auf Kontaminierung des TSH mit LH-Aktivität beruhen, läßt sich jedoch nicht sicher beweisen, da man TSH von LH bis heute noch nicht zu trennen vermochte.

Diskussion

E. Tonutti (Bonn):

Leblond u. Mitarb. haben gezeigt, daß bei thyreoidektomierten und gleichzeitig jodarm ernährten Ratten die Entwicklung des Hodens und der accessorischen Genitaldrüsen auf infantiler Stufe stehen bleibt. Nach diesen Untersuchungen ist also doch ein gewisser Einfluß der Schilddrüsenhormone auf die Gonadenfunktion wahrscheinlich.

Hals-Nasen-Ohren-Klinik der Universität Zagreb, Jugoslawien

Über die kochleovestibulären Veränderungen beim endemischen Kropf

Von

B. Gušić

Die Gehörschädigungen beim endemischen Kropf sind schon seit altersher bekannt und in den ältesten Beschreibungen der Alpenkretinen erwähnt. Es ist das große Verdienst von Nager, daß er uns die knöchernen Veränderungen beschrieben hat, die bei Kretinen die Ursache dieser Gehörabnahme darstellen. Daß aber die Gehörschädigungen und Vestibularisausfälle auch bei aquirierter Struma im Endemiegebiet häufig vorkommen und einen großen Prozentsatz der befallenen Bevölkerung umfassen können, dieser Tatsache wurde bisher kaum nachgegangen. Zwar haben schon vor 90 Jahren Baillarger in seiner «Enquête sur le goitre et le crétinisme» und dann 10 Jahre später Hans Bircher in seinem klassischen Werk „Der endemische Kropf und seine Beziehungen zur Taubheit und zum Kretinismus" auf diese Tatsache hingewiesen, doch hat diese Äußerung bisher kaum Beachtung gefunden. Etwas mehr wurde in neuester Zeit über solche Vorkommnisse bei sporadischer Struma berichtet.

Jugoslawien ist ein Land mit weit verbreiteter endemischer Struma. Die Endemiegebiete umfassen nicht nur die bis vor kurzem noch entlegenen Gebirgstäler, sie breiten sich auch in der Panonischen Ebene entlang der großen Flüsse Save, Drau und Donau aus. Reste einstiger größeren Endemiegebiete finden wir auch auf einigen Adriainseln, besonders auf der Insel Krk. Bei der medizinischen Bearbeitung dieser Endemiegebiete, die schon teilweise vor dem Kriege angefangen, aber erst nach dem letzten Weltkrieg systematisch durchgeführt wird und wo bei dieser Arbeit nicht nur Mediziner, sondern auch Tierärzte, Genetiker und andere Fachleute mitarbeiten, fiel uns die große Zahl der kochleovestibulären Störungen auf, die in gewissen Gegenden auch bis 80% der Strumatragenden betrug. Die audiologische Untersuchung, die wir an einigen Tausend solcher Kropfträger durchführten, zeigte uns ein äußerst buntes Bild von Veränderungen, die von ganz leichter Gehörabnahme oder Hyporeflexie des Vestibularapparates bis zur völligen Taubheit bzw. Areflexie des Gleichgewichtsorganes schwankten. Diese Befunde sprechen entschieden für eine zentrale Genese dieser Störungen. Wir konnten weiter feststellen, daß die Schwere dieser Veränderungen nicht so sehr von der Größe des Kropfes, sondern vielmehr von der Dauer der vorhandenen Struma abhängig war. Daß es sich dabei um eine Veränderung handelt, die dem pathologischen Substrat des Kropfes gleichzusetzen ist, beweist unter anderem ihr häufiges Vorkommen bei maligner Struma.

Die Zeit erlaubt mir nicht näher auf diese Fragen einzugehen. Ich möchte darum heute aus diesem weiten Fragekomplex nur zwei Tatsachen beleuchten, die, wie ich glaube, nicht nur für den Audiologen sondern auch für alle, die sich mit dem Strumaproblem befassen, von Interesse sein dürften.

Zuerst die Frage der Differenzierung der kongenitalen Fälle von denen, die ihren Kropf erst im späteren Leben erworben haben. Dabei müssen wir uns aber vorerst in dem Begriff der Bezeichnung Kretin einigen. Wenn wir nämlich diesen Namen nur für diejenigen Fälle behalten wollen, die in den Endemiegebieten von einer strumatragenden Mutter geboren, mit dem bekannten Symptomenkomplex behaftet sind, und ich glaube, daß gerade für solche Fälle auch diese Bezeichnung von den alten Autoren geprägt wurde, dann fragt es sich, sind wir in der Lage, in der großen Zahl der leichteren oder auch der ganz leichten Fälle, der sog. Kretinoiden, solche von den Fällen des aquirierten postnatalen Kropfes und seiner Folgen zu unterscheiden. In den schweren Fällen der vollausgebildeten Kretine ist dies natürlich ohne weiteres leicht, da ja die Größe der zentral bedingten Störungen von dem Zeitpunkt abhängt, in dem der pathologische Prozeß das Zentralnervensystem im Laufe seiner intrauterinen Entwicklung angreift. Es gibt aber in den schweren Endemiegebieten, und auch nicht nur dort, eine große Zahl von Fällen, bei denen die Schwere der Veränderungen sehr verschieden ausgebildet ist und oft auch nur ganz leichte Symptome verursacht, die dann mehr im psychologischen Bereich als in irgendwelchen organischen Störungen sich bemerkbar machen. Solche Fälle sind klinisch sehr schwer zu umfassen und noch schwerer von jenen ganz ähnlichen postnatal erworbenen zu trennen. Die Trennung aber dieser beiden Gruppen ist für uns von außerordentlicher Bedeutung, da die kongenitalen ja durch keine Therapie beeinflußbar sind, wogegen die später erworbenen meistens auf diese gut ansprechen. Das ist ja auch vollkommen verständlich, wenn wir bedenken, daß es sich bei der ersten Gruppe um Fälle handelt, wo gewisse hochdifferenzierte Teile des Zentralnervensystems überhaupt nicht oder auch nur ungenügend sich entwickelt haben, wogegen sich bei der zweiten Gruppe um degenerative Prozesse handelt, die mehr oder weniger die schon einmal entwickelten Zellelemente befallen haben. Und diese Unterscheidung ermöglicht uns gerade die audiologische Analyse.

Es ist ja bekannt, daß die intrauterinen Veränderungen am Kinde bei einer kropftragenden Mutter bei endemischer Struma schon sehr früh eintreten. Es sind zwei Vorgänge, die auf die Menge der in den Geweben vorhandenen Schilddrüsenhormone äußerst empfindlich sind; der Verknöcherungsprozeß und die Entwicklung der zentralen Ganglienzellen. Darum sind auch beide gleichzeitig befallen. Die Ossifikationsänderungen zeigen sich in einer mehr oder weniger persistierenden fetalen Platybasie und am abnormalen Verknöcherungsprozeß im Bereiche des Mittelohres besonders der Gehörknöchelchenkette. Als Folge davon meldet sich dann eine Mittelohrschwerhörigkeit unterschiedlichen Grades. Die Störungen in der Entwicklung der zentralen Ganglien führen wieder ihrerseits, neben anderen Symptomen, auch zu zentralen Gehör- und Vestibularisstörungen. Wir finden also bei intrauterinen Veränderungen neben Vestibularis- und Gehörstörungen von zentralem Typ immer auch solche von seiten des Leitungsapparates, die in der Regel bei postnatal erworbenen Veränderungen immer fehlen. Es ist also gerade die audiologische Untersuchung, die uns in allen Grenzfällen einen genauen Unterschied erst ermöglicht.

Die zweite Frage, die ich hier besprechen wollte, ist die Wichtigkeit der audiologischen Untersuchung für die Bewertung des Augenblickes, wann bei einem Fall eines endemischen Kropfes eine entsprechende Therapie nicht weiter aufgeschoben werden sollte. Es ist ja ohne weiteres klar, daß die alleinige Erscheinung eines Kropfes nicht gleichbedeutend mit dem Auftritt eines Krankheitszustandes zu bewerten ist. Wir sehen ja das am besten bei jugendlicher Struma, die nach der Vollendung der Pubertät wieder verschwindet und niemals zu irgendwelchen Krankheitssymptomen führt und darum auch keine kochleovestibulären Ausfälle aufweist. Dagegen konnten wir aber in unseren Reihenuntersuchungen der Kropftragenden mit endemischer Struma feststellen, daß die Erscheinung dieser kochleovestibulären Veränderungen in der Regel das erste und das früheste Zeichen der Dysharmonie darstellt, die zwischen der Produktion der Schilddrüsenhormone und ihres Bedarfes in jedem konkreten Falle entstanden ist. Dabei sind es gerade die Störungen des Gehörs, die weit öfters als jene des Gleichgewichtsapparates auftreten. Ob dies nun durch unsere empfindlicheren und feineren Untersuchungsmethoden am Gehör bedingt ist oder dadurch, daß die Möglichkeit der Kompensation der leichten Störungen im reichverzweigten Vestibularisgebiet ungemein groß ist, bleibe für jetzt dahingestellt. Es ist aber Tatsache, daß wir in der Lage sind, solche anfänglichen Ausfälle bei sofort eingeleiteter entsprechender Therapie leicht zu beseitigen und was noch viel wichtiger erscheint, jedes weitere Fortschreiten der Krankheitssymptome zu verhindern, was natürlich bei richtigen Kretinoiden, also solchen, wo diese Veränderungen schon intrauterin entstanden sind, nicht der Fall ist.

Wir wollten durch diese kurze Mitteilung Ihre Aufmerksamkeit auf die Wichtigkeit der audiologischen Untersuchung hinlenken, die wir bei der Behandlung des endemischen Kropfes nicht mehr missen möchten.

Literatur

1. Baillarger, J. G. F.: Enquete sur le goitre et le cretinisme. Paris 1873.
2. Bircher, H.: Der endemische Kropf und seine Beziehungen zur Taubstummheit und zum Cretinismus. Basel 1883.
3. Gušić, B.: I Jugosl. simpozij o gušavosti, p. 160. Beograd 1959.
4. — Pract. oto-rhino-laryng. (Basel) 19, 531 (1957).
5. Nager, F.: Z. Ohrenheilk. 75, 349 (1917).
6. — I Jugoslac. Simpozij o gušavosti, p. 172. Beograd 1959.
7. Pražić, M., o B. Salaj: II Jugoslav. Simpozij o endemskoj gušavosti, p. 139. Zagreb 1961.

Aus der Hals-Nasen-Ohren-Klinik der Universität Zagreb, Jugoslawien

Schädigung des statoakustischen Apparates bei Hyperthyreosen

Von

M. Pražić

Anknüpfend an die Auslegungen meines Vorsprechers Gušić haben wir audiologische Untersuchungen auch bei Hyperthyreosen durchgeführt und konnten wir bei etwa 25% der untersuchten Fälle Störungen im Bereich des Gehörs und Vestibularapparates feststellen. Die Art der Störungen war ihrem Charakter nach gleich jenen bei der gewöhnlichen endemischen Struma, mit dem einzigen Unterschied, daß diese Veränderungen eine geringere Intensität besaßen und seltener vorkamen.

Die Schädigungen des Gehörs präsentieren sich als perzeptive Läsionen, also als die Läsionen in den Haarzellen des Cortischen Organs. Sie zeichnen sich im Anfangsstadium durch eine typische Gehörsabnahme im oberen Areal des Hörspektrums aus, und darum können die Kranken lange Zeit symptomlos bleiben.

Erst im fortgeschrittenen Stadium, wenn die Schädigung auch auf die mittleren Frequenzen übergeht, werden sich die Kranken ihrer Schwerhörigkeit bewußt. So z. B. eine Hyperthyreose, die keine Gleichgewichtsstörungen, aber eine Verschlechterung des Gehörs bemerkt hatte. Die audiologische Analyse ergab normale Werte der Erregbarkeit des Vestibularapparates und eine beidseitige Läsion des Cortischen Organs.

Bei den Schädigungen des Gehörs handelt es sich um einen degenerativen Prozeß an den Haarzellen des Cortischen Organs, oder genauer, an Mitochondrien in diesen Zellen und an Mitochondrien der dendritischen Endelemente des Hörnervs, welche die Haarzellen umschlingen. Wenn diese Schädigungen der Haarzellen des Cortischen Organs einmal etabliert sind, sind sie als ein progressiver und degenerativer Prozeß irreparabel. In einigen Fällen ist Tinnitus das einzige Symptom, das die Kranken auf den Prozeß im Ohre aufmerksam macht.

Die Vorgänge im Bereich des Vestibularapparates können bei den Kranken für eine Zeit unbemerkbar sein, und erst später bei der weiteren Progression der Läsion bekommen die Kranken die Gleichgewichtsstörungen.

Die kochleovestibulären Störungen bei Hyperthyreosen scheinen die ersten Befunde zu sein, die den toxischen Verlauf einer Hyperthyreose anzeigen. Ihre frühe Entdeckung ermöglicht uns die entsprechende Therapie bei Zeiten einzuleiten und dadurch größeren Schädigungen vorzubeugen. Die audiologische Analyse sollte deswegen bei Hyperthyreosen einen Teil der nicht zu unterlassenden typischen Untersuchungsmethoden darstellen.

Thyroninderivate in der Behandlung
der Hypercholesterinämie

Von

J. Hoeflmayr, München

Die Zusammenhänge Schilddrüsenfunktion — Erhöhung des Cholesterinspiegels
und damit rasches Fortschreiten atherosklerotischer Veränderungen der Gefäße,
traten mit besonderer Deutlichkeit hervor, als vor fast genau 30 Jahren in
Amerika Blumgart u. Mitarb., hier in Wien Scherf, Winkelbauer u. Mitarb.
zur Behebung oder Besserung schwerster Angina pectoris-Anfälle die totale
Schilddrüsenexstirpation durchführten. Die Kontrollen nach der Operation
zeigten in allen Fällen außer myxödematösen Erscheinungen einen zunehmenden
Anstieg des Serum-Cholesterinspiegels auf 500 mg-% und mehr. Die durch die
totale Entfernung der Schilddrüse notwendig gewordene Substitutionstherapie
mit Schilddrüsenextrakten oder mit dem synthetischen Thyroxin beeinflußte
in deutlichem Maße auch den Serum-Cholesterinspiegel im Sinne einer Senkung.
Gleichzeitig konnte ein Hintanhalten atherosklerotischer Gefäßveränderungen
beobachtet werden.

Trotz der Beobachtung, daß das natürliche Hormon den Serum-Cholesterinspiegel beeinflußt, konnte das Thyroxin zur Therapie wegen seiner bekannten
unerwünschten Nebenwirkungen im Sinne einer Hyperthyreose nur in vorsich-
tiger Handhabung bei den Patienten eingesetzt werden, bei denen eine Unterfunktion der Schilddrüse bestand. Die Therapie, den Serum-Cholesterinspiegel
mit Schilddrüsenhormonen zu senken, änderte sich auch nicht durch die Entdeckung des 3,5,3'-Trijodthyronin durch Gross und Pitt-Rivers. Der Unterschied dieser beiden Hormone besteht vor allem in Eintritt und Dauer der Wirkung.

In zahlreichen Untersuchungen konnte in den vergangenen Jahren nachgewiesen werden, daß Thyroxin, aber auch dessen Vorstufen den Serum-Cholesterinspiegel zu senken vermögen (*1, 2, 3, 4, 5, 6, 7*), wobei die Unterschiede auf der
Beeinflussung des Grundumsatzes und des Sauerstoffverbrauchs des Herzens
beruhen. Diese beiden Faktoren stellen deshalb ein Maß für die therapeutische
Verwendbarkeit dar.

Zu dem in den letzten Jahren am intensivsten untersuchten Thyroninderivat
gehört sicherlich das rechtsdrehende Thyroxin.

Die natürlichen, in der Schilddrüse gefundenen Hormone sind optisch aktiv
und drehen das polarisierte Licht nach links. Nun wissen wir aus zahlreichen
Beispielen, daß die Richtung der optischen Aktivität bei derselben Substanz für
bestimmte Eigenschaften maßgeblich sein kann.

Untersuchungen einer großen Anzahl von Autoren ergaben, daß eine Reihe
von Eigenschaften, die dem natürlichen L-Thyroxin anhaften, in therapeutisch

wirksamen Dosen dem D-Thyroxin praktisch fehlen und nur bei Überdosierung in weit milderer Form auftreten.

Die hauptsächlichsten Unterschiede zwischen dem L- und dem D-Thyroxin seien in Kürze hervorgehoben. Dem D-Thyroxin wird eine größere Affinität zur Leber zugeschrieben, denn nach der Verabreichung von Dextrothyroxin findet sich eine vermehrte Ausscheidung von Cholesterin in der Galle. Diese tierexperimentellen Untersuchungen decken sich mit einer Beobachtung von Owen (8), der einem Patienten mit Gallengangsfistel über 10 Tage Dextrothyroxin verabreichte. Die durch die Totaldrainage abgesonderte Galle wurde jeweils vor und nach der Therapie mit D-Thyroxin über 3 Tage gesammelt und der Cholesteringehalt bestimmt. Die Verabfolgung von D-Thyroxin bei gleichbleibender Fettzufuhr hatte eine Erhöhung der Cholesterinausscheidung um etwa 200% zur Folge. Nach Absetzen der Medikation fiel die Cholesterinausscheidung innerhalb von 4 Tagen rasch auf den Ausgangswert ab.

Unterschiede zwischen den beiden Isomeren bestehen auch hinsichtlich ihrer Anreicherung in den verschiedenen Geweben. In Leber und Niere ist die Konzentration von D-Thyroxin höher als die von L-Thyroxin (9). Umgekehrt verhält es sich in den peripheren Geweben wie Muskel, Gehirn und Haut. Hier zeigte L-Thyroxin eine höhere Konzentration. Einige Autoren sehen in dieser Tatsache eine Erklärung für das unterschiedliche Verhalten auf den Grundumsatz, denn gemessen an der Sauerstoffatmung der Maus und der Ratte beträgt die stoffwechselsteigernde Wirkung von D-Thyroxin nur $^1/_{50}$ derjenigen des L-Thyroxin. So bleibt eine genügende therapeutische Breite, um den gleichen cholesterinsenkenden Effekt zu erzielen, obwohl D-Thyroxin 10mal höher als L-Thyroxin dosiert werden muß. Grundumsatzbeobachtungen beim Menschen ergaben eine Steigerung um etwa 2% (10). Die Gefahr einer ungünstigen Beeinflussung des Herzens und des Kreislaufes scheint nur bei höherer Dosierung beim Menschen gegeben zu sein.

Da eine Erhöhung des Serum-Cholesterinspiegels in unseren guten Zeiten jenseits des 35.—40. Lebensjahres gar nicht so selten ist, war die Möglichkeit gegeben, D-Thyroxin an Patienten zu erproben, deren Herz- und Kreislaufsystem noch keinen Anhalt für einen krankhaften Befund boten. Die Ergebnisse, über die kurz berichtet werden soll, wurden an 23 Patienten gewonnen. Diese 23 Patienten konnten über 20 Wochen hin kontrolliert werden. 11 Patienten davon unterziehen sich seit 11 Monaten einer regelmäßigen Kontrolle.

Das Alter dieser 23 Patienten lag zwischen 42 und 61 Jahren. Das Durchschnittsalter betrug 48 Jahre. An hier interessierenden Untersuchungen wurden durchgeführt: einmal der Gesamt-Cholesterinspiegel und zweitens, weil ihm heute erhöhte Bedeutung zugemessen wird, der β-Lipoproteidspiegel. Regelmäßig kontrolliert wurden Blutdruck und Puls.

Der durchschnittliche Cholesterinspiegelwert der genannten Patientenzahl betrug vor der Behandlung 295 mg-%. Unter einer durchschnittlichen Anfangsdosierung von 6 mg D-Thyroxin sank der Gesamtcholesterinspiegel innerhalb von 3 Wochen auf durchschnittlich 220 mg-%. Als dieser Wert bei einer durchschnittlichen Dosierung von 3,2 mg erreicht war, kam es erneut zu einer Anstiegszacke. Mit der Dosierung wurde nach den individuellen Gegebenheiten variiert. Das Ergebnis war, daß sich der Gesamtcholesterinspiegel über eine längere Zeit auf ein erniedrigtes Niveau einspielte. Nach der 13. Woche kam es, obwohl die Medikation im Gegensatz zur Anfangsdosierung erheblich reduziert worden war, nochmals zu einem Abfall. Nach 20 Wochen betrug der Gesamtcholesterinspiegel im Durchschnitt 238 mg-%. Fast parallel zur Kurve des Gesamtcholesterins verlief die Kurve der β-Lipoproteide.

Um Verträglichkeit und evtl. Nebenwirkungen besser beurteilen zu können, nahmen 10 Patienten die vorgeschriebene Dosis über den Tag verteilt, die restlichen Patienten die Dosis auf einmal am Morgen ein. Nach meinen Erfahrungen besteht hier kein Unterschied und ich glaube, aus praktischen Gründen ist es empfehlenswert, die Patienten die vorgeschriebene Dosis am Morgen einnehmen zu lassen.

Die Untersuchungen über die Anwendbarkeit der Thyroninderivate in der Behandlung der Hypercholesterinämie sind noch nicht endgültig abgeschlossen. Die mitgeteilten Beobachtungen sollen einen Beitrag zu diesen Untersuchungen darstellen.

Literatur

1. Boyd, G. S., and M. F. Oliver: J. Endocr. 21, 25—32 (1960).
2. — J. Atheroscler. Res. 1, 26—35 (1961).
3. —, and M. F. Oliver: Brit. med. Bull. 16, 138 (1960).
4. Chiu, G. C.: Arch. intern. Med. 108, 717 (1961).
5. Love V. Logan: Arch. intern. Med. 108, 833 (1961).
6. Mantz O. R.: Med. Welt 24, 1382—1383 (1962).
7. Schindler H.: Med. Klin. 44 (1866—1868).
8. Owen W. R., J. C. Owens and W. B. Neely: Angiology 13, 75 (1962).
9. Davis O., N. Sloan, Ch. Beck, M. Bergal: Méd. et Hyg. (Genève) 19, 455—458 (1961).
10. Owen W. R., J. C. Owens and W. B. Neely: J. Amer. med. Ass. 178, 1036 (1961).

Diskussion

H. W. Bansi (Hamburg):

Alle Thyroninderivate zeigen Dosis-abhängig eine gewisse Dissoziation zwischen der stoffwechselsteigernden und der den Cholesterinspiegel senkenden Wirkung. Bei den echten Hypercholesterinämien, die man mit Zöllner streng von den vorübergehend meist alimentär bedingten geringgradigen Erhöhungen des Serumcholesterins abtrennen sollte, werden die Cholesterinwerte unter der Therapie um etwa 100 mg/100 cm³ gedrückt. Dabei besteht eine gewisse Abhängigkeit vom Ausgangswert. Das Serumcholesterin steigt nach Absetzen der Hormonanaloge schnell wieder an. Man muß leider sagen, daß bisher alle Thyroxinanaloge und metaboliten für die Therapie nicht voll geeignet sind. Dies trifft meiner Ansicht nach auch auf das D-Thyroxin in der Dosis 2—6 mg zu, da auch trotz geringer Stoffwechselwirkung leicht Herzbeschwerden (Angina pectoris-Anfälle) auftreten.

J. Hoeflmayr:

1. Nach Untersuchungen und Beobachtungen von Bernheim et al. werden nicht nur alimentäre sondern auch essentielle Hypercholesterinämien mit ausgeprägter Xanthomatosis günstig beeinflußt. Die Xanthome bildeten sich zurück.

2. Die Beimengung von L-Thyroxin beträgt nach Angaben des Herstellers und Untersuchungen von Owen 2%.

Über den Einfluß bestimmter Serumeiweißfraktionen auf endokrine Vorgänge

Von

H. BENNHOLD, Tübingen

Mit 1 Abbildung

Die *Transportvorgänge* im menschlichen Körper werden durch eine aus *drei Komponenten* bestehende Apparatur geregelt. Das *Herz* steuert als Pumpwerk die *Motorik* bei; die *Vasomotoren* sorgen für eine durch zahlreiche Regulationsmechanismen und Regelkreise gesicherte *rationelle Verteilung des Minutenvolumens* im riesenhaften Gebiet der Kreislaufperipherie. Das „*Transportmilieu*" trägt als dritte Komponente der Transportapparatur wesentliches zu der *lokalen Abgabedosierung* an die einzelnen Zellen und Gewebselemente bei (BENNHOLD 1930, 1932, 1938, 1960—1963). Unter Transportmilieu ist ein bewegtes Milieu zu verstehen, in welchem — über die Summe der zu transportierenden Stoffe hinausgehend — auch Substanzen oder biologische Einheiten enthalten sind, welche dem Transportvorgang *als solchen* dienen, ohne daß sie dem Transportgut selbst zuzurechnen sind. In erster Linie sind also dem Transportmilieu zuzurechnen die *Erythrocyten*, wahrscheinlich auch die Leukocyten, ferner die *Blutplättchen* und in besonders großem Umfang die *Serumeiweißkörper*. Ihre riesengroße Grenzfläche und ihre in den letzten 3 Jahrzehnten festgestellte Aufteilung in vielen Fraktionen (nach SCHULTZE etwa 75) eröffnen besonders ausgedehnte Möglichkeiten für differenzierte Vehikelfunktionen (BENNHOLD 1929, 1930, 1932, 1938, 1960—1963).

In Abb. 1 sind in einem Elektrophoreseschema die Bindungsplätze, welche verschiedene körpereigene und körperfremde Substanzen besetzen, eingezeichnet (Lit. vgl. BENNHOLD und OTT 1961—1963). Sehr selten finden sich transportierte Stoffe in physiologischen Konzentrationen nur in *einem* Zustand, wie z. B. das Eisen, welches normalerweise ausschließlich an Transferrin (Siderophilin) gebunden zirkuliert (SCHADE 1946, LAURELL 1947). Bei den meisten Stoffen des Transportgutes bestehen Gleichgewichtszustände zwischen einer fixen und einer gebundenen Komponente (z. B. bei Phenolrot) oder auch Gleichgewichtszustände zwischen Komponenten, welche an ein oder zwei oder noch mehr Eiweißfraktionen — oftmals mit verschiedenen Bindungsintensitäten — haften. Die Bindung des Wassers an die hydrophilen Bluteiweißkörper und die Bindung des Sauerstoffs an das Hämoglobin der Erythrocyten, welcher sich dabei im Gleichgewichtszustand mit dem im Plasma gelösten Sauerstoff befindet, sind klassische, längst bekannte Beispiele. Analoge Vehikelfunktionen der Serumproteine haben sich nun für Farbstoffe, für Medikamente (z. B. Sulfonamide und Antibiotika), für Gallenfarbstoff, für Vitamine und für zahlreiche Metalle ergeben [Lit. vgl. BENNHOLD und OTT (1961)]. Es ließ sich auch zeigen, daß spezifische Insuffizienzen des Transportmilieus zur Entstehung schwerer Krankheiten entscheidend beitragen können [Kern-Ikterus der Frühgeburten, Wilsonsche Krankheit, primäre Hämochromatose (BENNHOLD 1960 u. 1963)].

Besonderes Interesse verdienen der Transport der Hormone und die Bindungen, welche sie dabei mit Serumeiweißfraktionen eingehen. Vom *Thyroxin* weiß man seit längerer Zeit, daß es am stärksten von α-Globulinen (zwischen α_1 und α_2)

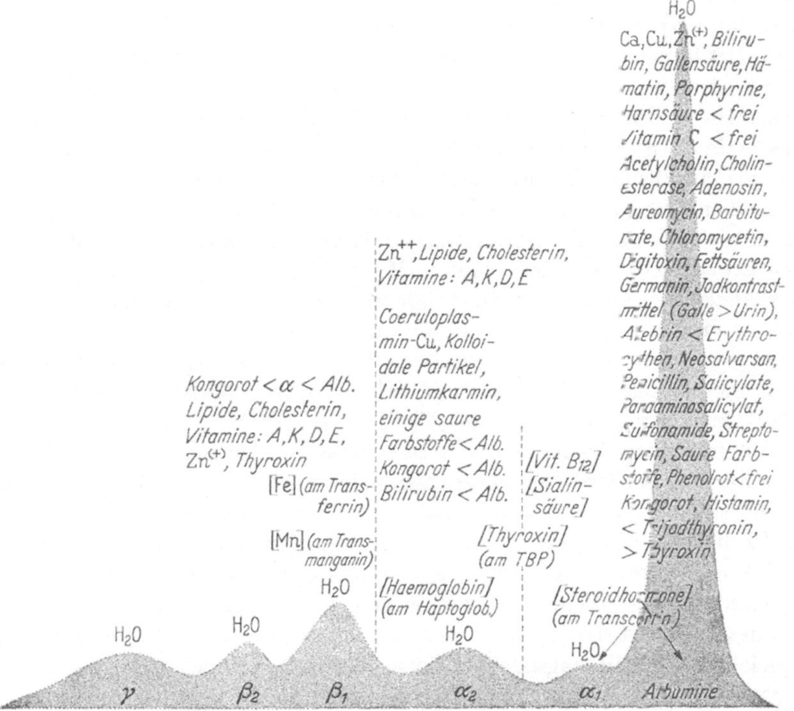

Abb. 1. Proteinbindung im Blutplasma nach hauptsächlichen Haftpunkten angeordnet. Die eingezeichneten Bindungen sind schematisch aufzufassen; viele Stoffe weisen in ihrer Bindung Gleichgewichtszustände, z. B. zu ungebundenen oder zu an bestimmte Globulinfraktionen gebundenen Anteilen auf. Am deutlichsten ist dies bei der Bindung des Wassers an allen Serumproteinfraktionen festzustellen. Bei anderen Substanzen besteht nur ein Bindungsgleichgewicht zwischen freien und an Albumin gebundenen Anteilen in Abhängigkeit von der im Serum vorhandenen oder zum Serum zugesetzten Substanzmenge. Bei wieder anderen Stoffen besteht ein Bindungsgleichgewicht zwischen Albuminen und α-Globulinen oder auch zu α- sowie β-Globulinen. In solchen Fällen wurde im obigen Schema meistens nur das hauptsächliche Trägerprotein eingezeichnet. Nur bei einzelnen besonders prägnanten Beispielen (Vitamin C, Harnsäure, Atebrin, Kongorot, Bilirubin) wurde das Gefälle zu freien Anteilen oder zu Anteilen, welche an andere Blutproteine gebunden sind, angegeben. So z. B. Harnsäure: Albumin < frei; Vitamin C: Albumin < frei; Atebrin: Albumin < Erythrocyten; Kongorot: Albumin > α-Globulin > β-Globulin; Phenolrot: Albumin < frei; Bilirubin: Albumin > α- > β-Globulin (im Vollserum); Zink: fest am α_1 und α_2, lockerer am Albumin und am β-Globulin (+) (Hund). Die mit eckigen Klammern eingefaßten Substanzen sind solche, von denen bekannt ist, daß sie nur an einer eng begrenzten Teilfraktion haften, welche im elektrischen Feld im Raum der α_1-, α_2-, β_1- oder β_2-Globuline wandert: z. B. das Vitamin B₁₂-bindende Globulin, welches im Rahmen der α_1-Glucoproteide wandert und dabei wahrscheinlich nur etwa 0,003% der α-Globuline ausmacht (vgl. Klin. Wschr. *1963*, S. 111)

gebunden wird (GORDON 1952, LARSON 1952, ROBBINS 1952, WINZLER 1952); außerdem geht es auch noch weniger feste Bindungen mit Präalbumin (ALY 1958, INGBAR 1958) und Albumin ein. Beide Komponenten stehen im Gleichgewichtszustand zueinander.

Die Oestrogene haften fast nur am Albumin und nur zu ganz geringen Anteilen auch an anderen Serumeiweißkörpern (BRUNELLI 1935, WEST 1951, ROTHCHILD 1952, ANTONIADES 1957, BISCHOFF 1957 u. 1958, SANDBERG u. Mitarb. 1957), in

etwas geringerem Maße bevorzugen *Progesteron* (WESTPHAL 1955 u. 1957, ANTO-
NIADES 1957) und *Testosteron* (WEST 1951, ROTHCHILD 1952, ANTONIADES 1957)
die Albumine gegenüber den α-Globulinen (WESTPHAL 1955 u. 1957, DAUGHADAY
1960). Im Gegensatz dazu haftet *Cortisol* mit großer Intensität an einem wahr-
scheinlich sehr kleinen Teil der α-Globuline, welcher von DAUGHADAY u. Mitarb.
(1958, 1959, 1961, 1962) als *C. B. G.* ("Cortisol Binding Globulin") und von
SANDBERG und SLAUNWHITE (1959) als Transcortin bezeichnet wird. DAUG-
HADAY (1960) schätzt den Transcortingehalt auf etwa 3 mg in 100 ml Plasma.
Corticosterone in hohen Konzentrationen können Cortisol aus dieser Bindung am
Transcortin verdrängen. *Aldosteron* haftet offenbar ebenfalls am intensivsten am
Transcortin (SANDBERG mit CARTER 1960, MEYER 1961), sehr viel schwächer am
Albumin; aus seiner Transcortin-Bindung wird es jedoch schon von relativ
kleinen Konzentrationen Cortisol verdrängt. *Spirolacton*, ein weitgehend antago-
nistisch wirkender Stoff, verdrängt erst in hohen Konzentrationen Aldosteron aus
seinen Eiweißbindungen (DAVIDSON u. Mitarb. 1962). Verhältnismäßig leicht wird
die an Albumin gebundene Cortisolkomponente von Oestrogenen und in geringerem
Maß von Progesteron und Testosteron aus dieser Bindung verdrängt. Auch die
Erythrocyten adsorbieren offenbar etwa 25% des gesamten, im Transportmilieu
enthaltenen Cortisols; die Glucoronidverbindungen befinden sich demgegenüber
zu 100% im Plasma (MIGEON 1959, VERMEULEN 1961).

Bei Betrachtung des Elektrophoreseschemas mit den eingetragenen Bindungs-
plätzen der verschiedenen zu transportierenden Stoffe muß die Frage auftauchen,
ob nicht viel häufiger, als oben ausgeführt, *Bindungskonkurrenzen* zu erwarten
sind. Es liegen bisher nur wenige Untersuchungen zu diesen Problemen vor.
Salicylsäure verdrängt in vitro *Thyroxin* aus der *Präalbuminbindung* (AUSTEN
1958, CHRISTENSEN 1959, WOLFF u. Mitarb. 1961) und führt in vivo zu einem
Abfall des PBI und des EOIP. Das stoffwechselsteigernde *2,4-Dinitrophenol* hat
den gleichen Verdrängungseffekt (WOLFF 1950, GOLDBERG 1955, CASTOR 1956,
CHRISTENSEN 1959, WOLFF 1961). Im Gegensatz hierzu wird das Thyroxin durch
Diphenylhydantoin aus seiner *α-Globulinbindung* verdrängt (OPPENHEIMER 1961);
ebenso durch DL-*Tetrachlorothyronine*. Letzteres kann in höheren Konzentrationen
sogar zusätzlich die *Thyroxinplätze im Präalbumin* besetzen. *Methylorange* und
Thiocyanate können *Testosteron* aus seiner Albuminbindung verdrängen (EIK-NES
1954). *Zinkionen* verdrängen Cortisol und Testosteron aus seiner Albuminbindung
(SLAUNWHITE in ANTONIADES 1960).

Die Wechselwirkung zwischen Bluteiweiß und Hormonen scheint sich nun,
wie in den letzten Jahren gefunden wurde, in beiden Richtungen auswirken zu
können. Einmal, wie wir oben sahen, in dem Sinne, daß die Bluteiweißkörper
durch Bindungen von Hormonen deren Aktivität und lokale Abgabe aus dem
Blute beeinflussen; andererseits kennen wir neuerdings auch Beobachtungen,
welche eine *Beeinflussung der Zusammensetzung des Bluteiweißbildes durch bestimmte Hormone* aufzeigen. Die *Oestrogene*, in hohen Dosen appliziert, führen
schon nach 3—7 Tagen zu einem starken *Anstieg von Transcortin* (MILLS u. BARTTER
1959, SANDBERG u. CARTER 1960), und zwar erfolgt dieser Transcortinanstieg
bereits *vor* dem Cortisolanstieg. Auch bei Addison-Patienten läßt sich dieser
Transcortinanstieg auf diese Weise auslösen. Beides weist darauf hin, daß der
Anstieg des Transcortinspiegels auch unabhängig von einer Erhöhung des Cortisol-

spiegels erzeugt werden kann. Der gleiche Transcortinanstieg findet sich regelmäßig in der *Schwangerschaft*; im fetalen Blut ist keine Erhöhung des Transcortinspiegels festzustellen. Im Blut der Mutter ist die Halbwertszeit für Cortisol verlängert, die Glucuronisierung des Cortisols ist verlangsamt. Post partum sinkt der Transcortinspiegel vom 5. Tage ab bis zur 7. Woche wieder allmählich zur Norm ab (DAUGHADAY und MARITZ 1960). *Aldosteron* scheint in der Schwangerschaft nicht stärker an Serumeiweiß gebunden zu sein.

In ähnlicher Weise steigert *Oestrogen-Applikation* auch die *Thyroxinbindungsfähigkeit* der α-Globuline (ENGSTROM 1954, DOWLING 1958); diese Bindungsfähigkeit ist in ähnlicher Weise temperaturabhängig wie die des Transcortins; sie ist bei 4° am stärksten und fällt bis 37° deutlich ab. Gegen eine daraus evtl. zu vermutende Identität des Transcortins mit dem TBG (Thyroxine Binding Globulin) spricht jedoch, daß BEISEL u. Mitarb. 1962 im Blute eines Indonesiers völliges Fehlen des TBG bei normaler Cortisolbindung feststellen konnten. Auch in der Schwangerschaft steigt das TBG an (DOWLING 1956).

Nach Untersuchungen von DOE und ZINNEMANN (1960) scheint ein übermäßig hoher Cortisolspiegel nur dann zu einem *Cushing-Syndrom* zu führen, wenn große Mengen *freien* Cortisols im Blut kreisen. Dieses kommt in der Schwangerschaft und bei Oestrogenkuren (z. B. bei Patienten mit Prostatacarcinom) *durch die gleichzeitig eintretende Transcortinvermehrung* nicht zustande. Diese von mehreren Seiten bestätigten Beobachtungen lassen eine vor Jahren empfohlene *Behandlung des M. Cushing* unter einem neuen Aspekt plausibel erscheinen. Zuerst LAQUEUR und DEELEN (1936), später DUNN (1938) empfahlen 1936 und 1938 für die Beobachtung des M. Cushing eine Kur mit Oestrogenen, wobei sie von der Vorstellung ausgingen, daß durch das periphere Eierstockshormon die Aktivität der Hypophyse – auch betreffs der ACTH-Abgabe – rückwirkend gedrosselt würde. MEYLER und HOMMES (1937) sowie SANSONE (1937) berichteten ebenfalls über gewisse Erfolge bei Progynonbehandlung eines M. Cushing.

Daß man mit dieser Behandlung einen überraschenden Heilerfolg erzielen kann, sah ich (BENNHOLD 1941) in den Jahren 1939—1941 bei einer 31 jährigen Patientin, die nach einem 2. Partus mit typischer Symptomatik erkrankte.

Eine Hypophysenbestrahlung ergab keine Besserung und auch die Verabreichung von Stilbenen (2 mal wöchentlich 3 mg Oestrostilben intramuskulär (7. 6. 1939—10. 7. 1939) hatte zunächst keinerlei Erfolg. Deshalb ging ich Mitte Juli 1939 zu einem Oestradiolester über und gab 2 mal wöchentlich je 5 mg (50000 E) Progynon B intramuskulär. Nach 8 Injektionen deutliche subjektive Besserung; es traten wieder unregelmäßige Mensesblutungen auf, und im Februar 1941 waren keine Cushing-Symptome mehr nachweisbar.

8 Jahre später, nachdem ich die Patientin wegen meiner Übersiedlung nach Tübingen aus den Augen verloren hatte, bekam sie ein offenbar schweres, von JORES beobachtetes Rezidiv; anläßlich einer explorativen Laparotomie erlitt sie eine Lungenembolie, der sie erlag. Eine Krankengeschichte war durch die kriegerischen Ereignisse nicht mehr vorhanden. Ob wieder ein Versuch mit Progynon gemacht worden war, ließ sich deshalb leider nicht mehr feststellen.

Durch die Untersuchungen von SELYE (1942), der im Tierversuch nach Oestron keinerlei Atrophie der Nebennierenrinde, sondern eher sogar eine Vergrößerung derselben feststellen konnte, ist heute erwiesen, daß Oestrogene keinerlei Rückkoppelungseffekt auf die Hypophyse ausüben im Sinne einer verminderten ACTH-Ausschüttung. In gleiche Richtung zu deuten sind Metapironversuche von GÖBEL.

Nachdem Doe und Zinnemann (1960) gezeigt haben, daß bei M. Cushing nur die starke Erhöhung des *freien* Cortisols ausschlaggebend für das Zustandekommen des Krankheitsbildes ist und nachdem die ausgesprochene Transcortinvermehrung durch Oestrogene bewiesen ist, erscheint es überwiegend wahrscheinlich, daß der therapeutische Effekt des Oestrogens in unserem Falle auf die vermehrte Bindung des pathologisch erhöhten *freien* Cortisols im Blut der Cushing-Patientin zurückzuführen ist.

Diese Beobachtungen zeigen wohl zum ersten Mal, daß durch ein Hormon über eine therapeutisch erzielte Vermehrung eines spezifischen Globulinvehikels ein mindestens längere Zeit anhaltender Heileffekt erzielt werden kann.

Zweck dieser Darlegungen war es, auf die klinisch wichtigen Wechselwirkungen von Hormonen und Plasmaeiweißkörpern hinzuweisen. Bestimmte Bluteiweißkörper können für den Transport und für die dosierte lokale Abgabe der Hormone von großer Bedeutung sein. Andererseits können manche Hormone – z. B. die Oestrogene – erheblichen Einfluß auf den Spiegel bestimmter Plasmaeiweißkörper haben (z. B. auf Transcortin und Thyroxinbindendes Globulin). Diese Befunde können für die Genese bestimmter endokriner Erkrankungen und für deren Beeinflussung von Bedeutung sein.

Literatur

Albright, E. C., F. C. Larson and W. P. Deiss: Proc. Soc. exp. Biol. (N. Y.) 84, 240 (1953).

Aly, F. W., u. K. H. Niederhellmann: Klin. Wschr. 36, 954 (1958).

Antoniades, H. N.: Hormones in Human Plasma. Boston 1960.

— J. W. McArthur, R. B. Pennell, F. M. Ingersoll, H. Ulfelder and J. L. Oncley: Amer. J. Physiol. 189, 445 (1957).

Austen, F. K., M. E. Rubini, W. H. Meroney and J. Wolff: J. clin. Invest. 37, 1131 (1958).

Beisel, V. R., K. Zainal, S. Hane, V. C. Di Raimondo and P. H. Forsham: J. clin. Endocr. 22, 1165 (1962).

Bennhold, H.: Wien. Arch. inn. Med. 35, 101 (1941).

— Verh. dtsch. Ges. inn. Med. 32, 353 (1930).

— Ergebn. inn. Med. Kinderheilk. 42, 273 (1932).

— Klin. Wschr. 38, 345 (1960).

— Klin. Wschr. 41, 109 (1963).

— E. Kylin u. St. Rusznyak: Die Eiweißkörper des Blutplasmas. Dresden: Theodor Steinkopff 1938.

—, u. H. Ott: Handbuch der allg. Pathologie v. Büchner, Letterer und Roulet, Bd. V 1 S. 166 ff. Berlin-Göttingen-Heidelberg: Springer-Verlag 1961.

Bischoff, F., and R. D. Stauffer: Amer. J. Physiol. 191, 313 (1957).

— J. G. Turner jr. and G. Bryson: Amer. J. Physiol. 195, 81 (1958).

Brunelli, B.: Arch. int. Pharmacodyn. 49, 262 (1935).

Castor, C. W., and W. Beierwaltes: J. clin. Endocr. 16, 1026 (1956).

Christensen, L. K.: Nature (Lond.) 183, 1189 (1959).

Daughaday, W. H.: J. clin. Invest. 35, 1428 (1956).

— J. clin. Invest. 36, 881 (1957).

— J. clin. Invest. 37, 519 (1958).

— Arch. intern. Med. 101, 286 (1958).

— Physiol. Rev. 39, No. 4, 286 (1959).

— In: Antoniades: Hormones in Human Plasma, S. 495. Boston 1960.

— R. E. Adler, I. Kozak Mariz and D. C. Rasinski: J. clin. Endocr. 22, 704 (1962).

—, and I. Kozak Mariz: Biological Activities of Steroids in Relation to Cancer. New York: Academic Press Inc. 1960.

— Metabolism 10, 936 (1961).

DAVIDSON, E. T., F. DE VENUTO and U. WESTPHAL: Endocrinology 71, 893 (1962).
DOE, R. P., H. H. ZINNEMAN, E. E. FLINK and R. A. ULSTROM: J. clin. Endocr. 20, 11 (1960).
DOWLING, J. T., N. FREINKEL and S. H. INGBAR: J. clin. Endocr. 16, 280 (1956).
— Progr. American Goiter Association, p. 11 (1958).
DUNN, H. W.: Endocrinology 22, 374 (1938).
EIK-NES, K., J. A. SCHELLMAN, R. LUMRY and L. T. SAMUELS: J. biol Chem. 206, 411 (1954).
ENGSTROM, W. W., and B. MARKARDT: J. clin. Endocr. 14, 215 (1954).
GOLDBERG, R. C., J. WOLFF and R. D. GREEP: Endocrinology 56, 560 (1955).
GORDON, A. H., J. GROSS, D. O'CONNOR and R. PITT-RIVERS: Nature (Lond.) 169, 19 (1952).
INGBAR, S. H.: Endocrinology 63, 256 (1958).
KALLEE, E.: Diskussionsbemerkung zum Vortrag von N. LANG u. K. H. GILLICH. In: Radio-
     aktive Isotope in Klinik und Forschung, Bd. 4, S. 378. München und Berlin: Urban
     & Schwarzenberg 1960.
LAQUEUR, E., u. TH. DEELEN: Ned. T. Geneesk. 1936, 743.
LARSON, F., W. P. DEISS and E. C. ALBRIGHT: Science 115, 626 (1952).
LAURELL, C. B.: Acta physiol. scand. 14, 1 (1947).
LEMARCHAND-BÉRAUD, A. VANOTTI et M. R. JEANNERET: Schweiz. med. Wschr. 93, 1, 7 (1963).
MEYER, CH. J., D. S. LAYNE, J. F. TAIT and G. PINCUSS: J. clin. Invest. 40, 1663 (1961).
MEYLER, L., u. M. HOMMES: Acta med. scand. 93, 253 (1937).
MIGEON, C. J., B. LAWRENCE, J. BERTRAND and H. HOLMAN: J. clin. Endocr. 19, No. 11,
     1411 (1959).
OPPENHEIMER, J. H., L. V. FISHER, K. M. NELSON and J. W. JAILER: J. clin. Endocr. 21,
     252 (1961).
ROBBINS, J., and J. E. RALL: J. clin. Invest. 34, 1331 (1955).
— J. clin. Invest. 36, S. 23 (1957).
— Recent Progr. in Hormone Research. Vol. 13, p. 161. New York: Academic Press Inc.1957.
— — D. V. BECKER and R. W. RAWSON: J. clin. Endocr. 12, 856 (1952).
— — and M. L. PETERMANN: J. clin. Invest. 36, 1333 (1957).
ROTHCHILD, J.: Endocrinology 50, 583 (1952).
SANDBERG, A. A., W. R. SLAUNWHITE and H. N. ANTONIADES: In: G. PINCUS (ed.) Recent
     Progr. Hormone Res. 13, 209 (1957).
— — J. clin. Invest. 38, 1290 (1959).
— W. R. SLAUNWHITE and A. C. CARTER: J. clin. Invest. 39, 1914 (1960).
SANSONE, L.: Arch. Soc. med. 64, 681 (1937).
SCHADE, A. L., and L. CAROLINE: Science 104, 340 (1946).
SELYE, A.: J. Pharmacol. exp. Ther. 75, 308 (1942).
SLAUNWHITE, W. R.: In: Antoniades: Hormones in Human Plasma, S. 478ff. Boston 1960.
SLAUNWHITE, W. R. JR., A. A. SANDBERG and H. N. ANTONIADES: In preparation.
VERMEULEN, A.: Acta Endocr. 37, 348 (1961).
WEST, C. D., F. H. TYLER, H. BROWN and L. T. SAMUELS: J. clin. Endocr. 11, 897 (1951).
WESTPHAL, U.: Endocrinology 57, 456 (1955).
— Arch. Biochem. 66, 71 (1957).
WINZLER, R. J., and S. R. NOTRICA: Fed. Proc. 11, 312 (1952).
WOLFF, J., L. RUBIN and J. L. CHAIKOFF: J. Pharmocol. exp. Ther. 98, 45 (1950).
— M. E. STANDAERT and J. E. RALL: J. clin. Invest. 40, 1373 (1961).

Diskussion

P. GÖBEL (Tübingen).

Zur Klärung der Frage, ob die von BENNHOLD soeben beschriebene Besserung eines Cushing-Syndroms nach Oestradiolverabreichung Folge einer hierdurch verursachten Bremsung der ACTH-Produktion des HVL sein könnte, haben wir Untersuchungen mit dem Metopiron-Test durchgeführt (Abb. 1).

Die Darstellung zeigt:

Nach Ausschüttung von ACTH durch den Hypophysenvorderlappen läuft die Synthese der Nebennierenrindenhormone an. Das Ausscheidungsprodukt des dabei im wesentlichen gebildeten Cortisol erfaßt man am besten als Porter-Silber-Chromogen (Reaktion der an C 17 befindlichen Seitenkette mit Phenylhydrazin in Schwefelsäure) im Urin. Die erste Säule zeigt die Ausscheidung bei 8 gesunden Versuchspersonen und die Schwankungsbreite. Nach Verabfolgung von exogenem ACTH als i.v.-Infusion steigt die Ausscheidung der Porter-Silber-Chromogene im Durchschnitt auf etwa das 3—4fache der Ausgangswerte an (zweite Säule). Die Ausscheidung der Porter-Silber-Chromogene bei einer Patientin mit Morbus Cushing (3. Säule) liegt etwa in der gleichen Größenordnung, da hier eine vermehrte ACTH-Produktion besteht.

Nach Gabe von Metopiron und Blockierung der C 11-Hydroxylase kann kein bzw. nur ganz wenig Cortisol gebildet werden. Danach fällt die „Cortisol-Bremse" weg, es kommt eine

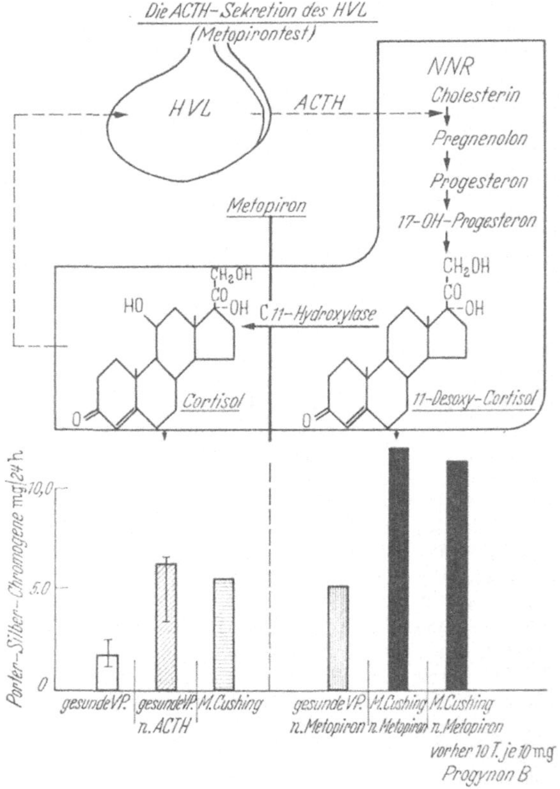

Abb. 1

vermehrte endogene ACTH-Sekretion in Gang. Die Porter-Silber-Chromogene im Urin steigen bei Gesunden etwa einem ACTH-Test entsprechend an, wie die 4. Säule zeigt. Dabei handelt es sich allerdings jetzt nicht um Ausscheidungsprodukte von Cortisol, sondern, da ja die C 11-Hydroxylierung blockiert ist, von 11-Desoxy-Cortisol (Reichsteins Compound S). Beim Morbus Cushing steigt die Ausscheidung der Porter-Silber-Chromogene auf etwa das Doppelte der Norm an (Säule 5). Man kann daraus schließen, daß die Aktivität der Hypophyse bei der ACTH-Ausschüttung gegenüber einer gesunden Versuchsperson verdoppelt ist. Nach Gabe von Oestrogenen vor dem Metopiron-Test ergibt sich keine wesentliche Veränderung (Säule 6). Die endogene ACTH-Produktion des Morbus Cushing ist also durch Oestrogene nicht zu beeinflussen.

Aus dem Pathologischen Institut der Universität Hamburg

Die primäre Atrophie der Nebennierenrinde

Von

J. KRACHT

Mit 2 Abbildungen

Die Einteilung der Nebennierenrindenatrophie in primäre und sekundäre Formen beruht auf einem für die gesamte glandotrop gesteuerte Peripherie gültigen Prinzip, wonach der Organausfall ursächlich entweder im glandotropen Erfolgsorgan selbst lokalisiert oder durch ein Defizit an adäquatem Tropin bedingt ist. Pathologisch-anatomisch sind beide Varianten durch charakteristische Strukturänderungen unterschieden. Der primären Atrophie liegt stets ein numerischer Parenchymschwund zugrunde und sie ist irreversibel, während die sekundäre Form als Beispiel für eine einfache Atrophie gilt und deshalb auch durch corticotrope Impulse zur Norm rücktransformiert werden kann. Aus therapeutischen, regulativen und aus Gründen der Häufigkeit stehen derzeit Fragen über sekundäre Nebennierenrindenatrophie im Vordergrund des Interesses. Die primäre Rindenatrophie ist demgegenüber selten. Sie wird in erster Linie durch die bilaterale Nebennierentuberkulose repräsentiert, obwohl bereits TH. ADDISON auf andere Ursachen hingewiesen und in seiner Originalarbeit einen Fall mit vermutlich entzündlicher Atrophie mitgeteilt hatte. Hierfür sind später Begriffe wie primäre Atrophie, idiopathische oder genuine Schrumpfnebenniere, cytotoxische Atrophie, adrenocortical contraction u. a. geprägt worden. Während früher die Tuberkulose Hauptursache des M. Addison war und die sog. idiopathische Atrophie eine deutlich niedrigere Frequenz aufwies, liegen die Verhältnisse heute eher umgekehrt, wie dies aus größeren Sammelstatistiken und aus dem Material unseres Instituts hervorgeht. Wir stellten fest, daß der prozentuale Anteil cytotoxischer Rindenatrophien an der Summe aller Fälle von Nebennierentuberkulose und primärer Atrophie im Laufe der letzten Jahrzehnte ständig gestiegen ist (1923–1932 11%, 1933–1942 33%, 1943–1952 50%, 1953–1962 67%). Die Gründe hierfür liegen vor allem im allgemeinen Rückgang der Tuberkulose und sind weniger in einer echten Zunahme der cytotoxischen Atrophie zu suchen. Gegenüber diesen beiden Schwerpunkten des primären Rindenschwundes sind andere Ursachen chronischer primärer Nebennierenrindeninsuffizienz bei uns von untergeordneter Bedeutung (Blastomykose, Coccidiomykose, Cryptococcose, Histoplasmose, Torulose, Infarktschrumpfnebenniere, Riesenzellengranulom, angeborene primäre Hypoplasie, Lymphogranulomatose, Echinococcus) oder sogar fraglich (Amyloidose, Tumormetastasen, Lues).

In diesem Zusammenhang sind folgende syndromartigen Varianten der primären Rindenatrophie zu erwähnen:

1. Thyreosuprarenaler Symptomenkomplex (Schmidt-Syndrom).

2. Idiopathischer Hypoparathyreoidismus, Nebennierenrindenatrophie und Moniliasis (SUTPHIN u. Mitarb. u. a.).

Das Substrat der cytotoxischen Nebennierenrindenatrophie besteht in einem progredienten diffusen entzündlich-degenerativen Schwund des Rindengewebes, der bis zur völligen Entrindung reicht. Das Mark bleibt dagegen stets intakt und ist allenfalls mit lockeren Rundzellinfiltraten durchsetzt. Formalgenetisch ist ein Initialstadium mit Parenchymschwund und entzündlicher Infiltration von einem Spätstadium zu unterscheiden, in dem der bindegewebige Ersatz und unter Umständen auch knotige Regenerate im Vordergrund stehen. Während für die floride Phase die Gleichmäßigkeit der Strukturänderungen kennzeichnend ist und damit die Abgrenzung gegenüber primären Atrophien anderer Genese erleichtert, wird die Beurteilung der Spätstadien im Hinblick auf die auch bei tuberkulöser Schrumpfnebenniere oder nach Gefäßverschluß vorkommenden Rindenregenerate erschwert. Trotzdem ist das Substrat der cytotoxischen Atrophie so charakteristisch, daß unter Zugrundelegung verschiedener Kriterien eine Abgrenzung sowohl von der sekundären Atrophie als auch von primären Unterfunktionszuständen anderer Genese in der Regel möglich sein sollte (WIEBE).

Zur Ätiologie sind anfänglich besonders die Lues und später infektiös-toxische Schädigungen angeschuldigt worden. HEDINGER wie FASSBENDER nehmen Endzustände verschiedener degenerativer und entzündlicher Schädigungen bzw. sogar narbige Restzustände von Blutungen an. Unter immunopathologischen Gesichtspunkten wurde ein von KOVACS postuliertes selektives Cytotoxin aktualisiert, zumal Schilddrüsenveränderungen vom Typ der Struma lymphomatosa bei cytotoxischer Atrophie nicht selten sind und auch im eigenen Material in etwa zwei Drittel der Fälle gefunden wurden. Der Nachweis von gegen Nebenniere gerichteten Antikörpern oder von Nebennieren- und Schilddrüsenantikörpern (ANDERSON u. Mitarb., MEAD, BLIZZARD u. Mitarb.) läßt daran denken, daß der cytotoxischen Atrophie ähnlich wie der chronischen Thyreoiditis immunpathologische Vorgänge nach Art eines Autoaggressionsschadens zugrunde liegen könnten. Es war daher naheliegend, die sich hieraus ergebenden Fragestellungen tierexperimentell anzugehen, zumal bisher experimentelle Modelle für eine primäre Nebennierenrindenatrophie mit Ausnahme des Adrenostaticums DDD fehlen.

Mit autologen und homologen Nebennierenhomogenaten in FREUNDS Adjuvans erzielten wir (KRACHT, FISCHER u. MÖBIUS) bei Meerschweinchen ähnlich wie COLOVER und GLYNN sowie STEINER u. Mitarb. im Bereich der Mark-Rinden-Grenze beginnende und sich später über die Rinde herdförmig und diffus ausbreitende Infiltrate aus histiocytären, lymphoreticulären und plasmacytoiden Elementen, die das Parencham aufsplittern, inselförmig einschließen und schließlich zum Schwund bringen. Das Mark und die inneren Rindenschichten sind dabei durchschnittlich stärker befallen als die äußere Rinde. Der Parenchymausfall betrug bis zu einer Beobachtungszeit von 150 Tagen maximal 40%, durchschnittlich etwa 20%. Eine Rindenatrophie wurde nicht erzielt, ebenso fehlten Rindenregenerate. Die Unterschiede zur cytotoxischen Atrophie des Menschen liegen

a) in dem bevorzugten Befall von Mark und innerer Rinde, während bei cytotoxischer Atrophie die Rinde gleichmäßig befallen ist und das Mark so gut wie unverändert bleibt,

b) im Ausbleiben einer Rindenatrophie im Tierexperiment (Abb. 1).

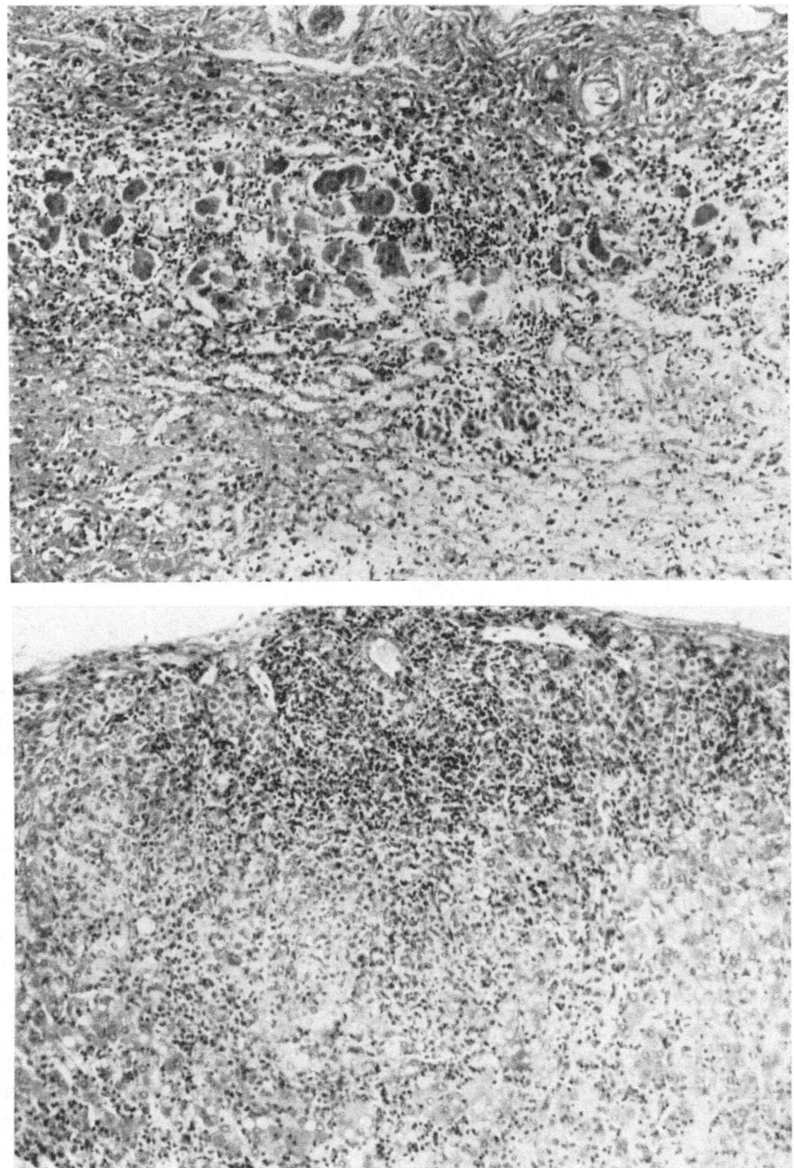

Abb. 1. *Oben:* Cytotoxische Schrumpfnebenniere (646/55, ♀ 64 Jahre). Verdämmerndes Rindenrestgewebe, lockere Rundzellinfiltrate und bindegewebiger Ersatz unter der fibrös verdickten Kapsel. *Unten:* Isoimmunoadrenalitis beim Meerschweinchen 65 Tage nach viermaliger Applikation von je 30 mg homologem Nebennierenhomogenat in FREUNDs Adjuvans complete, im Verlauf von 4 Wochen. Fleckförmige und diffuse lympho-histiocytäre Infiltration. Aufsplitterung und partielle Degeneration des Rindenparenchyms. H-E, Vergrößerung 130fach

Hierfür könnten Speciesunterschiede und im speziellen Fall auch die Angio-
architektonik der Meerschweinchennebenniere mit einer unterschiedlichen Reaktionsbereitschaft des aktiven Mesenchyms im Reticularis-Markkomplex einerseits
und in der Außenzone andererseits verantwortlich sein. Zur Deutung dieser
organspezifischen und weder durch Nebennierenhomogenat noch durch Freunds
Adjuvans allein erzielbaren Veränderungen nehmen wir einen durch Nebennieren-
antikörper ausgelöste und durch Freunds Adjuvans potenzierte immunopathische
Reaktion an, zumal uns serologisch im Antiglobulinkonsumptionstest und im

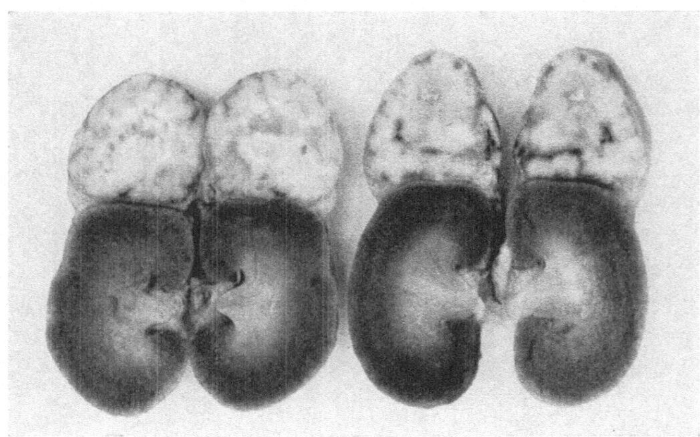

Abb. 2. Verkäste Nebennierentuberkulose der Ratte bds. 17 Mon. nach i.v. Infektion mit einem aviären Myco-
bakterienstamm aus tuberkulösem Material vom Schwein (Nr. 3751)

Boydentest der Nachweis von autoaggressiven Substanzen mit Autoantikörper-
charakter gelungen ist. Obwohl dieses Modell noch unvollkommen ist und trotz
mancher Parallelen auch trennende Kriterien gegenüber dem menschlichen
Krankheitsbild aufweist, ergeben sich Ansatzpunkte für die weitere Bearbeitung.
　　Alle Bemühungen zur Erzeugung eines der Nebennierentuberkulose des
Menschen vergleichbaren Substrats im Experiment waren bisher ergebnislos,
insbesondere durch Direktapplikation von Tuberkelbakterien in die Nebenniere.
Dieser Infektionsmodus ist einer i.v. Infektion vergleichbar und führt beim
Meerschweinchen zur generalisierten Tuberkulose. In Zusammenarbeit mit G.
Meissner stellten wir fest, daß für Hühner pathogene Mycobakterien aus tuber-
kulösem Material vom Schwein 12—18 Monate nach i.v. Infektion (5 mg) bei
Ratten Nebennierentuberkulose bewirken. Dabei ist die Nebenniere bevorzugt
befallen, während andere Organveränderungen vergleichsweise geringfügig sind
und sich möglicherweise erst im Rahmen einer Generalisation nach Verkäsung der
Nebennieren manifestieren. Die Veränderungen sind stets doppelseitig, beginnen
herdförmig in den inneren Rindenzonen oder an der Mark-Rinden-Grenze,
konfluieren später und treiben die Nebenniere bis auf ein Vielfaches ihrer normalen
Größe auf. Die Oberfläche ist fein- oder grobhöckerig beschaffen, die Schnittfläche
entweder homogen verkäst, kavernisiert oder gelegentlich auch fleckförmig ver-
kalkt (Abb. 2). Je nach Ausbreitung der Veränderungen ist das Mark-Rinden-
gewebe partiell erhalten oder ganz zerstört. Am längsten halten sich Glomerulosa

und äußere Fasciculata. Bei fortgeschrittener Zerstörung des Parenchyms können knotige Rindenregenerate auftreten, werden schließlich aber auch in die Verkäsung mit einbezogen. Während in lymphatischen Geweben (Milz, Lymphknoten) die epitheloidzellige Reaktion, in Lunge und Nieren dagegen gemischtförmige exsudativ-granulierende Veränderungen vorherrschen, verläuft die Nebennierentuberkulose vorwiegend parasitär. Es handelt sich z. T. um mit Kerntrümmern beladene reaktionslose Nekrosen, besonders in jenen Arealen, die unmittelbar an Rindengewebe angrenzen. Als besondere Reaktion werten wir eine in dieser Form nur in der Nebenniere auftretende und vielfach den Übergang zwischen Verkäsung und Rindenrestgeweben bildende Proliferation großer an Speicherzellen erinnernder mesenchymaler Zellen. Sie enthalten massenhaft Tuberkelbakterien. Im Rahmen der insgesamt spärlichen Ansätze zu einer Defektheilung bilden diese Zellen später Fasern, so daß schließlich ein sklerosiertes Bindegewebe entsteht. Die in Spätstadien mit 90–100% Parenchymausfall einhergehende experimentelle Nebennierentuberkulose der Ratte bietet wie Nebennierennekrosen nach Infektion mit Besnoitia jellisoni oder Histoplasma capsulatum beim Goldhamster (Frenkel) nicht nur die Möglichkeit, Beziehungen zwischen Erreger und Gewebssubstrat und die Modifikationen spezifisch entzündlicher Reaktionen durch steroidbildendes Gewebe, sondern auch andere inkretorische Regulationen bei experimentellem M. Addison zu verfolgen.

Literatur

Addison, T.: Lond. med. Gaz. **43**, 517 (1855); reprinted in Med. Classics **2**, 244 (1937).

Anderson, J. R., R. B. Goudie, K. G. Gray and G. C. Timburg: Lancet 1957 I, 1123.

Blizzard, R. M., R. W. Chandler, M. A. Kyle and W. Hung: Lancet 1962 II, 901.

Colover, J., and L. E. Glynn: Immunology **2**, 172 (1958).

Fassbender, H. G.: In: E. Kaufmann, Lehrbuch der speziellen pathologischen Anatomie, 11. u. 12. Aufl. Berlin: W. de Gruyter & Co. 1956.

Frenkel, J. K.: J. exp. Med. **103**, 375 (1956).

— In: H. D. Moon, The Adrenal Cortex. New York: P. B. Hoeber, Inc. 1961.

Hedinger, C.: In: A. Labhart, Klinik der inneren Sekretion. Berlin-Göttingen-Heidelberg: Springer-Verlag 1957.

Kovács, W.: Beitr. path. Anat. **79**, 213 (1928).

Kracht, J., K. Fischer u. G. Möbius: Verh. dtsch. Ges. Path. **46**, 152 (1962).

Mead, R. K.: New Engl. J. Med. **266**, 583 (1962).

Schmidt, M. B.: Verh. dtsch. Ges. Path. **21**, 212 (1926).

Steiner, J. W., B. Langer, D. L. Schatz and R. Volpe: J. exp. Med. **112**, 187 (1960).

Sutphin, A., F. Albright and D. J. McCune: J. clin. Endocr. **3**, 625 (1943).

Wiebe, V.: Inaug. Diss., Hamburg 1963.

Diskussion

E. F. Pfeiffer (Frankfurt):

40% NNR-Schwund bei Meerschweinchen sind ein durchaus befriedigendes Ergebnis, wenn man sich der Schwierigkeiten erinnert, die andere Autoren hatten, um pathologisch-anatomische Veränderungen hervorzurufen. Antikörper (humorale, zirkulierende) sind relativ leicht nachzuweisen, nicht dagegen Gewebsläsionen. Hinsichtlich der in vitro-Nachweise von Serumantikörpern erscheint überhaupt Vorsicht geboten. Wenn es sich wirklich um ein experimentelles Autoimmunleiden handelt, sollte der pathogene Antikörper an Zellen gebunden sein (vgl. isoallergische Encephalomyelitis, Autoimmunthyreoiditis und Nephritis-Nephrose). Vielleicht sollte man auch hier an Übertragungsversuche evtl. mit Hilfe der Parabiose denken, wie wir sie bei der nephrotoxischen Glomerulonephritis mit Nutzen verwandt haben [Übersicht E. F. Pfeiffer: Verh. Dtsch. Ges. inn. Med. (1962)].

J. Kracht:

Trotz der eindeutigen und teilweise recht ausgedehnten Rindenveränderungen nach Verabfolgung von Nebennierenhomogenaten in Freunds Adjuvans ist uns bisher der fluoroskopische Antikörpernachweis mit der indirekten Coons-Technik nicht gelungen. Dies dürfte teilweise auf dem Lipoidgehalt der Rinde beruhen, teilweise aber auch mit dem derartige Nachweise beeinträchtigenden steroidbildenden Substrat zusammenhängen.

Aus der Medizinischen Universitätsklinik Erlangen
(Direktor: Professor Dr. N. Henning)

Untersuchungen über Stoffwechseleffekte und die Wirkungsdauer von Metopiron

Von

L. Zicha, F. Scheiffarth, D. Bergner, A. Christmann und G. Poser

Mit 1 Abbildung

Das von Bencze und Allen (*1*) synthetisierte 1,2-Bis (3 Pyridyl)-2-Methyl-1 Propanon, das auch unter der Prüfungsnummer SU 4885, bzw. als Metopiron bezeichnet wurde, gilt als nicht toxisch (*14*). Es hemmt bekanntlich die 11-β-Oxydation und wird in Kombination mit ACTH-Belastungen in der Nebennierenrindendiagnostik verwendet (*2—14, 16—18, 20, 21*). Während sein Einfluß auf den Steroidstoffwechsel in zahlreichen Arbeiten analysiert werden konnte, liegen bisher kaum Untersuchungen darüber vor, inwieweit außer einer Hemmung der Synthese des Hydrocortison, Corticosteron und Aldosteron weitere davon abzutrennende Wirkungen nachweisbar sind. Im Ablauf von Metopirontesten war uns vor einiger Zeit aufgefallen — und auch Weissbecker hatte kürzlich darüber berichtet —, daß Metopiron bei Diabetikern den Blutzuckerspiegel zu senken vermag. Es tauchte nun die Frage auf, ob dieser Effekt auf den Zuckerstoffwechsel allein über eine Hemmung der Glucocorticoidsynthese zu erklären ist. Wir haben daher den Einfluß von 1 g Metopiron i.v. auf die blutzuckersteigernde Wirkung von 25 IE ACTH untersucht. Zu diesem Zweck wurden bei 5 Patienten intravenöse sowie bei einer Gruppe von 20 Patienten eines unausgewählten Krankengutes orale Glucosedoppelbelastungen ohne Hormonapplikation sowie mit ACTH und schließlich mit ACTH und Metopiron vorgenommen. Bis zu einem Gewicht von 70 kg wurden jeweils 1 g/kg Körpergewicht Glucose appliziert. Die Menge von 70 g Glucose als Einzelgabe wurde nicht überschritten. Die Bestimmungen des Blutzuckers erfolgten fermentativ. ACTH sowie ACTH + Metopiron wurden jeweils nach Abnahme des Nüchternblutzuckers in einem 1 Std-Tropfer mit physiologischer Kochsalzlösung infundiert. Beim Kontrollversuch wurden lediglich 100 cm³ physiologischer Kochsalzlösung appliziert. Zwischen den einzelnen Staub-Traugottschen Versuchen blieb jeweils ein 3 tägiges Intervall, die Reihenfolge der einzelnen Glucosetoleranzteste wurde variiert (Abb. 1a). Bei den intravenösen Glucosebelastungen konnten die relativ hohen Blutzuckergipfel durch die Applikation von Metopiron um etwa 150 mg-% gesenkt werden. Da die Applikation von ACTH + Metopiron den gleichen niedrigeren Kurvenverlauf zeigte, muß hierbei Metopiron die bereits früher von uns dargestellte (*19*) Wirkung von ACTH blockiert haben. Bei den oralen Glucosebelastungen gelang es, durch Metopiron den glucosesteigernden Effekt des ACTH während eines Zeit-

15*

raumes von 60—120 min deutlich zu reduzieren, nach 90 min ließ sich diese
Wirkung des Metopiron mit einem P von 0,05 sichern. Da die ACTH-bedingte
Zunahme der Blutzuckerwerte nicht in jedem Falle verhindert werden kann,
tauchte nun die Frage auf, ob exogen zugeführte Glucocorticoide durch Metopiron
in ihrer Wirkung gehemmt werden können. Diese Untersuchungen dienten der
Feststellung, ob Metopiron möglicherweise periphere Angriffspunkte im Zuckerstoffwechsel besitzt. Um die Prednisolon- mit den ACTH-Gruppen vergleichen zu

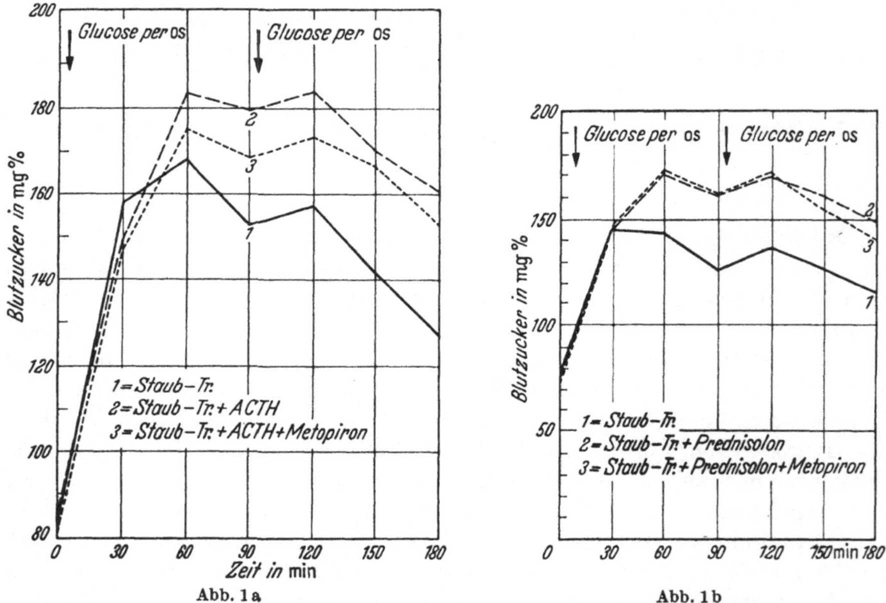

Abb. 1a   Abb. 1b

Abb. 1a und b. a Vergleichende Untersuchungen über den Einfluß von 25 IE ACTH i.v. und 1 g Metopiront
25 IE ACTH auf Glucosedoppelbelastungen nach Staub-Traugott (20 Fälle); b Vergleichende Untersuchungen
über den Einfluß von 25 mg Prednisolon i. v. und 1 g Metopiron + 25 mg Prednisolon auf Glucosedoppelbelastungen nach Staub-Traugott (20 Fälle)

können, haben wir bei insgesamt 70 Patienten Vergleichsuntersuchungen wischen
ACTH und Prednisolon vorgenommen. Hierbei zeigte sich, daß Prednisolon-Na-
hemisuccinat (25 mg) einen signifikant geringeren Effekt auf die Blutzuckerwerte
besitzt als ACTH. Bei 20 weiteren Fällen (Abb. 1b) konnte nachgewiesen werden,
daß die Prednisolonwirkungen auf die Glucosewerte des Blutes durch Metopiron
nicht verändert werden. Vergleichsuntersuchungen an 10 Patienten zwischen
Metopiron und ACTH + Metopiron ergaben, daß die Metopironkurven, insbesondere zwischen 60—120 min wesentlich niedriger liegen als die der Belastungen mit
ACTH + Metopiron. Beim Vergleich von ACTH und Metopiron zeigt sich im
Ablauf der Wirkungen ein signifikanter Unterschied nach 90 min., wobei sich nach
diesem Zeitpunkt die Metopironkurven praktisch nicht von denen der Kontrollen
unterscheiden. Während wir mit Hilfe des Glucosetoleranztestes mit ACTH oder
Prednisolon aus einem unausgewählten Krankengut von 220 untersuchten Fällen
44 Patienten mit einer prädiabetischen Stoffwechsellage erfassen konnten, gelang
nun durch Metopiron eine weitere Aufgliederung. 68% der Fälle mit einer prädiabetischen Stoffwechsellage und nahezu 10% der Patienten mit sonst noch

normalen Glucosetoleranztesten zeigten bei einer zusätzlichen Metopironapplikation keine Senkung der Glucosewerte nach ACTH-Applikation, vereinzelt kam es sogar zu einem Anstieg über den ACTH- und insbesondere den Prednisoloneffekt hinaus. Bei diesen Fällen fiel auf, daß es sich meist um ältere Patienten, einen Leberparenchymschaden, Pankreatitis oder übergewichtige Patienten handelt. Über die Ursache dieses Phänomens lassen sich verschiedene Vermutungen anstellen, z. B. die Mobilisierung gegenregulatorischer Systeme durch Metopiron. Untersuchungen zur Klärung dieser Frage sind zur Zeit noch im Gange.

Die Häufigkeit einer prädiabetischen Stoffwechsellage nimmt im übrigen mit steigendem Alter zu, erreicht mit 50 Jahren bereits zwei Drittel und nach dem 70. Lebensjahr 87% (250 Glucosetoleranzteste).

Neben den bekannten Wirkungen auf die 17-ketogenen Steroide im Harn und einem statistisch nicht zu sichernden Einfluß auf die 17-Ketosteroide besitzt Metopiron einen signifikanten Effekt auf die Stickstoffbilanz. Die N-Elimination nimmt zu. Natrium, Kalium, Kreatin, Kreatinin und auch Calcium ändern sich dagegen nur unwesentlich. Bei einer fraktionierten Sammlung des Harns sowie bei 4—6facher Kontrolle der Plasma 17-OHCS, des Hydrocortison sowie vor. Desoxyverbindungen haben sich große Schwankungen bei einzelnen Patienten im Ablauf der Metopironhemmung gezeigt. Die Wirkungsdauer schwankte zwischen 10 und 36 Std, das Maximum des Effektes zwischen 6 und 12 Std. Beim 4 Std-Tropfer war die Wirkungsdauer gegenüber dem 1 Std-Tropfer erhöht. Lediglich eine mehrmalige Kontrolle der Plasmawerte sowie eine fraktionierte Sammlung des Harns erlaubt einwandfrei diagnostisch zu verwertende Aussagen. Bereits KLEINFELDER, BRACHARZ und GEBERT (15) konnten eine unterschiedliche Wirkungsdauer des Metopiron nachweisen. Auf Grund dieser Beobachtungstatsachen sind wohl auch manche klinisch rätselhaften Steroidbefunde zu erklären, die den Wirkungsablauf des Metopironeffektes im Einzelfalle nicht erfassen.

Literatur

1. BENCZE, W. L., and M. J. ALLEN: J. med. pharm. Chem. 1, 395 (1959).
2. BROWNIE, A. C., and J. G. SPRUNT: Lancet 1962, 773.
3. BUUS, O., C. BINDER and F. PETERSEN: Lancet 1962, 1040.
4. CHART, J. J., H. SHEPPARD, M. J. ALLEN, W. L. BENCZE and R. GAUNT: Experientia (Basel) 14, 151 (1958).
5. CLEVELAND, W. W., M. NIKEZIC and C. J. MIGEON: J. clin. Endocr. 22, 281 (1962).
6. EBERLEIN, W. R., and A. M. BONGIOVANNI: J. clin. Endocr. 15, 1531 (1955).
7. FRANKEN, F. H., K. IRMSCHER u. H. A. v. SCHWEINITZ: Klin. Wschr. 40, 137 (1962).
8. GOLD, E. M., V. C. DI RAIMONDO and P. H. FORSHAM: Metabolism 9, 3 (1960).
9. HOLUB, D. A., E. Z. WALLACE and J. W. AILER: J. clin. Endocr. 20, 1294 (1960).
10. — J. W. JAILER, J. I. KITAY and A. G. FRANTZ: J. clin. Endocr. 19, 1540 (1959).
11. JENKINS, J. S., J. W. MEAKIN, D. H. NELSON and G. W. THORN: Science 128, 478 (1958).
12. — L. POTHIER, W. J. REDDY, D. H. NELSON and G. W. THORN: Brit. med. J. 1959, 398.
13. JENNY, M., A. M. RIONDEL et A. F. MULLER: Schweiz. med. Wschr. 92, 311 (1962).
14. KALLIOMÄKI, J. L., N. T. KÄRKI, H. A. SAARIMAA and E. TALA: Ann. rheum. Dis. 20, 244 (1961).
15. KLEINFELDER, H., H. BRACHARZ u. E. GEBERT: Klin. Wschr. 39, 1153 (1961).
16. LIDDLE, G. W., D. ISLAND, E. M. LANCE and A. P. HARRIS: J. clin. Endocr. 18, 906 (1958).
17. — H. L. ESTER, J. W. KENDALL JR., W. C. WILLIAMS JR. and A. W. TOWNES: J. clin. Endocr. 19, 875 (1959).
18. — D. ISLAND u. A. WALSER: Schweiz. med. Wschr. 90, 1351 (1960).

19. Scheiffarth, F., L. Zicha, D. Bergner u. R. Krämer: Internat. Steroidsymp. Ghent September 1962.
20. Solem, J. H., and T. Brinck-Johnson: Acta med. scand. 170, 89 (1961).
21. Tomkins, G. M.: Zit. nach G. W. Liddle, D. Island u. A. Walser: Schweiz. med. Wschr. 90, 1351 (1960).

Diskussion

K. Oberdisse (Düsseldorf):

Gemeinsam mit H. Zimmermann beobachtete ich eine 30jähr. Patientin mit dem Vollbild des Cushing-Syndroms (bilaterale Hyperplasie der Nebennierenrinden; operativ bestätigt). Bei dieser Patientin bestand ein Steroid-Diabetes. Bei einer Zufuhr von 220 g Kohlenhydraten und einer Insulindosis von 40 E Depot-Insulin Hoechst lagen die Blutzuckerwerte an drei aufeinanderfolgenden Tagen bei 142, 156 und 101 mg-%. An diesen Tagen betrug die Zuckerausscheidung 68, 72 und 75 g täglich. Wir behielten die Insulindosis und die Gesamt-KH-Zufuhr bei und verabfolgten täglich 3000 mg Metopiron. Dabei sank der Blutzucker auf subnormale Nüchternwerte ab, nämlich 95, 61 und 58 mg-%. Die Zuckerausscheidung lag an diesen Tagen bei 8,4 und 5,4 g. Wir setzten darauf unter Weitergabe von Metopiron die Insulindosis auf 36 E herab. Die Nüchternblutzuckerwerte betrugen jetzt 87 und 82 mg-%, während die Zuckerausscheidung an allen Tagen negativ war. Als wir das Metopiron absetzten, stiegen die Nüchternblutzuckerwerte auf 70, 109, 155 und 148 mg-% an, die Harnzuckerausscheidung auf 12,4, 18,4 und 37,2 g bei 36 E Depot-Insulin Hoechst und unveränderter Kost.

Eine deutliche Beeinflussung der Stoffwechsellage unter Metopiron ist demnach zu erkennen. Die Bilanz hat sich gebessert, während es nach Absetzen des Metopirons wieder zu einer Verschlechterung der Stoffwechsellage kam. Bei der Patientin wurde später eine totale Adrenalinektomie durchgeführt. Dadurch verschwand der Diabetes völlig. Der Blutzucker blieb normal. Die Harnzuckerausscheidung hörte völlig auf. Insulingaben waren nicht mehr notwendig.

E. F. Pfeiffer (Frankfurt):

Auch bei unseren Bestimmungen der Aktivität des endogenen ACTH nach Metopiron wurde ein sicherer Anstieg erst 6—8 Std, maximal 16 Std nach Beginn der Metopironzufuhr gefunden.

L. Zicha:

Der Unterschied zwischen dem erst später einsetzenden Anstieg des endogenen ACTH und dem raschen Metopironeffekt auf den Zuckerstoffwechsel kann zwei Ursachen haben: 1. Die ACTH-Mobilisierung kommt nach Blockade der Glucocorticoidsynthese erst relativ spät zustande. 2. Metopiron besitzt neben der Hemmung des ACTH-bedingten Einflusses auf den Zuckerstoffwechsel zusätzliche Wirkungen in der Peripherie, die allerdings nur das ACTH-mobilisierte Hydrocortison, nicht dagegen das Prednisolon betreffen.

Aus der I. Medizinischen Universitätsklinik Frankfurt am Main
(Direktor: Prof. Dr. F. Hoff)

Untersuchungen über den Transport und die Tagesrhythmik von endogenem ACTH im Blut bei Stoffwechselgesunden und Cushing-Kranken

Von

K. Retiene, A. Espinoza, Y. Abdel Rahman, K. H. Marx und E. F. Pfeiffer

Mit 2 Abbildungen

Die hypophysäre Pathogenese des Morbus Cushing auf dem Boden einer bilateralen NNR-Hyperplasie ist bekanntlich immer noch umstritten, weil eine Erhöhung des ACTH-Blutspiegels bei den meisten Kranken nicht nachgewiesen werden kann (Nelson u. Mitarb.). Von Liddle wurde vorgebracht, daß alle Cushing-Kranken eine vermehrte ACTH-Sekretion hätten, die nur durch die stark erhöhten Cortisolspiegel in den Normalbereich gesenkt werden würde. Der verstärkte Sekretionsdruck der Hypophyse werde erst nach der operativen Adrenalektomie sichtbar, wenn deutlich höhere ACTH-Spiegel als bei Addison-Kranken gemessen werden könnten.

Aus Experimenten von Nugent u. Mitarb. wissen wir, daß Dauerinfusionen von 1,5—5,0 E ACTH/Tag, die keine meßbare Erhöhung des ACTH im Blut bewirken, bereits genügen, um erhöhte Cortisolspiegel wie beim Morbus Cushing zu erzeugen. Bei so vorbehandelten Patienten fiel eine ganz gleichmäßige, konstante Erhöhung des Cortisolspiegels im Verlauf von 24 Std auf, was in gleicher Weise beim Morbus Cushing von Laidlaw u. Mitarb. sowie von Ekmann u. Mitarb. gesehen wurde. Der bei Stoffwechselgesunden beobachtete physiologische Abfall während der Nachtstunden war nicht mehr nachweisbar (Perkoff u. Mitarb.). Berechnet man das Integral der in diesen Arbeiten abgebildeten Tagesverlaufskurven von Cortisol, so resultiert beim Cushing-Kranken sogar ohne absolute Erhöhung der Einzelwerte allein durch die Konstanz der Sekretion eine Verdoppelung der Cortisolproduktion des Normalen.

Sollten mit verbesserten Meßverfahren ähnliche Verhältnisse für das ACTH beim Morbus Cushing nachgewiesen werden können, so wäre der in den meisten Fällen fehlende Nachweis absolut erhöhter ACTH-Werte erklärt.

Voraussetzung für solche Untersuchungen war die exakte Messung des normalen ACTH-Spiegels im 24 Std-Verlauf. Unser früher von Pfeiffer u. Mitarb. mitgeteiltes Verfahren, das auf dem Corticosteronanstieg im peripheren Blut der mit Dexamethason hypophysenblockierten Ratte beruht, war dafür unzureichend. Größtmögliche Empfindlichkeit und Genauigkeit wurde durch Messung des ungleich höheren Corticosteronanstieges im NNV-Blut hypophysektomierter Ratten erreicht (Retiene u. Mitarb.). Die unterste Empfindlichkeit dieser Methode liegt bei 0,01 mE ACTH, so daß bei Injektion von 5 ml pro Tier, ACTH-Spiegel von 0,2 mE/100 ml menschliches Plasma gerade erfaßt werden. Im unveränderten Plasma konnten wir maximal 0,8 mE/100 ml messen, was in guter Übereinstimmung zu den Ergebnissen anderer Autoren steht, die 0,4—1,0 mE/100 ml Plasma als normalen ACTH-Blutspiegel angeben (Vance u. Mitarb., Hale u. Mitarb.).

Die vermutete Tagesrhythmik der ACTH-Sekretion konnte tatsächlich nachgewiesen werden. Im unteren Teil der Abb. 1 sehen wie den Cortisolspiegel bei 3 Stoffwechselgesunden mit einem Hauptgipfel in den frühen Morgenstunden, einem kleineren Gipfel am späten Nachmittag und dem stärksten Abfall um

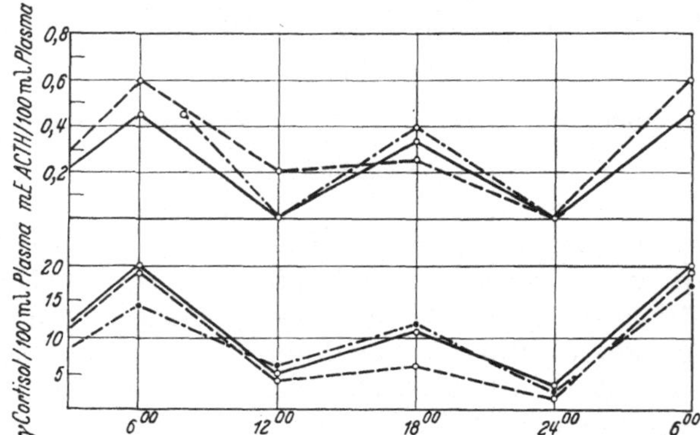

Abb. 1. Verhalten von ACTH und Cortisol im Blut über 24 Std bei Stoffwechselgesunden

Mitternacht. Im oberen Teil der Abbildung haben wir die durch Mehrfachbestimmung gesicherten ACTH-Werte von den gleichen Patienten aufgetragen. Der höchste Gipfel fand sich in den Morgenstunden. Um Mitternacht konnte bei allen 3 Probanden keine ACTH-Aktivität nachgewiesen werden. Es ergibt sich eine komplette Parallele des Verhaltens von ACTH und Cortisol. Diese Tagesrhythmik ist allerdings nur dann zu sehen, wenn der Patient Bettruhe einhält. Andererseits ist sie so konstant, wie Lipscomb uns kürzlich mitteilte, daß genau dieselbe Tagesrhythmik bei amerikanischen Soldaten sogar noch für mehrere Tage nach dem Flug nach Japan trotz des Zeitunterschiedes beibehalten wurde.

Die gleichen Untersuchungen erfolgten bei Cushing-Kranken vor und nach subtotaler Adrenalektomie. Abb. 2 zeigt die Befunde bei einem Cushing-Patienten vor Therapiebeginn.

Klinisch und steroidchemisch lag eine doppelseitige NNR-Hyperplasie vor. Cortisol war in dem Bereich erhöht, wie er häufig beim Morbus Cushing gefunden wird. Im Gegensatz zu den Befunden verschiedener Voruntersuchter (Nelson u. Mitarb., Pfeiffer u. Mitarb.) waren die ACTH-Spiegel bei diesen Patienten nun sogar ebenfalls erhöht. Bedeutend wichtiger erscheint jedoch der konstant hohe, gleichmäßige Blutspiegel sowohl von ACTH als auch von Cortisol im Verlauf von 24 Std. Die physiologische Tagesschwankung ist tatsächlich nicht mehr erkennbar. Bei einer Patientin mit operativ bestätigter NNR-Hyperplasie war es postoperativ zu keiner Remission der in diesem Fall sehr eindrucksvollen klinischen Symptome gekommen. Eine unzureichende Adrenalektomie mußte angenommen werden. Auch in diesem Fall fiel ein erhöhter, völlig gleichmäßiger Tagesverlauf von Cortisol auf. Leider wurde die Patientin zu einem Zeitpunkt operiert, als wir die jetzige, sehr empfindliche ACTH-Meßmethode noch nicht beherrschten. Mit der weniger empfindlichen Dexamethason-Blockade konnten nur fragliche ACTH-Aktivitäten nachgewiesen werden, Vielleicht ist diese Kranke jedoch als Beispiel für die von LIDDLE beschriebenen Fälle mit bilateraler NNR-Hyperplasie aufzufassen. Wären die ACTH-Aktivitäten hier im Normbereich, dann müßten sie bei dem erhöhten Cortisolspiegel als pathologisch angesehen werden.

Bei einer anderen Kranken mit operativ bestätigter NNR-Hyperplasie kam es zu einer fast völligen NNR-Insuffizienz nach der subtotalen Adrenalektomie. Unmittelbar nach der Operation lagen die ACTH-Werte bei nicht meßbarem Cortisol konstant um 500 mE/100 ml Plasma im 24 Std-Verlauf, und es fehlte jede Tagesschwankung. Erst nach einem halben Jahr waren wieder geringe Cortisolspiegel zu messen, und das ACTH lag nur noch bis auf das

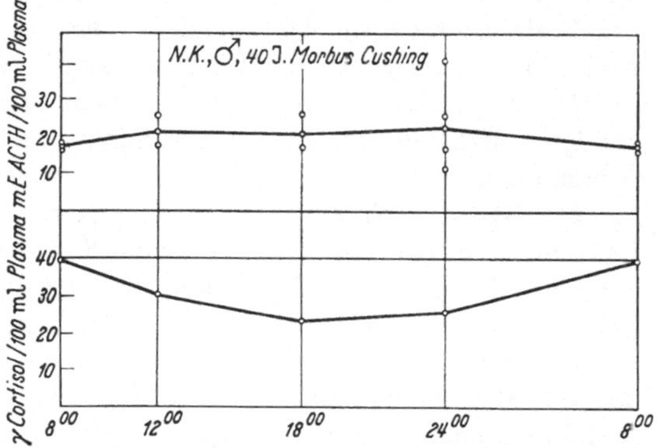

Abb. 2. Verhalten von ACTH und Cortisol im Blut über 24 Std bei einem unbehandelten Cushing-Patienten mit bilateraler NNR-Hyperplasie

200fache über der Norm. Überraschenderweise war die physiologische Tagesschwankung jetzt wieder nachweisbar.

Damit konnte eine sichere Tagesrhythmik von ACTH beim Stoffwechselgesunden nachgewiesen werden, die bei Morbus Cushing fehlte. Berechnet man die Mehrproduktion von ACTH bei völlig gleichmäßiger Sekretion des in den Morgenstunden gemessenen Normalwertes (Abb. 1), so kommt man auf 1,5 E ACTH/24 Std. Dies ist exakt die Menge, die in den Experimenten von NUGENT ausreichte, um Cortisolspiegel wie beim Cushing-Kranken zu erzeugen.

Der absolut erhöhte ACTH-Spiegel eines unserer Cushing-Patienten stellt sicher die Ausnahme (vgl. NELSON) dar. Es errechnet sich bei diesem Fall sogar eine Mehrproduktion von 25 E ACTH in 24 Std, eine Menge, die wir in der Klinik zur Funktionsprüfung der NNR infundieren.

Eine gegenseitige Zügelung von ACTH und Cortisol auf einem starren, im Einzelfall auch erhöhten Niveau kann somit für Cushing-Kranke mit bilateraler NNR-Hyperplasie angenommen werden. Fällt nach der Operation die periphere Bremsung der ACTH-Sekretion weg, so wird nach einiger Zeit die vom Hypothalamus ausgehende Tagesrhythmik von ACTH wieder erkennbar.

Beim Cushing-Syndrom soll weiterhin eine von der Norm abweichende Bindung von Cortisol an Plasmaeiweiß bestehen (SLAUNWHITE und SANDBERG). In früheren Untersuchungen über die biologische Halbwertszeit von exogenem ACTH im Blut des Menschen hatten wir auch für ACTH eine unterschiedliche Bindung an gewisse Trägerproteine diskutiert (RETIENE u. Mitarb.). Je nach der Geschwindigkeit der Infusion oder Injektion hatte das zugeführte ACTH eine sehr kurze oder verlängerte Halbwertszeit.

Je 10 cm³ Serum von Stoffwechselgesunden wurden jetzt mit und ohne Zusatz von exogenem ACTH sowie von einer Cushing-Patientin der präparativen Zonenelektrophorese in Polyvinylchlorid unterworfen. Die in den einzelnen Serumeiweißfraktionen vorhandenen ACTH-Aktivitäten wurden dann, wie vorher beschrieben, bestimmt.

Ein qualitativer Vergleich der in den verschiedenen Eiweißfraktionen gemessenen ACTH-Aktivitäten ist wegen der völlig unterschiedlichen Größenordnung der ACTH-Werte bei Normalen, dem exogenen Zusatz und der ACTH-Werte bei der Cushing-Patientin nicht möglich. Die prozentuale Verteilung der in allen Fraktionen gemessenen ACTH-Aktivitäten zeigte überraschenderweise ganz signifikante Unterschiede bei den bisher untersuchten Seren. Während das endogene ACTH des Stoffwechselgesunden vornehmlich in den schnell wandernden Albumin- und α_1-Globulinfraktionen nachgewiesen werden konnte, war die Hauptaktivität nach Zugabe von 5,0 mE exogenem ACTH in der β-Globulinfraktion zu messen. Bei einer Cushing-Patientin wanderte die Hauptaktivität dagegen mit der α_2-Globulinfraktion, in der bei den bisher untersuchten Normalfällen niemals ACTH nachgewiesen werden konnte.

Die ersten Befunde bedürfen der weiteren Bestätigung. Interessant scheint uns die Möglichkeit, endogenes ACTH überhaupt in einzelnen Serumeiweißfraktionen nachweisen zu können. Die Frage nach einem freien, aktiven ACTH und einem biologisch inaktiven, gebundenen ACTH läßt sich noch nicht beantworten. Sollte sich die Bindung des ACTH von Cushing-Kranken an spezielle Serumeiweißfraktionen bestätigen, so käme ein neuer Gesichtspunkt zu den quantitativen Überlegungen hinzu.

Literatur

EKMAN, H., B. HAKANSSON, I. D. McCARTHY, I. LEHMANN and B. SJÖGREN: J. clin. Endocr. **21**, 684 (1961).

HALE, H. B., G. SAYERS, K. L. SYDNOR, M. L. SWEAT and D. D. VAN FOSSAN: J. clin. Invest. **36**, 1642 (1957).

LAIDLAW, J. C., W. J. REDDY, D. JENKINS, N. ABU HAJDAR, A. E. RENOLD and G. W. THORN: New Engl. J. Med. **253**, 747 (1955).

LIDDLE, G. W., W. C. WILLIAMS JR. u. A. WALSER: Schweiz. med. Wschr. **90**, 1325 (1960).

LIPSCOMB, H. S.: Persönliche Mitteilung.

NELSON, D. H., J. W. MEAKIN, J. B. DEALY, D. D. MATSON, K. EMERSON and G. W. THORN: New Engl. J. Med. **259**, 161 (1958).

— Clinical Endocrinology I., 626—636, E. B. ASTWOOD Ed. New York-London: Grune and Stratton 1960.

NUGENT, CH. A., K. EIK-NES, L. T. SAMUELS and E. H. TYLER: J. clin. Endocr. **19**, 334 (1959).

PERKOFF, G. T., K. EIK-NES, C. A. NUGENT, H. L. FRED, R. A. NIMER, L. RUSH and F. H. TYLER: J. clin. Endocr. **19**, 432 (1959).

PFEIFFER, E. F., W. E. VAUBEL, K. RETIENE, D. BERG u. H. DITSCHUNEIT: Klin. Wschr. **38**, 980 (1960).

— F. GARMENDIA, W. E. VAUBEL u. K. RETIENE: Ergebn. inn. Med. Kinderheilk. (im Druck).

RETIENE, K., M. FISCHER, K. KOPP u. E. F. PFEIFFER: 8. Symp. Dtsch. Ges. Endokrinol. 1.—3. 3. 1961, München.

— — H. DITSCHUNEIT u. E. F. PFEIFFER: 9. Symp. Dtsch. Ges. Endokrinol. 3.—5. 5. 1962, Wiesbaden/Mainz (im Druck).

SLAUNWHITE, W. R. JR., and A. A. SANDBERG: J. clin. Invest. **38**, 384 (1959).

VANCE, V. K., W. J. REDDY, D. H. NELSON and G. W. THORN: Programm der 42. Tagung der American Endocrine Society, Miami, 9.—11. Juni 1960, Abstr. Nr. 28.

Aus der Medizinischen Klinik mit Poliklinik der Universität Erlangen-Nürnberg
(Direktor: Prof. Dr. N. Henning)

Untersuchungen über die Transcortinbindung mittels C¹⁴-Hydrocortison

Von

F. Wolf, L. Zicha, D. Bergner, G. Poser und G. Kleyensteiber

Mit 2 Abbildungen

Die Eiweißbindung von Glucocorticoiden ist von wesentlicher Bedeutung für die Pathophysiologie endokrinologischer Erkrankungen des Hypophysen-Nebennierenrindensystems · einerseits, für die therapeutische Anwendung der verschiedenen verfügbaren Corticoidderivate andererseits. Nachdem eine derartige Bindung bereits früher angenommen worden war, beschrieben Sandberg und Slaunwhite sowie Daughaday 1956/1957 das im einzelnen noch nicht definierte Transcortin als Träger dieser Bindung. Es handelt sich dabei um einen in der α-1-Globulinfraktion des Serums wandernden Eiweißkörper mit der etwa 3000-fachen Affinität zu Hydrocortison als andere Proteine. Das Bindungsgleichgewicht ist nach den bisher vorliegenden Untersuchungen erheblich von der Einführung bestimmter Gruppen im Steroidmolekül abhängig. Chemische Verfahren zur Bestimmung der Bindungskapazität für Glucocorticoide, d. h. der Transcortinaktivität, erfordern einen großen zeitlichen und apparativen Aufwand (de Moore u. Mitarb.). Einen wesentlichen methodischen Vorteil stellt die Verwendung radioaktiv markierter Substanzen dar, die noch in den geringsten Mengen (bis wenigstens 10^{-9} g) mit der erforderlichen Genauigkeit gemessen werden können.

In unseren Versuchen gelangte eine modifizierte Dialysiertechnik mit C¹⁴-markiertem freien Alkohol des Hydrocortisons zur Anwendung. 10 ml des zu untersuchenden Serums werden im Dialysierschlauch (Dicke 50 μ, Porengröße 30 A) mit physiologischer Kochsalzlösung auf 50 ml aufgefüllt. Da die einzelnen Substanzen nicht in markierter Form zur Verfügung standen, gaben wir in Verdrängungsversuchen das interessierende inaktive Corticoid in mehreren Ansätzen in verschiedenen Dosen in den Dialysierschlauch. Die Dialyse erfolgte gegen 50 ml physiologischer NaCl-Lösung, der zu Versuchsbeginn 0,1 μC markierten Hydrocortisons (entsprechend einer Gewichtsmenge von 1,45 g) zugesetzt wurde. Aktivitätsbestimmungen von jeweils 1 ml der Umgebungslösung wurden 0, 1, 3, 6, (12), 24 und 48 Std nach Versuchsbeginn ausgeführt. Nach Infrarottrocknung in 30 mm-Probenschälchen zählten wir je Probe 10^4 Impulse im Methandurchfluß-Probenwechsler mit Zeitdrucker[1] und erhielten so einen konstanten statistischen Fehler von 1%. Bei der Auswertung erfolgte eine Korrektur für die Volumenabnahme durch die Entnahmen und — wenn erforderlich — einen Verdunstungsverlust.

---

[1] Fa. Frieseke und Hoepfner, Erlangen-Bruck.

Haben wir im Inneren des Dialysierschlauches eine gegenüber Corticoiden indifferente Lösung, so stellt sich lediglich das Diffusionsgleichgewicht zwischen der Umgebungslösung und dem Inhalt des Dialysierschlauches ein, die Impulsrate sinkt außen auf 50% des Ausgangswertes ab und steigt innen entsprechend an. Bei vorhandener selektiver Corticoidbindung dagegen kommt es zur Anreicherung der Aktivität im Inneren, die Impulsrate der Umgebungslösung fällt auf weniger als 50% des Ausgangswertes ab. Dieser Abfall muß um so ausgeprägter sein, je stärker die Transcortinaktivität bzw. die nicht belegte Kapazität ist.

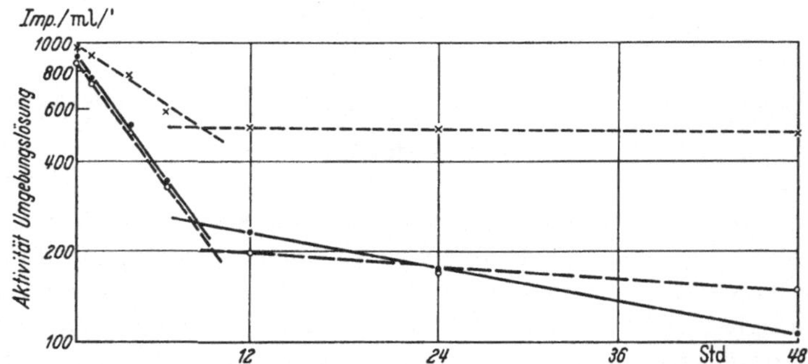

Abb. 1. Radioaktivität in der Umgebungslösung im Dialysierversuch mit Mischplasma von Normalpersonen (— · — · — · — 3 Fälle), mit Mischserum von Normalpersonen (— — o — — o — — o 3 Fälle) sowie mit einer Galleprobe (— — x — — x — — x)

Zunächst erfolgte die Prüfung des zeitlichen Ablaufes und der Temperaturabhängigkeit des Diffusionsvorganges einerseits und der Eiweiß-Bindung andererseits. Bei Vergleich zwischen 24 und 37°C zeigt sich ein deutlicher Einfluß der Temperatur hinsichtlich der Kurvenform und der Höhe des nach 24 (bis 48) Std erreichten Endzustandes. Einer Aktivitätsabnahme auf durchschnittlich 20% bei 37° steht eine solche auf nur 30% bei 24°C gegenüber. Auf Grund dieser Befunde wurden sämtliche weiteren Dialyse-Versuche bei 37°C ausgeführt.

Weiter wurde geprüft, ob die Methode ein unterschiedliches Verhalten von Plasma, dessen Verwendung ausländische Autoren bevorzugen, und Serum erkennen läßt. In Abb. 1 ist in halblogarithmischer Darstellung die Aktivität der Umgebungslösung gegen die Zeit aufgetragen. Eingezeichnet sind jeweils die Mittelwerte aus drei Doppelbestimmungen gesunder Probanden. Der initiale Abfall ist für die Plasma- und Serumwerte in der Steilheit identisch. Nach der 12. Std verlaufen die Serumwerte wesentlich flacher als die des Plasmas. Ob diese Veränderung durch Heparin bedingt ist, wäre zu diskutieren. Aus dem Diagramm ist ersichtlich, daß die Verwendung von Serum als Untersuchungsgut eine Standardisierung der Methode erleichtert.

In Abb. 1 ist noch ein Versuchsansatz mit Galle in einer Verdünnung 1:5 dargestellt. Wir sehen den der Diffusion der Aktivität in das Schlauchinnere entsprechenden exponentiellen Abfall und ab der 12. Std den besprochenen konstanten Verlauf bei der 50%-Linie. Die untersuchte Galle zeigte somit keine Transcortinaktivität.

Eine größere Zahl von Befunden ist in Abb. 2 zusammengefaßt. Die weiße Säule gibt den Mittelwert von 10 Kontrollseren gesunder männlicher Probanden

(Durchschnittsalter 31 Jahre) an. Die vertikale Linie kennzeichnet die Standard-
abweichung. Ausgehend von der Gleichgewichtseinstellung zwischen Umgebungslösung und Inhalt des Dialysierschlauches bei Fehlen einer Corticoidbindung gibt
der Ordinatenmaßstab die Differenz der Impulsrate gegen den diffusionsbedingten
50%-Wert der Ausgangsaktivität an. Der Mittelwert beträgt 26,4 ±3,6%. Über-
trägt man diese aus der Messung der Radioaktivität unmittelbar erhaltenen
Konzentrationswerte auf die Volumina des Gesamtsystems, so ist lediglich eine

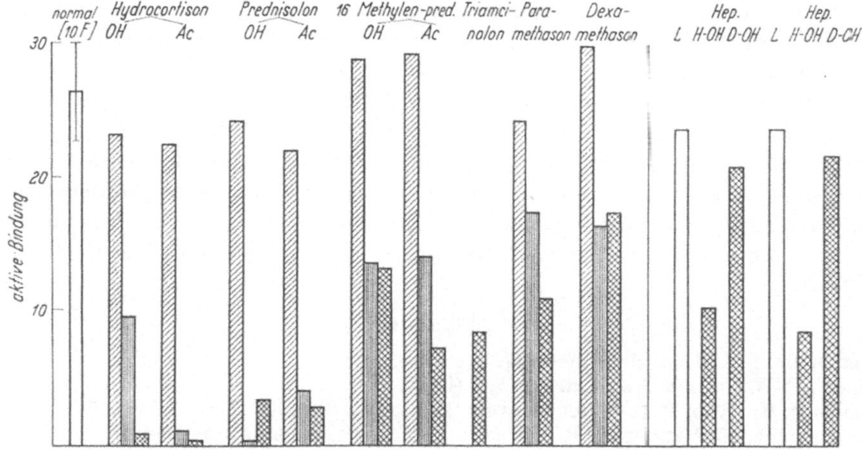

Abb. 2. Aktive C¹⁴-Hydrocortisonbindung von normalen Mischseren im Verdrängungsversuch mit verschiedenen
Corticoiden in einer Menge von 1 γ ▨, 10 γ ▥ und 100 γ ▩ sowie von 2 Hepatitis-Seren

Multiplikation mit dem Faktor 2 (50 ml: 100 ml) erforderlich. Unter Berücksichtigung der spezifischen Aktivität entspricht dann der genannte Mittelwert einer
C¹⁴-Hydrocortisonbindung von 0,75 γ/10 ml Serum.

Wie die weiteren Säulen zeigen, führt der Zusatz von 1 γ der acht untersuchten
verschiedenen Glucocorticoidverbindungen in keinem Falle zu sicheren Veränderungen des Gleichgewichtszustandes und damit der durch Radiohydrocortison
belegbaren Transcortinkapazität. Zusätze in Höhe von 10 γ der verschiedenen
Verbindungen bedingen z. T. bereits eine signifikante Hemmung der C¹⁴-Hydrocortisonbindung und lassen untereinander deutliche Unterschiede erkennen,
wobei der Zusatz von inaktivem Hydrocortison sowie Prednisolon den ausgepräg-
testen Effekt zeigt. Noch deutlicher treten diese Unterschiede bei den Zusatz-
versuchen mit 100 γ hervor. Dabei fällt besonders auf, daß 16-Methylen-Predni-
solon als freier Alkohol einen relativ geringen Hemmeffekt auf die Radiohydrocortisonbindung besitzt und quantitativ in dieser Reihe zusammen mit Para-
methason nach Dexamethason an zweiter Stelle liegt. Dieser Befund dürfte von
klinischem Interesse sein, da man vermutet, daß die Wirkung von Glucocorticoiden umgekehrt proportional ihrer Eiweißbindung sei.

MARGRAF und WEICHSELBAUM fanden, daß wenigstens 50% des Hydrocortisons
im Plasma als Acetat vorkommen. Unsere Arbeitsgruppe beschrieb die Acety-
lierung von synthetischen Präparaten. Deshalb wurde bei verschiedenen Deri-
vaten (Hydrocortison, Prednisolon, 16-Methylen-Prednisolon) die Eiweißbindung

der freien Alkohole und Acetate verglichen. Unter Berücksichtigung der verschiedenen Zusatzmengen gewinnt man aus den bisherigen Versuchen den Eindruck, daß Acetate durchschnittlich etwas stärker an Transcortin gebunden sind als die freien Alkohole der entsprechenden Verbindung.

Die — in der Abbildung nicht dargestellten — zur maximalen Unterdrückung der Radiohydrocortisonbindung notwendigen Dosen erwiesen sich als sehr unterschiedlich, sie betragen z. B. bei Hydrocortisonacetat 100 γ, bei 16-Methylen-Prednisolon und Dexamethason nahezu 50 mal mehr.

Besonders interessante Befunde ergab schließlich die orientierende Untersuchung von Hepatitisfällen und anderen Lebererkrankungen. Hier lassen sich keine wesentlichen Änderungen der Transcortinbindung im Leerversuch zeigen, es findet sich aber eine deutlich höhere C¹⁴-Hydrocortisonbindung gegenüber Normalseren bei Zusätzen von 100 γ Hydrocortison und 16-Methylen-Prednisolon. Inwieweit diese vermehrte Transcortinkapazität mit der klinischen Beobachtung zusammenhängt, daß die erforderliche initiale Glucocorticoiddosis in derartigen Fällen relativ hoch liegt, während die Erhaltungsdosen mit den bei anderen Erkrankungen üblichen übereinstimmen, wird noch an größeren Versuchsreihen geprüft.

Literatur

Daughaday, W. H.: J. clin. Invest. **37**, 511 (1958).

Funck, F.-W., u. L. Zicha: Med. exp. **7**, 1 (1962).

Margraf, H. W., u. T. E. Weichselbaum: 1. Internat. Stereoidkongr. Mailand 1962.

de Moor, P., K. Heirwegh, R. Deckx u. O. Steeno: Internat. Symposium on Adrenal Cortex Ghent 1962.

Sandberg, A. A., and W. R. Slaunwhite: J. clin. Invest. **37**, 1290 (1959).

Scheiffarth, F., u. L. Zicha: Acta endocr. (Kbh.) Suppl. **67**, 93 (1962).

Slaunwhite, W. R., and A. A. Sandberg: J. clin. Invest. **38**, 384 (1959).

Zicha, L., F. Scheiffarth, D. Bergner u. M. Engelhard: Acta endocr. (Kbh.) Suppl. **67**, 94 (1962).

Diskussion

H. J. Karl (München):

Bei den methodischen Angaben wurde nicht erwähnt, ob bei den Dialysen ein Zusatz gemacht wurde, um das Bakterienwachstum im Plasma zu hemmen. Nach eigenen Untersuchungen, sowie nach Angaben von Peterson, wird nämlich durch bakterielle Verunreinigung die Bindung von ¹⁴C-Hydrocortison ganz erheblich beeinflußt.

Wolf:

Bei der erforderlichen Versuchszeit bleibt das Bakterienwachstum in physiol. Kochsalzlösung unerheblich; Parallelversuche mit Antibiotica-Zusatz zeigten kein unterschiedliches Verhalten.

Aus dem staatlichen Institut für Rheumatologie, Budapest

Die Wirkung von Hydrocortison auf die Aldosteronproduktion der Nebennieren unter experimentellen Bedingungen

Von

P. Vecsei/Weisz, K. Farkas, V. Kemeny und D. Tanka

Mit 1 Abbildung

Die Wirkung von Hydrocortisongaben auf die Aldosteronproduktion gehört zu den Fragen, die in bezug auf die Tätigkeit der Nebennierenrinde noch unklar sind. Bei sekundären Aldosterosen wie Nephrose, Lebercirrhose und nach experimentell durch Zusammenschnüren der V. cava inferior entstandener Hyperaldosterose, vermindert die exogene Steroidverabreichung, gleichzeitig mit der eintretenden therapeutischen Wirkung, die endogene Aldosteronproduktion. Über den Einfluß auf die endogene Aldosteronproduktion der unter physiologischen, normalen Verhältnissen, also bei nicht pathogen erhöhter Aldosteronproduktion, von außen zugeführten Glykocorticoide, sind die Literaturangaben nicht so einheitlich. Sowohl die theoretische, als auch die praktische Bedeutung dieser Frage ist groß. Theoretisch wurde die Frage von Farrel (1) aufgeworfen, der bei Versuchen an Hunden nachwies, daß die chronische Cortisonbehandlung die Aldosteronproduktion unbeeinflußt läßt. Aus diesem Befund — gemeinsam mit anderen Daten — schloß er, daß ACTH (dessen Sekretion von Cortisongaben blockiert wird) in der Regelung der Aldosteronproduktion keine Rolle spielt. Klinisch wird die Frage infolge der Auffassung über die einzelnen Erscheinungen des „Steroidentziehungssyndroms" aktuell.

Bekanntlich entwickelt sich nämlich in seltenen Fällen nach Abbruch einer längeren Steroidbehandlung eine Nebenniereninsuffizienz, die manchmal von Störungen des Salz- und Wasserhaushaltes begleitet ist, die nur mit der Verminderung der Aldosteronsekretion erklärt werden können. Unter den Sektionsbefunden finden wir Beschreibungen, wonach neben der allgemein beobachteten Atrophie der Zona fasciculata auch eine Atrophie der Zona glomerulosa nachgewiesen werden konnte. Diese Beobachtungen weisen darauf hin, daß man, im Gegensatz zur allgemeinen Auffassung, bei exogener Glykocorticoidverabreichung mit der hemmenden Wirkung auf die Aldosteronproduktion gleichfalls rechnen muß.

Um diese Frage zu klären, führten wir Versuche mit Ratten durch. 80—120 g schweren männlichen Ratten gleicher Zucht, verabreichten wir 5 Tage hindurch täglich zweimal 5 mg Hydrocortison. Nach Beendigung der Hydrocortisonverabreichung wurde zu verschiedenen Zeitpunkten die Aldosteronproduktion der Nebennieren untersucht. Die Ratten wurden dann durch Dekapitation getötet,

die Nebennieren entfernt (gereinigt und mit einer Genauigkeit von 0,1 mg gewogen, in vier Teile geschnitten und nach der Beschreibung von Giroud (2) in
einer 200 mg-% Glucose enthaltenden, mit einer Mischung von 95% O_2 und
5% CO_2 durchströmten Krebs-Ringer-Bicarbonatlösung bei einer Temperatur
von 38°C inkubiert. Die Inkubationslösung wurde dann mit Chloroform extrahiert
und der Corticosteroidgehalt des Extraktes nach Reaktion mit Tetrazoliumblau

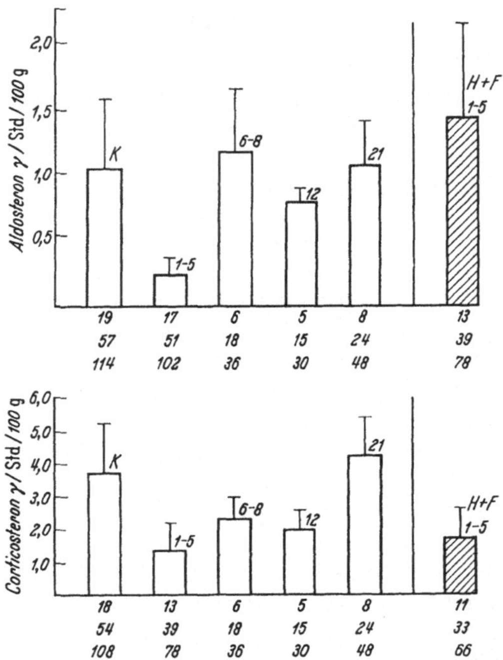

Abb. 1. Verhalten der Aldosteron- und Corticosteronproduktion bei Kontrollratten in verschiedenen Zeitabständen
nach Hydrocortisonentzug. *K* Kontrollratten. Nummer über den Säulen = Tage nach dem Hydrocortisonentzug,
H + F = Hydrocortison + Formalinverabreichung. Weitere Erklärung im Text

und nachfolgender Elution des entstandenen Formasans mittels spektrophoto-
metrischer Ablesung chromatographisch bestimmt. In je einem Röhrchen wurden
von wenigstens 3 Ratten mindestens 6 Nebennieren inkubiert. Aus der Aldosteron-
und Corticosteronproduktion der überlebenden Nebennieren folgerten wir auf die
in vivo Verhältnisse. Die Richtigkeit des Verfahrens wird durch Experimente
unterstützt, die van der Vies (3) und auch wir (4) schon früher durchführten.

Die erhaltenen Ergebnisse sind in Abb. 1 veranschaulicht, in der die Säulen
die Mittelwerte, die horizontalen Linien die quadratische Abweichung anzeigen. Unter den Säulen sind untereinander stehend, 3 Zahlen angeführt. Die
oberste Zahl ist die der Versuchsgruppen, die darunterstehende die der angewen-
deten Versuchsratten und die unterste die der inkubierten Nebennieren. Im
oberen Teil der Abbildung sehen wir die Mittelwerte der Corticosteronproduktion.
Diese entsprechen dem aus der Literatur bekannten und erwarteten Bild. In den
ersten Tagen ist eine merkliche Verminderung zu sehen. Später nähern sich die Werte
den Kontrollwerten und am 21. Tag nach Abbruch der Hydrocortisonverabreichung ist sogar eine gewisse Erhöhung der Corticosteronproduktion zu beobachten.

Im unteren Teil der Abbildung sehen wir die Aldosteronwerte.

In den ersten Tagen zeigt auch die Aldosteronproduktion eine Verminderung, die interessanterweise noch merklicher ist als die der Corticosteronproduktion. Später wird das Ausmaß der Verminderung geringer und nicht signifikant. Eine vollkommene Regeneration setzt erst am 21. Tag ein.

In der Abbildung haben wir auch die Ergebnisse eines anderen Versuches angeführt. Sofort nach Beendigung der Hydrocortisonbehandlung untersuchten wir auch solche Ratten (schattierte Säule), die gleichzeitig mit der Hydrocortisonbehandlung (also ebenfalls 5 Tage lang) einer Formalinbehandlung unterzogen worden sind. Von einer 2%igen Formalinlösung wurden täglich 0,5 ml/100 g Körpergewicht i.m. verabreicht. Es ist gut sichtbar, daß die Formalinbehandlung die Aldosteronproduktion vermindernde Wirkung der gleichzeitigen Hydrocortisongaben nicht nur abwehrte, sogar eine kleine Erhöhung verursachte.

Aus diesen Ergebnissen geht hervor, daß Hydrocortison, zumindest bei Anwendung von relativ großen Dosen, die Aldosteronproduktion gleichfalls vermindert. Der genaue Mechanismus dieser Wirkung ist noch ungeklärt, und hier weise ich auf die noch ungelösten Fragen der Aldosteronregelung hin. Möglicherweise übte die von uns verabreichte, verhältnismäßig große Hydrocortisongabe, zufolge ihrer Hydrocortison-Mineralcorticoidwirkung, auf die Aldosteronproduktion eine "feed back"-Wirkung aus.

Die Formalinverabreichung benutzten wir als Modell der chronischen „Stress"-Einwirkungen. Es ist ein sehr wichtiges Problem praktischer Natur, wie nach Steroidentziehung das Auftreten der verminderten Nebennierentätigkeit verhindert werden könnte. Diese Frage ist trotz mancher Versuche, z. B. Verabreichung von ACTH usw., bisher noch nicht gelöst. Auf der Basis unserer Versuche kann angenommen werden, daß „Stress"-Einwirkungen unmittelbar vor der Entziehung günstig wirken. Natürlich müssen unsere mit Formalin erzielten Resultate auch mit anderen klinisch ebenfalls anwendbaren „Stress"-Einwirkungen anderen Typs experimentell wiederholt werden.

In Zusammenhang mit unseren Formalinergebnissen zeigten weitere Untersuchungen, daß die Formalinbehandlung die nach Hydrocortisongaben eingetretene Atrophie der Nebennieren nicht verminderte. Diese Befunde sind ein neuer Beweis für die von uns und auch anderen Forschern beobachtete Erscheinung, daß das Gewicht der Nebennierenschichten mit ihrer Funktion in keiner unmittelbaren Beziehung steht.

Unsere bisherigen histologischen Untersuchungen stehen mit den funktionellen Resultaten in besserem Einklang. Die mit Hydrocortison und auch mit Formalin behandelten Ratten zeigten eine Verbreiterung der Zona glomerulosa und Verengung der chromophoben Zone, welch letztere sogar fallweise ganz verschwand.

Unsere Ergebnisse zusammenfassend, läßt sich sagen, daß unter gewissen Verhältnissen die Verabreichung von Hydrocortison nicht nur die Glykocorticoid-, sondern auch die Aldosteronproduktion vermindern kann.

Literatur

1. Farrell, G.: Recent Progr. Hormone Res. 15, 275 (1959).
2. Giroud, C. J. P., M. Saffran, A. V. Schally, J. Stachenke and E. H. Venning: Proc. Soc. exp. Biol. (N. Y.) 92, 855 (1956).

3. van der Vies, J.: Acta Endocr. **33**, 59 (1960).
4. Vecsei/Weisz, P. A.-né Kemény, I. Purjesz, L. Ritter, J. Márton és T. Gosztonyi: Orv. Hetil. **103**, 1607 (1962).

Diskussion

H. J. Karl (München):

Bekanntlich wird von der Nebennierenrinde der Ratte kein Cortisol, sondern Corticosteron produziert. Die Verabreichung von Cortisol führt bei den Tieren zu einer verminderten Corticosteronsekretion. Da aber Corticosteron zumindest teilweise Vorstufe von Aldosteron ist, wäre auch denkbar, daß exogen zugeführtes Cortisol bei den Tieren die Aldosteronsekretion durch Veränderung der Corticosteronproduktion beeinflußt.

P. Vecsei-Weisz:

Die Aldosteronproduktion nahm stärker ab als die von Corticosteron. Daher ist es unwahrscheinlich, allein mit dem Mangel an Corticosteron (als Precursor) den Aldosteronabfall zu erklären. Zwei weitere Möglichkeiten:

1. "Feed-back"-Wirkung von Hydrocortison selbst.
2. "Feed-back"-Wirkung wegen der Mineralocorticoideigenschaften der angewandten, relativ großen Hydrocortisondosen.

Aus der I. Medizinischen Universitätsklinik Hamburg-Eppendorf
(Direktor: Prof. Dr. H. BARTELHEIMER)

Über den Einfluß anaboler Hormone auf das Steroidulcus der Ratte

Von

J.-G. RAUSCH-STROOMANN

Mit 1 Abbildung

Es darf als gesicherte Tatsache gelten, daß das Ulcus eine recht häufige Komplikation der Behandlung mit Nebennierensteroiden darstellt.

In einer eigenen Zusammenstellung des Weltschrifttums mit 5285 behandelten Fällen wurde über 448 Ulcera und 225 mal über das Auftreten von Oberbauchbeschwerden berichtet. 45 mal kam es zu Blutungen, 41 mal zu Perforationen, 15 Fälle verliefen tödlich. Jeder Arzt, der einmal das Erlebnis einer solchen Komplikation hatte, wird in Zukunft größere Vorsicht bei der Indikationsstellung zur Steroidtherapie walten lassen und vor allem bei Patienten, die bereits eine Ulcusanamnese haben, vor Beginn einer solchen Therapie eine Röntgenuntersuchung des Magens vornehmen.

Über die Ätiologie des Steroidulcus herrscht keineswegs Klarheit, vielmehr sind verschiedene Theorien aufgestellt worden.

Ein Weg zu ihrer Erforschung besteht in der Durchführung von Tierversuchen, wiewohl solche immer nur bedingt auf den Menschen übertragbar sind. Wie von verschiedenen Autoren gefunden worden ist, kann man durch Gabe von Nebennierensteroiden im Magen der Ratte Ulcera erzeugen. Das gelingt aber nur mit Hilfe der Technik von SHAY, also indem zusätzlich eine Pylorusligatur vorgenommen wird, oder aber wenn man die Tiere für einige Tage hungern läßt.

Wir haben den zweiten Weg gewählt. Bei weiblichen Wistar-Ratten wurde ein Stress (6 Tage Hungern) ausgeübt und die Ulcusentstehung im Drüsenmagen und im Vormagen nach dem Töten der Tiere beurteilt, und zwar je nach Zahl und Größe der Ulcera bewertet von 0 bis $+++$. Von den einzelnen Tiergruppen ($n = 4$) wurden der Mittelwert und die Streuung berechnet und graphisch dargestellt.

Außerdem haben wir die Nebennieren der Tiere histologisch untersucht und nach dem Grade der progressiven bzw. der regressiven Transformation (TONUTTI) beurteilt. (Für die Unterstützung bei dieser Beurteilung sind wir Herrn Prof. KRACHT zu besonderem Dank verpflichtet).

Schließlich wurden das Gewicht beider Nebennieren festgestellt sowie die Gewichtsabnahme der Tiere während des Versuches. Uns kam es besonders darauf an, die Wirkung der einzelnen gebräuchlichen Steroidpräparate vergleichend in dieser Versuchsanordnung zu prüfen und dann in einer weiteren Versuchsreihe den Effekt eines anabolen Hormones, des SH 601 (1-Methyl-Δ-1-androstenolonönanthat) zu untersuchen.

                                          16*

Zunächst wurden die verschiedenen Hormone in einem sog. Kurzversuch während einer 6 tägigen Hungerperiode gegeben. Es bestand eine gewisse Beziehung der Ulcushäufigkeit zum Stresseffekt, aber nicht in allen Fällen. Besonders bemerkenswert ist, daß unter den Glucocorticoiden die Ulcera im allgemeinen im Drüsenmagen auftreten, bei den Kontrolltieren, bei ACTH-Gabe und bei den Mineralocorticoiden mehr im Vormagen.

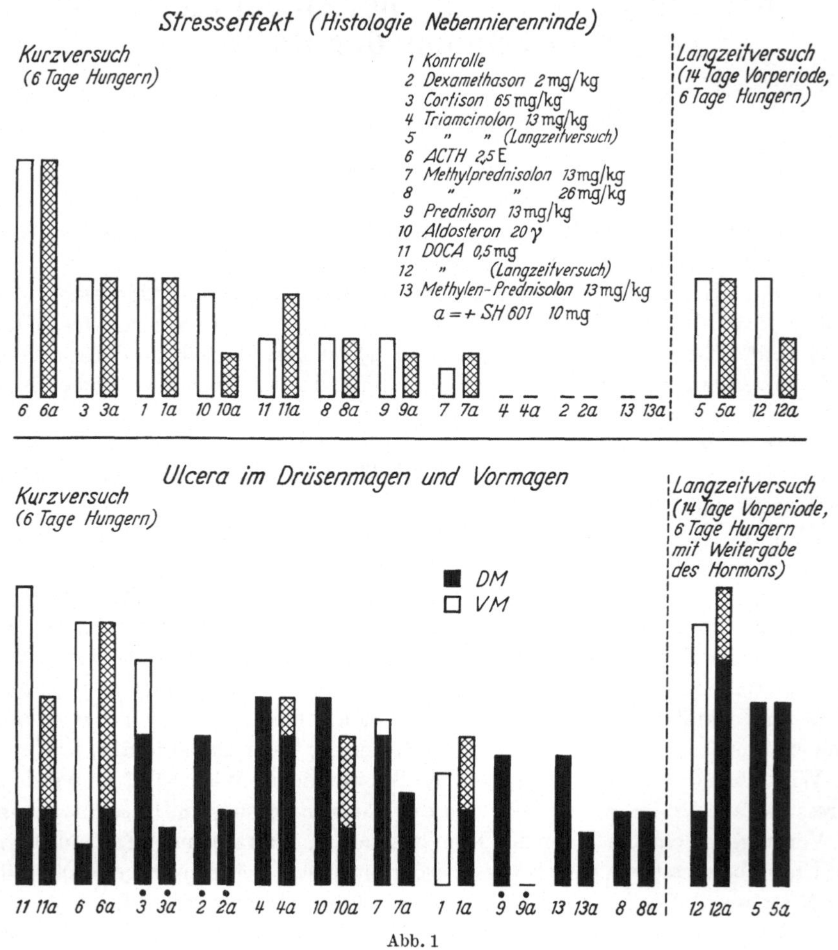

Abb. 1

Das ist auch nach Adrenalektomie der Fall. Interessant ist, daß nach Adrenalektomie sowohl die Gabe eines Glucocorticoids, wie auch die eines Mineralocorticoids die Ulcushäufigkeit wieder auf niedrigere Werte senkt.

In einem sog. Langzeitversuch unterschieden wir dann jeweils eine Vorperiode mit 14 tägiger Gabe des betreffenden Hormones und anschließend die Hungerperiode, entweder ohne oder mit Weitergabe des Mittels bzw. eines anderen Hormones. Dieser Versuch sollte als Modell für den Fall dienen, daß die Steroidbehandlung plötzlich abgesetzt wird. Es ergab sich, daß die Ulcusgefährdung be-

sonders groß ist, auch z. B. nach Absetzen von SU 4885, während z. B. die Ulcusgefährdung viel geringer ist, wenn man SU 4885 weitergibt. Interessant ist auch
ein Fall, wo nach Vorbehandlung mit Prednison während der Hungertage SU 4885
gegeben wurde. Mit dem Stresseffekt besteht keine Korrelation.

Und nun zur Behandlung mit anabolen Hormonen (Abb. 1). Das 1-Methyl-
Δ-1-androstenolonönanthat wurde bei dem Kurzversuch einen Tag vor den
Hungertagen i. m. gegeben, im Langzeitversuch jeweils vor Beginn einer Ver-
suchswoche. Ein Einfluß auf den Stresseffekt ergab sich nicht; auch auf das Neben-
nierengewicht und das Gewicht der Tiere ließ sich kein Effekt feststellen.

Bei den Kontrolltieren, bei ACTH-Gabe und bei Gabe von Mineralocorticoiden
fand sich keine Beeinflussung der Ulcushäufigkeit. Ein statistisch signifikanter
Unterschied ergab sich jedoch bei der Behandlung mit Cortison, Dexamethason
und Prednison, wahrscheinlich auch bei Methylenprednisolon. Bei diesen Hormonen, die zu den am häufigsten in der Therapie verwendeten gehören, scheint
nach dem Tierversuch eine Hemmung der Ulcusbildung im Drüsenmagen der
Ratte stattzufinden, wenn man ein anaboles Hormon gibt.

Ähnliche Beobachtungen machten KOWALEWSKI und SUCHOWSKY und JUNK-
MANN mit etwas anderer Versuchsanordnung.

Über die Ursache des Effektes herrscht keine klare Vorstellung, möglicherweise handelt es sich um die anabole Wirkung, einen capillarschützenden Effekt,
oder um einen Einfluß auf den allgemeinen Körperzustand der Tiere. Wir möchten
auf jeden Fall in Analogie zu unseren Ergebnissen die Meinung äußern, daß ein
Versuch der Verhütung des Steroidulcus durch anabole Hormone auch beim
Menschen gemacht werden sollte.

Literatur

1. SHAY, W., S. A. KOMAROV, S. S. FELS, D. MERANLE, M. GRUENSTEIN and H. SIPLET:
   Gastroenterology 5, 43 (1945).
2. KOWALEWSKI, K.: Proc. Soc. exp. Biol. (N. Y.) 101, 1 (1959).
3. SUCHOWSKY, G. K., u. K. JUNKMANN: Klin. Wschr. 39, 369 (1961).

Diskussion

G. VOGEL (Hoechst):
   A. ROBERT u. Mitarb. fanden bereits vor einigen Jahren, daß der Vormagen und der
pylorusnahe Teil (Hauptmagen) bei nach SHAY operierten oder hungernden Ratten mit oder
ohne Steroidbehandlung eine ganz verschiedene Ulcushäufigkeit aufweisen. Unbehandelte
Kontrollratten zeigten gehäufte und z. T. perforierte Ulcera im Vormagen, durch Cortisol
wurde deren Häufigkeit vermindert. Umgekehrt hatten unbehandelte hungernde Ratten kaum
Ulcera im pylorusnahen Teil, wohl dagegen zeigten dies in Abhängigkeit von der Dosis und
dem Präparat die mit Corticosteroiden behandelten Tiere.

W. HOHLWEG (Graz):
   Ich kann es mir nicht erklären, daß einerseits durch Zufuhr von ACTH, andererseits durch
Adrenalektomie — also direkt gegensätzliche Maßnahmen — die Ulcusentstehung bei den
Ratten am stärksten gefördert werden kann.

Aus dem Institut für Hygiene und Mikrobiologie der Universität des Saarlandes, Homburg

Isolierung lipophiler C_{18}- und C_{21}-Steroidconjugate aus peripherem Plasma

Von

G. W. OERTEL und E. KAISER

Mit 1 Abbildung

In früheren Mitteilungen berichteten wir bereits über das Vorkommen von lipophilen und solvolysierbaren 17-Ketosteroidconjugaten in peripherem menschlichen Plasma, die vornehmlich in α_1-globulinhaltigen Proteinfraktionen enthalten waren. Aufgrund der Zusammensetzung hochgereinigter Conjugatfraktionen aus rund 1 Mol 17-Ketosteroid, 1 Mol anorganischer Säure, 1 Mol Glycerin und 2 Mol Fettsäure schrieben wir dem isolierten Material die Struktur von 17-Ketosteroidestern einer Diglyceridschwefelsäure bzw. Diglyceridphosphorsäure zu. Da nach chromatographischen Untersuchungen der weitaus größte Teil der Plasma-17-ketosteroide in einer derartigen Conjugationsform vorzuliegen scheint, erhob sich die Frage, ob nicht auch andere, im Harn teilweise als Sulfat ausgeschiedenen C_{18}- oder C_{21}-Steroide im Plasma als lipophile Conjugate vorliegen. Wir unternahmen daher folgende Experimente: Sammelplasma von gesunden Schwangeren im 1. bis 3. Trimenon, welches uns z. T. Dr. HAMMERSTEIN, Berlin, zur Verfügung stellte, wurde zunächst dreimal mit je 2 Vol. eiskalten Methylenchlorids extrahiert, um freie Steroide zu entfernen. Es schloß sich die Extraktion der gesamten Conjugate mittels 5 Vol Äthanol-Aceton (1:1 v/v) an. Der Extrakt wurde im Rotationsverdampfer bei maximal 40° C zur Trockne gebracht und der Rückstand mittels Chloroform-Methanol-Wasser (1:9:2 v/v) auf eine mit dem gleichen Lösungsmittelgemisch vorbehandelte Säule aus aktivierter DEAE-Cellulose oder aktiviertem DEAE-Sephadex A-25 aufgetragen. Die Elution der einzelnen Fraktionen erfolgte mit je 200 ml Chloroform-Methanol-Wasser (1:9:2 v/v), 90%, 75%, 50%, 25% Methanol, Wasser und saurer Ammoniumsulfatlösung. Enthielt die mit saurer Ammoniumsulfatlösung eluierte Fraktion stets sämtliche Steroidsulfate, so fanden sich die lipophilen Conjugate ausschließlich in den mit organischen Lösungsmitteln eluierten ersten beiden Fraktionen. Die Entfernung der hierin gleichfalls enthaltenen Steroid-glucuronoside gelang durch Lösungsmittelverteilung zwischen Äthylacetat und 1 n Natronlauge. Während die in der Natronlauge befindlichen Steroid-glucuronoside einer Bebrütung mit β-Glucuronidase zugeführt wurden, reinigten wir die in der organischen Phase auftretenden lipophilen Steroidconjugate durch eine zweite Säulenchromatographie an Aluminiumoxyd, zerlegten sie durch Solvolyse und analysierten die freigesetzten Steroide nach mehrfacher Papierchromatographie in verschiedenen Lösungsmittelsystemen. Wie Tab. 1 zeigt, konnten alle drei, bisher in Schwangerenplasma nachgewiesenen Oestrogene: Oestron, Oestradiol und Oestriol in der als Sulfatidylsteroide bezeichneten Conjugatfraktion aufgefunden werden. Der Anteil der

Sulfatidyl-oestrogene an den gesamten Conjugaten betrug bei Oestron 75%, bei Oestradiol 68% und bei Oestriol 51%. Demgegenüber belief sich die Konzentration der in der Sulfatfraktion enthaltenen Oestrogenconjugate auf lediglich 20, bzw. 24 und 37% der solvolysierbaren Konjugate. Von den Oestrogen-glucuronosiden erwies sich nur das Oestriol-glucuronosid mengenmäßig von Bedeutung. Der Nachweis der einzelnen Oestrogene geschah vermittels bekannter, mehr oder

Tabelle 1. *Konzentration von Oestron, Oestradiol und Oestriol*
in einzelnen Fraktionen (μg/440 ml)

	Frei	Glucuro-nocide	Sulphat	Sulphatid	Gesamt
Oestron. . . .	0,82	1,18	2,76	11,52	16,28
Oestradiol. . .	0,42	0,46	0,91	2,89	4,68
Oestriol. . . .	1,26	2,16	3,21	5,49	12,12

weniger spezifischer Farbreaktionen, die im Verein mit den zur Isolierung benutzten chromatographischen Verfahren eine ausreichende Sicherung der Identität gewährleisten sollten.

In ähnlicher Weise wurde die Isolierung von C_{21}-Steroiden aus der lipophilen Conjugatfraktion von ACTH-Sammelplasma versucht. Wiederum bildeten Extraktion freier Steroide, Chromatographie der Conjugate an DEAE-Sephadex oder DEAE-Cellulose, Lösungsmittelverteilung, Chromatographie an Aluminiumoxyd und Analyse der mittels Solvolyse freigesetzter Steroide die einzelnen Schritte, die zur Isolierung von Cortisol und Tetrahydrocortisol führen sollten. Der Identifizierung der beiden Corticosteroide dienten mehrere der bekannten Nachweisverfahren. Außer der Anwendung bekannter Farbreaktionen, wie der Porter-Silber-Reaktion oder der Tetrazoliumblau-Reaktion hielten wir eine Überführung der freien Steroide in geeignete Derivate für notwendig, deren qualitativer Nachweis nach wiederholter Papierchromatographie in verschiedenen Lösungsmittelsystemen vermittels des Schwefelsäureabsorptionsspektrums erfolgte. Die Konzentration der als Cortisol und Tetrahydrocortisol angesehenen C_{21}-Steroide in der lipophilen Conjugatfraktion bewegte sich zwischen 60 und 40% der gesamten jeweiligen Conjugate. Besteht früheren Versuchen zufolge eine bevorzugte Bindung der als Sulfatidyl-17-ketosteroide angesehenen lipophilen Conjugate an α_1-Globuline des Plasmas, was durch Isolierung signifikanter Mengen von 17-Ketosteroiden aus α_1-Lipoproteinen bestätigt wurde, so sollten die isolierten C_{21}-Steroide gleichfalls in derartigen Plasmafraktionen zu finden sein. Die Chromatographie von Plasmaproteinen an DEAE-Sephadex, wie sie bereits im Falle der 17-Ketosteroid-conjugate durchgeführt wurde, diente der Überprüfung einer solchen Hypothese. Es zeigte sich, daß der größte Teil der conjugierten Porter-Silber-chromogene ebenso wie die lipophilen 17-Ketosteroidconjugate in einer vornehmlich aus α_1-Globulinen zusammengesetzten Proteinfraktion enthalten waren. Versuche zur Isolierung von C_{21}-Steroiden aus α_1-Lipoproteinen sind noch nicht abgeschlossen. Desgleichen ist das Vorkommen von Corticosteron in der Fraktion der sogenannten Sulfatidyl-steroide noch nicht erwiesen, wenngleich verschiedene Befunde auf das Vorhandensein dieses Corticosteroids in der lipophilen Konjugatfraktion hindeuten.

Zusammenfassend darf gesagt werden, daß in der großen Fraktion der lipophilen und solvolysierbaren Steroidconjugate, wie sie unter schonenden Bedingungen aus Plasma isoliert werden können, nicht nur die mengenmässig vorherrschenden 17-Ketosteroide, sondern auch C_{18}- und C_{21}-Steroide enthalten sind. Gelang doch die Isolierung von Oestron, Oestradiol und Oestriol, sowie von Cortisol und Tetrahydrocortisol aus dem Gemisch der „Sulfatidyl-steroide".

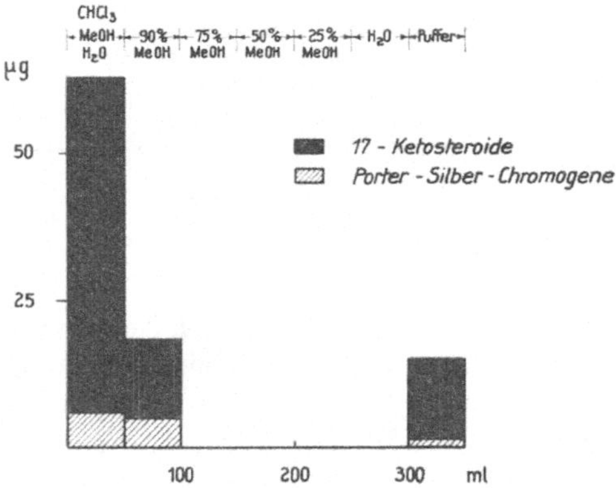

Abb. 1. Chromatographie einer lipophilen Conjugatfraktion aus vornehmlich α_1-globulinhaltigem Serumprotein an DEAE-Sephadex

Was die physiologische Bedeutung solcher Conjugate angeht, so ist diese bedeutsame Frage noch völlig offen. Handelt es sich bei Sulfatidylsteroiden um die Transportform der im Organismus benötigten Steroidsulfate oder dient diese Conjugatform dem Eintritt des Steroids in die Zelle. Eine Beantwortung dieser Frage bleibt weiteren Untersuchungen vorbehalten.

Aus dem Institut für Hygiene und Mikrobiologie der Universität des Saarlandes, Homburg

Zur Biogenese lipophiler 17-Ketosteroidconjugate

Von

G. W. OERTEL

Mit 2 Abbildungen

Die Isolierung verschiedener 17-Ketosteroid-sulfate aus peripherem Blut und Nebennierenvenenblut durch BAULIEU und die Untersuchungsergebnisse von PUCHE und NES, welche eine reversible, anionische Bindung von Dehydroepiandrosteron-sulfat an Serumalbumin befürworten, entsprachen den bisherigen Vorstellungen über das Vorkommen von 17-Ketosteroid-sulfaten im menschlichen Plasma. Demgegenüber zeigten chromatographische Versuche, daß bei der Säulenchromatographie von Plasmaextrakten an DEAE-Cellulose oder DEAE-Sephadex der weitaus größte Teil der vorhandenen 17-Ketosteroidconjugate sich deutlich von authentischen 17-Ketosteroid-sulfaten unterschied. Auch bei Lösungsmittelverteilung der in lipoidhaltigen Fraktionen enthaltenen 17-Ketosteroidconjugate zwischen Äthylacetat und Natriumbicarbonat blieb die Hauptmenge der 17-Ketosteroidconjugate in der organischen Phase. Da weiterhin im Verlaufe einer Dünnschichtchromatographie auf Kieselgel G und einer Papierchromatographie auf Kieselgelpapier Schleicher & Schüll Nr. 289 die aus Plasma isolierten, lipophilen 17-Ketosteroidconjugate die gleiche Wanderungsgeschwindigkeit besaßen wie synthetische Sulfatidyl-17-ketosteroide, erscheint die Frage nach der ursprünglichen Conjugationsform der Plasma-17-ketosteroide noch keineswegs befriedigend geklärt. Außer der Isolierung lipophiler Steroidconjugate und ihrer Strukturermittlung galt unser Interesse vor allem der Bildung solcher Conjugate.

Da die Leber bekanntlich über die für eine Bildung von Phosphatiden und neutralen Lipoiden notwendigen Enzymsysteme in reichlichem Masse verfügt, sollte eine Umwandlung von 17-Ketosteroid oder 17-Ketosteroidsulfat in lipophile Conjugate durch Bebrütung mit Lebergewebe theoretisch möglich sein. Für unsere Inkubationsversuche wählten wir daher jeweils 5 ml eines 20% Homogenats von Meerschweinchenleber in 0.1 M Phosphatpuffer von p_H 7,0, wobei die Zelltrümmer durch 10 minütiges Zentrifugieren bei 3000 g entfernt wurden. Als Substrat dienten 500 μg 7-Tritium-markiertes Dehydroepiandrosteron bzw. Dehydroepiandrosteron-sulfat, als Coenzyme 2—4 μM ATP, Coenzym A, CTP und DPN, entweder einzeln oder in Kombination. Bei Verwendung von freiem Dehydroepiandrosteron als Substrat fügten wir außerdem 10 μM Magnesiumchlorid und 100 μM Kaliumsulfat hinzu. Nach dreistündiger Bebrütung bei 37° C an der Luft wurden die Inkubate dreimal mit je 2 Vol. eiskalten Methylenchlorids extrahiert zwecks Entfernung freien Dehydroepiandrosterons. Es folgte die Extraktion der gesamten Conjugate mittels 5 Vol. Äthanol-Aceton (1:1 v/v). Der Rückstand des im Rotationsverdampfer zur Trockne gebrachten Extraktes unterwarfen wir sodann einer Säulenchromatographie an DEAE-Sephadex A-25, wodurch sich eine einwandfreie Trennung von lipophilen, solvolysierbaren 17-Ketosteroidconjugaten und

17-Ketosteroidsulfaten erreichen läßt. Die in der lipophilen Conjugatfraktion
möglicherweise enthaltenen Steroid-glucuronoside wurden durch Lösungsmittelverteilung zwischen Äthylacetat und Natriumbicarbonat entfernt und die 17-
Ketosteroidconjugate in der organischen Phase sodann durch Solvolyse zerlegt.
Für die Abtrennung des freigesetzten Dehydroepiandrosterons empfahl sich eine
zweimalige Papierchromatographie in verschiedenen Lösungsmittelsystemen. Die

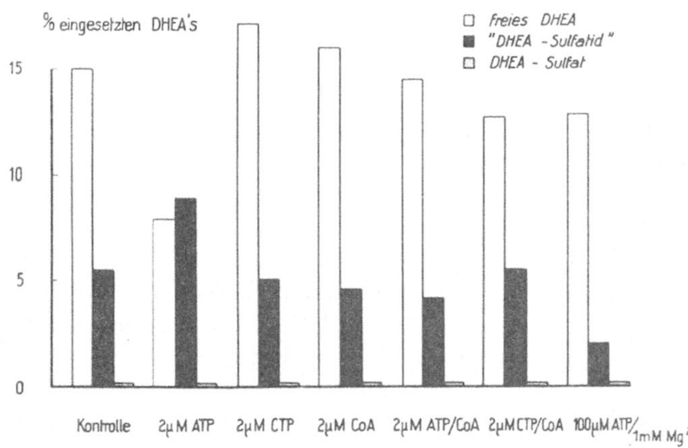

Abb. 1. Bebrütung von Leberhomogenat mit freiem Dehydroepiandrosteron

quantitative Bestimmung des isolierten Dehydroepiandrosterons erfolgte vermittels Zimmermann-Reaktion und Allen-Reaktion, sowie Messung der vorhandenen Radioaktivität im Packard-Tricarb-Szintillationszähler. Die Festlegung
der spezifischen Radioaktivität nach zusätzlichen Reinigungsschritten durch
Derivatbildung und Papierchromatographie derartiger Derivate gestattete eine
Aussage über die Reinheit bzw. die Identität des isolierten Materials. Wie Abb. 1
zeigt, führte die Bebrütung von Leberhomogenat mit freiem, markiertem Dehydroepiandrosteron zu einer Ausbeute von maximal 8% an dem gewünschten, lipophilen Conjugat. Von zugesetzten Coenzymen brachte nur ATP eine gewisse,
wenngleich begrenzte Wirkung, welche vielleicht auf die Rolle dieses Coenzyms bei
der Sulfurylierung, d. h. der Bereitstellung „aktiven Sulfats" zurückgeführt
werden könnte. Bei der Verwendung von markiertem Dehydroepiandrosteron-
sulfat als Substrat beobachteten wir in Gegenwart von Coenzym A oder Coenzym A
und ATP eine annähernd 17% Umwandlung des Substrats in lipophiles Conjugat.
Abb. 2. Hier wäre es denkbar, daß die durch Coenzym A und ATP beeinflußte
Konzentration an Diglycerid umsatzbestimmend ist. Bei dem Vergleich der
chromatographischen Eigenschaften einer aus Plasma isolierten, lipophilen Conjugatfraktion und dem aus Inkubaten gewonnenen lipophilen Dehydroepian-
drosteron-conjugat ergab sich eine völlige Übereinstimmung, was die Wanderungsgeschwindigkeit auf Dünnschichtplatten und Kieselgelpapier betraf. Des weiteren
glichen sich die aus Plasma isolierten oder durch Inkubation gebildeten 17-
Ketosteroidconjugate in ihrer Unbeständigkeit, die sich durch Zerfall in 17-
Ketosteroid-sulfat und Diglycerid offenbarte. Da außerdem im Ultraviolett-
absorptionsspektrum beider Substanzen ein Absorptionsmaximum bei 235—237 mμ
zu erkennen war, und das Schwefelsäureabsorptionsspektrum Absorptionsmaxima
bei 300 und 410 mμ aufwies, nehmen wir an, daß es sich bei dem biosynthetischen

Material und der aus Plasma abgetrennten lipophilen Conjugatfraktion um die gleiche Conjugationsform handelt, für welche wir die Struktur von Sulfatidylsteroiden vorgeschlagen haben.

Die Biosynthese des lipophilen Dehydroepiandrosteron-conjugats durch Bebrütung von Dehydroepiandrosteron oder Dehydroepiandrosteron-sulfat in

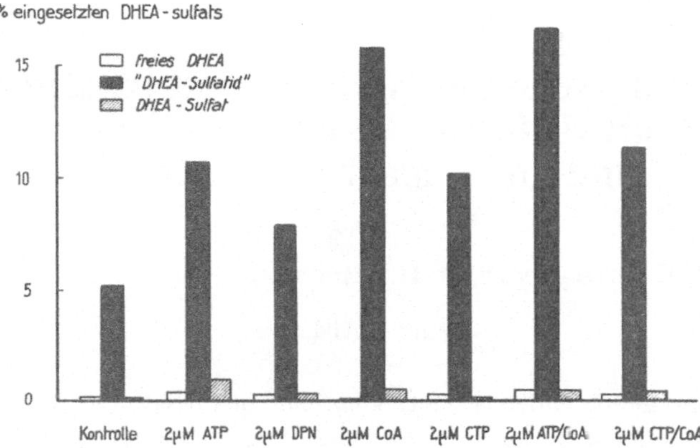

Abb. 2. Bebrütung von Leberhomogenat mit Dehydroepiandrosteron-Sulfat

Leberhomogenat sollte uns in die Lage versetzen, genügend Material für eine einwandfreie chemische Analyse bereitzustellen. Scheiterte doch die Strukturermittlung der aus Plasma isolierten lipophilen 17-Ketosteroidconjugate bisher letztlich an der geringen Menge verfügbaren Ausgangsmaterials, wie auch der Anwesenheit zahlreicher anderer, nur in ihrer Steroidkomponente unterscheidbaren Conjugate.

Ob die Biogenese solch lipophiler 17-Ketosteroidconjugate auf Lebergewebe beschränkt ist, erscheint angesichts der Isolierung derartiger Conjugate aus Nebennierenvenenblut in vergleichsweise höheren Konzentrationen fraglich. Vielmehr sind wir der Ansicht, daß die hier durch Inkubation von Lebergewebe mit 17-Ketosteroid erhältlichen, lipophilen 17-Ketosteroidconjugate die allgemeine Transportform der physiologisch wirksamen 17-Ketosteroid-sulfate darstellen.

Diskussion

W. Teller (Marburg):

Zu Ihren Untersuchungen hätte ich zwei Fragen:

1. Haben Sie im Plasma neben Hydrocortison und Tetrahydrocortisol noch andere C_{21}-Metaboliten, z. B. Tetrahydrocortison, als lipophile Conjugate nachweisen können?

2. War es Ihnen mit Ihren relativ schonenden Aufarbeitungsverfahren möglich, die Sulfatidyl-Steroidconjugate kristallin aus Plasma darzustellen und Infrarotspektren davon aufzuzeichnen, die mit den synthetischen Präparaten übereinstimmten?

G. W. Oertel:

1. Bei ACTH-Gabe beobachtet man eine höhere Konzentration von Sulfatidylsteroiden sowie einer nicht-solvolysierbaren Fraktion, welche wir als Phosphatidyl-dehydroepiandrosteron ansehen.

2. Die Infrarotspektren der angenommenen Sulfatidyl-17-Ketosteroide stehen noch aus und werden erschwert durch die relative Unbeständigkeit der natürlichen Sulfatidyl-17-Ketosteroide, die der von synthetischen vollkommen entspricht. Analysen von UV-Absorptionsspektren und Schwefelsäureabsorptionsspektrum sprechen allerdings für die von uns angenommene Struktur der lipophilen Conjugate. Die biosynthetische Gewinnung von „Sulfatidyldehydroepiandrosteron" sollte eine Infrarotanalyse durch ausreichende Bereitstellung notwendigen Ausgangsmaterials ermöglichen.

Aus der I. Medizinischen Universitätsklinik Frankfurt am Main
(Direktor: Prof. Dr. F. Hoff)

Immunologische Bestimmung von Insulin im Blut mit Hilfe von Insulinantikörpern und Jod[131]-markiertem Insulin

Von

F. Melani[1], H. Ditschuneit, H. H. Ditschuneit, A. Mucci[2], E. F. Pfeiffer*

Mit 2 Abbildungen

Die heute gebräuchlichen Methoden zur quantitativen Bestimmung von Insulin im Blut beruhen auf dem Vergleich bestimmter biologischer Wirkungen von Serum oder Plasma mit den entsprechenden Wirkungen von kristallisiertem Insulin auf den Stoffwechsel isolierter Gewebe. Von einigen Autoren wird die Glucoseaufnahme des Rattendiaphragma als Parameter der Insulinwirkung verwandt, von anderen die direkte Glucoseoxydation radioaktiver Glucose durch das isolierte epididymale Rattenfettgewebe (*2, 3, 5, 6*).

Zu diesem Verfahren sind in letzter Zeit immunologische Bestimmungsmethoden hinzugetreten, bei denen die neutralisierenden (*1, 7*) oder bindenden (*4, 8*) Eigenschaften von Insulinantikörpern zur quantitativen Bestimmung kleinster Insulinmengen ausgenutzt werden. Die Verfahren, bei denen die Bestimmung auf den neutralisierenden Antikörpereigenschaften beruhen, sind spezifisch und nur mit einem kleinen Fehler behaftet. Sie sind jedoch für die Messung von Insulin im Blut zu unempfindlich. Bei Ausnutzung der bindenden Antikörpereigenschaften, auf denen die von Grodski und Forsham (*4*) sowie Yalow und Berson (*8*) ausgearbeiteten Verfahren beruhen, konnte die Empfindlichkeit bis auf weniger als 1 μE/ml gesteigert werden. Dabei wird die kompetitive Hemmung der Bindung von Jod[131]-markiertem Insulin an Insulinantikörper durch steigende Mengen von nicht markiertem Insulin benutzt. Durch Erhöhung der Konzentration von nicht markiertem Insulin wird bei konstanter Menge von J[131]-Insulin und konstanter Antikörpermenge das Verhältnis von gebundenem zu nicht gebundenem Jod[131]-Insulin umgekehrt proportional beeinflußt. Das Problem dieses Verfahrens liegt in der Trennung von gebundenem und freiem Insulin und deren quantitativer Erfassung. Yalow und Berson benutzen hierfür die Papierelektrophorese mit anschließender Radiochromatographie. Die dazu erforderlichen spezifischen Aktivitäten von Jod[131]-Insulin müssen aber außerordentlich hoch sein (150—300mC/mg). Dadurch ist aber nicht nur die Gefahr der

---

[1,2] Stipendiat der A. v. Humboldt-Stiftung.

* Durchgeführt mit Unterstützung der Deutschen Forschungsgemeinschaft, Bad Godesberg.

Zerstörung des Insulinmoleküls gegeben, sondern die Herstellung und der Umgang mit diesem stark markierten Insulin erfordern spezielle Isotopenlaboratorien mit besonderen Sicherheitsmaßnahmen.

Die folgenden Untersuchungen verfolgten das Ziel, ein Verfahren zur Trennung von freiem und gebundenem Insulin auszuarbeiten, bei dem auch geringere und kommerziell leicht erhältliche spezifische Insulinaktivitäten verwandt werden können.

Methodik

Die Trennung von freiem und gebundenem Insulin führten wir im Agar-Gel auf einem Objektträger durch. Die spezifische Aktivität des verwandten Jod^{131}-Schweineinsulins betrug nur 6–10 mC/mg. Als Antiserum wurde ein Meerschweinchen-anti-Insulin-Serum benutzt.

0,5 ml verdünntes Antiserum wurde zusammen mit 0,5 ml Serum oder 0,5 ml Standardlösung aus Schweine-Insulin unterschiedlicher Konzentration (10 bis 500 μE/ml) und 50 μE Jod^{131}-Schweine-Insulin 3–4 Tage lang bei + 4° C aufbewahrt. Anschließend wurde mit Hilfe eines kleinen Filterpapierstreifens eine kleine Probe dieses Ansatzes auf einen mit einer Agargelschicht bedeckten Objektträger aufgebracht und das gebundene und freie Insulin elektrophoretisch getrennt. Nach der Trennung wird die Agargelschicht unmittelbar an der kathodischen Seite des kleinen Filterpapierstreifens in zwei Hälften zerschnitten und die Radioaktivität eines jeden Agargelstückes nach Frieren und Auftauen zwecks Zerstörung des Gels mit Hilfe eines Flüssigkeitsszintillationzählers gemessen.

Ergebnisse

Infolge der starken Elektroendosmose im Agargel wandern die β- und γ-Globuline im elektrischen Feld zur Kathode und die Albumine zur Anode. Das an die Antikörper-Globuline gebundene Insulin befindet sich demnach vom auftragenden Filterpapierstreifen aus gesehen, dem Startpunkt, auf der Seite der Kathode, das freie Insulin, das sich zusammen mit der langsam wandernden Albuminfraktion bewegt, auf der Seite der Anode. Ein geringer Anteil des freien Insulins wird vom Filterpapierstreifen adsorbiert, wodurch im Bereich der Auftragstelle ein kleiner radioaktiver Gipfel verursacht wird (Abb. 1).

Mit verschiedenen Antiserumverdünnungen ergibt das Verhältnis von gebundenem zu freiem Insulin (B/F) in Abhängigkeit von der Konzentration nicht markierten Insulins unterschiedliche Kurvenverläufe. Mit dem von mehreren Meerschweinchen gemischten Antiserum war mit einer Serumverdünnung von 1: 2500 und 50 μE/ml Jod^{131}-Schweineinsulin die größte Empfindlichkeit für den gewünschten Bereich zwischen 5 und 200 μ E/ml Insulin zu erreichen.

Infolge der hyperbolischen Gesetzmäßigkeit zwischen dem Verhältnis von gebundenem zu freiem Insulin und der Insulinkonzentration ergibt die graphische Darstellung bei doppelt logarithmischer Koordinatenteilung eine Gerade (Abb. 2). Aus den einzelnen um die Regressionsgerade sich gruppierenden Meßwerten mehrerer Versuchsansätze mit einer Antiserumverdünnung von 1: 2500 und 50 μE/ml Jod^{131}-Insulin errechnet sich ein Genauigkeitsindex von 0,24. Damit ist die Genauigkeit dieser immunologischen Methode nicht größer als die der von uns bisher verwandten Insulinbestimmung mit dem isolierten Rattenfettgewebe.

Sie ist aber empfindlicher und gestattet noch Insulinkonzentrationen unter 10 μ E/ml zu messen, bei denen die Rattenfettgewebsmethode bereits versagt.

Bei der Bestimmung des Insulingehaltes von Serumproben von 5 nüchternen Stoffwechselgesunden ergaben sich Werte zwischen 12 und 90 μE/ml und ein

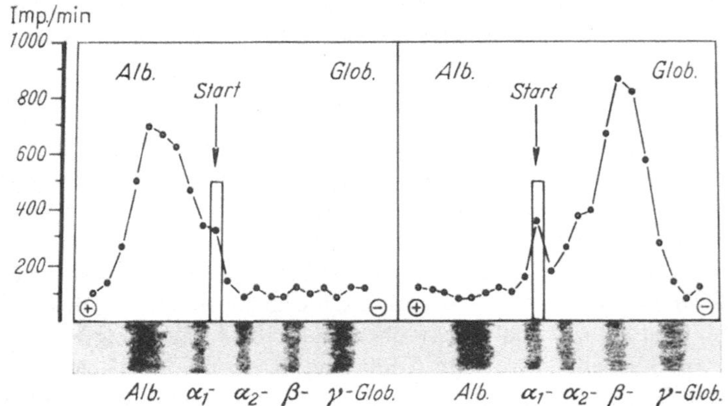

Abb. 1. Verteilung der Radioaktivität von J^{131}-Schweine-Insulin nach zonenelektrophoretischer Trennung mit Agargel zusammen mit normalem Meerschweinchenserum und Meerschweinchen-Antiinsulinserum

Mittelwert von 37 μE/ml. Von Yalow und Berson (9) werden die gleichen Werte für Stoffwechselgesunden angegeben. Mit der Rattenfettgewebsmethode fanden wir dagegen in den gleichen Seren eine höhere mittlere Insulinwirkung von 290 μE/ml.

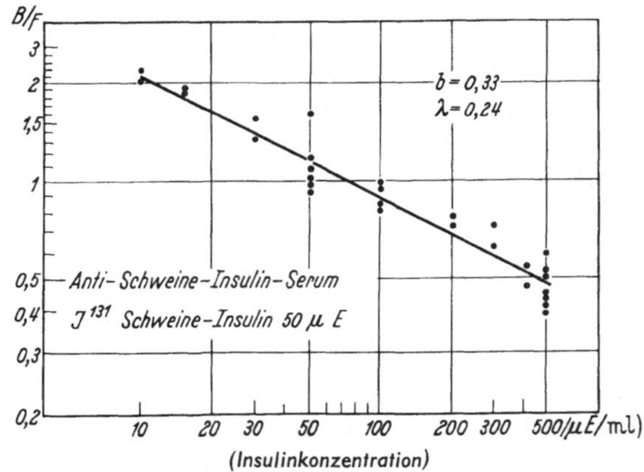

Abb. 2. Einfluß steigender Konzentration von nicht markiertem Schweine-Insulin auf das Verhältnis von gebundenem zu freiem J^{131}-Schweine-Insulin. b = Regressionskoeffizient, λ = Genauigkeitsindex

Auch bei den anderen beiden Gruppen, den Prädiabetikern und Diabetikern, besteht eine nahezu gleichgroße Differenz zwischen den immunologisch und biologisch mit dem Rattenfettgewebe gemessenen Insulinwerten im Nüchtern-serum. Die Insulinwerte der Prädiabetiker liegen im Bereich zwischen 45 und 240 μE/ml, und der Mittelwert von 102 μE-ml dieser Gruppe überragt deutlich den der Stoffwechselgesunden. Die mit der Rattenfettgewebsmethode bestimmten Insulinwirkungen der gleichen Seren sind wiederum nahezu fünffach höher.

Den höchsten mittleren Insulinwert weist mit 125 μE/ml die Gruppe der 6 Diabetiker auf, bei der auch mit der Rattenfettgewebsmethode der höchste Mittelwert von 570 μE/ml im Nüchternserum bestimmt wurde.

Nach Injektion von Glucose steigen die immunologisch gemessenen Insulinkonzentrationen bei den Stoffwechselgesunden nach 15 min auf 80, und nach 30 min auf 93 μE/ml an, und fallen nach 60 min bis auf 63 μE/ml zurück. Einen korrespondierenden Anstieg bei den gleichen Probanden in den gleichen Serumproben wurde auch mit der Rattenfettgewebsmethode gemessen. Bei den Prädiabetikern und Diabetikern finden sich dagegen nach intravenöser Glucosebelastung mit beiden Meßverfahren keine wesentlichen Änderungen der Insulinkonzentrationen.

Das gleichsinnige Verhalten der Insulinkonzentrationen im Nüchternserum und auch nach Glucosebelastungen in den verschiedenen Gruppen läßt vermuten, daß mit dem immunologischen Verfahren ein geringerer Anteil des gesamten Blutinsulingehaltes erfaßt wird als mit dem Rattenfettgewebe.

Literatur

1. ARQUILLA, E. R., and A. B. STAVITSKY: The production and identification of antibodies to insulin and their use in assaying insulin. J. clin. Invest. 35, 458 (1956).
2. DITSCHUNEIT, H., J. AHN-CHANG-SU, M. PFEIFFER u. E. F. PFEIFFER: Über die Bestimmung von Insulin im Blute am epididymalen Fettanhang der Ratte mit Hilfe markierter Glucose. Klin. Wschr. 37, 1234 (1959).
3. — J. D. FAULHABER u. E. F. PFEIFFER: Verbesserung der Methode zur Bestimmung von Insulin im Blut mit Hilfe radioaktiver 1-C^{14}-Glucose und dem epididymalen Rattengewebe. Atompraxis 8, 172 (1962).
4. GRODSKY, G. M., and P. H. FORSHAM: An immunochemical assay of total extractable insulin in man. J. clin. Invest. 39, 1070 (1960).
5. MARTIN, D. B., A. E. RENOLD and Y. M. DAGENAIS: An assay for insulin like activity using rat adipose tissue. Lancet 1958 I, 76.
6. VALLANCE-OVEN, J., and B. HURLOCK: Estimation of plasma-insulin by the rat diaphragm method. Lancet 1954 I, 68.
7. WARDLAW, A. C., and P. J. MOLONEY: The assay of insulin with anti-insulin and mouse diaphragm. Canad. J. Biochem. 39, 695 (1961).
8. YALOW, R. S., and S. A. BERSON: Immuno-assay of endogenous plasma insulin in man. J. clin. Invest. 39, 1157 (1960).
9. — — Plasma insulin concentrations in nondiabetic and early diabetic subjects. Determinations by new sensitive immuno-assay technic. Diabetes 9, 254 (1960).

Aus der I. Medizinischen Universitätsklinik Frankfurt am Main
(Direktor: Prof. Dr. F. Hoff)

Der Einfluß der Leber auf die Transportform von endogenem Insulin und die Wirkung von endogenem Insulin auf den Leberzellstoffwechsel

Von

J. M. Abdel Rahman[1], A. Mucci[2], R. Morcos[3], R. Petzoldt, G. Macht,
H. Ditschuneit und E. F. Pfeiffer*

Mit 1 Abbildung

Die Beziehungen zwischen Leber und körpereigenem Insulin sind charakterisiert einmal durch den Einfluß der Leber auf das Pankreashormon, das immer zuerst das Leberbett passieren muß, ehe es die periphere Zirkulation erreicht, zum anderen durch den Effekt, den das endogene Insulin bei seiner primären Leberpassage auf den Intermediärstoffwechsel der Leber ausübt.

Eine der ersten Untersuchungen über den Einfluß der Leber auf endogenes Insulin stammt von Meythaler und Stahnke (1930). Nach direkter Einleitung des venösen Pankreasblutes in die Vena cava beobachteten sie abnorm niedrige Blutzuckerwerte. Frühere Untersuchungen aus unserem Laboratorium [Pfeiffer u. Mitarb. (1959), Pfeiffer u. Mitarb. (1961)] wiesen in die gleiche Richtung.

Die früheren quantitativen Befunde, die den Einfluß der Leber auf die *Gesamtaktivität* des Insulins im Blute betreffen, werden nun ergänzt durch Veränderungen, die die *Transportform* des endogenen Insulins bei seiner Passage erfährt.

Die ersten Untersuchungen unserer Gruppe [Pfeiffer u. Mitarb. (1962)] haben einen derartigen Effekt nicht nachweisen können.

Die Untersuchungen, über die ich jetzt berichten werde, ergaben ein anderes Bild: Im Gegensatz zu den früheren Untersuchungen wurden Blutproben über den Bereich der damals untersuchten Gefäße hinaus, gleichzeitig aus der A. femoralis, der V. portae, der V. pancr.-duodenalis, der V. hepatica, sowie der V. femoralis bei 6 Hunden vor und nach Rastinon-Injektion entnommen. Das Serum der verschiedenen Proben wurde wieder mit Hilfe der Zonenelektrophorese präparativ in die 4 Fraktionen der γ-, β-, α_2- und α_1-Globuline und Albumine aufgetrennt und die Insulinwirkung der Einzelfraktionen am Rattenfettgewebe und Rattenzwerchfell gemessen.

Abb. 1 zeigt ein repräsentatives Resultat: Der Einfachheit halber wurden auf der Abbildung nicht die verschiedenen Eiweißfraktionen mit den in ihnen enthaltenen Insulinaktivitäten angegeben, sondern die der zu gleichen Teilen ge-

---

[1, 2, 3] Stipendiat der A. v. Humboldt-Stiftung.

* Durchgeführt mit Unterstützung der Deutschen Forschungsgemeinschaft Bad Godesberg.

mischten 1. und 2. Fraktion schraffiert als „gebundene" Insulinaktivität, die der 3. und 4. Fraktion unschraffiert als „freie" aufgetragen. Wie bei den früheren Untersuchungen, lag auch jetzt der größere Teil des Insulins bei Ruhesekretion vor Rastinon im Pankreasvenenblut in der „gebundenen" Form vor. Im Gegensatz zu früher wurde jetzt jedoch schon 5 min nach der Rastinon-Injektion Blut abgenommen. Bei Anstieg der „gebundenen" Form lag nunmehr der weitaus größte Teil des endogenen Insulins als „freies" Hormon vor. 15 min nach Rastinon war dagegen wie früher kein sicherer Unterschied mehr zu erkennen.

In der V. hepatica ist der Anstieg der Insulinaktivitäten erst zum 15 min-Termin zu messen, und hier überwiegt immer das „gebundene" Hormon. Das gleiche Verhältnis ist in der Peripherie zu beobachten. Über eine Bindung von Insulin in der Peripherie berichteten auch SAMOLS und RYDER (1961).

Damit ist es wahrscheinlich, daß nach Stimulierung der Insulinsekretion vornehmlich „freies" Insulin sezerniert, und dann in der Leber zu einem erheblichen Prozentsatz in die „gebundene" Form übergeführt wird. Dieses Resultat deckt sich mit den Ergebnissen von SAMAAN u. Mitarb. sowie von ANTONIADES und seiner Gruppe (1962).

Wenn aber das primär in die Leber nach Stimulierung einströmende Pankreasinsulin vornehmlich aus der „freien" Komponente besteht, dann erscheint es sinnvoll, diesen Effekt des „freien" endogenen Insulins auf den Leberstoffwechsel mit dem des jenseits der Leber in „gebundener" Form vorliegenden Hormons zu vergleichen. Hier gewannen wir eine Anregung durch Untersuchungen

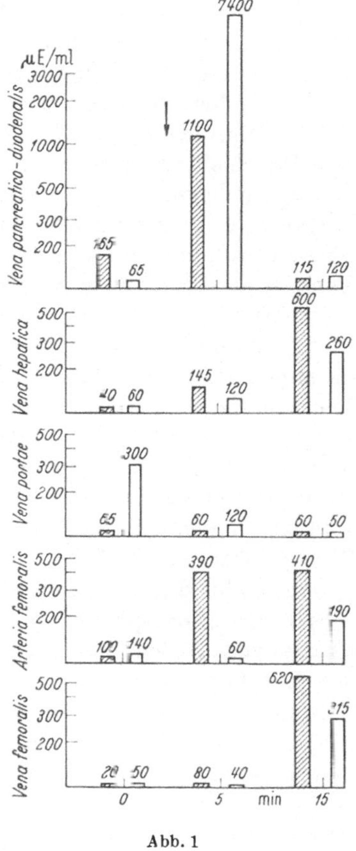

Abb. 1

MEYTHALERs [MEYTHALER und SCHÜRGER (1963)], der sich bereits vor Jahren die getrennte Gefäßversorgung der Leber zunutze gemacht hatte.

In Anlehnung an die Versuchsanordnung von MEYTHALER ließen wir im akuten Versuch bei 3 Hunden, durch Anastomose zwischen V. femoralis und einem Ast der V. portae, einem Leberlappen insulinhaltiges Pankreasvenenblut über die Pfordader, dem anderen peripheres Blut aus der V. femoralis zufließen. Unmittelbar vor sowie 5 und 15 min nach Stimulation der endogenen Insulinsekretion mit 100 mg/kg Rastinon, wurden gleichzeitig in beiden Leberlappen, unter Anwendung des Frierstoppverfahrens und enzymatisch optischer Testverfahren nach WARBURG verschiedene Zwischenstoffkonzentrationen des glykolytischen Kohlenhydratabbaues sowie Pyridinnucleotide und energiereiche Adenosinphosphatverbindungen gemessen. Außerdem bestimmten wir den Glykogengehalt der beiden Leberlappen.

In dem Leberlappen, dem Pankreasvenenblut zuströmte, fand sich nach Stimulierung der endogenen Insulinsekretion ein Abfall der Brenztraubensäure um 57% von 10,8 auf 5,4 γ/g Frischgewicht und auch ein nahezu gleichstarker Abfall des Milchsäuregehaltes innerhalb von 5 min. In dem aus der normalen Pfortaderblutversorgung ausgeschalteten und mit peripherem venösem Blut durchströmten Leberanteil wurde dieser Abfall vermißt. Es erfolgte eher ein Anstieg, der besonders deutlich die Milchsäure betrifft. Triose- und Hexosephosphate, Dioxyacetonphosphat und Fructose-1,6-diphosphat steigen in dem ausgeschalteten Leberlappen geringfügig an, während im normalen Leberlappen nach Stimulierung keine Änderung nachweisbar ist.

Bei den Adenosinphosphatverbindungen tritt im ausgeschalteten Leberlappen eine Verschiebung zu der energieärmeren Adenosinmonophosphatverbindung auf. In dem anderen, portal versorgten Leberanteil sind die unwesentlichen Änderungen nach 10 min wieder ausgeglichen. Der Glykogengehalt des von der Peripherie versorgten Leberlappens zeigt dagegen im Verhältnis zu dem mit portalem Pankreasblut durchströmten eine signifikante Verminderung, wie sie auch von Meythaler bei der chronischen Präparation gefunden wurde.

Damit wurde gezeigt, daß das aus dem Pankreas sezernierte „freie" Insulin einen unmittelbaren Effekt auf den glykolytischen Kohlenhydratstoffwechsel der Leber im Sinne einer Steigerung ausübt, und daß umgekehrt bei Durchströmung mit peripherem Blut, in dem das Insulin vorwiegend in „gebundener" Form vorliegt, der Glucoseabbau über die Glykolysekette bis zur Brenztraubensäure beeinträchtigt ist. Die stationären Zwischenstoffkonzentrationen stauen sich an.

Einen wesentlich stärkeren Einfluß scheint aber das freie Insulin auf den Glucoseabbau in der Leber über den Pentosephosphat-Cyclus auszuüben. Als Coferment für diesen im Cytoplasma der Zelle ablaufenden Abbaumechanismus wirken die Triphosphopyridinnucleotide. Die Unterbrechung des direkten Einstromes von „freiem" Pankreasinsulin in die Leber führte zu einer Verminderung des Reduktionsgrades dieser Triphosphopyridinnucleotide und damit zu dem gemessenen Anstieg der Konzentration von oxydiertem TPN um das 5fache des Ausgangswertes (von 27 auf 156 γ/g Frischgewicht). Eine besonders starke Drosselung des Pentosephosphatcyclus wurde auch von Siperstein u. Mitarb. (1958) bei Untersuchungen entsprechender Enzyme beim Alloxandiabetes der Ratte nachgewiesen. Damit gleicht die Drosselung des direkten Zuflusses von „freiem" Insulin aus dem Pankreas trotz genügender Menge „gebundenen" Insulins einem Insulinmangelzustand.

Zusammenfassung

A. Die Vff. haben bei 6 Hunden Blutproben aus der Vena pankreatica, v. portae, v. hepatica, Arteria und Vena femoralis jeweils vor und 5 und 15 min nach Tolbutamidinjektion entnommen. Das gewonnene Serum wurde präparativ elektrophoretisch getrennt und in den einzelnen Fraktionen das Insulin bestimmt. Die Vff. beobachteten:

1. Das Pankreasveneninsulin ist vor der Tolbutamidstimulierung meistens gebunden, nach der Stimulierung meistens frei.

2. Das Leberveneninsulin ist meistens gebunden.

3. Auch das periphere Insulin ist meistens gebunden.

B. Im Lebergewebe von Hunden, bei denen ein Leberlappen mit peripherem Blut (Verbindung einer v. femoralis mit einem Ast der Pfortader durch einen Katheter), der andere Leberlappen mit normalem Portalvenenblut durchströmt worden war, wurden Milch- und Brenztraubensäure, Dioxyacetonphosphat, Fructose-1,6-diphosphat, ATP, ADP, AMP, TPN und DPN und Glykogengehalt vor und 5 und 10 min nach Tolbutamidinjektion bestimmt.

Es hat sich ergeben, daß in dem ausgeschalteten Leberlappen (zu dem peripheres, also gebundenes Insulin kam) die Kurven von MS und BTS, Triose- und Hexosephosphaten höher nivelliert waren als in dem normal durchströmten Leberlappen (zu dem Pankreasinsulin, also freies Insulin kam). Bei dem Adenosinphosphatsystem tritt im ausgeschalteten Leberlappen eine Verschiebung zu der energieärmeren Adenosinmonophosphatverbindung auf, desgleichen beobachtet man einen verminderten Reduktionsgrad der TPN und des Glykogengehaltes.

Diese Ergebnisse werden kurz diskutiert.

Literatur

1. ANTONIADES, H. N., J. A. BOUGAS and H. N. PYLE: Studies on the state of insulin in blood: Examination of splenic, portal and peripheral human blood sera of diabetic and non-diabetic subjects for "free" insulin and insulin complexes. New Engl. J. Med. **267**, 218—222 (1962).
2. MEYTHALER, F., u. E. STAHNKE: Die Wirkung des Pancreashormons bei experimenteller Umgehung der physiologischen Leberpassage. Naunyn-Schmiedeberg's Arch. exp. Path. Pharmak. **152**, 185 (1930).
3. —, u. R. SCHÜRGER: Zur Frage der endogenen Insulinwirkung auf die Leber. Ärztl. Forsch. 17, 57 (1963).
4. PFEIFFER, E. F., M. PFEIFFER, H. DITSCHUNEIT u. AHN-CHANG-SU: Über die Bestimmung von Insulin im Blute am epididymalen Fettanhang der Ratte mit Hilfe markierter Glukose. Klin. Wschr. **37**, 1239 (1959).
5. — — — — and AHN-CHANG-SU: Clinical and experimental studies of insulin secretion following tolbutamide and metahexamide administration. Ann. N. Y. Acad. Sci. **82**, 479 (1959).
6. — Grundlagen und Perspektiven der oralen Diabetestherapie mit Sulfonyharnstoffen. 4. Congr. Int. Diab. Fed., 10—14. Juli 1961, p. 671, Genf.
7. — Dynamic der Insulinsekretion. I. Symp. der Deutschen Diabetes-Komitee 25/26. 10. 1962.
8. SAMOLS, E., and J. A. RYDER: Studies on tissue uptake of insulin in man using a differential immunoassay for endogenous and exogenous insulin. J. clin. Invest. **40**, 2092/2102 (1961).
9. SIPERSTEIN, M. D., and V. M. FAGEN: J. chem. Invest. **37**, 1196 (1958).
10. SAMAAN, N., D. STILLMAN and R. FRASER: Abnormalities of serum insulin-like activity in liver disease. Lancet **1962 II**, 1287.

Diskussion

O. SCHEIBE (Hamburg):

Haben Sie bei Ihren Untersuchungen zum Leberzellstoffwechsel auch ATP-Bestimmungen im Lebervenenblut durchgeführt unter der Fragestellung, ob der ATP-Abfall in der Leberzelle auch zu einem ATP-Abfall im Lebervenenblut führt?

J. M. A. RAHMAN:

Nein.

Untersuchungen zur Regulation des Kohlenhydratstoffwechsels beim Prädiabetes

Von

H. Ditschuneit, H. Kolb, Ch. Wahl, R. Morcos, W. H. Rott u. E. F. Pfeiffer*

Mit 2 Abbildungen

Zahlreiche klinische und experimentelle Beobachtungen lassen erkennen, daß für die diabetische Stoffwechselstörung wahrscheinlich auch Störungen des peripheren Regulationsmechanismus pathogenetische Bedeutung haben (*1, 2, 3, 4, 5, 6, 7*). Zur Erkennung eines Diabetes mellitus in der prädiabetischen Phase, in der definitonsgemäß ein normaler Blutzuckerspiegel und keine Glucosurie bestehen und auch mit den üblichen oralen Zuckerbelastungs- und i. v. Rastinontesten keine Störungen der Blutzuckerregulation zu erkennen sind, erschien es uns daher besonders erfolgversprechend, Untersuchungen über regulative Störungen der peripheren Wirkung von Insulin auf den Stoffwechsel durchzuführen.

Über das Ergebnis dieser Untersuchungen soll im folgenden berichtet werden.

Untersuchungsanordnung und Methodik

Für eine große Zahl von Probanden bestimmten wir die Assimilationsgeschwindigkeit intravenös injizierter Glucose während eines Zeitraumes von einer Stunde, führten Bestimmungen der Seruminsulinwirkung im Nüchternserum durch und prüften außerdem den Einfluß der intravenösen Glucosebelastung auf die Seruminsulinwirkung. Bei einigen Probanden führten wir zusätzlich Untersuchungen über Bindung und Transport von Insulin im Blut und ihre Beeinflussung durch orale Glucosebelastungen durch.

Einzelheiten der Methodik werden an anderer Stelle ausführlich beschrieben werden.

Ergebnis und Diskussion

Intravenös injizierte Glucose benötigt ungefähr 10 min bis zur vollständigen Diffusion in den extracellulären Verteilungsraum. Der Blutzucker fällt anschließend, vorwiegend infolge Assimilation durch das periphere Gewebe (*8*), nach einer exponentiellen Gesetzmäßigkeit ab, so daß er sich graphisch bei semilogarithmischer Koordinationsteilung als Gerade darstellen läßt und durch eine *Konstante* [Assimilationskonstante (k)] eindeutig bestimmt ist.

Bei Stoffwechselgesunden erfolgt der Abfall der Blutzuckerkonzentration sehr schnell, und der Assimilationskoeffizient erreicht mit $2,38 + 0,56$ den größten

* Durchgeführt mit Unterstützung der Deutschen Forschungsgemeinschaft, Bad Godesberg.

Wert aller Probandengruppen. Bei den Diabetikern, die je nach Behandlungsart in drei verschiedene Gruppen aufgeteilt wurden, vollzieht sich der Blutzuckerabfall als Ausdruck einer langsameren Assimilation verzögert, so daß der Kurvenverlauf flacher und der Assimilationskoeffizient signifikant kleiner wird.

Zwischen die Gruppe der Diabetiker und die der Stoffwechselgesunden ordnet sich eine Gruppe aus 34 Probanden ein, die wir im folgenden als Prädiabetiker bezeichnen wollen und bei denen allen bei den nächsten Familienangehörigen, bei Eltern oder Kindern, mindestens ein Erkrankungsfall an Diabetes aufgetreten ist und in der ferneren Verwandtschaft bei den meisten von ihnen weitere Diabetiker bekannt sind. Diese Gruppe zeigt den gleichen Blutzuckerausgangswert und auch den gleichen Blutzuckerspiegel 15 min nach Glucoseinjektion, die Assimilation erfolgt aber deutlich langsamer, so daß der Blutzucker nach 60 min mit $86{,}6 \pm 3{,}0$ mg% den Ausgangswert noch nicht wieder erreicht hat und signifikant über dem Blutzuckerspiegel der Stoffwechselgesunden Kontrollgruppe liegt.

Prinzipiell gleichartige Ergebnisse wurden auch von FRANCKSON u. Mitarb. (9) mitgeteilt. Auch CAMERINI-DAVALOS u. Mitarb. (10) fanden in einem hohen Prozentsatz bei Angehörigen von Diabetikern eine langsamere Glucoseassimilation.

Zwischen den in den einzelnen Gruppen umgesetzten Glucosemengen und den Assimilationskoeffizienten ergeben sich exponentielle gesetzmäßige Beziehungen. Erwartungsgemäß nähert sich die Umsatzkurve mit steigenden Assimilationskoeffizienten asymptotisch einem Grenzwert, der u.a. auch durch die endliche Oberfläche der assimilierenden Körperzellen verursacht wird. Der Umsatz in der stoffwechselgesunden Kontrollgruppe kommt mit $103{,}5 \pm 2{,}8\%$ diesem Grenzwert sehr nahe. Die Glucoseassimilation ist also bei Stoffwechselgesunden nahezu maximal und nur noch geringfügig steigerungsfähig. Entsprechend kann auch die biologisch aktive Insulinmenge, die im extracellulären Raum zur Überwindung der Zellmembran von der Glucose benötigt wird, als optimal angenommen werden.

Die pro Zeiteinheit assimilierte Glucosemenge ist direkt von der Größe der Insulinwirkung abhängig. Zwischen Geschwindigkeit des Blutzuckerabfalls nach der Glucoseinjektion und der extracellulären, biologisch aktiven Insulinmenge müßte demnach ein Zusammenhang aufzuzeigen sein. Vergleicht man aber das Ergebnis unserer Seruminsulinbestimmungen im Nüchternserum bei den einzelnen Gruppen mit unterschiedlich schneller Glucoseassimilation miteinander, dann ergibt sich ein anderes als das erwartete Bild.

Die Stoffwechselgesunden mit dem größten Assimilationskoeffizienten haben mit $167 \pm 123\ \mu$E/ml $(M + \sigma)$ die kleinste Seruminsulinwirkung, und die Diabetiker, die die injizierte Glucose wesentlich schlechter assimilieren, zeigen alle signifikant höhere Seruminsulinwirkungen im Nüchternserum. Bei der Gruppe der 45 insulinbehandelten Diabetiker beträgt der Mittelwert $507 \pm 348\ \mu$E/ml und bei den 21 mit D 860 behandelten Diabetikern $317 \pm 200\ \mu$E/ml. Auch die Seruminsulinwirkung der leichtesten, nur mit Diät behandelten Diabetiker überragt mit $466 \pm 260\ \mu$E/ml die der Stoffwechselgesunden. Am stärksten wird aber der Normalbereich durch die Prädiabetiker überschritten, deren Mittelwert $813 \pm 136\ \mu$E/ml beträgt. Von RENOLD und seinem Arbeitskreis (7) sowie VALLENCE-OWN u. Mitarb. (4) wurden gleichartige Beobachtungen mitgeteilt. Zwischen der Höhe des Insulinspiegels im Nüchternserum und der peripheren Regulation des Kohlenhydratstoffwechsels lassen sich offenbar keine Beziehungen herstellen.

Bei der Bestimmung der Seruminsulinwirkung unmittelbar nach der Glucoseinjektion während der Assimilationsphase ergeben sich ebenfalls deutliche Unterschiede zwischen den einzelnen Gruppen. Bei Stoffwechselgesunden ist eine Steigerung der Seruminsulinwirkung mit einem Maximum 15— 30 min nach der Glucoseinjektion zu beobachten (Abb. 1). Die Prädiabetiker lassen dagegen bei dem gleichen Glucosereiz keine Steigerung der Seruminsulinwirkung erkennen (Abb. 1). Die hohen Ausgangswerte dieser Gruppe haben eher eine abfallende als ansteigende Tendenz.

Eine Änderung des Gehaltes an biologisch aktivem Insulin im extracellulären Raum bei Stoffwechselgesunden erfordert auch der beobachtete Blutzuckerverlauf. Bei dieser Gruppe erfolgt nämlich die Assimilation nicht mit gleichbleibender Geschwindigkeit wie bei den Prädiabetikern, denn der Mittelwert des Blutzuckerspiegels 30 min nach Glucoseinjektion weicht signifikant von der Geraden ab, und außerdem wird der Blutzuckerausgangswert nach 60 min unterschritten. Zu diesem Zeitpunkt wird damit zeitlich mehr Glucose assimiliert als zu Beginn des Versuches, eine Tatsache, die ebenso wie die Beschleunigung des Assimilationsvorganges innerhalb der ersten halben Stunde des Versuches eine Steigerung der Insulinwirkung erfordert.

Bei den Gruppen mit manifester diabetischer Stoffwechselstörung wurde die hohe Seruminsulinwirkung des Serums durch den Reiz der injizierten Glucose ebenfalls nicht verändert.

Alle Seruminsulinwirkungen wurden mit dem Rattenfettgewebe gemessen. Damit könnten aber die hohen Insulinwirkspiegel bei Diabetikern und Prädiabetikern ebenso wie die fehlende Reaktion der Seruminsulinwirkung nach intravenöser Glucosebelastung bei diesen Probanden darauf zurückzuführen sein, daß mit dem isolierten Rattenfettgewebe auch das in vitro inaktive Insulin erfaßt wird und Rückschlüsse auf die Menge des extracellulären wirksamen Insulins daraus nicht zu ziehen sind. Als Inaktivator sind neben den von Vallence-Owen (4) beschriebenen Antagonisten besonders die von Antoniades u. Mitarb. (5) nachgewiesene Komplexbindung mit einem basischen Protein zu dikutieren. Eine derartige Bindung wird auch durch unsere weiteren Untersuchungen wahrscheinlich gemacht. Nach zonenelektophoretischer Auftrennung von Serum mit Hilfe eines speziellen Verfahrens fanden wir bei 10 Stoffwechselgesunden 73% der gesamten endogenen Insulinwirkung in der γ- und β-Globulinfraktion lokalisiert (Abb. 2). Die α_2-Globuline enthielten nur 3% und die mit den α_1-Globulinen gemischten Albumine 24% der gesamten Insulinwirkung.

Nach Glucosebelastung mit 100 g Glucose p. o. ändert sich die Verteilung der Insulinwirkung auf die vier verschiedenen Fraktionen deutlich. Die Insulinwirkung der Albuminfraktion steigt auf 48% an und die der γ- und β-Globuline geht auf 44% zurück (Abb. 2). Die gleichzeitig mit dem isolierten Rattenfettgewebe und Rattendiaphragma durchgeführten Untersuchungen zeigten, daß es sich bei dem im Albuminbereich wandernden Insulin um *freies* Insulin und bei dem im β-Globulinbereich lokalisierten um *gebundenes* handelt. Auch das Ergebnis der Untersuchungen mit Zusätzen von exogenem krist. Rinderinsulin ist in diesem Sinne zu interpretieren.

Damit entsprechen unsere Beobachtungen vollständig denen von Antoniades u. Mitarb. (5), die mit Hilfe von Ionenaustauschern nachwiesen, daß durch

Verabreichung von Glucose der Anteil des freien Insulins ansteigt und der des gebundenen abfällt.

Bei den Serumfraktionierungen von 6 Prädiabetikern mit verschlechterter Glucoseassimilation und hohen Insulinwirkungen ergibt sich vor der Glucosebelastung eine nahezu gleichartige Verteilung der Seruminsulinwirkung auf die einzelnen Eiweißfraktionen (Abb. 2). Aber die bei den Stoffwech-

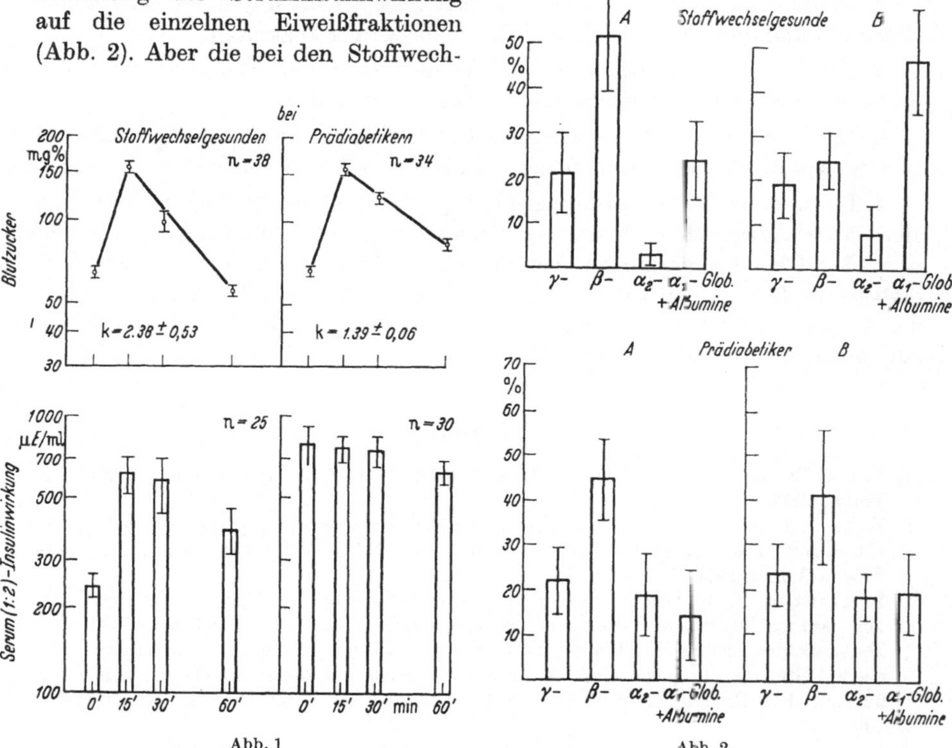

Abb. 1

Abb. 2

Abb. 1. Blutzuckerverlauf (mg-%) und Seruminsulinwirkung (μE/ml) nach i.v.-Glucosebelastung (0,3 g/kg)

Abb. 2. Prozentuale Verteilung der Insulinwirkung von zonenelektrophoretisch getrennten Serumeiweißfraktionen von Stoffwechselgesunden und Prädiabetikern. *A* 3 Std nach Nahrungsaufnahme, *B* 30 min nach Glucosebelastung (100 g p.o.)

selgesunden zu beobachtende Verschiebung zum Albuminbereich nach oraler Glucosebelastung bleibt bei den Prädiabetikern aus, so daß nach der Verabreichung der Glucose der größte Anteil der Insulinwirkung unverändert im γ- und β-Globulinbereich zu finden ist.

Dieser Defekt, von ANTONIADES u. Mitarb. (5) bereits bei Diabetikern mit manifester Stoffwechselstörung nachgewiesen, ist also auch bei den Prädiabetikern vorhanden. Diese unterscheiden sich von den manifesten Diabetikern im wesentlichen nur dadurch, daß sie einen höheren Seruminsulinwert aufweisen und dadurch wahrscheinlich in die Lage versetzt werden, den Stoffwechsel voll zu kompensieren.

Wie weit diese periphere Störung bei der Freisetzung von gebundenem Insulin mit der Starre der Insulinsekretion und der mangelhaften Insulinproduktion in

Zusammenhang steht und für die Pathogenese des Diabetes mellitus von Bedeutung ist, läßt sich heute noch nicht überblicken.

Zusammenfassung

1. Prädiabetiker lassen sich von Stoffwechselgesunden durch eine langsamere Glucoseassimilation bei intravenöser Glucosebelastung abgrenzen.

2. Die Seruminsulinwirkungen der Nüchternseren von Prädiabetikern liegen weit oberhalb des Streubereichs von Stoffwechselgesunden.

3. Nach intravenöser Glucosebelastung reagieren nur Stoffwechselgesunde mit einer Steigerung der Seruminsulinwirkung, nicht aber Prädiabetiker und Diabetiker.

4. Durch orale Glucosebelastungen (100 g p. o.) tritt bei Stoffwechselgesunden eine elektrophoretisch nachweisbare Verschiebung der Insulinwirkung von der γ- und β-Globulinfraktion zu der Albumin α_1-Globulinfraktion ein. Bei Prädiabetikern läßt sich diese Verschiebung nicht nachweisen. Die Insulinwirkung der Albumin-α_1-Globulinfraktion ist auf „freies" und die der β-Globulinfraktion auf „gebundenes" Insulin zurückzuführen.

Literatur

1. Falta, W., u. F. Högler: Die Zuckerkrankheit, 4. Auflage. Halle (Saale): C. Marhold Verlag 1953.
2. Hoef, J. J., A. Gommers and J. P. Hoef: Clinical Data on selected Cases of Prediabetes, III. Kongreß der Internat. Diabetes Federation, Düsseldorf, 1958. Stuttgart: Georg Thieme Verlag 1959.
3. Pfeiffer, E. F., H. Ditschuneit u. R. Ziegler: Über die Bestimmung von Insulin im Blut am epididymalen Fettanhang der Ratte mit Hilfe markierter Glukose, IV: Die Dynamik der Insulinsekretion des Stoffwechselgesunden und des Altersdiabetikers nach wiederholter Belastung mit Glukose, Sulfonylharnstoffen und menschlichem Wachstumshormon. Ein Beitrag zur Pathogenese des menschlichen Altersdiabetes. Klin. Wschr. **1961**, 415—426.
4. Vallence-Own. J., and M. D. Lilley: Further Studies on Insulin Antagonism associated with Plasma Albumin. 4. Kongreß der internat. Diabetes Federation, Genf, 10.—14. 7. 1961. Genéve: Editions Médicine et Hygiène.
5. Antoniades, H. M., K. Gunderson, P. M. Beigelman, H. M. Pyle and J. A. Bougasy: Studies on the State, Transport and Regulation of Insulin in Human Blood. Diabetes **11**, 261—270 (1962).
6. Wrenshall, G. B., A. Bogach and R. C. Ritchic: Extractable Insulin of Pancreas, Correlation with Pathological and Clinical Findings in Diabetic and non Diabetic Cases. Diabetes **1**, 87 (1962).
7. Renold, A. E.: Metabolic Consequences of Insulin Lack. 4. Kongreß der internat. Diabetes Federation, Genf, 10.—14. 7. 1961. Genéve: Editions Médecine et Hygiène.
8. Conard, V., J. R. M. Franckson, P. A. Bastenie, J. Kestens et L. Kovac: Mesure de l'assimilation du glucose, bases theoriques et application cliniques. Acta med. belg. ed Bruxelle, 1955, Vol. 1.
9. Franckson, J. R. M., H. A. Ooms, R. Bellens, V. Conard and P. A. Bastenie: Physiologie Significance of the Intravenous Glucose Tolerance Test. Metabolism **11**, 482—499 (1962).
10. Camarini-Davalos, R. A., A. Marble, M. Dhamdhere, S. B. Rees, D. G. Cawrence and A. Freedlander: Development of Methods for early Detection of Prediabetes. 4. Kongreß der Internat. Diab. Federation, Genf, 10.—14.7. 1961. Genève: Editions Medecine et Hygiène.

Diskussion

W. Teller (Marburg):

Amerikanische Autoren (Antoniades, Renold, Cahill u. a., s. "Hormones in Human Plasma", Little, Brown and Company, Boston 1960) haben in ähnlichen Versuchen die elektrophoretisch aufgetrennten Serumfraktionen auf ihre Insulinwirkung am Fettgewebe von Ratten-Nebenboden untersucht und dabei bewußt nicht von „Insulin" sondern von „*insulinähnlicher Aktivität*" (insulin-like activity) (I.L.A.) gesprochen, da ihnen bisher die Isolierung oder der chemische Nachweis von genuinem Insulin nicht gelang. Solange auch bei Ihnen dieser Nachweis noch aussteht, sollte man sich vielleicht in Ihren soeben geschilderten schönen Untersuchungen statt Insulin ebenfalls einer der I.L.A. ähnlichen Bezeichnung bedienen, um Mißverständnisse zu vermeiden.

Haben Sie Gelegenheit gehabt, gewisse retroperitoneale Fibrosarkome auf den Gehalt an I.L.A. hin zu untersuchen? Steinke (Peter Bent Brigham Hospital, Boston) fand in einigen dieser Tumoren abnorm hohe Mengen von I.L.A. Aus der Pädiatrie ist das Krankheitsbild der *idiopathischen Hypoglykämie* bei Säuglingen bekannt, welches pathogenetisch nicht einheitlich zu sein scheint und verschiedene Verlaufsformen hat. In einem solchen Fall konnte Antoniades vermehrt „freie" I.L.A. im Plasma nachweisen, die meines Wissens nach Pankreatektomie nicht verschwand und somit höchstwahrscheinlich *kein* Insulin darstellte.

E. F. Pfeiffer (Frankfurt):

Definiert den Begriff des „gebundenen" Insulins und macht die methodische Genese dieses Begriffs deutlich (Rattendiaphragma versus Rattenfettgewebe) und zitiert Versuche von Schöffling et al. (in Vorbereitung), die nach Hypophysektomie + Pankreatektomie immer noch insulinähnliche Aktivität nachweisen konnten.

Aus der II. Medizinischen Klinik der Universität München
(Direktor: Prof. Dr. Dr. G. BODECHTEL)

Über die Wirkung des Insulins auf die Fettaufnahme durch das Fettgewebe

Von

K. SCHWARZ und P. BOTTERMANN

Mit 1 Abbildung

Das Fettgewebe (FGW) ist nach unseren derzeitigen Kenntnissen ein über den Organismus verteiltes Organ, das einen sehr lebhaften intermediären Stoffwechsel besitzt, auf den das Insulin direkt einwirkt. Tierexperimentell konnten in vivo und in vitro im FGW die Glykogensynthese aus Glucose (12), die Oxydation von Acetat, Pyruvat und Glucose (6) und auch die Synthese langkettiger Fettsäuren (FS) aus Glucose, Acetat und Propionat nachgewiesen werden (14, 7, 4, 5). Die Störungen im Stoffwechsel des FGW unter Insulinmangel, die bei alloxandiabetischen Tieren auftreten und die durch Insulin vollkommen beseitigt werden können (5, 6), beweisen die direkte Insulinwirkung auf den Stoffwechsel des FGW. In vitro konnte der direkte Insulineffekt auf das FGW auch an der Steigerung der Glucoseaufnahme von WINEGARD und RENOLD (14, 9), der Fettsynthese (8) und des O_2-Verbrauches (13) gezeigt werden.

Nach Untersuchungen von RODBELL (10) werden nicht nur Kohlehydrate oder deren Metaboliten, sondern auch die als Emulsion im Blut vorhandenen Triglyceride (TG) vom isolierten FGW aufgenommen.

Im Rahmen klinischer Probleme über hormonale Einflüsse auf die Lipogenese und Lipolyse untersuchten wir zunächst experimentell die Frage, ob Hormone die Aufnahme von TG durch das isolierte FGW stimulieren können. Unser besonderes Interesse galt der Wirkung des Insulins, jenem Hormon, welches bekanntlich die Lipogenese aus Glucose sehr intensiv fördert.

Methodik

Als Versuchsmodell diente das für solche Untersuchungen geeignete epididymale FGW nüchterner Ratten, das in einer Krebs-Ringer-Pufferlösung mit 2%igem Albuminzusatz im Warburg-Gerät während 3 Std bei 37 Grad inkubiert wurde.

Dem Inkubationsmedium wurden Zusätze verschieden variierter Dosen von Glucose, in Alkohol gelöstem Triolein und kristallinem Insulin[1] zugeführt.

Die Messung der Triglyceride bzw. der veresterten Fettsäuren erfolgte nach der Methode von ALBRINK (1) und die der nichtveresterten Fettsäuren (NFS) nach DOLE (3), wobei jeweils Doppelbestimmungen ausgeführt wurden. Die Fehler-

---

[1] Für die Überlassung von kristallinem Insulin in Reinstform sei den Farbwerken Hoechst (Frankfurt a. M.) gedankt.

breite lag unter 3% und Recovery-Versuche im Serum mit bekannten Trioleinzusätzen ergaben Werte von 98 — 102%.

Ergebnisse

In 32 Doppelversuchen wurde isoliertes, pro Versuch von mindestens 3 Ratten gepooltes, FGW jeweils mit einem Zusatz von 0,5, 1,0 bzw. 2,0 μÄ/ml Triolein ohne und mit Insulin in einer Dosis von 1,1 mE/ml inkubiert. Nach orientierenden Versuchen hielten wir die Glucosekonzentration von 200 mg-% konstant.

Ohne Insulin nimmt das FGW bei einem Zusatz von 1 μÄ/ml Triolein im Mittel 199 μÄ/g/h $\pm$ 61 an VFS auf, das entspricht bei einem Angebot von 100% einer TG-Aufnahme von 36,5%. Nach Zugabe von 1,100 μE/ml Insulin steigt die Aufnahme von TG im Mittel auf 395 μÄ/g/h $\pm$ 77 bzw. auf 71 % an. Die Differenz der gesteigerten Trioleinaufnahme in das FGW mit Insulin ist mit einer Wahrscheinlichkeit P 0,02 signifikant.

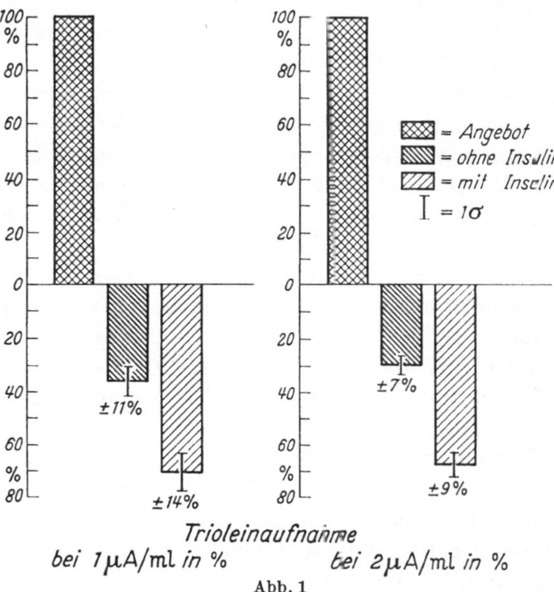

Abb. 1

Erhöht man das Angebot des zugesetzten Trioleins mit der Inkubationsflüssigkeit auf das Doppelte, nämlich auf 2 μÄ/ml, dann nimmt auch ohne Insulin die Aufnahme der TG zu, sie beträgt im Mittel 259 μÄ/g/h $\pm$ 62,6, entsprechend 30%. Nach Insulin erfolgt wiederum eine vermehrte Aufnahme von TG im Mittel von 585 μÄ/g/h $\pm$ 78,7 und einem Anstieg von 67,7%.

Auch bei erhöhtem Trioleinangebot verhalten sich die Werte der TG-Aufnahme nach Insulin sigifikant höher als bei den Versuchen ohne Insulin.

In der Abb. 1 sind die Werte der Aufnahme in Prozent vom Ausgangswert graphisch dargestellt.

Die Verteilung de Werte in Gaußschen Kurven zeigt, daß das Maximum der TG-Aufnahme ohne Insulin bei 200μÄ/g/h und mit Insulinzusatz bei 400μÄ/g/h liegt.

Unter ähnlichen Versuchsbedingungen konnten wir keinen Einfluß auf die Trioleinaufnahme nach direkter Einwirkung anderer Hormone, z. B. Glukagon, STH und Noradrenalin beobachten, ebensowenig wie nach Änderung der Glucosekonzentration.

Diskussion

Die vorliegenden experimentellen Ergebnisse berechtigen zu der Annahme, daß das FGW unter physiologischen Bedingungen TG auf nimmt und daß das fettstoffwechselaktive Hormon Insulin diesen Effekt signifikant stimuliert. Insulin vermag demnach nicht nur die Lipogenese aus Glucose spezifisch zu fördern, sondern auch den Eintritt und die Deponierung der als Triglyceride im Blut kreisenden Fette in das Fettgewebe direkt zu stimulieren. Die Vorstellung einer extracellulär oder an der Membran der Fettzellen stattfindenden Hydrolyse durch Aktivierung einer Lipase bzw. einer Lipoproteinlipase erscheint nicht wahrscheinlich, da wir in der Inkubationsflüssigkeit keine vermehrte Freisetzung von Glycerin und von NFS nachweisen konnten.

Untersuchungen von Rodbell (*10*) stützen die Annahme, daß die Lipoproteinlipase zwar für die Aufnahme der TG nicht notwendig, für den intracellulären Stoffwechsel der Hydrolyse und Resynthese in der Fettzelle jedoch von Bedeutung ist. Shafrir (*11*) und seine Arbeitsgruppe kamen nach experimentellen Untersuchungen mit radioaktivem L-C^{14}-Tripalmitin zu der gleichen Auffassung. Hemmt man nämlich die Lipoproteinlipase durch Enzymgifte, dann wird der Eintritt der TG in das FGW nicht verhindert, wohl aber die intracelluläre Hydrolyse und der energieverbrauchende Prozeß der Resynthese von α-Glycerophosphat und der FS-CoA-Verbindung zu Fett.

Der genaue Wirkungsmechanismus der TG-Aufnahme durch das FGW ist bisher noch unklar. Ob hierbei die der Phagocytose ähnlichen Prozesse eine Rolle spielen, wie das bei Chylomikronen beobachtet wurde, ist noch nicht zu entscheiden. Von Interesse sind hierzu Befunde von Barrnet und Ball (*2*), die am FGW einen als Pinocytose sehr charakteristischen Zellmembranvorgang morphologisch festhalten konnten.

Der von uns beobachtete Insulineffekt auf die Aufnahme von TG durch das FGW scheint nach eigenen Berechnungen ein aktiver Transportmechanismus zu sein, ähnlich dem der Glucoseaufnahme durch das FGW, weil die Kurve nach der Formel von Lineweaver flacher wird, wenn die Affinität des Transportsystems unter Insulin zunimmt.

Diese experimentell gewonnenen Befunde eines die Fettaufnahme stimulierenden Insulineffektes durch das FGW eröffnen neue Gesichtspunkte über den Stoffwechsel des Fettgewebes. Solche Aspekte gewinnen vielleicht für die Klinik ihre Bedeutung, zumal die hormonalen Einflüsse in der Pathogenese der Fettsucht ein aktuelles Problem der klinischen Endokrinologie bedeuten.

Literatur

1. Albrink, M. J.: J. Lipid. Res. 1, 53 (1959).
2. Barrnett, R., and F. G. Ball: Abstr. Ann. Meet. Nat. Acad. of Science, April 1959.
3. Dole, V. P.: J. clin. Invest. 35, 150 (1956).
4. Favarger, P. J., u. I. Gerlach: Helv. physiol. pharmacol. Acta 13, 96 (1955).
5. Feller, D. D., and E. Feist: J. biol. Chem. 228, 275 (1957).
6. Hausberger, F. X., S. W. Milstein and R. J. Rutman: J. biol. Chem. 208, 431 (1954).
7. — — J. biol. Chem. 214, 483 (1955).
8. Krahl, M. E.: Ann. N. Y. Acad. Sci. 54, 649 (1951).
9. Milstein, W. S., and F. X. Hausberger: Diabetes 5, 84 (1956).
10. Rodbell, M.: J. biol. Chem. 235, 1613 (1960).
11. Shafrir, B., A. Gutman and S. Landau: Bull. Res. Coun. Israel 11A, 91 (1962).
12. Shapiro, B., and E. Wertheimer: Metabolism 5, 79 (1956).
13. Sidman, R. L.: Anat. Res. 124, 723 (1956).
14. Winegrad, A. T., and A. E. Renold: J. biol. Chem. 233, 267 (1958).

Aus der Frauenklinik der Medizinischen Akademie Düsseldorf
(Direktor: Prof. Dr. med. ELERT)

Der Einfluß einer Kombination von Präparaten mit follikelstimulierender Aktivität (FSH) und luteinisierender Aktivität (LH) auf den Maus-Uterus-Test

Von

H. SCHMIDT-ELMENDORFF

Mit 2 Abbildungen

Kürzlich untersuchten P. S. BROWN und BILLEWICZ die Wirkung von follikelstimulierendem und luteinisierendem Hormon aus Schafshypophysen auf den Maus-Uterus-Test. Die Autoren fanden, daß diese beiden Hormone, für sich allein, eine sehr unterschiedliche Dosenwirkungskurve zeigten. Wenn FSH- und LH-Präparate jedoch kombiniert verabreicht wurden, so zeigte sich bei einem bestimmten Mischungsverhältnis, nämlich 80% FSH zu 20% LH, eine synergistische Wirkung auf den Maus-Uterus-Test.

Es wird im folgenden über einige Untersuchungen berichtet, bei welchen in ähnlicher Weise wie BROWN und BILLEWICZ einige bekannte Gonadotropine mit vorwiegender FSH-Wirkung mit Präparaten kombiniert wurden, die eine deutlich luteinisierende Eigenschaft zeigen.

Folgende Gonadotropine wurden verwandt:

1. *Follikelstimulierendes Hormon (NIH-FSH-S1) aus Schafshypophysen.*
2. *Luteinisierendes Hormon (NIH-LH-B1) aus Schafshypophysen.*
3. *Menschliches Menopause-Gonadotropin (HMG-24) aus dem Harn klimakterischer Frauen.*
4. *Serum Gonadotropin (PMS-G) aus dem Serum trächtiger Stuten.*
5. *Menschliches Chorion Gonadotropin (HCG) aus dem Harn schwangerer Frauen.*

Tabelle 1 zeigt die biologische Aktivität der untersuchten Gonadotropine, ausgedrückt in HMG-Einheiten.

Gonadotropin	FSH	LH	Gesamt	FSH/LH
NIH-FSH	68,1	28,7	15,7	2,37
NIH-LH	—	2051,0	—	—
HMG-24	1,0	1,0	1,0	1,0
PMS-G	1,3	0,62	2,9	2,10
HCG	—	1,7	—	—

In der letzten Spalte der Tab. 1 sind die Quotienten aus follikelstimulierender und luteinisierender Aktivität verzeichnet. NIH-FSH und PMS-G weisen Werte über 1,0 auf; dies spricht dafür, daß diese Präparate, verglichen mit HMG-24, mehr FSH- als LH-Aktivität enthalten.

Die Versuchsanordnung war wie folgt:

24 Mäuse wurden in 6 Gruppen zu je 4 eingeteilt; jede Gruppe erhielt eine andere Hormonkombination.

Der ersten und der letzten Gruppe wurden 100% des FSH-Präparates bzw. des LH-Präparates injiziert. Die übrigen Gruppen erhielten 80% FSH + 20% LH, 60% FSH + 40% LH usw.

| FSH [%] | 100 | 80 | 60 | 40 | 20 | 0 |
| LH [%] | 0 | 20 | 40 | 60 | 80 | 100 |

Bei der Untersuchung des synergistischen Effektes von NIH-FSH und HCG wurden zusätzlich die Quotienten 25/75, 20/80, 15/85, 10/90, 5/95 und 0/100 untersucht, während bei PMS-G/HCG die Quotienten 75/25, 80/20, 85/15, 90/10, 95/5 und 100/0 getestet wurden.

Abb. 1 zeigt die Dosenwirkungskurven des Maus-Uterus-Test, die entstehen, wenn das hochgereinigte NIH-FSH nach der oben beschriebenen Versuchsanordnung mit verschiedenen anderen Gonadotropin-Präparaten kombiniert wurde.

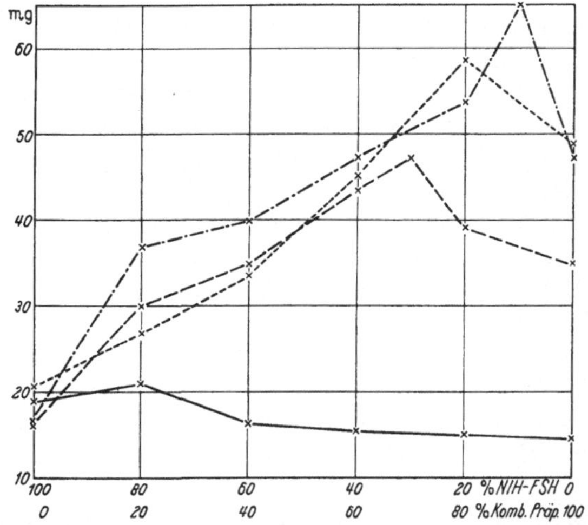

Abb. 1. ×——————× NIH—FSH (100 μg) + NIH—LH (100 μg); ×——× NIH—FSH (100 μg) + HMG—24 (0,5 mg); ×----× NIH—FSH (100 μg) + PMS + G (0,5 i.E.); ×—·—·—× NIH—FSH (100 μg) + HCG (0,5 i.E.)

In jeder dieser Kombinationen des NIH-FSH mit anderen Gonadotropinen war die NIH-FSH-Konzentration gleich, d. h. *100% NIH-FSH waren 100 μg, 80% waren 80 μg usw.*

Für die übrigen Gonadotropine wurden solche Konzentrationen gewählt, daß diese Hormone allein noch keine maximale Stimulation des Maus-Uterus-Gewichts hervorriefen und deshalb eine weitere Gewichtssteigerung durch den Synergismus zweier Gonadotropine möglich war. So waren *100% NIH-LH = 100 μg, 100% HMG = 0,5 mg, 100% PMS und = HCG entsprachen 0.5 iE.*

Es fällt auf, daß bei einer *Kombination von NIH-FSH mit NIH-LH* (ausgezogene Linie) reines FSH und reines LH (Gruppe 1 und 6) die geringste Wirkung auf den Maus-Uterus-Test haben. Eine Kombination der beiden Hormone im

Verhältnis 80:20 zeigt jedoch trotz gleichbleibendem Gesamtgewicht der Hormondosis eine angedeutet stärkere Wirkung.

Weiter ist bemerkenswert, daß — besonders wenn man die Gesamtdosis für NIH-FSH und NIH-LH erhöht — die Reaktion auf reines NIH-FSH signifikant größer ist als auf reines NIH-LH. Dies läßt vermuten, daß NIH-LH vollständiger von seiner FSH-Komponente befreit wurde als NIH-FSH von seiner LH-Aktivität. Bei NIH-FSH könnte bei höherer Dosierung die Kontaminierung mit LH-Aktivität ausreichen, um einen gewissen, wenn auch geringen FSH-LH-Kombinationseffekt zu erzeugen.

Schließlich fällt auf, daß das hochgereinigte NIH-FSH und das NIH-LH auch bei optimaler Kombination verhältnismäßig schwache Wirkung auf den Maus-Uterus-Test haben, obwohl die spezifische Aktivität von NIH-LH die LH-Aktivität der übrigen getesteten Präparate (HMG, PMS und HCG) weit übersteigt.

Hierfür könnte die geringere Depotwirkung des von inaktiven Begleitsubstanzen weitgehend befreiten NIH-LH verantwortlich sein.

Bei einer *Kombination von NIH-FSH mit HMG-24* (gestrichelte Linie) zeigt sich ein deutlicher Synergismus in der Wirkung auf den Maus-Uterus-Test bei einem Mischungsverhältnis von 30% NIH-FSH zu 70% HMG-24.

Hier bedurfte es eines größeren Prozentsatzes an LH-Aktivität in Form von HMG-24, um ein optimales Verhältnis zwischen FSH und LH herzustellen. Zwei Gründe könnten dafür verantwortlich sein:

1. Die geringere LH-Wirkung von HMG-24, verglichen mit NIH-LH.

2. Die begleitende FSH-Aktivität des HMG-24, die neben der FSH-Aktivität des NIH-FSH zur Verfügung steht.

Die absolute Wirkung einer Kombination von NIH-FSH und HMG-24 war signifikant größer als die von NIH-FSH und NIH-LH.

Interessant erscheint ferner die Tatsache, daß HMG-24 als menschliches Harngonadotropin noch nicht die optimale Kombination von FSH- und LH-Aktivität zur Uterusgewichtsvergrößerung und damit zur Oestrogenproduktion im Ovar der Maus hat, sondern daß es noch eines geringen Zusatzes von NIH-FSH bedarf, um diese Wirkung zu erzeugen.

Eine *Kombination von NIH-FSH mit PMS-G* zeigt die gepunktete Linie.

Hier wurden 2 Präparate kombiniert, die im Verhältnis zum HMG-24 vorwiegend FSH-Aktivität enthalten.

Es bedurfte eines Zusatzes von 20% NIH-FSH, um eine optimale Reaktion auf den Maus-Uterus-Test hervorzurufen. Das spricht ebenfalls dafür, daß das optimale FSH/LH-Verhältnis für den Maus-Uterus-Test leicht zu Gunsten der FSH-Aktivität liegt.

Schließlich zeigt die Abbildung die Dosenwirkungskurve einer *Kombination von NIH-FSH mit HCG*.

Bemerkenswert ist gerade hier der Synergismus der beiden Präparate bei einem Verhältnis von 10% NIH-FSH und 90% HCG.

Selbst Verschiebungen des Mischungsverhältnisses um 10%, also 20% NIH-FSH und 80% HCG, zeigten eine signifikant niedrigere Reaktion auf den Maus-Uterus-Test.

Allgemein läßt sich von dieser Abbildung sagen, daß das optimale Mischungsverhältnis mehr zugunsten des NIH-FSH nach links verschoben ist, je mehr LH-

Aktivität das Kombinationspräparat enthält, und umgekehrt nach rechts, je mehr FSH-Aktivität das Präparat besitzt.

Abb. 2 zeigt eine *Kombination von 0.5 iE PMS-G mit verschiedenen anderen Gonadotropinen.*

Es fällt auf, daß eine Kombination mit NIH-LH keine synergistische Wirkung hervorruft.

Die übrigen Präparate zeigen jedoch ausgeprägte Gipfel, insbesondere die Kombination von 90% PMS-G mit 10% HCG. Diese Tatsache ist bemerkenswert,

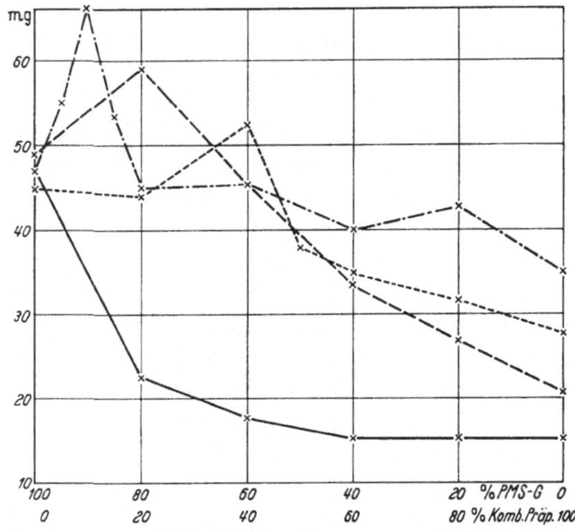

Abb. 2. ×————× PMS-G (0,5 iE) + NIH-LH (100 μg); ×— — —× PMS-G (0,5 iE) + NIH-FSH (100 μg); ×·····×PMS-G (0,5 iE) + HMG-24 (0,5 mg); ×—·—·—× PMS-G (0,5 iE) + HCG (0,5 iE)

denn beide Präparate sind besonders häufig zur Therapie bei Mann und Frau verwandt worden. Untersuchungen des synergistischen Effektes von FSH- und LH-Präparaten auf das menschliche Ovar werden zur Zeit durchgeführt.

Diskussion

E. Tonutti (Bonn):
   Nach Untersuchungen amerikanischer Autoren soll bei PMS je nach der angewandten Dosis mehr eine ICSH- bzw. FSH-Aktivität zu beobachten sein.

W. Hohlweg (Graz):
   Das Stutengonadotropin (PMS) kann man nicht als einen hauptsächlich follikelstimulierenden Faktor bezeichnen. Gemeinsam mit Dörner und Knappe konnte ich nachweisen, daß die Wirkung von PMS auf das Rattenovar durch FSH ebenso potenziert werden kann wie die von HCG aus Schwangerenharn oder von hypophysärem LH. PMS enthält nur einen etwas größeren Anteil an FSH als HCG.

A. Rockenschaub (Wien):
Mit dem Uterus-Test mißt man doch nur den LH-Effekt, der durch FSH potenziert bzw. ermöglicht wird. Mit reinem FSH entsteht doch kein Effekt am Uterus! Der Uterus-Test dürfte wohl so genaue Differenzierungen kaum zulassen. Wir messen damit nur qualitativ die Gonadotropine.

E. Daume (München):
   Das von Ihnen gefundene optimale Mischungsverhältnis von 10% FSH + 90% HCG für ein maximales Wachstum des Mäuse-Uterus ist nach unseren bisherigen Erfahrungen auch für Ovarstimulierungen beim Menschen sehr wirksam. Wir sahen nach 5—6 tägigen Gaben der Kombination 200 synergistische Einheiten FSH (aus Schweinehypophysen) + 2000 iE HCG bei 12 amenorrhoischen Frauen Oestrogenanstiege bis zu mg-Werten sowie auch deutliche Pregnandiolanstiege mit nachfolgenden Blutungen.

Aus der Medizinischen Universitätsklinik (Ludolf Krehl-Klinik) Heidelberg
(Direktor: Prof. Dr. G. SCHETTLER)

Methodik zur Routine-Gonadotropinbestimmung im Plasma des nichtschwangeren Menschen

Von

K. WALTER und M. HEGE

Mit 1 Abbildung

Der Nachweis von Gonadotropinaktivität im Blut des nichtschwangeren Menschen wurde bereits im Jahre 1929 durch FLUHMANN erbracht. Wirklich quantitative Gonadotropinbestimmungen sind seitdem nach unserer Literaturkenntnis nur von APOSTOLAKIS (1960a, b, c, 1962) mitgeteilt worden. Die nach dieser Methodik mittels Acetonfällung und anschließender Dialyse hergestellten Plasmaextrakte ermöglichten die Erfassung relativ hoher Blutgonadotropinspiegel, wie sie bei postklimakterischen Frauen und zum Zeitpunkt der Ovulation bei menstruierenden Frauen gefunden werden können.

Wir möchten hier eine von uns ausgearbeitete Bestimmungsmethode für Plasmagonadotropine beschreiben, mit welcher sich auch bei Männern sowie bei Frauen in jeglicher Cyclusphase biologische Titerbestimmungen durchführen lassen. Bei dem von uns verwendeten Plasmaextraktionsverfahren kommt ein Prinzip zur Anwendung, welches auch in der Gerbsäuremethode für die Gewinnung von Gonadotropinharnextrakten von JOHNSEN (1958) benutzt wird. Das aus dem Plasma hergestellte Eißweipräcipitat wird mit Hyflo Super Cell untermengt in einem Buchner-Trichter zu einem Filterkuchen geformt. Hierdurch ist es möglich, relativ rasch und ohne Zentrifugieren das Präcipitat in diesem Filterkuchen zu waschen und fraktioniert zu eluieren.

Für die Untersuchung wird Citratblut (1 Vol.-Teil 3,8%iges Natriumcitrat ad 10 Vol.-Teile Vollblut) abgenommen. 70 ml Citratplasma sind für die Aktivitätsbestimmung im Blut von Männern erforderlich, während bei postklimakterischen Frauen nur 20 ml Citratplasma benötigt werden. Das durch Zentrifugieren abgetrennte Plasma wird durch Zugeben von Essigsäure auf pH 5 eingestellt. Zu dem Plasma gibt man langsam und unter ständigem Rühren zunächst Aceton, dann Hyflo Super Cell und rührt das entstehende Gemisch anschließend etwa 1 min lang kräftig maschinell durch. Dann wird dieses Eiweißpräcipitat-Hyflo-Super-Cell-Gemisch auf den Buchner-Trichter gegeben, mittels des Vakuums einer Wasserstrahlpumpe werden die flüssigen Anteile abgesaugt. Es bildet sich damit der vorerwähnte Filterkuchen, welcher dann mit Aceton, absolutem Alkohol und ammoniakalischem 80%igem Alkohol gewaschen wird. Selbstverständlich muß Sorge getragen werden, daß hierbei keine Luft in den Filterkuchen eindringen kann.

Es folgt dann die Elution der gonadotropinhaltigen Fraktion mit ammoniakalischem 40%igem Alkohol, welche getrennt aufgefangen, ausgefällt und in üblicher Weise getrocknet wird[1].

Die Gewichte für die mit dieser Methode hergestellten rohen Trockenextrakte betragen durchschnittlich 4,8 mg/ml Plasma. Die Extrakte sind fast vollständig in Wasser löslich und werden in den praktisch notwendigen Dosen ohne erkennbare lokale oder allgemeine toxische Zeichen von infantilen Mäusen toleriert.

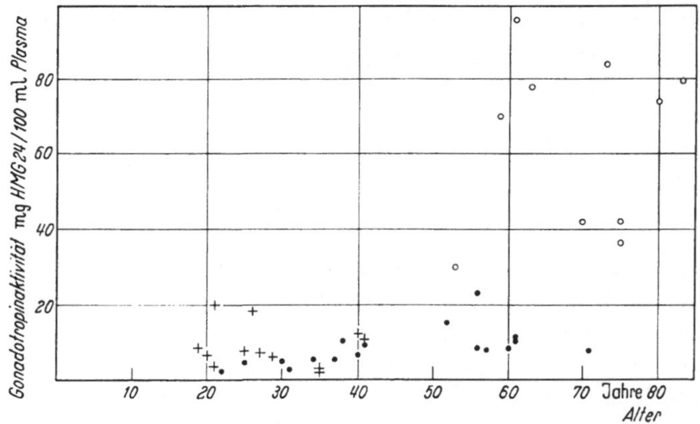

Abb. 1. Darstellung der Beziehung zwischen Alter und Plasma-Gonadotropintiter bei Männern sowie bei Frauen vor und nach der Menopause. ● Männer; ○ Frauen in der Menopause; + Frauen vor der Menopause

Um bei niedrigem Blutgonadotropintiter nicht zu große Plasmamengen zu benötigen, führen wir die Aktivitätsbestimmungen an infantilen Mäusen mit einer Augmentationstechnik durch, wie sie von DÖRNER, HOHLWEG und KNAPPE (1960) für die Bestimmung der Gonadotropinaktivität in Harnextrakten benutzt wurde. Wir setzen deshalb den Injektionslösungen 0,05 iE Choriongonadotropin pro

Tabelle 1. $n =$ Anzahl der bei den einzelnen Personengruppen durchgeführten Plasma-Gonadotropinbestimmungen. Weitere Erläuterungen siehe Text

	n	Gonadotropinaktivität mg HMG 24 / 100 ml Plasma	
		Arithmetisches Mittel	Streubereich
Männer	17	8,2	2,4—23,0
Frauen in der Menopause .	11	64,0	30,0—96,0
Frauen vor der Menopause	12	8,9	2,4—20,0

Dosis zu. Man erreicht damit nach unseren Erfahrungen eine Empfindlichkeitssteigerung um etwa einen Dosissprung bei einem Dosisintervall mit dem Faktor 2. Die Austestung erfolgte gegenüber unserem Laboratoriumsstandard, welcher aus dem Harn normaler Männer nach dem Permutit-Verfahren von JOHNSEN (1955) hergestellt wurde und dessen biologische Aktivität im gewöhnlichen Maus-Uterus-Test das 2,5fache des provisorischen Standardpräparates HMG 24 beträgt. Stets

---

[1] Einzelheiten der Plasmaextraktionsmethode werden an anderer Stelle mitgeteilt.

wurden sog. 5- bzw. 6-Punkte-Versuche angesetzt. Wegen der großen Steilheit der Dosiswirkungskurven war die mathematische Auswertung nur als 4 oder 3 Punkte-Versuche möglich. Die Dosiswirkungskurven für die Plasmaextrakte und den Laborstandard verlaufen innerhalb der statistischen Variation parallel. Bei Verwendung von zwei Tieren pro Dosis liegen die Werte für den Präzisionsindex λ um 0,1, also im brauchbaren Bereich. In jedem Fall war es möglich, in den Plasmaextrakten biologische Aktivitäten nachzuweisen.

In der Abb. 1 sind die Ergebnisse der Plasmagonadotropinbestimmungen bei 40 innersekretorisch normalen Personen in Abhängigkeit vom Lebensalter dargestellt. Erwartungsgemäß finden sich relativ hohe Werte bei postklimakterischen Frauen, während diejenigen für Männer sowie für Frauen vor der Menopause in etwa gleichem Bereich um 8 bis 9 mg HMG 24 pro 100 ml Plasma liegen. Tab. 1 zeigt die gefundenen arithmetischen Mittelwerte für die einzelnenPersonengruppen zusammen mit dem einfachen Streubereich der ermittelten Ergebnisse.

Zusammenfassung

Es wird eine Methodik beschrieben, mit welcher relativ stark angereicherte und wenig toxische Gonadotropinextrakte aus Plasma hergestellt werden können. Nach unserer Literaturkenntnis konnten hiermit erstmals die Plasmagonadotropinspiegel bei Männern und bei Frauen vor der Menopause quantitativ gemessen werden.

Literatur

Apostolakis, M.: J. Endocr. **19**, 377 (1960a).
—, and J. A. Loraine: J. clin. Endocr. **20**, 1437 (1960b).
— — In: C. H. Gray and A. L. Bacharach: Hormones in Blood. New York: Academic Press 1960c.
— Klin. Wschr. **39**, 9, 453 (1961).
Dörner, G., W. Hohlweg u. G. Knappe: Klin. Wschr. **38**, 17, 878 (1960).
Fluhmann, C. F.: J. Amer. med. Ass. **93**, 672 (1929).
Johnsen, S. G.: Acta endocr. (Kbh.) **20**, 101 (1955).
— Acta endocr. (Kbh.) **28**, 69 (1958).

Diskussion

H. Karg (München):

Die Toxicität von Plasmabereitungen für die Testtiere bei Gonadotropinbestimmungen ist besonders erheblich, wenn man — wie bei dem von uns geübten Ovar-Ascorbinsäure-Test — intravenös zu injizieren hat. Wir konnten feststellen, daß durch gleichzeitige Verabfolgung eines Rutinpräparates an die Testratten die toxischen Wirkungen praktisch auszuschalten sind.

Aus dem Physiologisch-chemischen Institut (Direktor: Prof. Dr. J. Kühnau)
und dem Hormonlabor der II. Medizinischen Klinik (Direktor: Prof. Dr. A. Jores)
der Universität Hamburg

Zur Wirkung von Testosteronpropionat auf Muskeln und Leber der Ratte

Von

D. Matzelt, M. Apostolakis und K. D. Voigt

Mit 3 Abbildungen

Die anabole Aktivität von Testosteron und einigen seiner Derivate scheint eine gut belegte Tatsache. Kritisch gesehen muß man aber festhalten, daß die Rückschlüsse auf die anabole Wirkung solcher Verbindungen letztlich auf Tierexperimenten, und zwar auf dem Gewichtsanstieg des M. Levator ani beruhen. Es mehren sich jedoch die Zweifel, ob dieser Test wirklich ein zuverlässiger Parameter der anabolen Potenz darstellt und insbesondere, ob ein Parallelismus zwischen dem Verhalten dieses Muskels und dem anderer Muskeln nachzuweisen ist. Hinsichtlich des Intermediärstoffwechsels können aus solchen Ansätzen natürlich keine Aussagen abgeleitet werden. Aus diesen Gründen entschlossen wir uns, den Einfluß von anabolen Substanzen auf Enzymaktivitäten zu untersuchen. Nach dem Vorhergesagten ist klar, daß in solche Studien nicht allein der M. Levator ani einbezogen werden darf, sondern gleichzeitig ein typischer Vertreter der quergestreiften Körpermuskulatur mituntersucht werden muß. Auf Grund früherer Erfahrungen schien es sinnvoll, zusätzlich der Leber Aufmerksamkeit zu widmen. Neben den Aktivitätsveränderungen der Enzyme erfaßten wir zusätzlich den Protein- und Glykogengehalt in den vorgenannten Organen. An dieser Stelle kann nur kurz auf die Planung und Durchführung der Experimente eingegangen werden. Eine ausführliche Darstellung findet sich an anderer Stelle (M. Apostolakis, D. Matzelt u. K. D. Voigt: Biochem. Z. **337**, 414 (1963).

Die Planung der Experimente geht aus der Abbildung 1 hervor. Die Untersuchungen wurden an männlichen Wistarratten mit einem durchschnittlichen Gewicht zwischen 119 und 132 g durchgeführt. Alle Tiere erhielten eine Standarddiät ad libitum. Das Kollektiv wurde in 6 Gruppen (CA = kastriert-adrenalektomiert, CU = kastriert-unbehandelt, NU = normale Vergleichsgruppe, NT_1 = normale Tiere mit 1 mg Testosteron/die behandelt, CT_1 = kastrierte Tiere mit 1 mg Testosteronpropionat/die behandelt und CT_2 = kastrierte Tiere mit 2 mg Testosteronpropionat/die behandelt) unterteilt, wobei die Anzahl der Tiere (n) in jeder mindestens 12 betrug. Die gesamte Beobachtungsperiode war 31 Tage lang. Die Kastration erfolgte am ersten Tage. Die Behandlung mit Testosteronpropionat begann am 21. und dauerte bis zum 31. Tag. In der Gruppe 1 wurde zusätzlich am 27. Tag eine Adrenalektomie vorgenommen. Am 31. Tag wurden die Tiere durch Nackenschlag getötet, dekapitiert und ausgeblutet. Unmittelbar anschließend wurden die Organgewichte bestimmt und die Organe für die verschiedenen Ansätze aufgearbeitet.

Die Auswahl und Art der durchgeführten Bestimmungen geht ebenfalls aus Abb. 1 hervor. Von den beiden Musculi Biceps femoris wurde jeweils nur einer (unilateral) in die Untersuchungen einbezogen.

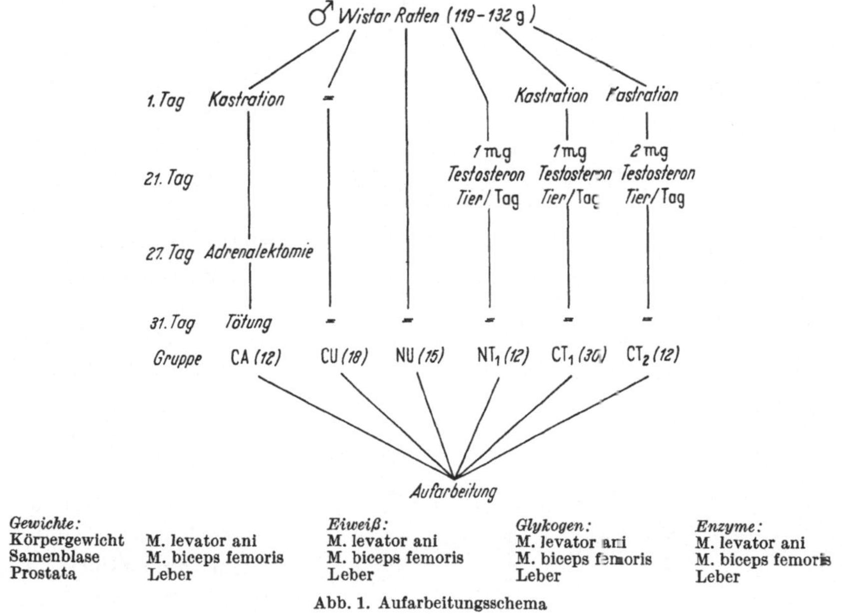

Abb. 1. Aufarbeitungsschema

Eine Aufgliederung der von uns erfaßten Enzyme und ihre Zuordnung zu den metabolischen Abläufen ist in Abb. 2 unternommen. Die gemessenen Enzymaktivitäten sind durch Unterstreichung hervorgehoben. Soweit es die schematische Darstellung erlaubt, haben wir ihnen die jeweiligen Substrate zugeordnet. Ein wichtiges Enzym beim Abbau der Glucose, die aus der Nahrung oder dem körpereigenen Glykogen stammt, über den Embden-Meyerhof-Weg ist die Fructose-1,6-diphosphoaldolase (ALD). Sie katalysiert die Bildung von 2 Triosen. Von der einen, dem Dihydroxy-aceton-phosphat (DHAP) gewinnt man über das Baranowski-Enzym (GDH) Anschluß an den Stoffwechsel der Neutralfette. Die zweite Triose, der 3-Phosphoglycerinaldehyd (3-PGA) wird von der Glycerophosphatdehydrogenase (GAPDH) katalysiert. Ein anderer Weg von der Glucose zum 3-Phosphoglycerinaldehyd führt über den Warburg-Dickens-Horecker-Shunt. Die 6-Phosphogluconatdehydrogenase (6-PGDH) steht hier als Typ solcher Enzyme, die den Pentosephosphatcyclus katalysieren. Ihre Erfassung erscheint von Interesse, weil dabei das für Synthesen erforderliche TPNH regeneriert wird. Über den Citronensäurecyclus, dem Sammelbecken des Intermediärstoffwechsels, sind Fette und Eiweißstoffwechsel mit dem Kohlenhydratabbau verbunden. Die Messung der Malatdehydrogenaseaktivität (MDH) gibt über die Umsatzgrößen im Citronensäurecyclus Aufschluß. Das Gleichgewicht der von diesem Enzym katalysierten Reaktion liegt

weitgehend auf der Seite der Oxalessigsäure. Diese Säure ist gleichzeitig Ausgangs-
substrat für die Bildung von Phospho-enolpyruvat, von wo aus der Glykolyseweg
rückwärts beschritten werden kann. Über die Glutamatpyruvat- (GPT) und die
Glutamatoxalacetat-Transaminasen (GOT) findet der Proteinstoffwechsel Anschluß
an den Krebscyclus. Gemessen wurde außerdem die Tryptophanpyrrolase (TP).
Parameter für den Nebenweg der Glykolyse von Pyruvat zum Lactat war die
Lactatdehydrogenase (LDH). Als muskelspezifisches Enzym wurde schließlich die
Kreatinphosphokinase in die Untersuchungen mit einbezogen. Sie ist auf diesem Schema nicht mit aufgeführt.

Aus der Vielzahl der Ergebnisse soll an dieser Stelle auf zwei besonders eingegangen werden:

1. Die Sonderstellung des M. Levator ani und

2. das Verhalten der GPT in Muskeln und Leber unter dem Einfluß von Testosteronpropionat.

Die Testosterongabe führte bei allen Tieren zu einem eindeutigen, allerdings verschieden starken Anstieg des Gewichtes von Samenblase, Prostata und M. Levator ani. Die Verdopplung der Dosis bei den kastrierten Tieren ergab

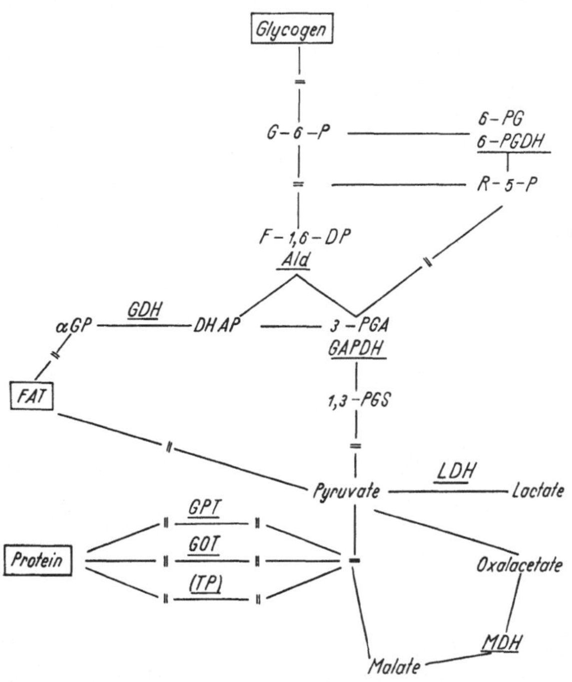

Abb. 2. Einordnung der gemessenen Enzyme in den grobschematisierten
Intermediärstoffwechsel

einen weiteren Gewichtsanstieg lediglich für den M. Levator ani. Bei Normaltieren
führt demgegenüber schon 1 mg Testosteronpropionat/die über 10 Tage zu signifikant
höheren Gewichten dieser Organe. Demgegenüber änderte sich das Gewicht des
M. biceps femoris in keiner Gruppe eindeutig. Auch die Lebergewichte wurden
weder durch Kastration noch durch Testosterongabe beeinflußt. Hier führte allein
die Adrenalektomie zu einem deutlichen Abfall. Das Studium des Eluat- und
Homogenateiweißes in den verschiedenen Organen ergab folgende Verhältnisse:
Vergleichbar zum Gewichtsanstieg führte die Testosterongabe zu einer signifikanten
Zunahme von Homogenat- und Eluateiweiß bei kastrierten und normalen Tieren
im M. Levator ani.

Im M. biceps femoris fand sich mehr Eluateiweiß dagegen nur, wenn man die
Werte der kastriert-unbehandelten Gruppe (CU) denen der normalen Vergleichsgruppe (NU) und der kastrierten Gruppe, die 2 mg Testosteronpropionat/die
(CT$_2$) erhielt, gegenüberstellt. Wichtiger für den Eiweißgehalt des M. biceps
femoris und insbesondere auch für den der Leber ist offensichtlich die Neben-

nierenrindenfunktion. Es ließ sich zeigen, daß Homogenat- und Eluat-Eiweiß des M. biceps femoris in der kastriert-adrenalektomierten Gruppe (CA) signifikant höher liegen als in der kastriert-unbehandelten Gruppe (CU). Die Leber dagegen weist einen gegenüber der CU- und NU-Gruppe signifikant niedrigeren Eluateiweißgehalt in der CA-Gruppe auf.

Unter anderem läßt sich aus den Resultaten die Sonderstellung des M. Levator ani ablesen. Sein Verhalten entspricht mehr dem der sekundären Geschlechtsorgane. Eine anabole Wirkung des Testosteronpropionats auf den M. biceps femoris dagegen findet sich nur, wenn man den Eluatproteingehalt normaler oder kastriert-behandelter Ratten in Beziehung zu dem kastriert-unbehandelter Tiere setzt.

Wie an anderer Stelle dargelegt, sind aus Enzymaktivitätsveränderungen bei sorgfältiger Berücksichtigung wesentlicher Prämissen bedingte Rückschlüsse auf den Intermediärstoffwechsel möglich. Unter diesem Gesichtspunkt verdienen die gegensätzlichen Bewegungen von GPT-Aktivitäten und Eiweißgehalt in Muskeln und Lebern besondere Aufmerksamkeit. Der Eiweißansatz in der Leber, der sowohl unter Testosteronpropionat als auch unter Corticosteron zu beobachten ist, steht im Einklang mit einer Aktivitätssteigerung dieses Enzyms. Wie zu erwarten, führen die Kastration bzw. die Adrenalektomie zu einem Verlust an Eiweiß und GPT-Aktivitäten in diesem Organ. Eine synergistische Wirkung von Testosteronpropionat und Corticosteron auf die GPT und den Eiweißaufbau in der Leber unterliegt somit keinem Zweifel. In der Muskulatur und besonders ausgeprägt im M. Levator ani finden wir dagegen eine antagonistische Wirkung auf Eiweiß und GPT-Aktivität: Nach Kastration ist der erniedrigte Eiweißgehalt begleitet von erheblich gesteigerten GPT-Aktivitäten. Testosteronverabreichung hebt die Eiweißwerte an und hemmt die GPT (Abb. 3). Eine Erklärung des unterschiedlichen Verhaltens der GPT in Leber und Muskulatur muß von der Annahme ausgehen, daß unter den gewählten experimentellen Bedingungen die Gleichgewichtslage dieses Enzyms in der Leber vorwiegend zur Glutamat-, in der Muskulatur dagegen zur α-Ketoglutaratbildung führt, es sich also bei der GPT in der Leber einerseits und in der Muskulatur andererseits um Hetero-Enzyme im Sinne WIELANDs und PFLEIDERERs handelt.

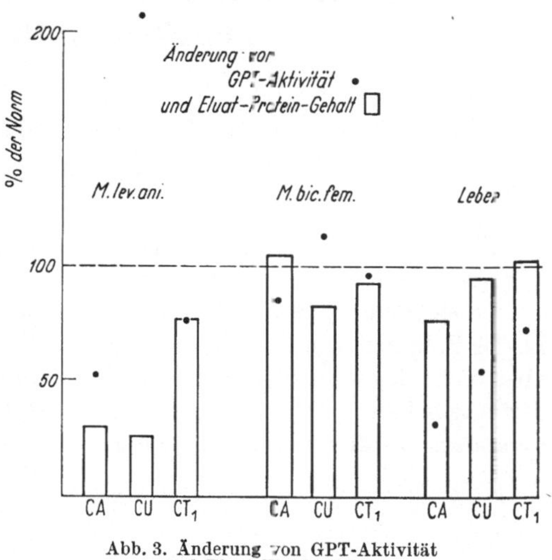

Abb. 3. Änderung von GPT-Aktivität und Eluat-Eiweiß-Gehalt

Aus dem Anatomischen Institut der Universität Bonn
(Direktor: Prof. Dr. med. E. Tonutti)

Prüfung eines im A-Ring erweiterten Testosteronderivates

Von

M. Herrmann und H.-G. Goslar

Mit 1 Abbildung

Nach der geglückten Strukturanalyse und Synthese der Steroidhormone wurde von vielen Autoren vorausgesetzt, daß die Struktur des Steroidmoleküls und die Unversehrtheit des Steranskeletes für die biologische Wirksamkeit unerläßlich sei. In der Folgezeit wurden viele Steroide synthetisiert, bei denen die Substituenten, aber nicht das Molekülgerüst, verändert wurden. So sind sehr viele Testosteronderivate bekannt geworden, bei denen die Substituenten des A-Ringes weitgehend verändert wurden, womit die androgenen Wirksamkeitskomponenten, anabole

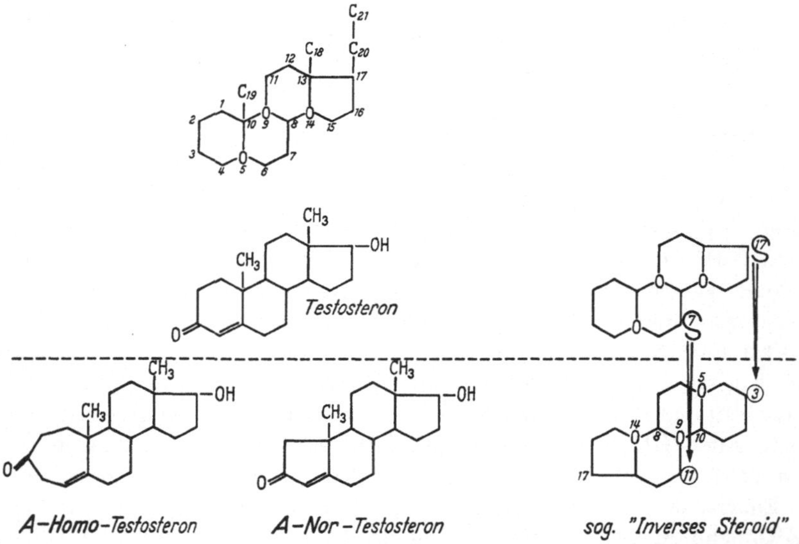

Abb. 1. Strukturformel der Steroide, normale Konfiguration des Testosterons, unter der gestrichelten Linie die synthetischen Steroide. Näheres siehe Text

Stoffwechselwirkung und Wirkung auf die Geschlechtsorgane, wesentlich beeinflußt werden konnten. Langecker hat in ihrem Referat auf dem letzten Symposion in Mainz (5) und in einer ausführlichen Publikation (6) einen umfassenden Überblick über diese Testosteronderivate gegeben.

Neuerdings wurden sogenannte „inverse" Steroide synthetisiert (Abb. 1), bei denen am spiegelbildlich verkehrten Steranskelet Substituenten des entsprechenden normalen C-Atoms eingeschleust werden (3). 1959 wurde über die Synthese eines sogenannten A-Nor-Testosterons berichtet (9), bei dem der Ring A des Steranskeletes zu einem 5-Ring verengert wurde (1, 8a—c). Diese genannten Testosteronderivate hatten keine androgene Wirksamkeit. MÜLLER u. Mitarb. (7) haben mit Diazomethan bei Testosteronacetat in Position 3,4 eine Ringerweiterung durchführen können. Auch im amerikanischen Schrifttum (4) wurde über diese Möglichkeit berichtet. Wir hatten Gelegenheit[1] bei einem in dieser Weise veränderten Testosteronacetat die Hemmwirkung auf die gonadotrope Partialfunktion der Hypophyse (HVL) beim Normaltier und die Substitutionswirkung beim kastrierten Tier zu prüfen (2).

Material und Methodik

75♂ weiße Mäuse aus einheitlicher Zucht, im Gewicht um 26 g, wurden bei 23 ± 1° C gehalten, mit „altromin"-R und Wasser ad libitum versorgt und wie folgt auf die Versuchsgruppen verteilt:

A. 35♂ Mäuse, von denen 10 Tiere 10 Tage 2 mg Testosteronpropionat in 0,2 ml Öl/die s. c., 5 Tiere 10 Tage 0,2 ml Sesamöl/die s. c., 5 Tiere 10 Tage 2 mg A-Homo-Testosteronacetat in 0,2 ml Öl/die s. c. erhielten und 15 Tiere unbehandelt als Kontrollen dienten.

B. 40♂ Mäuse wurden kastriert. 3 Wochen nach der Operation wurden 10 Tiere 5 Tage mit 2 mg Testosteronpropionat in 0,2 ml Öl/die s. c., 10 Tiere 5 Tage mit 0,2 ml Sesamöl/die s. c., 10 Tiere 5 Tage mit 2 mg A-Homo-Testosteronacetat in 0,2 ml Öl/die s. c. behandelt. 10 Tiere dienten unbehandelt als Kontrollen.

Die Tiere wurden zur gleichen Tageszeit 24 Std nach der letzten Injektion mit Chloroform abgetötet. Samenblasen und Präputialdrüsen sowie bei Gruppe A die Hoden und Nebenhoden wurden sofort entnommen und in Bouinscher Lösung fixiert. In fixiertem Zustand wurden diese Organe in 80%igem Alkohol gewogen und dann, wie die ebenfalls in Bouinscher Lösung fixierte Leber, Schilddrüse, Milz und Nebenniere, in üblicher Weise in Paraffin eingebettet. Nach Herstellung 7 μ dicker Schnitte, Färbung mit HE, HOPA (Hämalaun, Orange G, Phosphormolybdänsäure, Anilinblau) oder Goldner. Ausmessen des Kernvolumens der Leydigschen Zwischenzellen des Hodens, der Leberzellen, der Zellen der Zona fasciculata der Nebennierenrinde und der Follikelzellen der Schilddrüse nach Zeichnen der Kerne bei 2000facher Vergrößerung mit Hilfe eines Nomogrammes. Pro Tier und Organ wurden 200 Kerne gemessen.

Die formolfixierten Organe, Leber und Nebenniere, wurden auf ihren Gehalt an Sudanschwarz- und Scharlachrot-färbbaren Lipoiden und polarisationsoptisch auf ihren Gehalt an doppelbrechenden Substanzen untersucht.

Die Wolman fixierte Leber wurde mit der PJS-Reaktion vor und nach Diastaseeinwirkung auf ihren Glykogengehalt, mit dem histochemischen Nachweis der Orthodiacethylbenzolreaktion auf freie Aminogruppen untersucht.

---

[1] Wir danken Herrn Prof. MÜLLER, Direktor des Chemischen Instituts der Universität Tübingen, für die freundliche Überlassung der Substanz.

Ergebnisse

A. Hemmwirkung auf die gonadotrope Partialfunktion des HVL bei Normaltieren (s. Tab. 1).

Mit Testosteronpropionat wurden die bekannten Effekte an den Genitalorganen erzielt. Während das Hodengewicht abfiel, nahmen Samenblasengewicht und Präputialdrüsengewicht zu. Dementsprechend fand sich eine Verminderung des Kernvolumens der Leydigschen Zwischenzellen des Hodens, eine Vergrößerung des Samenblasenepithels und eine Aktivitätssteigerung der Präputialdrüsen. An den genannten Organen konnte bei den nur mit dem Lösungsmittel Öl behandelten Kontrolltieren keine Veränderung gegenüber Normaltieren festgestellt werden. Zufuhr von A-Homo-Testosteronacetat hatte weder auf Hodengewicht noch auf das Kernvolumen der Leydigschen Zwischenzellen des Hodens einen Einfluß, während Samenblasen- und Präputialdrüsengewicht abnahmen. Epithelhöhe der Samenblasen und Aktivität der Präputialdrüsen waren geringfügig vermindert.

Tabelle 1. Darstellung der Versuchsergebnisse aus Versuch A an Normaltieren.
Kursive Werte signifikant gegenüber Normal ($P < 0,01$)

Versuchsgruppe		Normal	Normal + Öl	Normal + A-Homo-testosteron	Normal + Testosteron
Organgewicht in mg ($m \pm \varepsilon$)	Hoden (Durchschnitt einseitig)	$85,5 \pm 1,8$	76 ± 14	$85 \pm 3,7$	*$63 \pm 6,2$*
	Samenblasen (Durchschnitt einseitig)	$71,3 \pm 3,4$	70 ± 20	$58 \pm 6,5$	*$115 \pm 7,5$*
	Präputialdrüsen	$87,5 \pm 5$	78 ± 20	64 ± 8	109 ± 12
Kernvolumen in μ^3/100 Kerne ($m \pm \varepsilon$)	Hoden, Leydigzellen	14311 ± 214	14854 ± 312	14439 ± 540	*7151 ± 155*
	Leber	21167 ± 1067	23572 ± 1068	*16470 ± 450*	30569 ± 2220
	Nebennierenrinde Fasciculatazellen	11144 ± 227	11390 ± 202	10946 ± 420	9963 ± 372
	Schilddrüse Follikelzellen	5981 ± 121	keine Messung	6380 ± 405	*7753 ± 240*
Körpergewicht	Durchschnittliche Zunahme pro Tier in g während der Behandlung	$3,6 \pm 0,4$	$3,8 \pm 0,5$	$1,9 \pm 1$	*$5,3 \pm 0,4$*
Histologie, Veränderungen gegenüber normal ($\pm$)	Hoden, Leydigzellgröße	$\pm$	$\pm$	$\pm$	—
	Samenblasen, Epithelhöhe	$\pm$	$\pm$	$\pm$	+
	Präputialdrüsen Aktivität	$\pm$	$\pm$	$\pm$	+
	Schilddrüse, Follikelzellhöhe	$8\,\mu$	keine Messung	$8\,\mu$	$9,5\,\mu$

Die durchschnittliche Gewichtszunahme der Tiere während des Versuches war bei unbehandelten Kontrollen und nur mit Öl behandelten Tieren fast gleich. Testosteron führte wie erwartet zu einem stärkeren Gewichtszuwachs, unter A-Homo-Testosteronacetat war die Zunahme geringer als normal. In diesem Zusammenhang ist das Ergebnis der Kernmessungen der Leberzellen interessant. Während die Normaltiere eine deutlich zweigipflige Kernverteilungskurve aufweisen, die durch alleinige Ölzufuhr nicht wesentlich verändert wird, wurde durch

Testosteron das Kernvolumen excessiv erhöht, es waren nur noch große Kerne zu finden. Zufuhr von A-Homo-Testosteronacetat führte zu einer signifikanten Verminderung des Kernvolumens gegenüber der Norm, es waren nur noch Kerne des kleinen Typs zu finden. Auf das Leberglykogen hatte die unterschiedliche Behandlung keinen merklichen Einfluß, ebenso ließ sich mit der o-Diacetylbenzolreaktion auf freie Aminogruppen keine Änderung des Eiweißstoffwechsels nachweisen. Die Schilddrüse zeigte unter Testosteronzufuhr eine deutliche Zunahme des Kernvolumens und auch der Epithelhöhe, während A-Homo-Testosteronacetat hier ohne deutlichen Effekt blieb. An der Nebenniere konnte unter Testosteronzufuhr eine Abnahme des Kernvolumens der Zellen der Zona fasciculata festgestellt werden, ebenso geringe Veränderungen im Sinne einer regressiven Transformation. Auch hier zeigte A-Homo-Testosteronacetat keinen wesentlichen Effekt.

B. Substitutionswirkung nach Kastration (s. Tab. 2).

Während die Behandlung der kastrierten Tiere mit Testosteron zu einer signifikanten Erhöhung des Samenblasen- und Präputialdrüsengewichtes führte, ebenso zu einer deutlichen Zunahme der Epithelhöhe der Samenblasen und der Präputialdrüsenaktivität, hatte die Zufuhr von A-Homo-Testosteronacetat keinen Einfluß auf die Kastrationsfolgeerscheinungen bei beiden Organen.

Tabelle 2. Darstellung der Versuchsergebnisse aus Versuch B an kastrierten Tieren. *Kursive Werte signifikant gegenüber kastriert* $(P < 0,01)$

Versuchsgruppe		Kastriert	Kastriert + Öl	Kastriert + A-Homo-testosteron	Kastriert + Testosteron
Organgewicht in mg $(m \pm \varepsilon)$	Samenblasen (Durchschnitt einseitig)	$5,0 \pm 0,3$	$4,15 \pm 0,4$	$6,1 \pm 0,4$	*33,6 $\pm$ 2,1*
	Präputialdrüsen	$29 \pm 2,2$	$26,8 \pm 2,2$	$31,1 \pm 2,1$	*58 $\pm$ 3,6*
Kernvolumen in μ^3/100 Kerne $(m \pm \varepsilon)$	Leber	$17\,679 \pm 2140$	$24\,540 \pm 2400$	$21\,012 \pm 1225$	*36 072 $\pm$ 3000*
	Nebennierenrinde Fasciculatazellen	$10\,959 \pm 212$	$11\,276 \pm 165$	$11\,110 \pm 260$	$10\,076 \pm 402$
Körpergewicht	Durchschnittliche Zunahme pro Tier in g während der Behandlung	$0,2 \pm 0,4$	$0,75 \pm 0,25$	$1.22 \pm 0,32$	$2,1 \pm 0,61$
Histologie, Veränderungen gegenüber normal $(\pm)$	Samenblasen, Epithelhöhe	—	—	—	$\pm$
	Präputialdrüsen Aktivität	—	—	—	$\pm$

Der durchschnittliche Gewichtszuwachs der mit Testosteron behandelten Tiere war gegenüber den Kontrollen erhöht. Die Gewichtszunahme unter der Behandlung mit A-Homo-Testosteronacetat war etwa halb so groß, damit zwar größer als bei den unbehandelten kastrierten Kontrollen, aber deutlich geringer als bei unbehandelten Normaltieren. Das Kernvolumen der Leberzellen zeigte ein ähnliches Verhalten. Kastration führte zu einer deutlichen Abnahme des Kernvolumens, Testosteronzufuhr zu einer deutlichen Erhöhung gegenüber den kastrierten Kontrollen und den unbehandelten Normaltieren. Im Glykogenbild war auch hier kein Unterschied zwischen den einzelnen Gruppen festzustellen. Ebenso ließ die o-Diacetylbenzolreaktion keine Differenzen im Verhalten der freien Aminogruppen bei den einzelnen Versuchsgruppen erkennen.

Diskussion der Ergebnisse

Wie aus den geschilderten Versuchsergebnissen deutlich wird, besitzt das untersuchte A-Homo-Testosteronacetat keine androgene Wirksamkeit. Daraus kann geschlossen werden, daß die Ringerweiterung in Position 3,4 des A-Ringes zu einem Verlust der spezifischen Hormonwirkung durch Veränderung der Sterankonfiguration führt. Dies ist aus dem Ausbleiben der Substitutionswirkung beim kastrierten Tier erkenntlich. Die Versuche an Normaltieren zeigen außerdem, daß die untersuchte Substanz keine Hemmwirkung auf die gonadotrope Partialfunktion des HVL besitzt. Aus dem Ausbleiben des Gewichtsanstieges kann auf eine fehlende anabole Wirkung geschlossen werden.

Damit entsprechen unsere Ergebnisse bei Ringerweiterung im Ring A durchaus denen, die bei Verengerung des A-Ringes (A-Nor-Testosteron) erzielt wurden (9). Auch der Wirkungsausfall bei „inversen" Steroiden (3) entspricht diesen Befunden. Somit ist für die genannten Veränderungen der Beweis erbracht, daß die Unversehrtheit des A-Ringes eine conditio sine qua non für die Erhaltung der spezifischen Hormonwirkung ist. Ob auch bei A-Homo-Testosteronacetat eine Hemmwirkung auf Testosteron vorliegt, bzw. eine antiandrogene Wirksamkeit besteht, kann noch nicht sicher ausgesagt werden. Neuere Befunde deuten darauf hin, doch bedarf es zu ihrer Sicherung weiterer Untersuchungen.

Zusammenfassung

An männlichen Mäusen wurde die biologische Wirksamkeit eines hochgereinigten A-Homo-Testosteronacetates geprüft. Die Substanz besitzt keine Hemmwirkung auf die gonadotrope Partialfunktion des Hypophysenvorderlappens. Im Substitutionsversuch an kastrierten Tieren zeigt sie keine androgene Wirksamkeit. Eine anabole Wirkung kann nicht nachgewiesen werden.

Literatur

1. Fieser, L., u. M. Fieser: Steroide. S. 655. Weinheim (Bergstraße): Verlag Chemie 1961.
2. Herrmann, M., u. H.-G. Goslar: Experientia (Basel) **19**, 76 (1963).
3. Jacques, J., and G. Pincus: International Congress of Hormonal Steroids, Mailand, 14.—19. 5. 1962. Excerpta med. (Amst.) International Congress Series **51**, 3—6 (1962), Abstract.
4. Johnson, W. S., M. Neeman, S. P. Birkeland and N. A. Fedoruk: J. Amer. chem. Soc. **84**, 989 (1962).
5. Langecker, H.: 9. Symposion dtsch. Ges. Endokrinologie, 3.—5. 5. 1962, Mainz. Berlin-Göttingen-Heidelberg: Springer-Verlag S. 171—173.
6. — Acta endocr. (Kbh.) **41**, 494—500 (1962).
7. Müller, Eu., u. B. Zeh: Z. Naturforsch. (im Druck).
8. Ourisson, G.: Bull. Soc. chim. Fr. **1962**, a) S. 331, b) S. 337, c) S. 341.
9. Weisenborn, F. L., and H. E. Applegate: J. Amer. chem. Soc. **81**, 1960 (1959).

Aus der Frauenklinik (Direktor: Prof. Dr. R. Elert) und dem Physiologisch-Chemischen Institut (Direktor: Prof. Dr. K. Hinsberg) der Medizinischen Akademie Düsseldorf

Vergleichende Untersuchungen über den Oestrogengehalt im fetalen und mütterlichen Blut

Von

W. Schild, K. Schürholz und A. Seuken

Die neuesten Erkenntnisse über die Biosynthese und den Metabolismus der Sexualhormone haben die Frage aufgeworfen, wie weit während der Schwangerschaft dieses Geschehen in der Placenta abläuft und in welchem Grade der Fet und auch die Mutter daran beteiligt sind. Die Bildung der Steroide Oestron, 17β-Oestradiol und Oestriol in der Placenta gilt als gesichert (Lit. bei 5). Durch in-vitro-Untersuchungen ist die Fähigkeit einzelner fetaler Organe, Oestrogene umzubauen, nachgewiesen worden (3, 4, 7). Gewisse Befunde geben zu der Vermutung Anlaß, daß eine Oestrogensynthese im Feten stattfindet (11, 13). Die unterschiedlichen Oestrogenspiegel im mütterlichen und kindlichen Blut haben weiterhin zu der Annahme geführt, daß eine besondere Placentaschranke vorhanden sei.

Eine weitere Klärung dieser Fragen bzgl. Synthese und Metabolismus der Oestrogene sowie Austausch dieser Hormone zwischen Fet und Mutter läßt sich durch Bestimmung der Oestrogenkonzentrationen in den Nabelschnurgefäßen und im placentanahen mütterlichen Blut erzielen. Es wurden daher getrennte Untersuchungen des Nabelvenen-, Nabelarterien- und Retroplacentarblutes durchgeführt und hierbei die drei „klassischen" Oestrogene qualitativ und quantitativ bestimmt und zueinander in Beziehung gesetzt.

Zur Aufarbeitung gelangten jeweils 40—62 ml Sammelblut der drei genannten Arten. Für die Isolierung von Oestron, 17β-Oestradiol und Oestriol wurden die von Diczfalusy u. Mitarb. (6) angegebenen methodischen Schritte zur Extraktion und Reinigung geringgradig modifiziert und mit der säulenchromatographischen Trennung und fluorimetrischen Bestimmung nach Ittrich (10) kombiniert. Auf die Trennung in freie und konjugierte Hormone wurde verzichtet.

In Tab. 1 sind die ermittelten Oestrogenspiegel aufgeführt. Die unterschiedlichen Oestronkonzentrationen mit einem höheren Wert in der Nabelschnurvene und einem niedrigeren in den Nabelarterien treten deutlich hervor, während der Gehalt an Oestradiol im arteriellen und venösen Nabelschnurblut nur eine geringe allerdings gleichsinnige Differenz aufweist. Beim Oestriol sind praktisch keine Unterschiede festzustellen.

Die Spiegel von Oestron und Oestradiol sind im arteriellen und venösen Nabelschnurblut deutlich niedriger als im Retroplacentarblut, wogegen sich beim Oestriol die umgekehrten Verhältnisse feststellen lassen. Von diesen verschiedenen Konzentrationen ist allerdings nur der Unterschied des Oestrongehaltes in Nabelarterien und Retroplacentarblut signifikant.

Der gegenüber dem Nabelvenenblut verminderte Gehalt an Oestron und Oestradiol im Nabelarterienblut weist auf einen Metabolismus dieser Oestrogene im Feten hin. Es läßt sich jedoch nicht sagen, ob die Umwandlung der genannten Hormone überwiegend in andere Substanzen als Oestriol erfolgt. Die Befunde sprechen gegen eine Biosynthese der Oestrogene im fetalen Organismus.

Tabelle 1. *Oestrogenkonzentrationen (unkorrigierte Werte) im Nabelschnurvenen-, Nabelschnurarterien- und Retroplacentarblut. I = Oestron, II = 17 β-Oestradiol, III = Oestriol. Untersuchte Sammelblutmengen 40—62 ml. Prüfung der Signifikanz der Mittelwertdifferenzen (n = 10)*

	Oestrogenkonzentration (μg/100 ml)		
	Nabelschnur-venenblut	Nabelschnur-arterienblut	Retroplacentar-blut
I	$3{,}2 \pm 1{,}3$	$0{,}3 \pm 0{,}1$	$7{,}2 \pm 1{,}9$
	$P = 0{,}05$	$P < 0{,}01$	
		$P > 0{,}1$	
II	$0{,}5 \pm 0{,}5$	$0{,}1 \pm 0{,}1$	$4{,}1 \pm 2{,}2$
	$P > 0{,}4$	$P > 0{,}05$	
		$P > 0{,}1$	
III	$51{,}2 \pm 19{,}9$	$45{,}1 \pm 10{,}3$	$18{,}5 \pm 7{,}0$
	$P > 0{,}7$	$P > 0{,}05$	
		$P > 0{,}1$	

Es ist daran zu denken, daß evtl. bestimmte Stoffwechselvorgänge in der Frucht durch die Produkte dieser metabolischen Reaktionen gesteuert werden. Den bei Konjugierungsvorgängen im Feten gebildeten Verbindungen dürfte eine ähnliche Bedeutung zukommen. Solche Umbaustoffe der Oestrogene gelangen durch die Nabelarterien in die Placenta. Da ihre Menge den Grad ihrer Funktion im Feten widerspiegelt, darf man annehmen, daß sie in der Placenta einen entsprechenden regulatorischen Einfluß auf die Hormonproduktion ausüben.

Solche Wechselbeziehungen würden dem Mechanismus einer Rückkoppelung ähnlich sein, d. h. einem System, das seine eigene Aktivität zu steuern vermag. In der Placenta müssen Reaktionen ablaufen, welche die in der Frucht gebildeten Umwandlungsprodukte beseitigen, sei es durch Hydrolyse, weiteren Abbau und/oder Ausscheidung zur Mutter hin.

Für eine Kontrolle oestrogenbedingter Fermentbeeinflussung durch Umwandlungsprodukte stark wirksamer Oestrogene sprechen die von Villee (*8, 15*) bei in-vitro-Untersuchungen gefundenen Ergebnisse. Danach läßt sich eine Stimulierung verschiedener Dehydrogenasen durch Oestron und Oestradiol bei nur unbedeutender Wirksamkeit des Oestriols feststellen, während bei gleichzeitiger Einwirkung von Oestron und Ostradiol zusammen mit Oestriol eine Hemmung der enzymstimulierenden Wirkung der beiden ersten Hormone zu beobachten ist.

Es ist auffällig, daß diesseits und jenseits der Placenta erhebliche Unterschiede der Oestrogenkonzentrationen vorhanden sind. Allerdings ist die bei solchen Untersuchungen nicht zu vermeidende ungleichzeitige Gewinnung des Nabelschnur-

und Retroplacentarblutes zu berücksichtigen, die evtl. geringe Konzentrations-
veränderungen der Hormone zur Folge hat. Diese können jedoch nicht die Ursache
der oben aufgezeichneten deutlich unterschiedlichen Oestrogenspiegel sein. Wie
weit durch das Geburtsgeschehen die Hormonmengen im fetalen und mütterlichen
Blut rein mechanisch, z. B. durch Auspressen der in der Placenta befindlichen
Oestrogene, verändert werden, ist unbekannt. Daher können aus den vorliegenden Befunden nur vorsichtige Rückschlüsse auf den Zustand in der Gravidität
gezogen werden.

Der im Retroplacentarblut gegenüber dem Nabelschnurblut erhöhte Gehalt
an Oestron und Oestradiol könnte an eine zusätzliche Hormonproduktion der
mütterlichen Ovarien denken lassen. Die Möglichkeit einer solchen Oestrogen-
bildung ist durch ZANDER u. Mitarb. (17) nachgewiesen worden, jedoch ist sie im
Vergleich zur Hormonsynthese in der Placenta so gering, daß sie bei Berücksichtigung der von PEARLMAN (14) errechneten Halbwertszeit der menschlichen
Blutoestrogene keine Rolle spielen kann. In diesem Sinne spricht auch die Beobachtung, daß in der Gravidität nach bilateraler Ovariektomie die Oestrogenausscheidung unverändert bleibt (Lit. bei 2, 12).

Bezüglich der freien Oestrogene scheint eine einfache Diffusion von der Placenta
in den kindlichen und mütterlichen Kreislauf möglich zu sein. Eine unterschiedliche Permeabilität der Placenta für freie Oestrogene und für wasserlösliche
Oestrogenglucuronoside wurde von DANCIS u. Mitarb. (1) bei Perfusionsstudien
an Meerschweinchen beobachtet. DICZFALUSY u. Mitarb. (3) glauben auf Grund
von Untersuchungen bei Interruptiones, daß dies auch für andere konjugierte
Oestrogene zutrifft. Somit dürfte die Placenta an der Aufrechterhaltung der
genannten Konzentrationsunterschiede mitbeteiligt sein.

Die Oestrogenspiegel im Retroplacentarblut können zum Teil darauf beruhen,
daß im mütterlichen Blut zusätzlich reichlich konjugierte Oestrogene vorhanden
sind, welche nicht ohne weiteres durch die Placenta zu gelangen vermögen und
sich daher im mütterlichen Blut anreichern. Die günstigen Ausscheidungsver-
hältnisse für Oestriolconjugate wären der Grund für den relativ niedrigen Oestriol-
spiegel im Blut der Mutter. Getrennte Bestimmungen von freien und konjugierten
Oestrogenen in analoger Weise wie oben angegeben könnten zur weiteren Klärung
dieser Fragen beitragen.

Die physiologische Bedeutung der im fetalen und mütterlichen Kreislauf
befindlichen großen Oestrogenmengen ist weitgehend unbekannt. Im Hinblick
auf die in vitro an verschiedenen Geweben erhobenen Befunde, die zu der Theorie
führten, daß die Steigerung im Pyridinnucleotid-Transhydrogenasesystem-
Durchsatz durch Oestradiol eine Energiezunahme zur Folge hat, welche sich in
einer gesteigerten Eiweiß-, Nucleinsäuren- und Fettsynthese zeigt (16), scheinen die Oestrogene besonders solche Reaktionen zu beeinflussen, die für
Wachstumsvorgänge bedeutungsvoll sind. Es sind mehrere Hypothesen aufgestellt worden, die die möglichen Funktionen der Oestrogene im Organismus
erklären sollen, jedoch stehen eindeutige Beweise noch aus (9). Um über die
Bedeutung der Produktion so großer Hormonmengen in der Placenta etwas Näheres
zu erfahren, sind weitere Untersuchungen von Stoffwechselvorgängen bei der
schwangeren Frau und auch beim Fetus wichtig, denn es ist anzunehmen, daß die
Hormone nicht nur Wachstum und Funktion der mit dem Gestationsgeschehen

zusammenhängenden mütterlichen Organe beeinflussen, sondern auch bestimmte Wirkungen auf die Frucht entfalten, die für deren Entwicklung unbedingt notwendig sind.

Literatur

1. Dancis, J., W. L. Money, G. P. Condon and M. Levitz: J. clin. Invest. 37, 1373 (1958).
2. Diczfalusy, E., and U. Borell: J. clin. Endocr. 21, 1119 (1961).
3. — O. Cassmer, C. Alonso and M. de Miquel: Acta endocr. (Kbh.) 37, 353 (1961).
4. — — — — and B. Westin: Acta Endocr. 37, 516 (1961).
5. — u. C. Lauritzen: Oestrogene beim Menschen. Berlin-Göttingen-Heidelberg: Springer-Verlag 1961.
6. —, and M. Magnusson: Acta endocr. (Kbh.) 28, 169 (1958).
7. Engel, L. L., u. M. Halla: Biochim. biophys. Acta 30, 435 (1958).
8. Hagerman, D. D., and C. A. Villee: In: Endocrinology of Reproduction. Edit. C. W. Lloyd. New York: Acad. Press 1959.
9. Hisaw, F. L., J. T. Velardo and C. M. Goolsby: J. clin. Endocr. 14, 1134 (1954).
10. Ittrich, G.: Z. physiol. Chemie 320, 103 (1960).
11. Lelong, M., S. Vandel, P. Borniche et M. F. Jayle: Ann. Endocr. (Paris) 12, 922 (1951).
12. Oettle, M.: Z. Geburtsh. Gynäk. 136, 294 (1952).
13. Parker, F., and B. Tenney: Endocrinology 23, 492 (1938).
14. Pearlman, W. H.: In: Ciba Found. Coll. on Endocrin. 11, 238, 245 (1957).
15. Villee, C. A.: J. biol. Chem. 215, 171 (1955).
16. — Klin. Wschr. 39, 173 (1961).
17. Zander, J., E. Brendle, A. M. v. Münstermann, E. Diczfalusy, B. Martinsen and K. G. Tillinger: Acta obstet. gynec scand. 38, 724 (1959).

Aus der Frauenklinik (Direktor: Prof. Dr. R. Elert), der II. Medizinischen Klinik und Poliklinik (Direktor: Prof. Dr. K. Oberdisse), und dem Pathologischen Institut (Direktor: Prof. Dr. H. Meessen) der Medizinischen Akademie Düsseldorf

Klinische, endokrinologische und morphologische Untersuchungen bei einem Fall von Gynandroblastom

Von

W. Nocke, H. Zimmermann, R. Buchholz und R. Poche

Mit 2 Abbildungen

Robert Meyer (*22*) berichtete 1930 erstmalig über einen virilisierenden Ovarialtumor, der neben den morphologischen Kriterien eines Arrhenoblastoms auch Strukturen eines Granulosazelltumors enthielt und führte für diesen Tumor die Bezeichnung „Gynandroblastom" ein (cf. *15*). Infolge der Schwierigkeit, wenig differenzierte Sertoli-Leydig-Zell- und Granulosa-Theca-Zell-Strukturen eindeutig voneinander zu unterscheiden, kann die Zuordnung „gemischter" Ovarialgeschwülste zu dieser Tumorklasse problematisch sein (*12, 23, 35*). Aus diesen Gründen können von den seit 1930 mitgeteilten etwa 60 Fällen bei kritischer Überprüfung offenbar nur 19 Fälle als sichere Gynandroblastome betrachtet werden (*11, 12, 15—17, 20, 21, 23, 23a, 29, 30, 33, 35*).

Die klinische Symptomatik wird wie beim Arrhenoblastom durch eine ausgeprägte Virilisierung bestimmt. Daneben können Zeichen vermehrter Oestrogenwirkung wie Uterushypertrophie (*12, 22, 30*), Uterus myomatosus (*33*), Metrorrhagien (*12, 30, 33*) sowie glandulär-cystische Hyperplasie (*12, 30, 33*), Polyposis (*33*), Carcinoma in situ (*12*) und Carcinom des Endometriums (*33*) auftreten.

Über Hormonuntersuchungen bei Gynandroblastomen liegen bisher nur einzelne Mitteilungen vor (*12, 20, 30*).

Fallbericht

Vorgeschichte. Die von uns beobachtete, 13³/₄jährige Patientin hatte nach spontaner Menarche im 11. Lebensjahr etwa 1 Jahr lang regelmäßig menstruiert. Seit dem 12. Lebensjahr bestand sekundäre Amenorrhoe. Gleichzeitig mit dem Auftreten der Amenorrhoe begannen sich stärkere Behaarung des Gesichts, des Unterbauchs und der Extremitäten sowie Acne auf Gesicht und Schultern zu entwickeln. Die Stimme wurde rauher und tiefer. Im 13. Lebensjahr traten einzelne rötliche Streifen in der Hüftgegend, Vergrößerung des Halsumfanges und mäßige Gewichtszunahme auf.

Klinische Befunde. Die Pat. hatte bei kräftigem Körperbau und angedeutet männlichen Körperproportionen eine Länge von 170 cm und ein Gewicht von 68,8 kg (P-Index > 97). Neben schwacher Oberlippenbehaarung und mäßiger Acne vulg. auf Gesicht, Schultern und Oberkörper bestand Hirsutismus an den Extremitäten und besonders im Wangen- und Kinnbereich. Im Hüftbereich bds. fanden sich blaurote Striae. Der Halsumfang betrug 39 cm, die Stimme war rauh und tief, und es bestand eine leichte, diffuse, weiche Struma. Das Knochenalter (re. Hand) war gegenüber dem chronologischen Alter um wenigstens 4 Jahre voraus.

Die *gynäkologische Untersuchung* ergab folgenden Befund: nur mäßig entwickelte Mammae, virile Pubes, Druckschmerz im li. Unterbauch; Clitorishypertrophie, Virgo intacta, Uterus hühnereigroß, anteflektiert, frei beweglich; enteneigroßer, beweglicher Tumor der li. Adnexe, etwa pflaumesgroßes re. Ovar.

Durch orientierende Steroidbestimmungen im Urin konnte ein extraadrenaler, androgen-produzierender Prozeß gesichert werden. Bei der daraufhin vorgenommenen *Laparatomie* wurde ein enteneigroßer, grauer, glatter Tumor des linken Ovars (74 g) gefunden. Auf der Schnittfläche zeigten sich in der Ovarialrinde vereinzelte kleine Cysten. Das Mark war hühner-eigroß, schwammig und teilweise cystisch aufgequollen. Die li. Adnexe wurden exstirpiert. Das gut pflaumengroße, graue, glatte re. Ovar zeigte auf der Schnittfläche polycystische Veränderungen und wurde zu zwei Dritteln keilreseziert.

Nach einer Entzugsblutung am 13. Tag post op. sind bei der Pat. bis heute in Abständen von 24—28 Tagen regelmäßige Blutungen mit biphasischen Basaltemperaturcyclen aufgetreten. Auch äußerlich stellte sich eine deutliche Verweiblichung ein (Rückgang von Acne und Hirsu-tismus, Ausbildung weiblicher Pubes, Mammawachstum mit Vergrößerung und Pigmentierung der Areolae, auffällige Veränderungen von Gesichtsausdruck und Körperproportionen).

Histologischer Befund (E-Nr. 11960/62). Teil eines stark vergrößerten Ovars. In der Rinde zahlreiche Primärfollikel. Dicht unterhalb der Rinde ein Tumorgewebe, das aus mehreren Anteilen besteht. In einem sehr zellreichen Stroma befinden sich große, helle, epithelähnliche Zellen mit runden oder ovalen, meist dunklen, teilweise auch etwas geblähten Kernen. Diese Zellen bilden dicht beieinanderliegende Stränge oder Schläuche mit kleinen Lichtungen, so daß hier das Bild eines tubulären Adenoms vorliegt. An anderen Stellen erkennt man große Bezirke eines Gewebes, dessen Zellen an Granulosa- und Thecazellen erinnern und die stellenweise luteinisiert sind. Die an Granulosazellen erinnernden Zellen bilden manchmal unscharf be-grenzte Stränge und formieren sich zu girlanden-, rosetten- oder follikelähnlichen Strukturen, so daß das Bild eines Granulosa-Theca-Zelltumors entsteht. Dieses Geschwulstgewebe verliert sich in ein lockeres, bindegewebiges Stroma, das herdförmig ödematös oder gallertig auf-gelockert sein kann und auch größere Gruppen von sehr weiten Blutgefäßen enthält, so daß an einzelnen Stellen angiomartige Strukturen entstehen. — *Diagnose:* Gynandroblastom.

Hormonuntersuchungen

Methodik. Die Sammlung und Aufbewahrung der Urine erfolgte wie an anderer Stelle beschrieben (*25*). Die biologische Bestimmung der hypophysären Gonadotropine erfolgte durch 6-Punkt-Bestimmung im Maus-Uterus-Test (5 Tiere/Dosis) aus Sammelurin von 7 Tagen (*1, 10, 14*). Die für die chemischen Steroidbestimmungen benutzten Methoden sind in den Legenden von Tab. 1, Abb. 1 und Abb. 2 angegeben.

Ergebnisse und Diskussion[1]

Die HPG-Ausscheidung der Pat. sprach mit < 2 HMG-E/24 Std für eine praktisch ruhende gonadotrope HVL-Funktion. Bestimmungen der 17-KS-

---

[1] Im Text werden folgende Abkürzungen benutzt:

ACTH	= 75 I.E. Corticotropin A/500 ml 5% Glucose / 8 Std i.v.
PMS	= Serumgonadotropin schwangerer Stuten, i. m.
HCG	= menschliches Choriongonadotropin, i. m.
HPG	= hypophysäre Gesamtgonadotropine (bezogen auf Standard HMG 20 A)
17-KS	= Neutrale Total-17-Ketosteroide
DHA	= Dehydro*epi*androsteron (3 β-Hydroxy-androst-5-en-17-on)
A	= Androsteron (3 α-Hydroxy-5 α-androstan-17-on)
Aet	= Aetiocholanolon (3 α-Hydroxy-5 β-androstan-17-on)
Adion	= Androstendion (Androst-4-en-3,17-dion)
11-Oxy-17-KS	= Summe aller 11-Keto- und 11 β-Hydroxy-17-Ketosteroide
11-O-A	= 11-Ketoandrosteron (3 α-Hydroxy-5 α-androstan-11,17-dion)
11-O-Aet	= 11-Ketoaetiocholanolon (3 α-Hydroxy-5 β-androstan-11,17-dion)
11-OH-A	= 11-Hydroxyandrosteron (3 α, 11 β-Dihydroxy-5 α-androstan-17-on)
11-OH-Aet	= 11-Hydroxyaetiocholanolon (3 α, 11 β-Dihydroxy-5 β-androstan-17-on)

Tabelle 1. *Chromatographische Fraktionierung von neutralen 17-Ketosteroiden im Plasma und im Urin bei einem Gynandroblastom des Ovars unter verschiedenen Bedingungen.*
(Abkürzungen vgl. Anm.[1], S. 290)

	Bedingungen	Total-17-KS	DHA	A	Aet	$5\alpha/5\beta$ (=A/Aet)	11-O-A	11-O-Aet	11-OH-A	11-OH-Aet	X	Adion
a) Plasma[1]	ohne Behandlung (17. 8. 62)	—	57,9	18,0	25,6	0,7	—	—	—	12,6	—	0,5
	unmittelbar ante op. (27. 8. 62)[3]	—	71,5	15,2	38,8	0,4	—	—	—	35,6	—	1,2
	unmittelbar post op. (27. 8. 62)	—	23,8	19,0	19,1	1,0	—	—	—	30,6	—	0
	10 Tage post op. (5. 9. 62)	—	53,4	29,9	23,2	1,3	—	—	—	21,4	—	0
	5 Monate post op. (1. 2. 63; 25. Tag post menstr.)	—	23,3	10,0	8,9	1,1	—	—	—	22,7	—	0
b) Urin[2]	ohne Behandlung (26. 5. 62)	13,5	0,78	6,70	2,30	2,9	0,56	1,11	0,65	0,21	1,20	—
	nach Dexamethason (5. 6. 62)	9,7	0	3,72	4,50	—	0	0,23	0,21	0,21	0,84	—
	nach HCG (17. 6. 62)	27,1	0,13	15,60	9,90	1,6	0,17	1,00	0,13	0,08	0,10	—

[1] Die Werte sind ausgedrückt als μg Dehydro*epi*androsteron-Äquivalent/100 ml Plasma. — Die Bestimmungen wurden ausgeführt im Laboratorium von Herrn Doz. Dr. G. W. OERTEL, Homburg/Saar.

[2] Die Werte sind ausgedrückt als mg Dehydro*epi*androsteron-Äquivalent/24 Std. — Die Bestimmungen wurden ausgeführt mit der Methode von STARKA (*34*) unter Benutzung des Hydrolyseverfahrens von JOHNSEN (*18*).

[3] 1 Tag nach Beendigung der Dexamethason/HCG-Behandlung (cf. Abb. 1 und 2).

Fraktionen im Plasma (Tab. 1a)[1] zeigten einen auffallend hohen Wert für Adion. Die Absolutwerte der übrigen Fraktionen lagen im Normbereich (*27, 28*). Jedoch war die relative Konzentration von Aet deutlich erhöht (A/Aet = 0,7; normal: 1,2—1,3). Nach Gabe von HCG unter gleichzeitiger Hemmung der NNR mit Dexamethason wurden noch am Morgen nach Absetzen der Behandlung erhöhte Werte für DHA, Aet, 11-OH-Aet und Adion beobachtet. Dabei wurde besonders Aet relativ stark mobilisiert (A/Aet = 0,4). Unmittelbar nach Exstirpation des Tumors zeigten DHA, Aet und 11-OH-Aet erniedrigte Werte, während Adion nicht mehr nachweisbar war. Der relativ starke postoperative Abfall von Aet bewirkte eine Normalisierung des Quotienten A/Aet.

Bei den Voruntersuchungen zur Klärung der Differentialdiagnose einer adrenalen oder extraadrenalen Virilisierung ergab sich eine gegenüber der mittleren

TTC-CS	= Triphenyltetrazoliumchlorid-reduzierende Corticosteroide (Steroide mit 20,21-Ketol- und 17α,21-Dihydroxy-20-Keto-Seitenkette)
17-OHCS	= Total-17α-Hydroxycorticosteroide
PD	= Pregnandiol (5β-Pregnan-3α,20α-diol)
PT	= Pregnantriol (5β-Pregnan-3α,17α,20α-triol)
Oestrogene	= Oestron + 17β-Oestradiol + Oestriol
Oe_1	= Oestron (3-Hydroxy-oestra-1,3,5(10)-trien-17-on)
Oe_2	= 17β-Oestradiol (Oestra-1,3,5(10)-trien-3,17β-diol)
Oe_3	= Oestriol (Oestra-1,3,5(10)-trien-3,16α,17β-triol)

[1] Für die Plasmasteroidbestimmungen sind wir Herrn Doz. Dr. G. W. OERTEL, Homburg (Saar), sehr zu Dank verpflichtet.

Altersnorm 2fach erhöhte mittlere 17-KS-Ausscheidung (13,4 mg/24 Std), während die TTC-CS (Mittelwert 8,8 mg/24 Std) im Normbereich für erwachsene Frauen lagen. Intravenöse Zufuhr von ACTH ergab mit Anstiegen der 17-KS um 56% und der TTC-CS um 171% keinen Anhalt für eine gestörte NNR-Funktion (cf. 4).

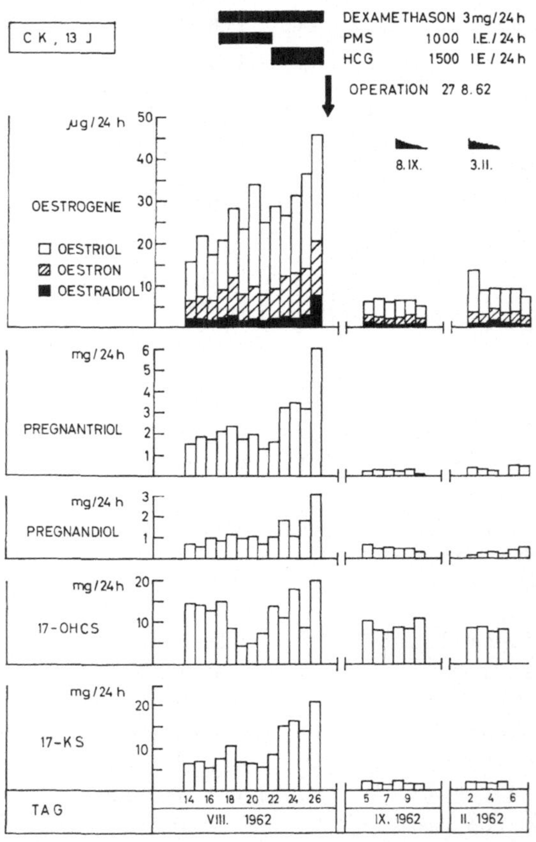

Abb. 1. Ausscheidung von neutralen 17-Ketosteroiden (17-KS)[1], 17 α-Hydroxycorticosteroiden (17-OHCS)[2], Pregnan-3 α, 20 α-diol, Pregnan-3 α, 17 α, 20 α-triol[3], Oestron, 17 β-Oestradiol und Oestriol[4] ohne Behandlung, nach Gabe von Dexamethason + PMS, Dexamethason + HCG sowie nach Exstirpation des Tumors.

Methoden:

[1] Norymberski, Stubbs u. West (26).
[2] Appleby, Gibson, Norymberski u. Stubbs (2).
[3] Nocke & Nocke (unveröffentlicht).
[4] Brown (6); Modifikation nach Brown, Bulbrook & Greenwood (7); Kober-Reaktion nach Nocke (24).

Dexamethason (3—5 mg/24 h) bewirkte lediglich eine Verminderung der TTC-CS um 36% und ließ die 17-KS-Ausscheidung unbeeinflußt. Injektionen von je 1000 I. E. HCG 4 Tage lang verursachten eine Verdoppelung der 17-KS-Ausscheidung, während die TTC-CS-Ausscheidung sich nicht veränderte. Wie die chromatographische Fraktionierung ergab (Tab. 1b), bestanden die von der Pat. ausgeschiedenen 17-KS zu 67% aus A + Aet (9,0 mg/24 Std). Nach Dexamethason war der absolute Wert für A + Aet (8,2 mg/24 Std) praktisch unverändert, während die relative Konzentration auf 85% anstieg. HCG bewirkte gegenüber dem Ausgangswert eine 2,8fache Erhöhung von A + Aet (25,5 mg/24 Std) und damit einen Anstieg der relativen Konzentration auf 94% der Total-17-KS.

Nähere Aufschlüsse über die Steroidproduktion des Tumors wurden aus den in Abb. 1 und Abb. 2 zusammengefaßten Untersuchungen gewonnen. Die mittlere 17-KS-Ausscheidung (6,3 mg/24 Std) war zwar gegenüber der mittleren Altersnorm auch hier 2fach erhöht, lag jedoch noch innerhalb der Vertrauensgrenzen für $P = 0,05$ (5). Bei Berücksichtigung des accelerierten Wachstumsalters der Pat. entsprach die Ausscheidung einem mittleren Normalwert (5). Andererseits lag die mittlere Ausscheidung von 17-OHCS (13,8 mg/24 Std) außerhalb der oberen Vertrauensgrenzen $(P = 0,05)$ und war gegenüber dem mittleren altersentsprechenden Normalwert 2,5fach erhöht (5).

Die mittlere Ausscheidung von PD zeigte mit 0,75 mg/24 Std keine Abweichung von den in der Proliferationsphase oder bei Amenorrhoe gewohnten Normalwerten, während PT mit einem Mittelwert von 1,70 mg/24 Std etwa 1,5fach darüber lag (8, 13).

Die Oestrogenausscheidung entsprach mit 18 μg/24 Std mittleren Normalwerten für die späte Proliferationsphase (9). Die relativen Konzentrationen der Oestrogenfraktionen zeigten deutliche Abweichungen von der Norm ($Oe_2:Oe_1:Oe_3$ $= 1:2,7:6,4$; Normalwerte $= 1:2:3$; $Oe_3/Oe_1 + Oe_2 = 1,73$; Normalwert $= 1$), aus denen eine relativ vermehrte Ausscheidung von Oestron und besonders von Oestriol hervorgeht. Obwohl diese Werte den Oestrogenmengen entsprechen, die bei Frauen mit anovulatorischen Blutungen und proliferiertem Endometrium gefunden werden (9), waren bei unserer Pat. seit 2 Jahren keine Durchbruchblutungen aufgetreten. Darüber hinaus ließen sich im Vaginalabstrich keine Oestrogeneffekte nachweisen. Diese Beobachtungen lassen auf eine Inhibierung der peripheren Oestrogenwirkung schließen, für die ein gestörtes Gleichgewicht zwischen Oestrogen- und Androgenproduktion verantwortlich sein dürfte.

Nach Gabe von Dexamethason, PMS und HCG war die Ausscheidung von 17-KS, PD und PT zunächst nicht oder kaum verändert, während die 17-OHCS als Ausdruck der NNR-Hemmung deutlich abfielen. Die Werte erreichten am 3. Tag nach Beginn der Dexamethasongabe mit $1/3$ der Basiswerte ein Minimum. PMS bewirkte danach eine Verdoppelung der Oestrogenausscheidung sowie 35—60%ige Erhöhungen der Ausscheidungswerte für 17-KS, PD und PT. Eine noch deutlichere Mobilisierung von Steroiden verursachte die Gabe von HCG. Die Stimulationswerte lagen für 17-KS 3fach, für 17-OHCS und PD 4fach, für PT 3,6fach und für Oestrogene 2,6fach über den Bezugswerten. Wie aus den Relationen der einzelnen Oestrogenfraktionen hervorgeht, wurden Oestron und Oestriol relativ stärker mobilisiert als Oestradiol ($Oe_2:Oe_1:Oe_3 = 1:3,4:7,5$; $Oe_3/Oe_1 + Oe_2 = 1,67$).

Nach der Exstirpation des Tumors waren alle untersuchten Steroide deutlich erniedrigt, am stärksten 17-KS, PT und Oestrogene. Auch eine 5 Monate nach der Operation vorgenommene Kontrolluntersuchung ergab unverändert niedrige Ausscheidungswerte für 17-KS, 17-OHCS, PD und PT. Die Oestrogene lagen mit etwa 10 μg/24 Std im mittleren Normalbereich für die frühe Proliferationsphase (9).

Die chromatographische Fraktionierung der 17-KS (Abb. 2) ergab keine erhöhte Ausscheidung der als Androgenmetaboliten anzusehenden 11-Desoxyverbindungen; die Werte für DHA lagen sogar deutlich unter dem bei gesunden Frauen gewohnten Bereich. Nach Gonadotropingabe unter gleichzeitiger NNR-Hemmung wurde

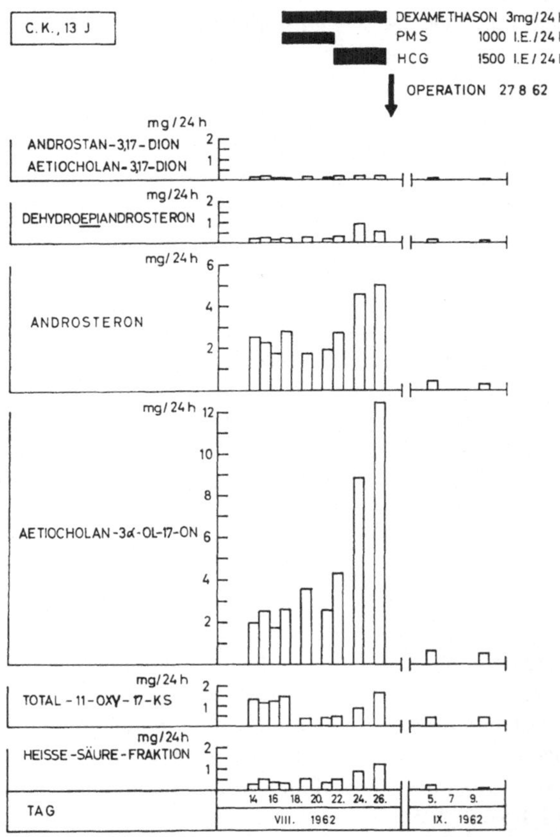

Abb. 2. Ausscheidung von sechs 17-Ketosteroid-Fraktionen (fraktionierte Hydrolyse, Gradientenelutionschromatographie an Aluminiumoxyd)[1]. Bedingungen wie Abb. 1

[1] Methode: Kellie & Wade (19).

jedoch eine überraschende Funktionsreserve des Tumors für die Biosynthese von 11-Desoxysteroiden sichtbar, die nach HCG in einer 1,6fachen bzw. 6fachen Erhöhung der Ausscheidungswerte von A und Aet ihren Ausdruck fand. Durch Dexamethason wurde lediglich die Ausscheidung der 11-Oxy-17-KS deutlich erniedrigt. Alle übrigen Fraktionen, insbesondere A und Aet, zeigten keine sichere Hemmung. Nach Exstirpation des Tumors fielen A und Aet auf $^1/_4$ bzw. $^1/_3$ der Bezugswerte ab. Aus diesem Verhalten ist zu folgern, daß die metabolischen Vorläufer von A und Aet überwiegend im Tumor produziert wurden und nur zu einem geringen Teil der NNR entstammten.

Von besonderem Interesse ist das Verhalten der 11-Oxy-17-KS (Abb. 2): nach einem deutlichen Abfall als Ausdruck der NNR-Hemmung erfolgte unter gleichzeitiger Gabe von Dexamethason und HCG ein stufenförmiger Anstieg und nach der Exstirpation des Tumors ein Abfall auf $^1/_3$ der Ausgangswerte. Ein sehr ähnliches Verhalten zeigten die 17-OHCS (Abb. 1), das nur z. T. durch die Miterfassung von PT in dieser Steroidgruppe erklärbar ist. Diese Befunde verdienen Beachtung im Zusammenhang mit der erhöhten Grundausscheidung der 17-OHCS, dem Konzentrationsanstieg von 11-OH-Aet im Plasma nach Dexamethason + HCG (Tab. 1a) und der Striaebildung bei unserer Patientin: sie werfen die Frage nach der Möglichkeit einer extraadrenalen 11β-Hydroxylierung von Steroiden auf, wie sie verschiedentlich in Testestumoren gefunden wurde (3, 31), für Ovarialtumoren jedoch bisher unbewiesen ist.

Zusammenfassung

Es wird über ein Gynandroblastom des Ovars bei einem 13jährigen, sekundär amenorrhoischen Mädchen berichtet. Nach Exstirpation des Tumors stellten sich regelmässige, ovulatorische Menstruationscyclen ein. Im Tumorgewebe wurden histologisch neben Granulosa- und Theca-Zell-Formationen tubuläre Strukturen nachgewiesen. Das andere Ovar war vergrößert und polycystisch verändert. Durch chemische Steroidbestimmungen im Urin und im Plasma vor und nach Exstirpation des Tumors und in Verbindung mit Funktionstests wurde eine beträchtliche, durch Gonadotropine stimulierbare Biosynthese von C_{18}-, C_{19}- und C_{21}-Steroiden im Tumorgewebe nachgewiesen. Es ergaben sich Hinweise, die eine 11β-Hydroxylierung von Steroiden im Tumor möglich erscheinen lassen.

Wir danken Frl. Dipl.-Chem. A. SEUKEN, Frau R. LINDECKE, Frl. B. RETZLAFF, Frau R. THEELEN, Frl. R. TÖNJES und Frau M. SCHÜTTE für ihre Mitarbeit. Vorliegende Untersuchungen sind Teil eines Forschungsprogramms, das an der Frauenklinik der Medizinischen Akademie Düsseldorf mit Unterstützung des Kultusministeriums des Landes Nordrhein-Westfalen durchgeführt wird.

Literatur

1. ALBERT, A.: Recent Progr. Hormone Res. 12, 227 (1956).
2. APPLEBY, J. I., G. GIBSON, J. K. NORYMBERSKI and R. D. STUBBS: Biochem. J. 60, 453 (1955).
3. BAGGET, B., L. L. ENGEL, L. L. FIELDING, K. SAVARD, R. I. DORFMAN, F. L. ENGEL and H. McPHERSON: Fed. Proc. 16, 149 (1957).
4. BIRKE, G., E. DICZFALUSY and L.-O. PLANTIN: J. clin. Endocr. 18, 736 (1958).
5. BORTH, R., A. LINDER and A. RIONDEL: Acta endocr. (Kbh.) 25, 33 (1957).
6. BROWN, J. B.: Biochem. J. 60, 185 (1955).
7. — R. D. BULBROOK and F. C. GREENWOOD: J. Endocr. 16, 49 (1957).
8. — A. KLOPPER and J. A. LORAINE: J. Endocr. 17, 401 (1958).
9. — R. KELLAR and G. D. MATTHEW: J. Obstet. Gynaec. Brit. Emp. 66, 177 (1959).
10. BUCHHOLZ, R.: Z. ges. exp. Med. 128, 219 (1957).
11. DOCKERTY, M. B.: Int. Abstr. Surg. 81, 179 (1945).
12. EMIG, O. R., A. T. HERTIG and F. C. ROWE: Obstet. and Gynec. 13, 135 (1959).
13. FOTHERBY, K.: Brit. med. J. 1960 i, 1545.
14. HEINRICHS, H. D., and F. EULEFELD: Acta endocr. (Kbh.), Suppl. 53 (1960).
15. HERTIG, A. T., and H. GORE: In: Atlas of tumor pathology, Sect. IX, Fasc 33. Tumors of the female sex organs. Part 3: Tumors of the ovary and Fallopian tube. Armed Forces Inst. of Pathology. Washington, D.C. 1961.
16. HOBBS, J. E.: Trans. Amer. gynec. Soc. 71, 57 (1948).

17. Hughesdon, P. E., and I. T. Fraser: Acta obstet. gynec. scand. **32**, Suppl. 4 (1953).
18. Johnsen, S. G.: Acta endocr. (Kbh.) **21**, 127 (1956).
19. Kellie, A. E., and H. P. Wade: Biochem. J. **66**, 196 (1957).
20. McBride, R. A., S. H. Sturgis and J. F. Crigler: Obstet. and Gynec. **19**, 814 (1962).
21. Mechler, E. A., and W. C. Black: Amer. J. Path. **19**, 633 (1943).
22. Meyer, R.: Beitr. path. Anat. **84**, 485 (1930).
23. Morris, J. M., and R. E. Scully: Endocrine Pathology of the Ovary. St. Louis: C. V. Mosby Co. 1958.
23a. Neubecker, R. D., and J. L. Breen: Am. J. clin. Path. **38**, 60 (1962).
24. Nocke, W.: Biochem. J. **78**, 593 (1961).
25. — R. Buchholz, R. Elert, L. Nocke u. J. Wennemann: 8. Symp. dtsch. Ges. Endokrinol. München 1961. Berlin-Göttingen-Heidelberg: Springer-Verlag 1962.
26. Norymberski, J. K., R. D. Stubbs and H. F. West: Lancet **1953 I**, 1276.
27. Oertel, G. W.: Chemische Bestimmung von Steroiden im menschlichen Plasma. Berlin-Göttingen-Heidelberg: Springer-Verlag 1962.
28. —, u. E. Kaiser: Clin. chim. Acta **7**, 221 (1962).
29. Plate, W. P.: J. Obstet. Gynaec. Brit. Emp. **45**, 254 (1938).
30. Ross, J. W., M. A. Weinberger and L. A. Desbordes: Amer. J. Obstet. Gynäk. **77**, 188 (1959).
31. Savard, K., R. I. Dorfman, B. Bagget, L. L. Engel, L. M. Lister and F. L. Engel: J. clin. Endocr. **16**, 970 (1956).
32. Schiller, W.: Disk. zu W. C. Black: Amer. J. Path. **18**, 766 (1942).
33. Scully, R. E.: J. clin. Endocr. **13**, 1254 (1953).
34. Starka, A. L.: Naturwissenschaften **45**, 240 (1958).
35. Teilum, G.: Cancer **11**, 769 (1958).

Aus dem Hauptlaboratorium der Schering AG., Berlin-West

Nachweis intrauteriner Virilisierung durch Sagittalschnitte von Rattenfeten

Von

F. Neumann

Mit 1 Abbildung

Die tierexperimentelle Prüfung neuer synthetischer Gestagene auf virilisierende Eigenschaften hat sich als notwendig erwiesen, nachdem in der Klinik in den letzten Jahren wiederholt über Virilisierungserscheinungen am Genitale neugeborener Mädchen berichtet wurde, deren Mütter in der Schwangerschaft mit synthetischen Gestagenen behandelt worden waren [K. Thomson u. J. H. Napp (1960), L. Wilkins (1960), L. Wilkins et al. (1958) u. a.].

Als Versuchstiere haben sich Ratten und Mäuse als geeignet erwiesen. Zur Beurteilung der Virilisierung wurden bisher die Messung des Anogenitalabstandes und die mikroskopische Anatomie des Genitales auf Querschnitten durch den Fetus herangezogen [R. Mey u. H. Scheid (1959), C. Revesz et al. (1960), H. F. L. Schöler u. A. M. de Wachter (1961), G. K. Suchowsky u. K. Junkmann (1960, 1961) u. a.].

Diese Art der Beurteilung, insbesondere die mikroskopische Anatomie, kann leicht zu Fehlinterpretationen führen, die durch unterschiedliche Lage der Schnittebenen bedingt sind. Außerdem können leichte Virilisierungsgrade nicht sicher erfaßt werden.

Aus diesem Grunde haben wir versucht, eine Methode zu entwickeln, mit der auch leichte Virilisierungserscheinungen sicher erfaßt und Fehlinterpretationen vermieden werden können.

Normale geschlechtsreife weibliche Ratten werden gedeckt. Der Schwangerschaftsbeginn wird durch Spermiennachweis im Vaginalsekret gesichert. Vom 16.–19. Tag erhalten die graviden Tiere täglich die Testsubstanz subcutan oder per os. Am 21. Tag werden die Feten durch Sectio caesarea entnommen, frontal in Nabelhöhe durchtrennt und in Bouinschem Gemisch fixiert. Nach 14 tägiger Fixierung wird zur groben Orientierung der Anogenitalabstand mit einer Schublehre gemessen. Zur histologischen Aufarbeitung wird eine etwa 2 mm dicke sagittale mediane Gewebsscheibe mit einer Rasierklinge herausgeschnitten. Nach der Paraffineinbettung werden aus dieser Gewebsscheibe Serienschnitte angefertigt. Jeder 10. Schnitt wird aufgezogen und mit der Hämatoxylin-Eosin-Methode gefärbt. Die histologische Sichtung nehmen wir mit einem Visopan-Sichtungsgerät vor und zeichnen die für die Auswertung interessierenden Organe bei 47 facher Vergrößerung auf Transparentpapier.

Zur Beurteilung der Virilisierung werden folgende Kriterien erfaßt: Länge des Septum urovaginale, Anogenitalabstand gemessen auf histologischen Präparaten, Mündungsform der Urethra, in zweiter Linie Verlauf und Länge der Urethra, Verhalten der Corpora cavernosa und Formänderungen der Klitoris.

Als erstes Anzeichen einer Virilisierung fällt eine dosisabhängige Verkürzung des Septum urovaginale auf. Den Grad der Verkürzung haben wir folgendermaßen erfaßt: Es wird eine Gerade gezogen, die etwa dem Verlauf der Wirbelsäule entspricht. Auf dieser Linie werden zwei Senkrechte errichtet, deren eine den kranialen Rand der Symphyse trifft, während die zweite die Spitze des „Septum" berührt. Der Abstand der beiden Senkrechten wird in cm gemessen. Gleichzeitig mit der Verkürzung des Septum findet eine Epithelwucherung im caudalen Bereich der dorsalen Kloakenwand statt. Außerdem zeigen sich im caudalen Vaginalteil zapfenartige Verdickungen, mitunter besteht die Verbindung zum kranialen Vaginalteil (Müllersche Vagina) nurmehr aus einer schmalen Zellbrücke. Bei stärkerer Virilisierung erreicht der caudale Vaginalanteil den kranialen nicht mehr.

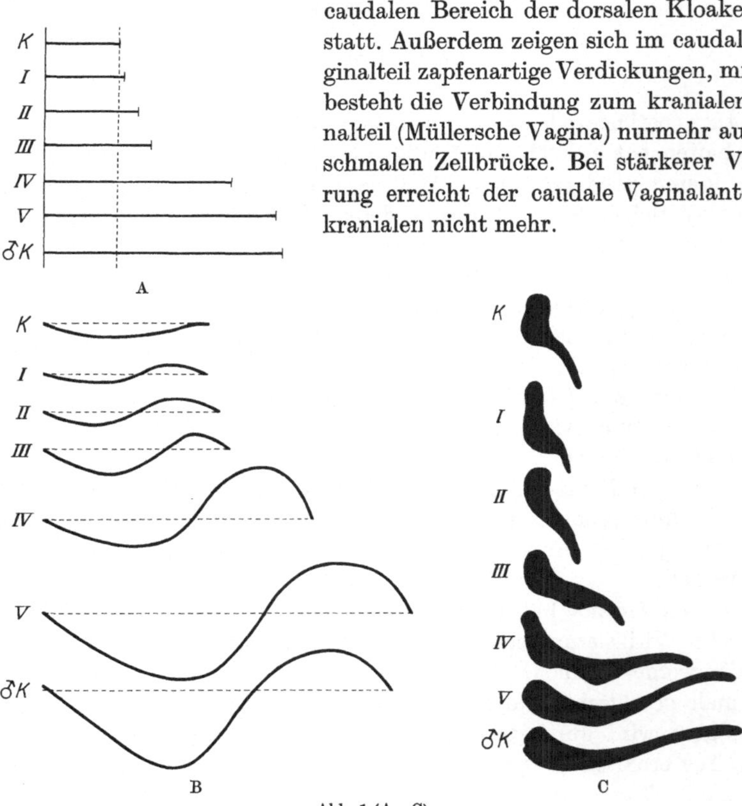

Abb. 1 (A—C)

Der Anogenitalabstand wird vom Ventralrand des Anus bis zum Orificium externum der Urethra gleichfalls bei 47facher Vergrößerung gemessen.

Das Orificium urethrae verschiebt sich mit fortschreitender Virilisierung immer mehr in Richtung auf die maskulin gestaltete Klitoris.

Unter Berücksichtigung der beschriebenen Punkte war es möglich, 5 verschiedene Grade der Virilisierung zu definieren. Alle Stadien wurden mit abgestuften Dosen von 17α-Methyltestosteron bei s. c. Verabfolgung hervorgerufen.

Abb. 1 zeigt das Verhalten des Anogenitalabstandes (A) der Corpora cavernosa (C) und der Urethra (B) bei den 5 definierten Virilisierungsstadien.

1. Stadium. Verkürzung des Septum urovaginale auf 4—2 cm

2. Stadium. Verkürzung des Septum urovaginale auf 2—0 cm

3. Stadium. Die Septumlänge erreicht nicht den kranialen Rand der Symphyse.

4. Stadium. Das Septum fehlt. Das Orificium externum der Urethra liegt analwärts der penisartigen Klitoris an.

5. Stadium. Äußeres Genitale wie beim männlichen Fet. Mündung der Urethra an der Spitze der penisartigen Klitoris.

Steroide, die intrauterin virilisieren, erzeugen qualitativ die gleichen Bilder wie das Methyltestosteron.

Wir haben virilisierte Rattenfeten aufwachsen lassen. Dabei blieben die Veränderungen bestehen. Bei der Sektion zeigt sich folgendes Bild: Die Ovarien waren stark luteinisiert und unterschieden sich in keiner Weise von denen normaler geschlechtsreifer weiblicher Ratten. Die Uteri waren stets stark entwickelt und i. d. R. prall mit Sekret gefüllt.

In Abhängigkeit von der Dosierung bestand eine totale oder partielle Vaginalatresie.

Bei der partiellen Atresie war der kraniale Vaginalteil gut entwickelt, es zeigte sich nach caudal eine spontane Verjüngung. Histologisch konnte an dieser Stelle ein Übergang von der i. d. R. mit stark verhorntem Plattenepithel ausgekleideten Vagina in eine Urethra festgestellt werden, wobei das Epithel polygonal wurde. Der entwickelte Vaginalteil dürfte Müllerschen Gängen entstammen, während die Bildung des caudalen Vaginalteils aus dem Epithel der dorsalen Kloakenwand unterblieben war. Bei solchen Tieren waren mitunter gut entwickelte Samenblasendrüsen sowie Prostataanlagen vorhanden. Sexuell verhielten sich Tiere mit solch schweren Veränderungen inaktiv. Waren jedoch die Maskulinisierungserscheinungen am äußeren Genitale nur wenig ausgeprägt und ein Introitus vaginae vorhanden, so waren die Tiere begattungsbereit und wurden gravid.

Tabelle 1. *Weibliche gravide Ratten vom 16.—19. Tag mit Methyltestosteron behandelt*

Dosis/mg/Tier/ Tag je 5 Tiere	Anzahl der Feten	Länge des Septum urovaginale	Anogenitalabstand mikrosk.	Virilisierungsstadien %-Werte					
				0	I	II	III	IV	V
3,0	15	—	$13,6 \pm 0,4$	—	—	—	—	—	100
1,0	11	—	$8,8 \pm 2,2$	—	—	—	—	73	27
0,3	12	—	$8,3 \pm 1,0$	—	—	—	—	100	—
0,1	12	$-1,3 \pm 2,0$	$6,2 \pm 0,7$	—	8	8	67	17	—
0,03	11	$2,8 \pm 1,7$	$4,5 \pm 0,6$	27	36,5	36,5	—	—	—
0,01	11	$5,0 \pm 1,3$	$4,3 \pm 0,5$	91	9	—	—	—	—
unbehandelte Kontrolle	43	$5,5 \pm 0,5$	$3,9 \pm 0,5$	91	9	—	—	—	—

$$\pm = \sqrt{\frac{\Sigma d^2}{n-1}}$$

Literatur

THOMSEN, K., u. J. H. NAPP: Geburtsh. u. Frauenheilk. **20**, 508 (1960).

WILKINS, L.: J. Amer. med. Ass. **172**, 1026 (1960).

— H. W. JONES, G. H. HOLMAN and R. S. STEMPFEL: J. clin. Endocr. **18**, 559 (1953).

Mey, R., u. H. Scheid: Geburtsh. u. Frauenheilk. **19**, 783 (1959).
Schöler, H. F. L., and A. M. de Wachter: Acta endocr. (Kbh.) **38**, 128 (1961).
Suchowsky, G. K., u. K. Junkmann: Geburtsh. u. Frauenheilk. **20**, 1019 (1960).
— — Endocrinology **68**, 341 (1961).

Diskussion

W. Hohlweg (Graz):

Wenn Mäuse — und ich glaube, auch Rattenweibchen — bis zum 5. Tag nach der Geburt einige mg Testosteron injiziert erhalten, so führt das zu einer irreversiblen Schädigung der gonadotropen HVL-Funktion, woraus eine Störung der Ovarialfunktion und Sterilität resultieren. Es ist erstaunlich, daß intrauterin virilisierte Rattenweibchen geschlechtsreif werden und eine normale Ovarialfunktion aufweisen, ja sogar fertil sind, wenn die Virilisierung keinen zu hohen Grad erreicht hat.

F. Neumann:

Mir sind die Arbeiten bekannt, in denen berichtet wird, daß Ratten, die in den ersten Lebenstagen mit androgenen und anderen Steroiden behandelt werden, später gestörte sexuelle Verhältnisse aufweisen. Diese Befunde müssen unseren Ergebnissen nicht unbedingt widersprechen. Entscheidend dürfte der Zeitpunkt der Steroideinwirkung sein (bei uns vor der Geburt, dort nach der Geburt).

W. Jöchle (Bergkamen):

Ergänzend zur Diskussionsbemerkung von Hohlweg sei auf jüngste Mitteilungen von Barraclough und Gorski [J. Endocr. **25**, 175 (1962)] verwiesen, wonach bei neugeborenen weiblichen Ratten bereits extrem niedrige Testosterondosen (10 γ) irreversible Zwischenhirnbeeinflussung und in der Folge Follikelpersistenz und Daueroestrus bewirken. Es berührt eigentümlich, daß die während der Gravidität verabreichten Androgene — die für die gezeigten Virilisierungen weiblicher Feten ausreichen — jene Zwischenhirnwirkung vermissen lassen. Es muß daher ein „Filter" postuliert werden, der im Fetus selbst bis zur Geburt das hypothalamische Sexualzentrum vor der unzeitgemäßen Einwirkung von Steroiden schützt.

Aus dem Hauptlaboratorium der Schering AG., West-Berlin

Intrauterine Feminisierung männlicher Rattenfeten durch das stark gestagen wirksame 6-chlor-Δ^6-1,2-methylen-17α-hydroxy-progesteronacetat

Von

F. NEUMANN und H. HAMADA

Mit 1 Abbildung

Bei der Prüfung eines neuen synthetischen Gestagens auf intrauterine Virilisierung, konnten wir mit der im vorangegangenen Vortrag beschriebenen Methode schwere Feminisierungserscheinungen an den männlichen Feten feststellen.

Das Steroid 6-chlor-Δ^6-1,2α-methylen-17α-hydroxyprogesteronacetat ist im Clauberg-Test an infantilen Kaninchen geprüft s. c. 250 mal, p. o. 1000 mal stärker gestagen wirksam als Progesteron.

GREENE u. Mitarb. (1938) sahen Feminisierung männlicher Rattenfeten nach Behandlung der Mütter mit Oestradioldipropionat. RAYNAUD und FRILLEY (1947) sowie JOST (1947, 1950) berichteten über Feminisierungserscheinungen nach Zerstörung der Gonaden durch Röntgenstrahlen bei Mäusefeten resp. nach Ausschaltung der Testes durch intrauterine Kastration bei Kaninchenembryonen.

Wir haben, ähnlich wie im letzten Vortrag beschrieben, die für die Auswertung interessierenden Organe bei 47facher Vergrößerung auf Transparentpapier gezeichnet und auf diesen Zeichnungen den Anogenitalabstand vom ventralen Rand des Anus bis zum Orificium ext. der Urethra, sowie mit einem Kurvimeter die Länge der Urethra vom Kranialrand der Symphyse bis zur äußeren Mündung gemessen (s. Tab. 1).

Aus der Tab. 1 ist ersichtlich, daß der Anogenitalabstand und die Urethralänge dosisabhängig verkleinert sind. Bei einer Dosierung von 10 mg/Tier/Tag werden beinahe die Werte norm. weiblicher Feten erreicht.

Auf Abb. 1 sehen Sie feminisierte Feten (A und B), deren Mütter vom 16. bis 19. Tag der Gravidität 10 bzw. 1 mg des Steroids s. c. erhielten.

Zum Vergleich sind unten links (C) ein normaler männlicher und rechts daneben (D) ein normaler weiblicher Fet abgebildet.

Der Penis ist bei feminisierten Feten gering entwickelt, klitorisähnlich, die Urethra weiblich, bei entsprechender Dosis ist ein Sinus urogenitalis wie bei weib-

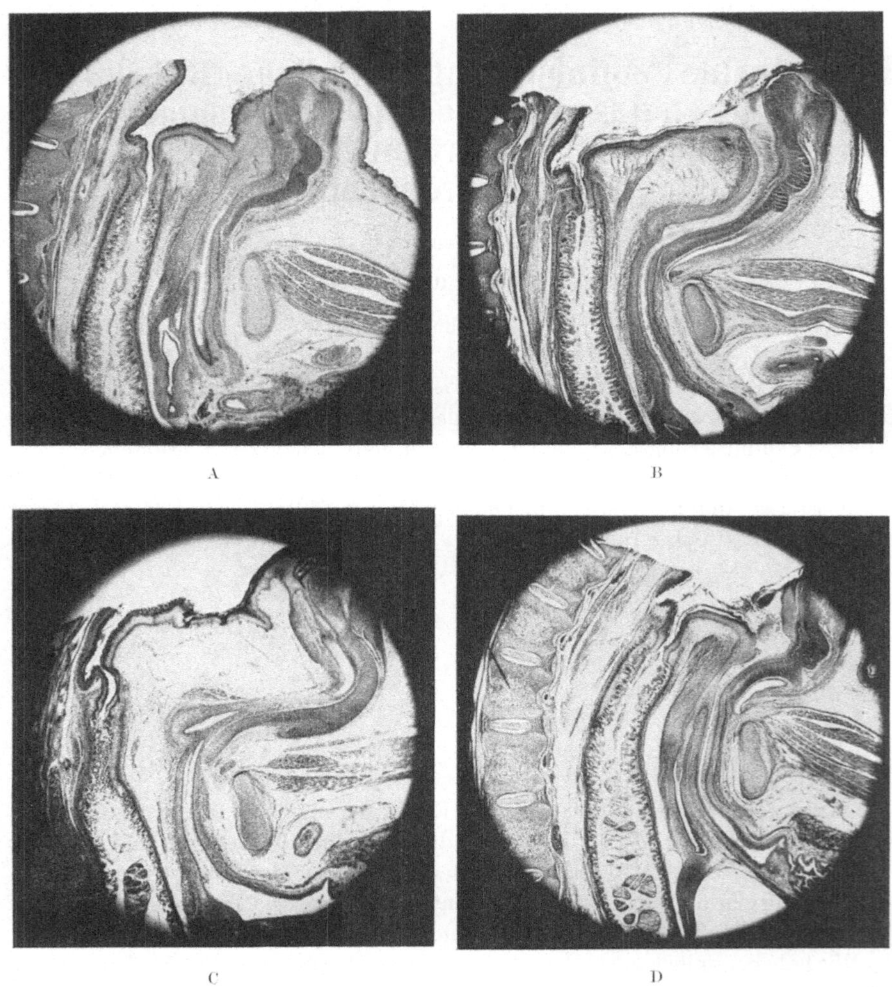

Abb. 1 (A—D)

lichen Feten vorhanden, kleinere Dosierungen bewirken eine Hypospadie. Die S-Form im Verlauf der Urethra fehlt völlig oder ist schwach ausgeprägt, die Corpora cavernosa sind klein. Bei höheren Dosen wird der Sinus urogenitalis durch ein Septum in einen ventralen Harntrakt und dorsalen Vaginalstrang getrennt.

Die Veränderungen bleiben im späteren Leben bestehen.

Der Gesamttyp des Tieres erscheint weiblich (grazile Kopfform, zartes Haarkleid). Das Tier ist kryptorch, die Testes lassen sich in der Inguinalregion palpieren, sind jedoch kleiner, als es dem Alter und Gewicht des Tieres entsprochen hätte. Ein Scrotum ist nicht angelegt, die Dammbreite entspricht der eines weiblichen Tieres, der Penis ist verkümmert, die Urethra mündet hypospadisch. Die Sexualbehaarung im Dammbereich fehlt.

Sexuell verhielt sich das Tier völlig inaktiv. Die Hoden und Samenblasen sind klein, der Penis ist verkümmert, klitorisartig, die Prostata fehlt fast vollständig. Bei der histologischen Untersuchung waren in der Prostata nur wenige Primärsprossen vorhanden.

Wir glaubten zunächst, daß die feminisierende Wirkung des Steroids auf eine Oestrogenwirkung zurückzuführen wäre. Im Allen-Doisy-Test an der kastrierten weiblichen Ratte und im Uteruswachstumtest an der infantilen Maus ist die Verbindung jedoch inaktiv.

Mit der Gestagenwirkung ist dieser Effekt sicher nicht gekoppelt, da eine Reihe von uns geprüfter gestagen gleich stark wirksamer Steroide diesen Effekt nicht zeigten.

Zur Diskussion stand noch eine starke zentrale Hemmwirkung und eine direkte Antiandrogenwirkung. Wir prüften die Antiandrogenwirkung an kastrierten männlichen Ratten im Gewicht von etwa 100 g nach tgl. s. c. Verabfolgung von 0,1 mg Testosteronpropionat und abgestuften Dosen der Testsubstanz über 7 Tage.

Tabelle 1. *Beeinflussung von Anogenitalabstand und Urethralänge bei männlichen Rattenfeten nach der Behandlung der Muttertiere mit 6-Chlor-Δ^6-1,2 α-methylen-17 α-hydroxyprogesteronacetat*

Verabreichungsart 16.—19. Tag an je 5 Tieren	Dosis mg/Tier pro Tag	Anzahl der Feten	Anogenitalabstand histolog. in cm gemessen bei 47facher Vergrößerung	Länge der Urethra in cm gemessen bei 47facher Vergrößerung
s. c.	30	21 ♂	4,5 ± 0,47	10,1 ± 0,82
s. c.	10	14 ♂	5,4 ± 1,08	11,4 ± 3,51
s. c.	3	27 ♂	9,1 ± 1,98	14,5 ± 3,14
s. c.	1	20 ♂	10,4 ± 1,57	17,1 ± 3,51
s. c.	0,3	9 ♂	13,0 ± 1,26	24,0 ± 1,06
s. c.	0,1	12 ♂	13,5 ± 0,40	24,0 ± 1,04
Kontrollen		30 ♂	13,4 ± 1,63	24,0 ± 1,86
Kontrollen		43 ♀	4,3 ± 0,68	9,8 ± 0,79

Tabelle 2. *Antiandrogenwirkung (geprüft an männlichen kastrierten Ratten über 7 Tage, pro dosi 5 Tiere, subcutane Verabfolgung)*

Anfangsgewicht	Endgewicht	Dosis mg/Tier pro Tag	Samenblase	Prostata	M. Lev. ani	Nebenniere
102	130	10,0 + 0,1 T.P.	14 ± 2,6	18 ± 1,0	15 ± 1,0	17
101	128	3,0 + 0,1 T.P.	19 ± 7,7	22 ± 4,7	16 ± 1,4	22
101	125	1,0 + 0,1 T.P.	32 ± 9,5	39 ± 4,9	15 ± 1,4	28
100	120	0,3 + 0,1 T.P.	59 ± 27	64 ± 8,2	17 ± 1,6	35
100	118	0,1 + 0,1 T.P.	88 ± 33	108 ± 20	20 ± 3,2	33
101	125	0,1 T.P.	116 ± 27	144 ± 40	23 ± 2,0	28
101	116	unbeh. Kontrolle	13 ± 2,7	19 ± 3,8	11 ± 1,7	39

In the table above, the first two columns "Anfangsgewicht" and "Endgewicht" are grouped under "Tiergewichte in g", and "Samenblase", "Prostata", "M. Lev. ani", "Nebenniere" are grouped under "Organdurchschnittsgewichte/100 g Tier".

$$\pm = \sqrt{\frac{\Sigma d^2}{n-1}}$$

Aus Tab. 2 ist ersichtlich, daß das durch T. P. stimulierte Samenblasen- und Prostatawachstum mit 3 mg der Testsubstanz noch völlig unterdrückt werden kann.

Zum Schluß möchte ich noch auf die weitgehende Übereinstimmung unserer Befunde mit dem klinischen Bild der testiculären Feminisierung beim Menschen hinweisen. Als mögliche Ursache dieser Intersexform wird eine Androgen-(Testosteron)resistenz vermutet. Es wäre möglich, daß das beschriebene Steroid in diesem Sinne wirkt. Außerdem erscheint es uns nötig, daß neue Steroidpräparate, die bei Schwangeren Anwendung finden sollen, auf diese Nebenwirkung hin untersucht werden.

Literatur

Greene, R. R., M. W. Burrill and A. C. Ivy: Science 88, 130 (1938).
Raynaud, A., et M. Frilley: Ann. Endocr. (Paris) 8, 400 (1947).
Jost, A.: Arch. Anat. micr. Morph. exp. 36, 242 (1947).
— Gynéc. et Obstét. 49, 44 (1950).

Diskussion

W. Hohlweg (Graz):

Da die Sexualhormone lokal wirksam sind und das 6-Chlor-6-Dehydro-1,2-Methylen-17 α-hydroxy-progesteron-acetat scheinbar lokal antiandrogen wirkt, könnte man versuchen, es kosmetisch bei Frauen anzuwenden, die einen Bartwuchs aufweisen, ohne daß besondere hormonelle Störungen vorhanden sind.

Wirkungen von Dauerbelichtung und Sulfonamid-Verabreichung auf Cyclus und spontanes Mammatumorwachstum bei 2 C₃H-Mäuseinzuchtstämmen

Von

W. JÖCHLE

Mit 2 Abbildungen

In der vergleichenden Tumorforschung fehlen bislang uneingeschränkt vergleichbare tierische Modelle für das Mammacarcinom des Menschen, aus denen pathogenetische Hinweise auf die Rolle des Neuro-Endokriniums und daraus resultierende therapeutische Konsequenzen abzulesen sind. Es erscheint darum erlaubt, trotz eingeschränkter Aussagemöglichkeit, auf bekannte tierische Modelle zurückzugreifen und ihre Beeinflußbarkeit auf der Basis neuro-endokriner Regulationen zu untersuchen.

Auf dem Symposium dieser Gesellschaft in Homburg/Saar war daher 1960 über die Wirkung lebenslanger Dauerbelichtung auf Cyclus und spontanes Tumorwachstum bei C₃H-Mäusen aus dem Inzuchtstamm des niederländischen Krebsforschungs-Institutes, Amsterdam (Professor O. MÜHLBOCK), berichtet worden. Entgegen den vielfach an Ratten erhobenen Befunden — die nach Dauerbelichtung permanenten Oestrus aufweisen (2, 3, 7) — vermochten diese Tiere den Cyclus aufrecht zu erhalten; die Oestrusphase war jedoch verlängert, das Auftreten von Mammatumoren und das tumorbedingte Absterben eindeutig acceleriert (4, 6).

Bisher unveröffentlicht blieben Untersuchungen am gleichen Tiermaterial, wonach — einer Anregung von Professor WARBURG (Berlin), folgend — Dauerfütterung eines Sulfonamids (Sulfamethoxypyrimidin) anscheinend auf Grund einer Cyclushemmung das Auftreten von Mammatumoren im Versuchszeitraum von 350 Lebenstagen verhinderte. Bei einem Drittel unbehandelter Kontrolltiere konnten während der gleichen Zeit spontan aufgetretene Mammatumoren nachgewiesen werden.

Diese Befunde veranlaßten, unter identischen äußeren Bedingungen einen Versuch anzusetzen, bei dem dauerbelichtete und in zwölfstündigem Licht-Dunkel-Wechsel gehaltene Tiere entweder 1,0 bzw. 0,1 mg Sulfamethoxypyrimidin pro die erhielten oder unbehandelt blieben. Für diese Untersuchungen wurden jedoch C₃H-Mäuse eines Inzuchtstammes aus dem R. B. Jackson-Institut, Bar Harbor, USA, verwendet. (Bezeichnung: C₃H-JAX). Die Versuche begannen am 100. Lebenstag der Tiere und wurden über 400 Tage fortgeführt; pro Versuchsgruppe wurden 30 Tiere eingesetzt.

Entgegen bisherigen Erfahrungen kam es bei allen dauerbelichteten Tieren der C$_3$H-Unterlinie-JAX zu rasch einsetzenden Cyclusstörungen mit lang anhaltenden Daueroestren, die etwa ab dem 300. Versuchstag in permanenten Dioestrus übergingen (Abb. 1). Gleichlaufend war unter Dauerlicht das Auftreten spontaner Tumoren der Mamma signifikant verzögert und das Tumorwachstum eindeutig verlangsamt: d. h. die Überlebenszeit nach Auftreten der Tumoren war um etwa 100% verlängert (Abb. 2).

Tägliche Fütterung von 1,0 mg Sulfamethoxypyrimidin hob diesen Unterschied zwischen dauerbelich-

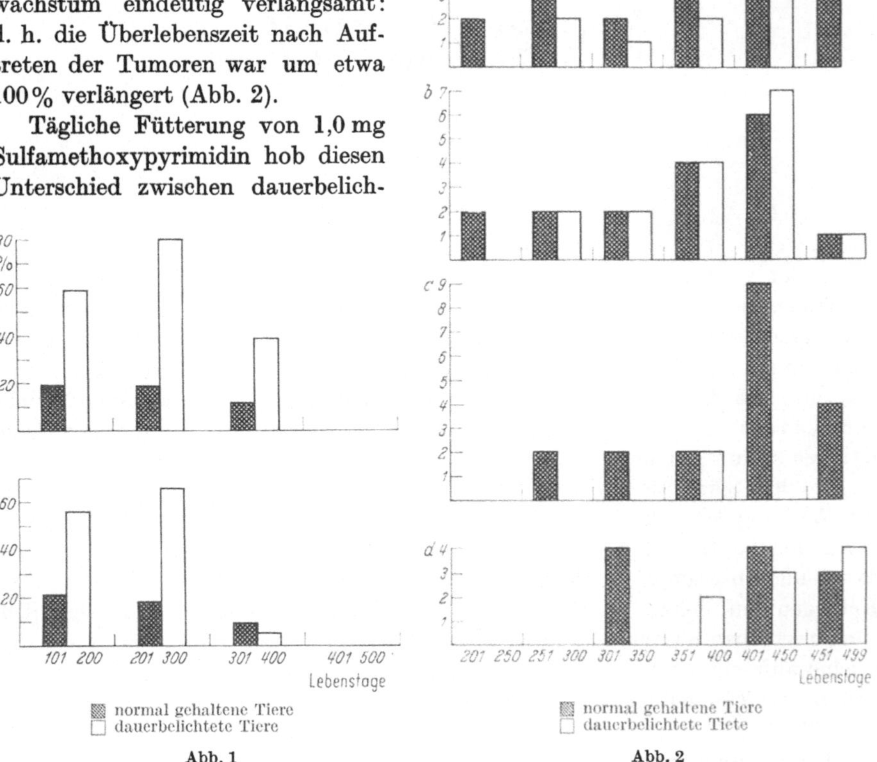

Abb. 1. Anteil der Oestrustage in % im täglichen Scheidenabstrichbild unbehandelter C$_3$H-JAX-Mäuse (oben) und mit Durenat® (Sulfamethoxypyrimidin) behandelter C$_3$H-JAX-Mäuse (unten)

Abb. 2a—d. a Auftreten von Mammatumoren bei unbehandelten C$_3$H-JAX-Mäusen; b Auftreten von Mammatumoren bei mit Durenat behandelten C$_3$H-JAX-Mäusen; c durch Mammatumoren bedingtes Absterben bei unbehandelten C$_3$H-JAX-Mäusen; d durch Mammatumoren bedingtes Absterben bei mit Durenat behandelten C$_3$H-JAX-Mäusen

teten und normal gehaltenen Versuchstieren weitgehend auf und induzierte ein intermediäres Verhalten (Abb. 2). Sulfamethoxypyrimidin in der Dosis von 0,1 mg pro die blieb dagegen weitgehend wirkungslos; die Versuchsgruppen reagierten ähnlich den unbehandelten Tieren.

Somit konnten die früher erhobenen, oben beschriebenen Befunde an C$_3$H-Mäusen mit den Tieren einer anderen Inzuchtlinie des gleichen Stammes nicht reproduziert werden. Primär andersartige Reaktionen dieser Tiere auf Dauerlicht — das Auftreten von Daueroestren — accelerierte nicht Tumorinduktion und Tumorwachstum, sondern verzögerte beides eindeutig. Sulfamethoxypyrimidin vermochte bei diesen Tieren wohl die Intensität der Daueroestren geringfügig zu inhibieren (s. Abb. 1), nicht jedoch die Ovarfunktionen auszuschalten, wie es eingangs für die damals verwendete C_3H-Inzuchtlinie nachgewiesen werden konnte. Daraus resultiert, daß nicht, wie früher angenommen, Speciesunterschiede zwischen Ratten und Mäusen in der Reaktion auf Dauerlicht bestehen, sondern Inzuchtlinien einzelner Tierrassen sich unter bestimmten vergleichbaren Versuchsbedingungen unterschiedlicher verhalten können als vergleichbare Rassen verschiedener Species; daß deshalb bei allen Veröffentlichungen exakte Angaben über die verwendeten Tierrassen einerseits gemacht werden sollten — wobei Begriffe wie C_3H, C 57 black, Sprague-Dawley, Wistar als Rassenbezeichnungen aufzufassen sind — und die in den einzelnen Rassen gezüchteten Unterlinien zu machen sind; daß die Resistenz gegenüber der cyclusaufhebenden Lichtwirkung gekoppelt mit der Empfindlichkeit gegenüber Sulfamethoxypyrimidin zu sein scheint.

Bezogen auf Tumorinduktion und Tumorwachstum kann jedoch aus den differierenden Ergebnissen der Schluß gezogen werden, daß nicht Oestrogenangebot allein, sondern erhöhtes Oestrogenangebot bei aufrecht erhaltenem Cyclus mit seiner rhythmischen Stimulierung der krebsgefährdeten Mammaanlage das Tumorgeschehen beschleunigt; durch stetes Oestrogenangebot allein wird es retardiert.

Ehe der Versuch unternommen wird, diese patho-physiologische Erfahrung mit epidemiologischen Erhebungen an Mammatumoren bei der Frau zu vergleichen, sei erwähnt, daß nach eigenen Erfahrungen die gleiche Situation — genetisch bedingt unterschiedliche Ansprechbarkeit auf tumorauslösende Stimulantien — für das derzeit bevorzugte Mammatumor-Tiermodell gilt: Für die durch cancerogene Kohlenwasserstoffe (3-Methylcholantren; 7—12 Dimethylbenzanthrazen) ausgelösten Mammatumoren bei Ratten (*1, 5, 8*). Hier ist die Reagibilität und die therapeutische Ansprechbarkeit auf Sexualhormone an spontanes Auftreten von Mammatumoren in selektierten Inzuchtlinien der Rassengruppe Sprague-Dawley gebunden, worüber bereits anderenorts berichtet wurde (*5*).

Versuchstier-Inzuchtlinien geben Aufschluß über ganz bestimmte Reaktionsweisen, die genetisch fixiert, durch Umwelteinflüsse realisiert werden. Sie geben vervielfacht über ein sonst nur individuell vorhandenes Reaktionsvermögen Aufschluß. Darum sind Modellaussagen von einer Inzuchtlinie beschränkt und nicht allseitig verwendbar. Untersuchungen an mehreren Inzuchtlinien ähnlichen Erbgutes runden jedoch das Bild und erlauben eher Vergleiche. Fragt man nun nach dem Modellwert des Aufgezeigten und vergleicht damit die statistisch hoch signifikanten Erfahrungen aus der Epidemiologie der Mammatumorgenese beim Menschen, so weist sich: Hier wie dort scheinen genetische Disposition ausschlaggebend für die Realisationsmöglichkeit eines Mammatumors zu sein (*12, 13*). Tumorrealisation ist abhängig vom individuellen neuro-endokrinen Reaktionsvermögen (*9, 10*) und der Art und Weise, wie dieses System auf belastende Umweltreize reagiert und wie es vor Tumorentstehung durch Fortpflanzungsfunktionen in Anspruch genommen wurde. (*11, 12, 13*).

Unter diesen Gesichtspunkten erscheint weitere Arbeit auch an tierischen Mammatumormodellen vertretbar.

Literatur

1. HUGGINS, CH., and N. C. YANG: Science **137**, 3526, 257 (1962).
2. JÖCHLE, W.: Endokrinologie **33**, 3—4, 130 (1956).
3. — 4. Symp. Dtsch. Ges. Endokrinologie. Berlin 1956, S. 284. Berlin-Göttingen-Heidelberg: Springer-Verlag 1957.
4. — 7. Symp. Dtsch. Ges. Endokrinologie, Homburg 1960. S. 96. Berlin-Göttingen-Heidelberg: Springer-Verlag 1961.
5. — Naturwissenschaften **48**, 13, 481 (1961).
6. — VII. Conf. Intern. Soc. Biol. Rhythm. Siena 1960; Edizioni Panminerva med. **1962**, p. 87.
7. — Zbl. Vet.-Med., Reihe A, 1963 (im Druck).
8. LANDAU, R. L., E. N. EHRLICH and CH. HUGGINS: J. Amer. med. Ass. **182**, 632 (1962).
9. SCHUBERT, K., u. G. BACIGALUPO: Arch. Geschwulstforsch. **19/3**, 230 (1962).
10. — Arch. Geschwulstforsch. **19/3**, 224 (1962).
11. VOSS, H. E.: Med. heute **9/8**, 313 (1960).
12. WILSON, R. A.: J. Amer. med. Ass. **182**, 327 (1962).
13. WYNDER, E. L., J. J. BROSS and T. HIRAYAMA: Cancer **13/3**, 559 (1960).